Drug and Alcohol Abuse Reviews • 5

Addictive Behaviors
in Women

Edited by

Ronald R. Watson

University of Arizona, Tucson, Arizona

Humana Press • Totowa, New Jersey

Library of Congress Cataloging-in-Publication Data

Addictive behaviors in women / edited by Ronald R. Watson.
     p. cm. — (Drug and alcohol abuse reviews)
  Includes index.
  ISBN 0-89603-257-4
  1. Women—Substance abuse. 2. Substance abuse—Sex differences.
3. Women—Substance use—Physiological aspects. I. Watson, Ronald R. (Ronald Ross) II. Series.
RC564.5.W65A33 1994
616.86'0082—dc20   93-48458
                                            CIP

Contents

Preface

Many lifestyle decisions made on a daily basis induce addiction to drugs, work, sex, gambling, or any of the many components of our lives. Some can have deleterious effects on survival and productivity. Some addictions are gender-specific or have special consequences for women, such as the effects of drug use on fetal growth and development. Therefore, research specialists were invited to provide concise reviews of addictive actions and behaviors as they particularly affect women.

Addictive Behaviors in Women is a unique collection of summaries of the effects of women's choices that produce various addictive behaviors and some of the consequences of these decisions. Fetal exposure to drugs of abuse, including alcohol and the nicotine in tobacco, produce a major component of all birth defects, and have long-term consequences on society's medical costs. Other behavioral decisions not usually involving drugs of abuse, such as gambling, overeating, and sexual activity, are also known to affect family health and medical costs. By understanding the causes and effects of such addictive decisions, they can be avoided and treated, thereby making women's lives safer, more productive, and healthier.

Ronald R. Watson

Contributors

Antonia Abbey • *Wayne State University, Detroit, MI*

Limor Azizy • *Research Institute on Addictions, Buffalo, NY*

Barbara A. Berman • *Division of Cancer Control, Jonsson Comprehensive Cancer Center, University of California, Los Angeles, CA*

Pamela Carlisle-Frank • *Research Institute on Addictions, Buffalo, NY*

Shoni Davis • *King County MOMS Research/Demonstration Project, Perinatal Treatment Program, Seattle, WA*

Myra Q. Elder • *The Diagnostic and Rehabilitation Center, Philadelphia, PA*

Judith S. Gavaler • *Oklahoma Transplantation Institute, Baptist Medical Center, Oklahoma City, OK; The Oklahoma Medical Research Foundation, Oklahoma City, OK*

Susan Goeters • *Association for Behavior Analysis, Western Michigan University, Kalamazoo, MI*

Blake Gosnell • *Department of Veterans Affairs, William S. Middleton Memorial Veterans Hospital, Madison, WI*

Ellen R. Gritz • *Department of Behavioral Science, M. D. Anderson Cancer Center, University of Texas, Houston, TX*

Charles J. Grossman • *Research Service, Department of Veterans Affairs Medical Center, Cincinnati, OH; Department of Biology, Xavier University, Cincinnati, OH; and Department of Physiology and Biophysics, College of Medicine, University of Cincinnati, OH*

Janice Haaken • *Portland State University, Portland, OR*

Deborah L. Haller • *Division of Substance Abuse Medicine, Medical College of Virginia, Virginia Commonwealth University, Richmond, VA*

Torild Hammer • *The Norwegian Youth Research Centre, Oslo, Norway*

Sydney L. Hans • *Department of Psychiatry, University of Chicago, IL*

Aaron T. Hogue • *The Diagnostic and Rehabilitation Center, Philadelphia, PA*

Patricia James • *Philadelphia Health Management Corporation, Philadelphia, PA*
Dean D. Krahn • *Department of Veterans Affairs, William S. Middleton Memorial Veterans Hospital, Madison, WI*
Candace Kurth • *Department of Veterans Affairs, William S. Middleton Memorial Veterans Hospital, Madison, WI*
Linda S. LaGrange • *Department of Behavioral Science, New Mexico Highlands University, Las Vegas, NM*
Barbara W. Lex • *Department of Psychiatry, Harvard Medical School, Alcohol and Drug Abuse Research Center, McLean Hospital, Belmont, MA*
Judith L. Marks • *Behavioral Medicine Program, Department of Psychiatry, School of Medicine, University of Michigan, Ann Arbor, MI*
Diane A. Mathis* • *Division of Addiction Research and Treatment, Hahnemann University School of Medicine, Philadelphia, PA*
Donna McDuffie • *Wayne State University, Detroit, MI*
Nancy K. Mello • *Department of Psychiatry, Harvard Medical School, Alcohol and Drug Abuse Research Center, McLean Hospital, Belmont, MA*
Jack H. Mendelson • *Department of Psychiatry, Harvard Medical School, Alcohol and Drug Abuse Research Center, McLean Hospital, Belmont, MA*
David S. Metzger • *Department of Psychiatry, Veterans Administration Hospital, University of Pennsylvania Medical School, Philadelphia, PA*
Helen A. Navaline • *Department of Psychiatry, Veterans Administration Hospital, University of Pennsylvania Medical School, Philadelphia, PA*
Mark Nienaber • *Department of Veterans Affairs Medical Center, Research Service, Cincinnati, OH*
Hilde Pape • *The Norwegian Youth Research Centre, Oslo, Norway*
Jerome J. Platt • *Division of Addiction Research and Treatment, Hahnemann University School of Medicine, Philadelphia, PA*
Cynthia S. Pomerleau • *Behavioral Medicine Program, Department of Psychiatry, School of Medicine, University of Michigan, Ann Arbor, MI*
Gary Roselle • *Medical Service, Department of Veterans Affairs Medical Center, Cincinnati, OH*

*Deceased.

Elaine R. Rosenblum • *Oklahoma Transplantation Institute, Baptist Medical Center, Oklahoma City, OK; The Oklahoma Medical Research Foundation, Oklahoma City, OK*

Lisa Thomson Ross • *Wayne State University, Detroit, MI*

Lisa Roth • *Philadelphia Health Management Corporation, Philadelphia, PA*

Gary Schmitt • *Research Service, Department of Veterans Affairs Medical Center, Cincinnati, OH*

Sidney H. Schnoll • *Division of Substance Abuse Medicine, Medical College of Virginia, Virginia Commonwealth University, Richmond, VA*

Irving W. Shandler • *The Diagnostic and Rehabilitation Center, Philadelphia, PA*

Thomas E. Shipley Jr. • *The Diagnostic and Rehabilitation Center, Philadelphia, PA*

Siew K. Teoh • *Department of Psychiatry, Harvard Medical School, Alcohol and Drug Abuse Research Center, McLean Hospital, Belmont, MA*

Janet M. Teets • *Department of Nursing, Miami University, Oxford, OH*

Per Vaglum • *Department of Behavioral Sciences in Medicine*

Barbara C. Wallace • *Department of Health Education, Teachers College, Columbia University, New York*

Michael Windle • *Research Institute on Addictions, Buffalo, NY*

Rebecca C. Windle • *Research Institute on Addictions, Buffalo, NY*

Charlene Woodard Motley • *Division of Substance Abuse Medicine, Medical College of Virginia, Virginia Commonwealth University, Richmond, VA*

Personality and Addiction

Focus on Women

Deborah L. Haller, Charlene Woodard Motley, and Sidney H. Schnoll

Psychopathology and Substance Abuse

Over the past few years, it has become increasingly clear that most drug treatment programs do not adequately address the psychiatric needs of the "dually diagnosed." This oversight may be presumed to be at least partially responsible for the high relapse rate in addicts. To better define the problem, researchers have attempted to identify the axis I and axis II disorders that exist in various subgroups of addicted persons. The underlying assumption is that the patient's treatment needs will be able to be effectively managed once diagnoses are known.

Prevalence studies have detected high rates of psychopathology in those suffering from substance use disorders. Most common are depressive and anxiety disorders[1-3] along with personality disorders.[3-5] It should be noted, however, that subpopulations of addicts (e.g., cocaine abusers, intravenous drug abusers (IVDAs), and methadone patients) generate different frequency distributions of psychiatric diagnoses.[6-8]

From: *Drug and Alcohol Abuse Reviews, Vol. 5: Addictive Behaviors in Women*
Ed.: R. R. Watson ©1994 Humana Press Inc., Totowa, NJ

It is unfortunate that few studies have focused on the female addict. However, those that have evaluated gender differences suggest that female substance abusers exhibit greater emotional disturbance, especially mood disorder, than do their male counterparts.[9–10] In our own work with pregnant and postpartum substance abusers,[11] the incidence of co-occurring nonsubstance use axis I disorders is approx 45%. The rate for lifetime occurrence of depression (based on the structured interview for DSM-III or SCID) is 28%, whereas that for anxiety disorders is 31%. Additionally, 75% have personality disorders that have been verified by multiple assessment methods (MMPI, MCMI, SIDP-R). The most common axis II disorder is antisocial personality disorder (approx 62%). Most of the other personality disorders have base rates of about 20%, although three are quite rare (schizoid, schizotypal, and obsessive compulsive). Many patients have multiple axis II disorders; in this sample, the range was 0–6/person. Of particular interest is the preponderance of axis II diagnoses falling in cluster B. Individuals with cluster B diagnoses (borderline, histrionic, narcissistic, and antisocial) are described as "dramatic, emotional, and erratic."[12] Before significance can be attached to these figures, however, it is important to compare them with those for nonaddicted female psychiatric patients, as well as for normal women with similar demographic characteristics.

The impact of psychopathology on treatment process and outcome has been addressed. Woody et al.[13] demonstrated that male addicts with antisocial personality disorder (ASP) typically do not do well in any treatment setting, although those with ASP plus depression do somewhat better. The additional diagnosis of mood disorder appears to attenuate the negative effects of the ASP diagnosis. In this instance, more pathology (in terms of number of diagnoses) is not necessarily a poor prognostic indicator. Somewhat surprisingly, our group has recently shown that ASP (in combination with other psychiatric diagnoses) is not a determinant of early dropout for female addicts enrolled in a comprehensive day treatment program.[14] Obviously, the relationship between presence of specific psychiatric disturbance(s) and treatment outcome is complex and bears further study.

The role that psychiatric and addiction severity plays in relation to treatment process and outcome has also been explored. McLellan et al.,[15,16] using the Addiction Severity Index (ASI), have repeatedly demonstrated a negative relationship between treatment outcome and level of psychiatric disturbance in male substance abusers. Others have also determined that the more severe the psychiatric illness, the poorer the outcome.[17] Degree or level of psychopathology thus appears to be a powerful determinant of treatment outcome.

The severity variable may be difficult to evaluate in a diagnostic system that assesses only for presence or absence of a disorder. Thus, when patients with severe disorders are assigned to treatment settings or modalities insufficient to meet their needs, poor outcomes occur. The larger issue is one of treatment matching. Once the patient has been diagnosed, the treatment prescription theoretically becomes easier. However, we do not yet know which treatments work for which patients. Individuals with different addictive problems may share DSM-III diagnoses in common. Should these other diagnoses or the substance use disorder guide treatment? Are there other dimensions, such as personality, that need to be considered? Just how significant is the overlap between personality, psychopathology, and addiction?

Theoretical Aspects of Substance Abuse

Diagnosis-related research, as discussed earlier, centers around detection of individuals who score above a certain threshold for specific forms of psychopathology. However, it tells us absolutely nothing about those who fail to meet the threshold criteria. In diagnosis-related research, the focus is on presence or absence of symptoms rather than on a description of the individual. Personality, in contrast, has been defined by Maddi in his classic *Personality Theories: A Comparative Analysis* as a "stable set of characteristics or tendencies that determine those commonalities and differences in the psychological behavior (thoughts, feelings, and actions) that have continuity in time and may or may not be easily understood in terms of the social and biological pressures of the immediate situation alone" (p. 10).[8] There is no apparent judgment as to relative psychological health or sickness implied by this definition. What is important to recognize, then, is that although personality bears a close relationship to psychopathology (including the personality disorders), these are not synonymous concepts and must remain distinct.

Indeed, persons with no detectable psychopathology still have personality. A personality description reveals more about an individual than does a list of symptoms or diagnoses. Personality type suggests personal strengths and weaknesses, adaptive coping strategies, and defense mechanisms. Knowledge of personality style not only facilitates prediction about how an individual might approach various situations, it also gives clues about how to intervene therapeutically when there are difficulties.

Alcoholism

With this in mind, an examination of the so-called "alcoholic personality" is in order. In his recent review article, Miller cited numerous studies that identify personality traits consistently attributed to alcoholics.[19] These include impulsivity, low frustration tolerance, passive-dependency, narcissism, and weak ego functioning. Alcoholics have also been described as neurotic, angry, and schizoid. Although psychoanalysts[21–23] approach alcoholism from slightly different perspectives, the defining personality features they address (including use of the splitting defense, disturbed object-relations, intensified affect, fluctuating self-esteem, impulsivity, and over- and undervaluation of others) are essentially descriptive of those suffering from borderline and narcissistic disorders. What is not clear, however, is whether these traits predate the addiction or whether use of alcohol, in fact, precipitated these behaviors.

Donovan identified depression and ASP as key elements in his etiological model of alcoholism.[24] However, these factors are not seen as relating directly to the development of the disorder. Instead, they are viewed as contributing to heavy drinking that unleashes a genetic vulnerability in an already "at risk" person. If this hypothesis is true, the search for the alcoholic personality cannot legitimately proceed without careful consideration of genetic, biological, and familial factors.

Cloninger had proposed two distinct types of alcoholism that appear phenotypically similar.[25] These are defined on the basis of a tridimensional model of personality. The three dimensions represented in this model are supposedly independent and are thought to be related to a heritable activity level in a central monoaminergic pathway. In fact, Cloninger's two types have been associated with differing neurophysiological and neurochemical characteristics. Type 2 is described as a "male-limited" form of alcoholism characterized by:

1. High novelty seeking;
2. Low harm avoidance; and
3. Low reward dependence.

Type 2 individuals have a basically antisocial presentation. In contrast, the type 1 "milieu-limited" group is comprised of both males and females. In order for type 1 individuals to be at risk for alcoholism, certain environmental circumstances must exist. Type 1 is characterized by:

1. High reward dependence;
2. High harm avoidance; and
3. Low novelty seeking.

The clinical presentation is essentially passive-dependent and anxious. Pertinent to this discussion is the fact that type 1 alcoholics show an increase in alpha activity and a corresponding decrease in tension as a function of use of alcohol. Type 1 alcoholics lend support to the self-medication hypothesis.[26]

Opioids

Opioid addiction has most frequently been associated with pathological drive states (particularly aggression), an inability to cope with negative affects, ego and superego deficiencies, narcissistic vulnerability, and an overall immaturity of the personality.[22,27] Opiate use has been seen as serving adaptive functions. Thus, narcotics have been viewed as a chemical defense,[22,28,29] as a means of preventing regression,[29,30] and as a means of self-regulation of negative affect states.[26,31–33]

Khantzian focused on the opioid addict's rage and aggressive impulses, which he sees as frequently stemming from a brutal childhood history.[31] Narcotics, including methadone, are viewed as a medication with a specific antiaggression action. This dynamic view is not incompatible with the belief that endorphins (endogenous opioids) play a role in the regulation of aggression. It may thus be hypothesized that a deficient level of endorphins may provoke supplementation from external sources.

Treece and Khantzian[33] and Wurmser[22,29] also addressed the narcissistic vulnerability of the opioid addict. However, this presentation is not limited to narcotics users. Narcissistic issues have also been emphasized by Hendrin[34,35] in relation to marijuana and amphetamine users, by Krystal and Raskin[36] in their work with sedative-hypnotic abusers, and by Nicholson and Treece[37] in their study of methadone-maintained polysubstance abusers. Finally, narcotic dependence has been associated with ASP.[38] It is interesting that Kernberg viewed the antisocial personality as a variant of narcissistic personality.[20]

Cocaine

Psychodynamic theory contends that cocaine addicts use this drug because of its specific psychotropic effects. Khantzian referred to this as a "self-selection" process. Theorists have hypothesized that cocaine:

1. Provides relief from dysphoric feelings;
2. Improves self-esteem;
3. Increases assertiveness;
4. Reduces feelings of boredom and emptiness; and
5. Increases attention and concentration, leading to more productive, purposeful work.[22,39,40]

Khantzian stated that cocaine is "compelling" for some because it helps them to overcome these symptoms. In relation to this hypothesis, it is interesting that some investigators have found adult ADD cocaine-dependent patients benefit greatly by being placed on therapeutic doses of stimulants. In such cases, cocaine use typically ceases.[41]

A different position was taken by Zinberg.[42] He felt that the addict's lifestyle and social setting are the main source of threat to the ego. As the addict regresses secondary to chronic drug use and gradually comes to rely more heavily on primitive defenses, the addict's capacity to perceive and integrate reality becomes impaired. To counteract this process, Zinberg proposed that treatment should focus on reality-based concerns as opposed to intrapsychic issues.

One recent study identified gender differences in relation to drug use patterns and psychiatric comorbidity for cocaine addicts.[10] Males were more likely to use cocaine as part of a larger pattern of social behavior and were more frequently diagnosed as antisocial. Females were more likely to be depressed. This suggests there may be differences in the underlying etiology for cocaine abuse in men and women.

Summary

The theoretical writings in the field of addiction suggest that substance abusers manifest a remarkably consistent constellation of personality problems. These are distinctly "characterological" in nature with antisocial, borderline, and narcissistic traits being the most evident. In addition, addicts experience uncomfortable mood states, such as rage, anxiety, and depression. Because of their personality problems, however, they have great difficulty tolerating and/ or defending against such emotions in an appropriate and effective way. The drugs they use may help to attenuate this discomfort to some degree.

The idea that personality characteristics determine drug of choice is an important concept. If this is so, then the users of different drugs would comprise relatively homogeneous subgroups and treatment efforts could be organized around the substance being used. This dynamic explanation for addiction is not in conflict with a more biological perspective. Genetic factors may predispose the individual to the type of character disturbance associated with a particular addiction.

The opposing idea, that distinct subtypes of addicts exist within a drug use category, is also of interest. If this is the case, then within drug-group treatments would need to vary depending on the presentation of the individual patient. Clearly, these two hypotheses have driven the empirical studies in the field of addiction. The emergence of thinking about addiction as a multifaceted, multidetermined disorder is thus essential to the rest of our discussion.

Empirical Studies of Personality and Addiction

What scientific evidence do we have of the existence of an addicted personality? In 1974, Retka and Chatam[43] described drug addicts in the following way: alienated, frustrated, passive psychopath, aggressive psychopath, emotionally unstable, nomadic, inebriate, narcissistic, dependent, sociopath, hedonistic, childlike, paranoid, rebellious, hostile, infantile, neurotic, overattached to mother, retreatist, cyclothymic, constitutionally immoral, hysterical, neurasthenic, hereditarily neuropathic, weak character and will, lack of moral sense, self-indulgent, introspective, extroverted, self-conscious, motivational immaturity, pseudo-psychopathic delinquent, and essentially normal. The descriptors are so many and so varied that they fail to give any clear impression. In order for a personality description to be meaningful, it must first discriminate addicts from nonaddicts and from other clinical groups. Second, it should demonstrate that these personality characteristics predispose a person to addiction (i.e., predate the addiction) and do not simply occur as a consequence of the disorder.[44]

The empirical literature is replete with studies on the relationship between personality and addiction. These studies have relied heavily on the use of psychological assessment techniques, including objective personality tests, projective personality tests, and measures of specific traits, such as anxiety and locus of control. There are a number of problems with the literature as a whole. Alcoholism has been the most thoroughly explored addictive disorder. Relatively few studies are available emphasizing drugs other than alcohol and heroin. Researchers have often lumped subjects with different addictive problems together, making the study groups extremely heterogeneous. The current epidemic of cocaine abuse has not yet impacted the literature in this area in a significant way. Furthermore, drugs, such as marijuana, seem to have been overlooked almost completely, despite their frequency of use. In sum, few contemporary substance abusers limit themselves to the use of a single drug and yet the literature is not reflective of the polysubstance abuse, which is the more typical clinical presentation.[2,45] A final difficulty with the literature is that few studies address females as the target population. Results must therefore be generalized to women only with extreme caution. In light of these limitations, the primary focus of this discussion will be on the personality typologies that have been empirically derived for specific subgroups of substance abusers. Efforts made to identify gender differences will be discussed where applicable.

The MMPI and Alcohol Abuse

A review of the literature reveals that the most frequently employed self-report measure used in the assessment of personality characteristics of substance abusers is the Minnesota Multiphasic Personality Inventory (MMPI). Graham and Strenger's 1988 review[46] emphasizes the consistency with which the 24 two-point code-type is found among alcoholic samples.[47–50] Several early studies[48,51] reported the 24 configuration as modal for males with the 46 being modal for females; more recent studies, however, have shown the

24 configuration to characterize the mean profiles for both sexes.[52,53] Differences have also been reported for various ethnic/cultural subgroups. For instance, Page and Boszlee[54] found the 49 code-type to characterize White alcoholics, the 24 to characterize Hispanics, and the 96 to characterize American Indians. Several investigators have noted that the 49 profile characterizes men who later develop alcoholism; once alcoholic, they generate a 24 mean profile.[55,56]

Numerous attempts have been made to discriminate between alcoholics, other substance abusers, and psychiatric patients using the MMPI. In 1958, Hoyt and Sedlacek demonstrated that alcoholics have significantly lower scores than psychiatric patients on the scales of the neurotic triad (scales 1, 2, and 3). This finding was later shown to be contingent on the subgroup of alcoholics being studied.[58] Zelen et al. found no differences for men and women on the individual scales of the MMPI; however, when they combined scales 1, 2, and 3 (the neurotic triad), clear differences emerged with the females scoring significantly higher on these scales.[59]

Attempts have likewise been made to discriminate alcoholics from drug addicts (and from criminals) based on the MMPI. In a study conducted by Hill et al.,[60] the similarities of these groups were found to far outweigh the differences, although several significant findings did emerge. First, both alcoholics and drug addicts scored higher on depression than did criminals. Second, alcoholics scored lower than the comparison groups on scales K and 4, whereas drug addicts scored higher on scales 5 and 9. Roth et al.[61] failed to replicate these findings; although differences were obtained on demographic variables for alcoholics and nonaddicted prisoners, no differences on the MMPI clinical scales were found. In 1973, however, Overall found that drug addicts scored higher on scales K and 9 than did alcoholics, who scored higher on scales L, F, 3, and 7.[62] Based on these findings, Overall concluded that alcoholics and drug addicts represent different personality types and that the only reason they have been viewed similarly is because of their uniformly high scores on scale 4.

One problem with the mean profile approach is that it tends to obscure information about homogeneous subgroups. Thus, Hodo and Fowler (1976) determined the mean MMPI profile for a sample of alcoholics under study to be 24.[49] However, <1/4 of the sample actually generated a 24 profile. The reality is that, although the 24 code-type is the most common one for alcoholics, others also occur with frequency including the 49, 27, 12, and 78.[48,63] This is quite important since the correlates of these code-types are very different. Some are suggestive of character pathology (24 and 49), whereas others are more suggestive of a neurotic adjustment (27, 12, and 78). Thus, treatment recommendations and prognosis for patients generating these code-types would be variable.

Another approach involves the use of cluster analysis. Blashfield meta-analyzed 11 cluster analytic studies employing the MMPI and concluded that there are only two types of alcoholics.[64] The first type is characterized by a rather low-elevation profile with a peak score on scale 4. The second type is more elevated overall and has peaks on scales 2, 7, and 8. Despite the simplicity of this model, Graham and Strenger argued that there is merit in studying more than just two types since the behavioral correlates of the subtypes can be clinically meaningful.[46]

As early as 1969, Goldstein and Linden identified four subtypes of male alcoholics (classifying 45% of patients) using the cluster methodology.[65] Their type I alcoholic was characterized by a primary elevation on scale 4 with a secondary elevation on scale 2 and no other significant scale elevations. This type has subsequently been identified by others including Donovan et al.,[66] Loberg,[67] and Nerviano et al.[68] The type I alcoholic has been described by Graham[69] and by Greene[70] as impulsive, angry, dissatisfied with his achievements, and poorly adjusted in terms of job and marriage. Guilt is experienced, but is insufficient to prevent further episodes of acting out. The prognosis for rehabilitation is poor. However, in terms of their drinking, type I alcoholics evidence less actual alcohol intake,[68] have fewer alcohol-related medical and social problems,[67] and are less likely to have received prior psychiatric services.[68] Finally, there appears to be a familial aspect to type I alcoholism with the fathers of these patients typically having serious alcohol problems themselves.

Type II alcoholics are described in Gilberstadt and Duker[71] and in Marks et al.[72] These individuals typically manifest a distress syndrome characterized by depression, anxiety, and attention and concentration difficulties. They are basically shy and introverted individuals who feel inadequate and insecure. They tend to remain in treatment longer than other alcoholic patients, and to evidence progress over time despite the fact they are prone to rehospitalization early in the course of treatment.[73] Their daily alcohol intake is the highest of all the groups identified. Additionally, type II alcoholics frequently experience alcohol-related physical problems, such as tremors and memory loss.[68]

The type III alcoholic is characterized by a primary elevation on scale 4 and by secondary elevations on scales 2 and 9. This type has also been confirmed by others, including Filstead et al.,[74] Pfost et al.,[75] and Svanum and Dallas.[73] These patients, who are viewed as "primary" alcoholics, have the heaviest absolute alcohol intake of the four types. They typically have long histories of alcoholism punctuated by acute alcoholic episodes. Their long-term prognosis is very poor, and their recovery attempts are characterized by multiple episodes of hospitalization and only brief periods of abstinence.

The type IV alcoholic is characterized by elevations on scales 4 and 9 but with no other scale elevations. This type has also been identified by others, including Nerviano et al.,[68] and is described by Graham,[69] Greene,[70] and Marks et al.[72] Type IV is the quintessential antisocial personality. These patients are in frequent trouble with the authorities. They are self-indulgent and self-centered. They manifest low frustration tolerance and express anger in inappropriate ways. Their relationships are typically shallow and superficial, although they may make a good initial impression. Their addiction tends to be characterized by chronic, excessive use of alcohol with intermittent "dry spells." These patients are quite likely to also abuse drugs.

Several additional alcoholic types have been identified since the pioneering work of Goldstein and Linden.[65] Nerviano et al.[68] and Pfost et al.[75] have both described a neurotic type characterized by elevations on the neurotic triad (scales 1, 2, and 3), with a possible secondary elevation on scale 4. These patients tend to exhibit difficulties with dependency and to be highly somatic, while lacking psychological insight into their difficulties. They are about average in their alcohol intake and alcohol-related problems, and are least likely to have alcoholic fathers.[68]

The final type, identified by Donovan et al.,[66] Filstead et al.,[74] Loberg,[67] Nerviano et al.,[68] and Svanum and Dallas,[73] is indicative of severe psychopathology. The modal profile has elevations on both scales 8 and F of 80–100. These patients are generally seen as psychotic. They typically require inpatient treatment and psychotropic medication. They do not do well in traditional substance abuse treatment. They have a high daily intake of alcohol and are most likely to have alcoholic fathers. Many are polysubstance abusers. Their personal histories are wrought with episodes of interpersonal difficulties, vocational problems, and prior episodes of psychiatric care.

A somewhat different approach was taken by Conley and Prioleau,[76] who classified slightly less than half of 2661 MMPI profiles using a system adapted from an earlier study.[77] This classification system was composed of profile types recurring in the literature in cluster-analytic, factor-analytic, and theoretical *a priori* studies. In this study, large profile differences were found for five basic types of alcoholism for both sexes. The distribution of personality types for males and females was also significantly different. The classic type was the most frequent for men (13.5%) with the psychopathic type being second (9.5%). The schizoform B type (elevations on scales 4 and 8) occurred least often (6.9%). In contrast, the schizoform B type was the most common form of alcoholism for women (10.8%) and the classic type was second (9.5%). The schizoform A type (elevation on scale 8 with 6, 7, or 9 also up) was least likely to occur. In terms of prognosis, the psychopathic and schizoform types are viewed as "essential" or "fast track" forms of alcoholism. For individuals in these categories, alcoholism typically has early onset and is quite socially disruptive. The neurotic and classic forms, in contrast, are typically associated with later onset and fewer social consequences to drinking.

Other strategies have been utilized to identify and classify alcoholics via the MMPI besides the mean profile and cluster methodologies. For instance, the MacAndrew Scale (MAC) was developed specifically to detect individuals with drinking problems. Although it has been relatively successful at differentiating alcoholics from normals and from psychiatric patients,[78,79] it has failed to consistently discriminate alcoholics from other substance abusers.[80,81] The MAC has been generally effective with males and females, inpatients and outpatients, Hispanics and American Indians. It does not, however, clearly distinguish Black alcoholics from Black nonalcoholics.[82] Furthermore, Preng and Clopton[83] have questioned whether it differentiates dual diagnosis alcoholics from psychiatric patients without alcohol problems.

MacAndrew himself[78,84] has identified a 15% false negative rate in identifying alcoholics when the usual cutoff of 24 is employed. He labeled the high scorers as "primary alcoholics" and the low scorers as "secondary alcoholics." Primary alcoholics typically have earlier onset of drinking and are less able to identify precipitants to abusive drinking. The low-scoring alcoholics represent an interesting subgroup. In general, those who score low on the MAC scale are less likely to act out, but more likely to be depressed.[75,85] Low scorers have also been shown to be more repressive (on the R scale); this finding has held up for females as well as for males.[86,87]

Allen et al. determined that the base rate for scoring high on the MAC was 91% for male alcoholics, but only 71% for female alcoholics.[88] They determined that MAC scores have different implications for the sexes. Thus, high-MAC men typically score higher on scales 4 and 9 than do low-MAC men. By contrast, high-MAC women score lower than low-MAC women on scales 2 and 0. The authors interpreted this to mean that high-MAC men but low-MAC women experience greater emotional distress; this is further reflected in their more elevated MMPI clinical profiles, where low-MAC women are characterized as depressed and introverted. The authors concluded that, although the MAC may not detect "atypical" alcoholics, it might serve a second purpose by facilitating the treatment planning process for homogeneous subgroups of problem drinkers.

MacAndrew summarized MMPI data for male alcoholics and nonsubstance-abusing psychiatric patients.[78] Both groups are more emotionally distressed and depressed than normals. Except for the items dealing specifically with alcohol-related content, the responses of nonmodal alcoholics (approx 15% of alcoholic men) are indistinguishable from those of the nonsubstance-abusing psychiatric outpatients. In contrast, the self-attributions of the modal alcoholics differ considerably from those of psychiatric outpatients with the alcoholics having an orientation toward the world as a place that is potentially rewarding (perhaps immediately gratifying).

In 1986, MacAndrew[89] turned his attention to a comparison of addicted women, their nonaddicted but psychiatrically impaired counterparts, and normals. Although small gender-specific factors relating to family dissatisfaction and irreligiosity were noted, the clinical samples characterized themselves as depressed and emotional, just as the men had. MacAndrew next extended his work in this area by extracting 41 MMPI items that differentiated female alcoholics from nonsubstance-abusing female psychiatric outpatients.[90] A principle factor analysis yielded three factors:

1. Deviant thrill-seeking;
2. Remorseful intrapunitiveness; and
3. Blackouts.

Approximately 20% of the female alcoholics were unable to be distinguished from the modal psychiatric patients. Accordingly, MacAndrew identified a nonmodal female alcoholic type. As previously with alcoholic males, he suggested that this minority type was representative of secondary or "reactive" alcoholism. He concluded:

1. There is no single alcoholic personality structure;
2. Ignoring individual differences in research by combining groups will inflate the error term; and
3. It is clinically inefficient to treat the alcoholic population as homogeneous.

Unfortunately, it is not known whether these subjects were pure alcoholics or whether they were, in fact, polydrug abusers.

Finally, MMPI studies on the alcoholic personality have been conducted at the item level. As early as 1963, MacAndrew and Geertsma factor-analyzed scale 4 in hopes of better understanding the contribution of the specific items of this scale to alcoholism. Their belief was that scale 4, as a whole, was measuring deviance from societal norms rather than alcoholism *per se*. The specific relationship between scale 4 elevation and alcoholism applies to women as well as to men.[58,91,92] Not only have peak scores on scale 4 repeatedly been reported for females, but these elevations have been found to be higher for women than for their male counterparts.[92] The MAC has also been factored and determined to be multidimensional. However, the number of factors identified varies considerably from study to study[84,93,94] suggesting, once again, heterogeneity of the alcoholic population.

In sum, there are MMPI single-scale elevations (particularly scale 4 and MAC) and two-point profile types (especially the 24) that occur with considerable frequency in alcoholic samples. With some exceptions, these profile characteristics differentiate alcoholics from other clinical and nonclinical groups although none is unique to alcoholics. Furthermore, the specifics are highly related to the subpopulation of alcoholics under study. Alcoholic women appear to differ from alcoholic men in that they are often more distressed and neurotic; nevertheless, the similarities for the sexes are much greater than the differences. One clear problem with most of these studies is their failure to give specific criteria for study inclusion. This makes it difficult to compare findings across studies.

The MMPI and Drug Abuse

MMPI studies addressing addictions other than to alcohol are equally complex. To start, investigators studying drug abuse have rarely operational-ized the term. Nor have they discussed the implications of concurrent alcohol abuse. Methadone patients have, at times, been referred to as ex-addicts and studied together with abstinent heroin addicts. It is thus difficult to ascertain the actual sample characteristics and, therefore, difficult to draw firm conclu-sions. Nevertheless, the MMPI has been employed in dozens of studies of personality and drug addiction, and some findings have been relatively stable.

Opioids

The mean profile approach, discussed with regard to alcoholism, has also been employed in research with drug abusers. Early on, Hill et al.[60] con-cluded that the profile type associated with heroin addiction is a 49. Craig, in his review of the empirical literature pertaining to personality of heroin addicts, cited numerous studies identifying significant elevations on scale 4 for narcotics abusers.[95] When scale 4 was factored by Astin in 1959, the mean T score for this population was found to be 75.[96] No fewer than 60% of the sample generated a profile with scale 4 as the highest score, and only 13% obtained a scale 4 score with a ranking lower than third. Craig noted that the median T score = 75 for opioid addicts was maintained across 21 studies and 51 different addict groups (a total of more than 3000 subjects).[95]

In 1964, Olson compared the MMPI profiles for male and female nar-cotics addicts.[97] The males scored higher on scales L, K, 4, and 9, whereas the females scored higher on scales 2 and 6. However, the mean profiles for both males and females evidenced peaks on scales 4 and 9. Thus, although there were gender differences noted, these were not the defining features of the profile. After administering the MMPI to more than 800 male and female addicts, Berzins et al. identified two main types of addicts.[98] However, since males and females were well represented in both groups, it was concluded that the similarities between the sexes far outweighed any differences. Sutker and Moan addressed within gender groupings by comparing female nonaddicted prisoners with their addicted imprisoned counterparts and with female street addicts.[99] The addict groups responded in a more deviant direction, regardless of whether or not they were incarcerated, and generated MMPI profiles with marked elevations on scales 4 and 9.

Craig cited a few studies attempting to differentiate opioid addicts from alcoholics.[95] In one, addicts and alcoholics were both shown to have higher scores on scale 2 than prisoners, whereas addicts and criminals had higher scores on scale 4 than did alcoholics.[60] The addicts also generated higher scores on scales 5 and 9 than did either of the other groups. Overall employed a discriminate analysis technique to determine that alcoholics score significantly higher than addicts on scales 2, 3, and 7, although they also evidence an elevation on scale 4.[62] By contrast, addicts scored highest on scales 4 and 9. The higher the elevations on scales 4 and 9, the more likely the subject was to be an addict. If scales 3 and 7 were also elevated, the profile was more likely to be that of an alcoholic.

Attempts have likewise been made to use the Heroin scale (He) to differentiate heroin addicts from other drug abusers and from alcoholics. However, findings have been inconsistent.[100,101] The ability of the MAC to differentiate drug addicts with and without concurrent alcoholism was demonstrated by Craig.[102] Interestingly, the severity of the alcohol problem (abuse vs dependence) was not a factor. Lachar et al. were unable to separate heroin addicts from psychiatric controls with the MAC, however.[80]

Again, the group comparison methodology (based on means) may be criticized because it assumes homogeneity within substance-abusing groups. To address the issue of heterogeneity, Collins et al. identified eight addict types via a factor analytic technique based on a sample of 59 attendees at a methadone maintenance clinic.[103] Three factors accounted for 60% of the variance. All three factors were characterized by MMPI profiles, with prominent elevations on scales 2, 4, 8, and 9. A more recent study comparing data from the MMPI and MCMI for 163 methadone-maintained opioid addicts revealed that the highest MMPI scores were found on scales 2, 4, 9, and 3, with the mean two-point code being 42.[104] The sample was about one-third female. When principle axis factor analysis was done, three MMPI factors emerged, accounting for 64% of the variance; however, the authors failed to either label or interpret the identified factors.

As is the case with alcoholics, scale 4 elevations are characteristic of opioid addicts. However, the simultaneous elevation of scale 9 rather than scale 2 is likely. As is the case with alcoholics, addicts are generally able to be differentiated from other clinical groups and from normals. Within-group types are also distinguishable. Although mean profiles for opioid users vary slightly as a function of gender, the defining features remain essentially the same for males and females.

The MMPI and Cocaine and Polysubstance Abuse

Craig assessed the MMPI profiles of smokers of cocaine freebase being treated at a VA hospital and found significantly elevated scores on scale 4.[105] Scores on scales 2 and 9 also approached clinical significance. The data are of limited utility, however, since the sample was all male and mostly Black.

In a recent article, the MMPI profiles of 268 patients entering treatment for cocaine addiction were examined.[106] MANOVAs were done to test for racial and gender differences but none were found. Again, a clinically significant elevation was detected on scale 4. Scale 9 was also elevated and the mean scores on scales 2, 7, and 8 approached significance. Although the elevation on scale 4 has also been consistently found in alcoholics,[46] it appears that scale 9, rather than scale 2, is most apt to be the next highest scale elevation for cocaine addicts. The authors noted their particular concerns for relapse in this population. It is their belief that the "sensation seeking" that is associated with elevations on both scales 4 and 9 is likely to place cocaine abusers in high-risk situations repeatedly. They also acknowledged the problems associated with posthoc analyses of personality. In this instance, it is unclear whether the elevation on scale 9 is a premorbid characteristic, or whether it is merely reflective of chronic stimulant use.

Dougherty and Lesswing studied 100 hospitalized cocaine users, 18% of whom were female.[4] As 72% were dependent on other substances in addition to cocaine (37% alcohol, 10% alcohol and marijuana, 11% marijuana, 15% multiple substances), the sample was essentially one of polysubstance abusers. Ninety percent generated significantly elevated MMPI profiles. Sixty-five percent of these were characterized by high points on either scale 4 or 9. The authors concluded that, as a group, cocaine abusers have poor impulse control and low frustration tolerance. They evidenced a "hedonistic approach with needs for excitement, stimulation, and immediate gratification" (p. 47). They further characterized the sample as angry and rebellious, while employing the defenses of acting-out, externalization, and rationalization.

Finally, a 1980 study by Rothauzer looked at the MMPI profiles of nonopioid dependent polysubstance abusers.[107] Although both male and female subjects were studied, data were combined for purpose of analysis. Cluster analysis yielded three distinct types, classifying 45% of profiles. Type II was similar to types previously found in other typological studies of alcoholics employing the MMPI.[98,103] The author thus hypothesized that this may be a generic addict type. However, the other two types were quite different from those previously detected. Both were characterized by extreme elevations despite the fact that the subjects were not exhibiting severe psychopathology. Rothauzer noted that many of these profiles would be discarded as invalid if traditional cutoffs were employed. He thus argued that traditional cutoffs may be too restrictive for use with polysubstance-abusing populations.

Pre- and Posttreatment Studies with the MMPI

None of these MMPI studies proves the existence of an addictive personality. Longitudinal studies will be required to demonstrate that identified personality traits are more than a consequence of addiction. True personality characteristics should endure despite treatment and subsequent sobriety.

With this in mind, several studies have addressed the issue of change in alcoholics' MMPI scores as a function of treatment.[108–110] The general finding is that scores on scales reflecting emotional distress (e.g., 2 and 7) typically improve after treatment; this suggests that the observed elevations were more a function of drug use than of "preaddictive" personality traits. Conversely, scores on scale 4 have generally been resistant to change despite treatment with few studies supporting scale 4 elevation as a transient characteristic.[108,110] Thus, the qualities associated with scale 4 elevation might be presumed to be independent of substance use and therefore more likely to reflect predisposing personality characteristics. Similarly, studies of the MAC pre- and posttreatment suggest that the scores are enduring despite abstinence of from 2–9 mo.[111,112] The conclusion is that the MAC is measuring personality characteristics associated with alcoholism rather than alcohol use.

Premorbid MMPI data are available for several samples. In one study, test–retest reliability, before and after onset of alcoholism was moderate (median, .39), suggesting that the prealcoholic personality was somewhat stable [55] In another study, male students who later developed alcoholism were found to score higher on scales F, 4, and 9 than their nonalcoholic counterparts.[56] A third study by these investigators[113] looked at the ability of some of the MMPI special scales to predict alcoholism. Although five scales were investigated, only the MAC and the Rosenberg scales were able to differentiate the prealcoholics, with the MAC correctly identifying 72% of those who would later develop problems with alcohol.

Summary of Findings for the MMPI

Alcoholics and drug addicts share in common an elevation on scale 4 of the MMPI. The fact that a scale 4 elevation figures prominently in the mean profiles of all drug-abusing groups (as well as those destined to develop addictive problems) suggests that it is measuring traits that are risk factors or cofactors for addiction. Mean profiles do vary, however, depending on drug of choice and a multitude of demographic variables. Alcoholics are most likely to generate a 24 profile type, whereas both heroin and cocaine abusers typically have the highest elevations on scales 4 and 9. In terms of discreet findings for women, there are relatively few. Although small differences frequently arise, these have few implications for treatment.

It has become abundantly clear, however, that there are subtypes of individuals within each drug-use group. A particular subtype may, in fact, be associated with several drug-use groups. The question thus arises as to whether drug of choice is the critical variable. Perhaps the concept of "addictive type" is more appropriate. The issue of group confounds must also be raised. Perhaps type 1 appears readily in samples of alcoholics and heroin and cocaine addicts because it is a generic personality type for substance abusers. On the other hand, type 1 may appear in all three populations because the subjects actually have similar drug use but have not been categorized according to standard criteria. In this age of polysubstance abuse, interactions between personality variables and drug-use variables must be more carefully considered if study outcomes are to be meaningful in a clinical sense.

The MCMI

Results on objective personality tests other than MMPI are fewer and, for the most part, less rigorous. However, the Millon Clinical Multiaxial Inventory (MCMI) has recently stimulated considerable interest. Craig et al. administered the test to several hundred opioid addicts and alcoholics in treatment at a VA hospital.[114] The alcoholics scored higher on the avoidant and dependent personality styles, all three pathological personality styles (schizotypal, borderline, and paranoid), and the clinical syndromes of psychotic thinking, psychotic depression, and alcohol abuse. Conversely, the opioid addicts scored higher on the narcissistic personality disorder scale and the drug abuse clinical syndrome.

Cluster analysis yielded two types of drug addicts. The first type was characterized by having the highest scores on the narcissistic and antisocial personality disorder scales and moderately high scores on both the alcohol and drug abuse scales. The second type had the highest scores on the passive–aggressive and avoidant personality disorder scales, along with high scores on the anxiety and depression scales.

Four alcoholic types were generated. The first was characterized by passive–aggressiveness. Subjects in this group also scored high on borderline and paranoid states, as well as on anxiety. Type 2 alcoholics had high scores on dependent, avoidant, passive–aggressive, and schizoid personality styles, and were also anxious and depressed. The third type was compulsive, with most other scores falling in the normal range. Type 4 alcoholics resembled the type 2 drug addicts. They scored high on the narcissistic and antisocial personality disorder scales. They also had the highest drug abuse scores among the alcoholic groups, and were moderately depressed.

In sum, Craig et al. pointed out that the continued search for differences between alcoholics and addicts is a reflection of the "uniformity myth." In fact, some alcoholics resemble some drug addicts, although there are also distinct types in both categories. They stressed the need to address questions, such as how does personality style effect treatment outcome, recidivism, and abstinence? In other words, any classification scheme should be clinically meaningful.

Marsh et al. obtained MCMIs from 159 opioid addicts maintained on methadone.[104] The highest mean scores for the clinical syndromes were on the drug abuse, alcohol abuse, anxiety, and dysthymia scales. The highest mean scores for the personality disorders were for the antisocial, narcissistic, histrionic, and paranoid personality disorders. Principle-axis factor analyses were able to account for all but 21% of the variance. Factor 1 had positive loadings on the passive–aggressive, alcohol abuse, drug abuse, psychotic thinking, and psychotic depression scales and a negative loading on the compulsive scale. Factor 2 had positive loadings on the dependent, borderline, anxiety, somataform, and dysthymia scales. Factor 3 had positive loadings on the schizoid, avoidant, and schizotypal scales and negative loadings on the histrionic, narcissistic, and hypomanic scales. Finally, factor 4 (accounting for only 6% of the variance) had positive loadings on antisocial, paranoid, and psychotic delusion scales. Marsh et al. concluded that there are multiple clinical syndromes associated with opioid dependence. The observation that opioid addicts manifest every one of the personality disorders is felt to have significant implications for treatment.

In an MCMI study comparing the scores of Black, male heroin and cocaine addicts, Craig and Olson[115] determined that the heroin abusers had significantly higher scores on the alcohol abuse, anxiety, and somataform clinical syndrome scales (perhaps as a function of residual withdrawal), whereas the cocaine abusers scored significantly higher on the antisocial dimension. Although these differences are of interest, the groups were actually quite similar in that the antisocial and narcissistic personality disorder scales were the two highest for both groups. Also, both groups demonstrated concurrent alcohol abuse, although drinking was more of a problem for the heroin addicts. Finally, as might be expected, the most elevated clinical syndrome scale for both groups was on the drug abuse scale, demonstrating concurrent validity.

In addition to performing univariate analyses, the data were analyzed via a multivariate approach. Four distinct clusters were identified, two for each group. The clusters formed around personality style, as opposed to drug of choice. The majority of cocaine addicts fell in cluster 1, which was dominated by elevations on the narcissism, antisocial, histrionic, paranoid, and drug abuse scales. This pattern corresponds to Millon's "interpersonally acting out" type.[116] Such individuals act out recurrently in response to stress. They are typically arrogant, self-centered, mistrustful, and impulsive; however they do experience frustration and guilt. The cocaine addicts in cluster 2 generated elevations on the passive–aggressive, antisocial, narcissistic, paranoid, avoidant, drug abuse, alcohol abuse, and dysthymia scales. This pattern has been labeled by Millon as "emotionally contemptuous."[116] Although such individuals evidence significant distress, they have little need for support from others. Their moods are erratic, and their behavior is characterized by manipulations. The heroin addicts in cluster 3 evidenced high scores on the narcissistic, antisocial, drug abuse, and alcohol abuse scales. This is reflective of a classic antisocial presentation. Finally, the cluster 4 heroin addicts (the majority of the group) were characterized by high scores on the passive–aggressive, alcohol abuse, and drug abuse scales. This pattern has been termed by Millon as "emotionally ambivalent." This group evidences erratic behavior characterized by angry outbursts, as well as by periods of remorse and guilt.

Finally, the authors performed ideographic analysis, comparing base rates for the personality disorders for the two groups of addicts. The heroin addicts evidenced prevalence rates >25% on narcissistic and antisocial personality disorders. The cocaine addicts had comparable findings for these two disorders, and also had a 30% prevalence rate for dependent personality disorder. In sum, the authors contended that heroin and cocaine addicts are quite similar in terms of personality style. They felt their findings refuted the "self-medication hypothesis,"[26] suggesting that addicts select a drug of choice because it has the capacity to ameliorate specific negative affect states (age in the case of heroin addicts, depression in the case of cocaine addicts).

Calsyn and Saxon also explored the issue of personality subtypes among opioid and cocaine addicts.[117] Subjects were 110 male veterans seeking outpatient drug treatment. MCMI profiles for all subjects were sorted multiple times to identify those with psychotic disturbances, affective disturbances, severe personality disorders, and basic personality disorders. The prevalence rates for the first three sorts were as follows: 10% psychotic, 47% depressed, 22% with severe personality disturbance. No differences existed for the opioid and cocaine abuse groups, although Blacks were more likely than Whites to receive severe personality disorder diagnoses (mostly as a function of higher paranoia scores). The results for the fourth sort (basic personality disorders) did yield group differences with 84% of subjects able to be classified according to a predetermined classification procedure. No racial differences occurred for this sort. Both groups were frequently classified as narcissistic and antisocial, however, cocaine addicts were more likely to be withdrawn/negativistic. Those subjects who were essentially without elevations on the basic personality scales were more likely to be opioid addicts. In sum, the MCMI detected high rates of psychopathology for both the opioid and cocaine dependent subgroups, particularly in relation to axis II disorders. Calsyn and Saxon felt that the study results support similarity as opposed to differences between groups.

Yet another MCMI study investigated the relationship between personality and alcoholism type.[118] Subjects, 250 male alcoholic veterans, were administered the MCMI and the Alcohol Use Inventory (AUI). Cluster analysis performed on mean scores of the MCMI scales resulted in identification of three factors. Cluster 1, the smallest, was characterized by an essentially normal MCMI profile. None of the scales reached a clinically significant elevation. These subjects were seen as functioning in the neurotic range. Cluster 2 evidenced "prominent" elevations on the narcissistic and antisocial personality disorder scales as well as on the alcohol and drug abuse scales. There was also a clinically significant elevation on the paranoid personality scale. These individuals were seen as basically narcissistic and antisocial. Cluster 3, the largest, evidenced prominent elevations on the passive–aggressive and avoidant personality scales as well as the anxiety, dysthymic, and alcohol abuse scales. Clinically significant scores were additionally obtained on the schizoid and dependent personality disorder scales. These individuals evidenced broad character pathology with the basic style being passive–aggressive and avoidant. Multiple one-way ANOVAs performed on the clusters yielded significant differences between the groups on all scales.

The three clusters were next compared in terms of their AUI findings. An ANOVA, based on the mean scores of the clusters, was performed for the AUI scales and significant differences were found on 18 of 21 drinking-related variables. However, the majority of the differences were owing to the significantly lower scores of those in cluster 1. Those in cluster 3 had the highest scores on the AUI scales, and evidenced significantly more anxiety and guilt about their drinking than did those in cluster 2. Cluster 3 alcoholics were also more likely to drink alone than those in cluster 2, who were more social in their drinking style. The authors concluded that there are distinct subgroups of alcoholics, and supported the concept of alcoholism as a "spectrum" disorder.

Flynn and McMahon analyzed 139 MCMI profiles obtained from a group of known drug abusers in treatment.[119] As a group, the subjects' scores on scale T (drug abuse) were indicative of the "presence" of symptomatology. These scores on scale T did not differ significantly at three test administration points (intake, 1 mo, 3 mo), suggesting that the scale was measuring traits not influenced by treatment efforts. Their findings appeared to be consistent with those found for Millon's standardization group.

However, the literature contains several studies that challenge the ability of the MCMI T scale to identify drug abusers successfully.[120,121] In the 1990 study, only 39.4% of a drug-abusing sample (75 White, male veterans) were correctly classified using the clinically relevant cutoff of 74. If the cutoff of 84, indicating "prominence" of the drug abuse syndrome is used instead, only 19.7% of profiles are correctly classified. This means that more than 60% of known heroin and cocaine abusers failed to be detected by means of the T scale. At the same time, only 12% of the comparison group (60 White, male veterans without drug dependencies who were receiving psychiatric care) was misclassified, suggesting that the false positive rate for the scale is relatively low.

In the 1991 study,[121] only 26% of 110 male veterans admitted to outpatient drug abuse treatment obtained base rate scores >84 (indicating prominence) whereas another 23% of the sample obtained scores of between 74 and 84 (suggestive of symptomatology). Thus, 51% of the sample received MCMI scale *T* scores that were below the clinical relevance cutoff point. Of additional concern was the finding that the T scale was more likely to detect Black drug abusers than White drug abusers. It is unclear whether this represents a racial bias in the test, or if the test is simply more valid for Blacks. Finally, addicts with severe psychopathology, and with narcissistic and antisocial personalities in particular, were more likely to have elevated scale T scores. The authors pointed out that this may be an artifact of item-overlap. However, it also seems plausible that, for those addicts correctly identified, the likelihood is greater that these disorders will coexist.

With regard to the low detection rate for scale T among known drug abusers, we have also found that only about half of a sample of drug-dependent pregnant and recently postpartum women were detected via the MCMI T scale.[122] A comparably low rate of detection for those with known alcohol problems via scale B (alcohol abuse) was also of concern.

Summary of Findings for the MCMI

Issues discussed in relation to research with the MMPI apply here as well. Investigators have focused on the output of their statistical manipulations without focusing as closely on the independent variable. In order for the relative contribution of personality and drug use to be understood, the drug-use groups must be better defined. In spite of this, the data available are interesting and appear to parallel those for the MMPI. "Types" are found both within and across drug-use groups. The "myth of heterogeneity" is again identified as causing problems. The consistent finding for an antisocial component is clear. Also, the extent to which narcissism plays a role supports the work of the dynamic theorists discussed earlier in this chapter.

Other Objective Tests

A fair number of studies have employed the 16 Personality Factor Questionnaire (16 PF) in the study of alcoholics. De Palma and Clayton were successfully able to differentiate alcoholics from controls on 14 of 16 scales.[123] The greatest difference for the two groups was found on the "emotional vs mature" subscale. They concluded that alcoholics are ruled by the "pleasure principle." Although studies have generally supported this finding,[124,125] differences have been found on an assortment of variables, including intelligence, impulsivity, and sensitivity.[125]

As with the MMPI and MCMI, many studies employing the 16 PF have focused on differentiating various clinical groups. Results have varied, depending on the sample being investigated. For instance, in comparing hospitalized and imprisoned alcoholics, Ross found a correlation coefficient of .91 suggesting few differences.[126] Ciotola and Peterson, however, in an attempt to distinguish alcoholics, opioid addicts, and polysubstance abusers, found significant differences for the three groups on seven lower-order factors and two higher-order ones.[127] The alcoholics were significantly shier, more apprehensive, more anxious, and more dependent than the opioid addicts. The polysubstance abusers fell in between the other two groups on all four scales. The 16 PF was also utilized to study two subgroups of alcoholics (gamma and delta) identified by Jellineck.[128] Results suggested that the gamma alcoholics were less emotionally stable, more depressed, more timid, and more independent than the delta alcoholics.[129]

The cluster methodology has also been used to identify subgroups of addicts using the 16 PF. Lawlis and Rubin performed cluster analyses and then computed a discriminate function to determine the statistical significance of the clusters obtained.[130] Three types of alcoholics emerged: an inhibited, maladaptive type, a sociopathic type, and an aggressive type. In another cluster analytic study, Nerviano and Gross found two types of alcoholics—

an anxious, introverted type and a dependent type.[131] However, in their 1983 review article, these authors asserted that there has been a major match for only one male type on the 16 PF.[132] They further noted that one typology involving women[133] failed to yield substantial scale deviations for any type. Thus only one type, resembling the replicated type for males, appeared viable. This type is characterized by rather severe anxiety and schizoid features.

As no longitudinal studies involving the 16 PF are available, it remains unclear whether any observed differences between and within groups are a function of personality or of drug use. However, as with the MMPI, changes in test findings typically occur following substance abuse treatment.[134,135] This suggests that findings may be more related to being an addict as opposed to being the kind of person who becomes one.

A recent investigation employed the NEO-Personality Inventory (NEO-PI) to evaluate the personality dimensions of male and female drug abusers with and without antisocial personality disorder.[136] It was reported that the antisocial personality disorder group was "significantly more vulnerable to stress, more prone to anger, more impulsive, more emotionally cold and distant, and more disagreeable and vindictive than the non-ASP group" (p. 232). Regarding gender comparison, the authors noted that male and female substance abusers obtained similar NEO-PI profiles, however males demonstrated significantly higher scores on the openness to experience and agreeableness factors. They concluded that females are less receptive to novel experiences and more antagonistic than males.

Knoblaugh, in a study employing college freshmen, isolated what he believed to be a "female component" of alcoholism.[137] Based on concepts of Eastern philosophy (Taoism), the Western translation of this component would roughly be one of depression, anxiety, and low self-esteem. The Ego Grasping Orientation (EGO) was used to differentiate among males and females without alcohol-related problems, those with alcoholic-related problems, and those belonging to alcoholic groups. Accordingly, subjects were divided into six groups based on their Michigan Alcohol Screen Test (MAST) scores and gender. Using the EGO score as dependent variable, ANOVA revealed significant differences for the three alcohol classifications and for the gender groupings. There was also a significant group × gender interaction. The author concluded that a high EGO score is "an antecedent or concomitant" of women's alcoholism. He found this to be consistent with Cloninger's groupings of male and female alcoholics.

Finally, with regard to Cloninger's tridimensional personality model, a recent study attempted to assess empirically construct validity of the Tridimensional Personality Questionnaire (TPQ).[138] Accordingly, the test was administered to 267 hospitalized substance abusers, 172 of whom were alcoholic. One-third of the sample was female. The authors found that the alcoholic patients were not classified into Cloninger's type 1 and type 2 groups according to the expected frequencies. A large number were, in fact, classified as low on both novelty seeking (NS) and harm avoidance (HA). This contradicts Cloninger's predictions that hospitalized alcoholic males will mostly fall into type 2 (high NS/low HA), whereas most females will exhibit type 1 (low NS/ high HA). Although MANOVAs failed to reveal any significant effects for drug of abuse, a significant gender effect was obtained. The specific difference was on HA, with females scoring higher than males.

The Rorschach

The Rorschach studies are open to challenge, in that most of the test protocols have been scored and interpreted in a subjective way. An early study described 12 heroin addicts as psychopathic, immature, and impulsive.[139] The authors further noted their subjects' distinct lack of affect, interests, and energy. Sixty-five adolescent addicts were described somewhat differently by Zimmerling et al.[140] As a group, they were seen as having weak ego development and as being prone to withdrawal into fantasy. However, they were not seen as either impulsive nor aggressive. Bleckner commented on the Rorschach records of 54 addicts, including 17 females.[141] A sense of impoverishment characterized their responses, which were few in number and which evidenced lack of attention to detail. Also, impulsiveness, immaturity, and escape into fantasy were noted. The female subjects, however, were seen as having somewhat better internal resources than the males.

Craig, in his review on personality characteristics of heroin addicts, identified several empirically based Rorschach studies.[96] Although both employed comparison groups, the investigators also served as examiners. Because they were not blinded, the possibility of examiner bias exists. Gerard and Kornetsky studied 32 drug-addicted and 22 drug-exposed (but nonaddicted) adolescents.[142] The experimental subjects generated constricted, impoverished responses that lacked "richness." Additionally, they evidenced poor object relations and had difficulty dealing with affect-laden material. The second study investigated "womb" fantasies among 30 adult, male heroin addicts.[143] Again, subjects were compared to heroin-exposed (but nonaddicted) controls. The addicts were shown to have a higher rate of such fantasies; this was interpreted as indicative of their primitive need for nourishment.

Although no scoring criteria or actual test data were presented, Dougherty and Lesswing described the Rorschach records of 100 cocaine abusers as indicative of narcissism, underlying anger, and diminished reality testing.[4] They attributed these characteristics, along with cognitive slippage, to chronic drug abuse. They further noted that, despite the presence of acute distress, subjects displayed normal levels of dysphoria and depression.

Finally, Blatt and Berman tested the hypothesis that there are three types of opioid addicts (those with sociopathic features, those with depressive features, and those with psychotic features).[144] Accordingly, they administered the Loevinger Sentence Completion Test, the Rorschach, and the Bellack Ego Functions Interview to 53 opioid addicts, and then submitted variables derived from the data to cluster and discriminate analyses. Three types were identified, one with predominantly impaired interpersonal relationships and affective lability (42%), one with predominantly impaired thought processes and ego functioning (30%), and one with predominantly diminished ideational and verbal function (28%). They concluded that this was evidence for three opioid addicted personality types, characterized as character disordered, borderline psychotic, and depressed, respectively.

The number of projective test studies employing the scientific method is so limited that it is impossible to draw any conclusions. From a clinical standpoint, however, the reports are not inconsistent with findings of objective test studies nor with underlying theoretical concepts. It will be interesting to see if, with the advent of the Exner scoring system for the Rorschach, a rash of well designed and controlled studies employing this instrument will now be done.

Summary

Researchers have taken a relatively consistent approach to describing and classifying substance abusers via objective personality tests. The mean profile approach gives a general picture and allows for comparisons across samples. Nevertheless, no profile is unique to substance abusers. Also, although mean profiles describe the group, as a whole, reasonably well, they tend to obscure the presence of homogeneous subgroups. These subgroups are important since they provide clinically relevant information that can be used in treatment planning.

Interestingly, many subtypes are not specific to drug of choice. This raises the question of relative importance of drug use patterns and psychopathology. In sum, the most definitive things that can be said are:

1. All substance abuse groups have features in common and the similarities are generally greater than the differences;
2. Depending on sample characteristics, there are also reliable test differences and clinical groups are thus able to be distinguished from one another;
3. There are homogeneous subgroups existing both within and across drug use groups; and

4. Although small gender related findings have been reported, male and female substance abusers have much in common and the similarities seem greater than the differences.

With regard to the projective tests, these are limited in their utility since they are few in number and lack scientific rigor. Nevertheless, the available studies also support the existence of multiple types of substance abuse.

In terms of whether the personality factors noted are predispositional or a function of chronic substance use, this question remains, to a large degree, unanswered. Carefully designed longitudinal research is necessary to resolve the issue. However, the fact that many of the identified characteristics of addicts change as a function of treatment and abstinence suggests that these are related to drug use, as opposed to being personality indicators. On the other hand, the single most robust finding, across tests and samples, is for an antisocial component. This element may therefore be hypothesized to be a necessary, although not sufficient, condition for the development of addictive illness.

Finally, in order to reach a more sophisticated understanding regarding addiction and personality, substance-abusing subjects must be better described from the outset. Nearly all of the studies reviewed suffer as a result of not having adequately defined their samples. The specifics of their drug use (including substance(s) used, amount and duration of use, route of administration, family history of addiction, severity of addiction, areas of functioning affected by drug use, and so forth) must all be taken into account. To date, researchers have focused heavily on test output, while being less than rigorous about defining their subjects. This pervasive methodological weakness has the potential to cause group contamination, perhaps leading to some of the confusing findings. Thus, future studies should be as meticulous about grouping individuals prior to analysis as they have been in trying to group them afterward. Such an approach should reduce confounds and allow for a clearer picture of the addicted person to emerge.

MMPI Data for 90 Addicted Women

The Virginia Commonwealth University, Medical College of Virginia Hospitals Center for Perinatal Addiction (CPA) is a NIDA-funded treatment research unit for female addicts and their children. In order to be admitted, a women must either be pregnant or recently postpartum. The majority of patients exhibit polysubstance dependence. Approximately 85% of the women are cocaine dependent, 40% percent are alcoholic, 40% are marijuana dependent, and 25% are heroin dependent. The picture is one of clear polysubstance abuse, with cocaine addiction most prominent. The sample is very treatment-experienced, with nearly 70% having had at least one inpatient admission. The mean age is 27 yr, and 80% of the women are Black and 20% are White. The women come from urban, suburban, and rural areas throughout the Commonwealth of Virginia. As a group, they are emotionally, cognitively, educationally, and financially impoverished, with few community resources available to them. Many are entangled with the criminal justice system as a function of their drug use, and nearly all are involved with social service agencies. The most common referral sources are healthcare professionals (medical and psychiatric) and the courts. Very few patients are self-referrals.

One of the major focuses at CPA during the past 3 yr has been on personality and psychopathology in addicted women, with particular attention being paid to axis II pathology. The larger goal of the project is to better understand treatment process and outcome for addicted women who evidence psychiatric comorbidity. To date, more than 100 women have been admitted to the study and have participated in an initial assessment. This comprehensive evaluation consists of a large number of measures of psychological functioning that are readministered periodically to assess for change as a function of treatment rendered. Multiple measures of disturbance have been employed, whenever feasible, in order to assess the reliability of measurement and to begin to look at the validity of the constructs associated with personality disorder.

MMPI-2 data have been analyzed for 90 women admitted to CPA. Corresponding MCMI-II data are available, but have not yet been reviewed. Table 1 depicts the full distribution of MMPI-2 code-types present in this sample of addicted women. The eight 2-point code-types describing >5% of the sample each are indicated by an asterisk. Table 2 gives comparative base rates for female psychiatric patients (based on the original MMPI) and for the MMPI-2 normative sample for these eight code-types.

Altogether, the eight 2-point code-types categorize about 70% of cases. Classification was made based on absolute high-points and without purification. The 24 type characterizes 18% of cases. The 24 code-type has previously been identified as the most frequently occurring profile type among addicted populations.[70] These data replicate this finding for a subsample of female, mostly Black, polysubstance abusers.

Several comments about the code-type distribution are in order. First, a number of the identified 2-point codes have previously been reported to have alcohol and drug abuse as common correlates, both for MMPI and MMPI-2. These include the 24, 47, 48, and 49, all of which have a common

Table 1
Distribution of MMPI Code Types
Center for Perinatal Addiction

Code-type	Percentage of sample
0–2–7	1.1
0–4/4–0	2.2
0–5/5–0	2.2
0–7–8	1.1
1–3/3–1	1.1
1–4–6	1.1
1–9/9–1	3.3
2–4/4–2	17.8*
2–5/5–2	1.1
2–7–8	2.2
3–4/4–3	4.4
4–5–9	1.1
4–6/6–4	8.9*
4–7/7–4	5.6*
4–8/8–4	7.8*
4–9/9–4	6.7*
5–6/6–5	1.1
5–8/8–5	1.1
5–9/9–5	6.7*
6–7–9	1.1
6–8/8–6	10.0*
7–8/8–7	2.2
8–9/9–8	5.6*
4	3.3
9	1.1

*>5% of sample.

elevation on scale 4. In this sample, an additional scale 4 type was identified (46). Interestingly, Graham once identified this as the modal profile for female alcoholics.[48] Thus, five of the eight most frequently occurring configurations, accounting for greater than two-thirds of the entire sample (and about three-fourths of the classified profiles), have a common elevation on scale 4.

In describing correlates of scale 4 for MMPI-2, Butcher noted that high scorers frequently have substance abuse as part of their symptom picture; he further urged that this be taken into account when treatment is being planned.[145] Those with elevations on scale 4 were described as experienc-

Table 2
Comparison of Base Rates for Selected MMPI Code Types

Code-type	Study sample $N = 90$ (females)	MMPI-2 normative,[a] $N = 1462$ (females)	Psychiatric (MMPI),[b] $N = 12,000$ (male and females)
2–4/4–2	17.8	3.1	7.5
4–6/6–4	8.9	3.8	5.1
4–7 (8)	5.6	1.7	2.3
4–8/8–4	7.8	3.0	8.7
4–9/9–4	6.7	5.8	6.7
5–9/9–5	6.7	—	.59 (high 5 only)
6–8/8–6	10.0	2.4	3.9
8–9/9–8	5.6	4.5	2.4

[a]Personal communication with Nathan Weed based on data collected by James Butcher.
[b]From ref. 144.

ing a variety of problems related to their impulsivity and poor judgment, including legal and interpersonal difficulties. This clinical picture is highly consistent with that observed in our female addicts at point of entry to treatment. Butcher further described high scale 4 individuals as treatment resistant; they did not come willingly to therapy and frequently left treatment prematurely. This is also true of the study participants. In terms of additional scale 4 correlates, Graham identified high scorers as rebellious, hostile, "refractory" individuals who demonstrate low frustration tolerance, excessive risk-taking behavior, and an inability to learn from past mistakes.[146] He further described high scorers as insensitive to the needs of others, self-centered, and immature. Their interpersonal relationships are typically shallow and reflect their inability to form meaningful attachments to others. All of these descriptors are consistent with our clinical experience in working with these women. For specific interpretive information for these five MMPI-2 profile configurations, please refer further to Butcher[145] and Graham.[146]

Three additional 2-point code types figured prominently in the sample (59, 68, and 89). The 68 type, accounting for 10% of profiles, and the 89 type are of considerable interest. Although these are "psychotic" profile types, few of the subjects exhibit this degree of overt psychopathology. Rather, they manifest characteristics normally associated with a less dramatic elevation on scale 8, such as alienation, identity problems, and extremely low self-worth. It may be that the ethnicity and socioeconomic status are having an influence, and that elevations on scale 8 for addicted women need to be interpreted with this in mind. Elevations on scale 8, $T >$ 80, in the absence of confusion and cognitive disorganization, is reminiscent of Rothauzer's finding for polysubstance abusers.[107] In this study also, disturbed-looking profiles appeared to be overpathologizing. Both the 68 and 89 profiles in the current study conform to Conley and Prioliau's schizoform A alcoholic personality.[77] This type has been associated with "fast track" (or essential) alcoholism, and is characterized by early onset, social disruption, and a familial pattern of substance abuse.

The 59 and 89 code types share scale 9 elevation in common. Butcher noted the usefulness of scale 9 as a predictor of "accessibility" for treatment.[145] Those individuals scoring above $T = 70$ (the majority of the patients in this sample) are seen as distractable and overactive, making them generally uncooperative in therapy. He noted their general disregard for regular session attendance coupled with an attitude of being too busy. This attitudinal stance, in conjunction with their characteristic narcissism, denial, and avoidance of self-reflection, combine to make the therapeutic endeavor difficult at best.

Of particular interest is the 59 two-point code that is sufficiently uncommon in females as to not have been considered in the renorming of the test. In 1971, Webb reported that only .59% of female psychiatric patients generate a profile with high-point scale 5.[147] Thus, the obtained study rate of 6.7% (11.1% when all two-point types with defining scale 5 elevations are considered) represents a dramatic and intriguing finding, bearing further investigation.

Relatively little has been written about high scale 5 females. What there is suggests that these are uninhibited, active, aggressive individuals who have rejected the traditional female role. As a group, their interests and activities tend to be stereotypically masculine, and they are seen as dominating and competitive in nature. Graham noted that, among hospitalized psychiatric patients, high scale 5 females are sometimes psychotic, manifesting suspiciousness, delusions, and even hallucinations.[146] However, the mean profile for the 59 patients in this study is relatively benign in terms of overall elevation. Indeed, the 59 and 49 types appear to represent the best-adjusted patients. Although the numbers are too small for statistical analysis, it is of clinical interest that, in a sample where abuse of all types (verbal, physical, and sexual) is highly prevalent, none of the 59 women reported themselves to be victims. Either their "toughness" in some way protects them from the likelihood of abuse, or their self-perception is one of relative invulnerability.

Summary

Psychopathology is extremely common among this sample of 90 cocaine-, alcohol-, and marijuana-dependent women. Both axis I and axis II disorders are present in significant numbers whereas personality disorder is a near universal phenomenon. The cluster B diagnoses are overrepresented.

In terms of personality type, a large proportion (about 70%) of these women were able to be classified on MMPI-2 into one of eight 2-point code-types. Each of these eight characterized >5% of the total sample. Five of the eight code-types had scale 4 as one of their defining high points, whereas three had scale 9 and two had scale 8 as defining high points. The 59 code-type represents an especially unusual finding, which should be further explored. Scale 5 may be making a significantly different contribution on MMPI-2 for women, especially addicted women, than it did on MMPI.

References

[1] F. H. Gavin and H. D. Kleber (1986) Abstinence symptomatology and psychiatric diagnosis in cocaine abusers. *Arch. Gen. Psychiatry* **43,** 107–113.

[2] B. J. Rounsaville, M. M. Weissman, K. Crits-Cristoph, C. H. Wilber, and H. D. Kleber (1982) Diagnosis and symptoms of depression in opiate addicts: Course and relationship to treatment outcome. *Arch. Gen. Psychiatry* **39,** 151–156.

[3] R. D. Weiss, S. D. Mirin, J. L. Michael, and A. C. Sollogub (1986) Psychopathology in chronic cocaine users. *Am. J. Drug Alcohol Abuse* **12,** 17–29.

[4] R. J. Dougherty and N. J. Lesswing (1989) Inpatient cocaine abusers: An analysis of psychological and demographical variables. *J. Subst. Abuse Treatment* **6,** 45–47.

[5] E. J. Khantzian and C. Treece (1985) DSM-III psychiatric diagnosis of narcotic addicts: Recent findings. *Arch. Gen. Psychiatry* **42,** 1067–1071.

[6] B. E. Havassy and D. A. Wasserman (1991) Prevalence of co-morbidity among cocaine users in treatment, in *NIDA Research Monograph Series, vol. 119, Problems of Drug Dependence: Proceedings of the 53rd Annual Scientific Meeting.* College on Problems of Drug Dependence, U.S. Government Printing Office, Washington, DC., 1992b, p. 227.

[7] L. B. Cottler, W. M. Compton III, D. Mager, G. A. Storch, and J. Hudziak (1991) Psychiatric histories among drug abusers: IVDA vs. non-IVDA, in *NIDA Research Monograph Series, vol. 119, Problems of Drug Dependence 1991: Proceedings of the 53rd Annual Scientific Meeting.* College on Problems of Drug Dependence, U.S. Government Printing Office, Washington, DC., 1992b, p. 228.

[8] B. J. Mason, J. H. Kocsis, D. Melia, E. T. Khuri, R. B. Millman, J. Sweeney, A. Wells, and M. J. Kreek (1991) Psychiatric comorbidity in methadone maintained patients, in *NIDA Research Monograph Series, vol. 119, Problems of Drug Dependence: Proceedings of the 53rd Annual Scientific Meeting.* College on Problems of Drug Dependence, U.S. Government Printing Office, Washington, DC., 1992b, p. 230.

[9] M. N. Hesselbrock, R. E. Meyer, and J. J. Keener (1985) Psychopathology in hospitalized alcoholics. *Arch. Gen. Psychiatry* **42,** 1050–1055.

[10]M. L. Griffin, R. D. Weiss, S. D. Mirin, and U. Lange (1989) A comparison of male and female cocaine abusers. *Arch. Gen. Psychiatry* **46**, 122–126.

[11]D. L. Haller, J. S. Knisely, K. S. Dawson, and S. H. Schnoll (1993) Perinatal substance abusers: Psychological and social characteristics. *J. Nerv. Ment. Dis.* **181**, 509–513.

[12]American Psychiatric Association (1987) *Diagnostic and Statistical Manual of Mental Disorders* (3rd ed., rev.) American Psychiatric Association, Washington, DC.

[13]G. E. Woody, T. A. McLellan, L. Luborsky, and C. P. O'Brien (1985) Sociopathy and psychotherapy outcome. *Arch. Gen. Psychiatry* **42**, 1081–1086.

[14]D. L. Haller, R. K. Elswick Jr., K. S. Dawson, J. S. Knisely, and S. H. Schnoll (1992) Retention in treatment of perinatal substance abusers, in *NIDA Research Monograph Series, vol. 132, Problems of Drug Dependence: Proceedings of the 54th Annual Scientific Meeting.* College on Problems of Drug Dependence, U.S. Government Printing Office, Washington, DC., p. 303.

[15]T. A. McLellan, L. Luborsky, G. E. Woody, C. P. O'Brien, and R. Kron (1981) Are the "addiction related" problems of substance abusers really related? *J. Nerv. Ment. Dis.* **169**, 232–239.

[16]T. A. McLellan, A. R. Childress, J. Griffith, and G. E. Woody (1984) The psychiatrically severe drug abuse patient: Methadone maintenance or therapeutic community? *Am. J. Alcohol Abuse* **10**, 77–95.

[17]T. R. Kosten, B. J. Rounsaville, and H. Kleber (1986) A 2.5-year followup of cocaine use among treated opioid addicts. *Arch. Gen. Psychiatry* **44**, 281–284.

[18]S. R. Maddi (1986) *Personality Theories: A Comparative Analysis.* Dorsey, Homewood, IL.

[19]L. Miller (1990) Neuropsychodynamics of alcoholism and addiction: Personality, psychopathology, and cognitive style. *J. Subst. Abuse Treatment* **7**, 31–49.

[20]O. F. Kernberg (1975) *Borderline Conditions and Pathological Narcissism.* Aronson, New York.

[21]H. Kohut (1971) *The Analysis of the Self.* International Universities, New York.

[22]L. Wurmser (1974) Psychoanalytic considerations of the etiology of compulsive drug use. *J. Am. Psychoanal. Assoc.* **22**, 820–843.

[23]H. Krystal (1977) Self representations and the capacity for self care. *Ann. Psychoanal.* **6**, 209–246.

[24]J. M. Donovan (1986) An etiological mode of alcoholism. *Am. J. Psychiatry* **143**, 1–11.

[25]R. Cloninger (1987) Neurogenic adaptive mechanism in alcoholism. *Science* **236**, 410–416.

[26]E. J. Khantzian (1985) The self-medication hypothesis of addictive disorders: Focus on heroin and cocaine dependence. *Am. J. Psychiatry.* **142**, 1259–1264.

[27]P. B. Sutker and R. P. Archer (1984) Opiate abuse and dependence disorders, in *Comprehensive Textbook of Psychopathology.* H. E. Adams and P. B. Sutker, eds., Plenum, New York, pp. 585–621.

[28]E. Glover (1956) The etiology of drug addiction, in *The Early Development of the Mind.* E. Glover, ed., International Universities, New York, pp. 187–215.

[29]L. Wurmser (1978) *The Hidden Dimension: Psychodynamics in Compulsive Drug Use.* Aronson, New York.

[30]O. Fenichel (1945) *The Psychoanalytic Theory of Neurosis.* Norton, New York.

[31]E. J. Khantizian (1978) The ego, the self, and opiate addiction: Theoretical and treatment considerations. *Int. Rev. Psychoanal.* **5**, 189–198.

[32]E. J. Khantizian (1982) Psychological (structural) vulnerabilities and the specific appeal of narcotics. *Ann. NY Acad. Sci.* **398**, 24–32.

[33]C. Treece and E. J. Khantizian (1986) Psychodynamic factors in the development of drug dependence. *Psychiatr. Clin. N. Am.* **9**, 399–412.

[34]H. Hendrin (1973) Marijuana abuse among college students. *J. Nerv. Ment. Dis.* **156**, 259–270.

[35]H. Hendrin (1974) Amphetamine use among college students. *J. Nerv. Ment. Dis.* **158**, 256–267.

[36]H. Krystal and H. A. Raskin (1970) *Drug Dependence Aspects of Ego Function.* Wayne State University, Detroit, MI.

[37]B. Nicholson and C. Treece (1981) Object relations and differential treatment response to methadone maintenance. *J. Nerv. Ment. Dis.* **169**, 424–429.

[38]R. J. Craig (1982) Personality characteristics of heroin addicts: Review of empirical research 1976–1979. *Int. J. Addict.* **17**, 227–248.

[39]E. J. Khantizian (1975) Self selection and progression in drug dependence. *Psychiatry Dig.* **10**, 19–22.

[40]H. Wieder and E. H. Kaplan. Drug use in adolescence: Psychodynamic meaning and pharmacogenic effect. *Psychoanal. Study Child* **24**, 399–431.

[41]E. J. Khantizian (1983) An extreme case of cocaine dependence and marked improvement with methylphenidate treatment. *Am. J. Psychiatry* **140**, 784–785.

[42]N. E. Zinberg (1975) Addiction and ego function. *Psychoanal. Study Child* **30**, 567–588.

[43]R. L. Retka and L. R. Chatam (1974) The addict personality. *J. Psychedelic Drugs* **6**, 15–20.

[44]G. E. Barnes (1979) The alcoholic personality. *J. Stud. Alcohol.* **40**, 571–634.

[45]S. Belenko (1979) Alcohol abuse by heroin addicts: A review of research findings and issues. *Int. J. Addict.* **14**, 965–975.

[46]J. R. Graham and V. E. Strenger (1988) MMPI characteristics of alcoholics: A review. *J. Consult. Clin. Psychol.* **56**, 197–205.

[47]R. D. Fowler and J. L. Bernard (1960) *MMPI Composite Profiles for Inpatient and Outpatient Alcoholics.* Studies in Alcoholism, Alabama Commission on Alcoholism, Montgomery, AL.

[48]J. R. Graham (1978) MMPI characteristic of alcoholics, drug addicts, and pathological gamblers. Paper presented at the 13th Annual Symposium on Recent Developments in the Use of the MMPI, University of the Americas, Puebla, Mexico.

[49]G. L. Hodo and R. D. Fowler (1976) Frequency of MMPI two-point codes in a large alcoholic sample. *J. Clin. Psychology* **32**, 487–489.

[50]R. Lanyon (1968) *A Handbook of MMPI Group Profiles.* University of Minnesota, Minneapolis, MN.

[51]C. C. Hewitt (1943) A personality study of alcoholic addiction. *Q. J. Stud. Alcohol* **4**, 368–386.

[52]D. M. Eshbaugh, D. J. Tosi, and C. N. Hoyt (1980) Women alcoholics: A typological description using the MMPI. *J. Stud. Alcohol* **41**, 310–317.

[53]T. McKenna and R. Pickens (1981) Alcoholic children of alcoholics. *J. Stud. Alcohol* **42**, 1021–1029.

[54]R. D. Page and S. Bozlee (1982) A cross-cultural MMPI comparison of alcoholics. *Psychol. Rep.* **50,** 639–646.

[55]M. L. Kammeier, H. Hoffmann, and R. G. Loper (1973) Personality characteristics of alcoholics as college freshmen and at time of treatment. *Q. J. Stud. Alcohol* **34,** 390–399.

[56]R. G. Loper, M. L. Kammeier, and H. Hoffmann (1973) MMPI characteristics of college freshman males who later become alcoholics. *J. Abnorm. Psychol.* **82,** 159–162.

[57]D. P. Hoyt and G. M. Sedlacek (1958) Differentiating alcoholics from normals and abnormals with the MMPI. *J. Clin. Psychology* **14,** 69–74.

[58]A. C. Rosen (1960) A comparative study of alcoholics and psychiatric patients with the MMPI. *Q. J. Stud. Alcohol* **21,** 253–266.

[59]S. L. Zelen, J. Fox, E. Gould, and R. W. Olson (1966) Sex-contingent differences between male and female alcoholics. *J. Clin. Psychol.* **22,** 160–165.

[60]H. E. Hill, C. A. Haertzen, and H. Davis (1962) An MMPI factor analytic of alcoholics, narcotics addicts, and criminals. *Q. J. Stud. Alcohol* **23,** 411–431.

[61]L. H. Roth, N. Rosenberg, and R. B. Levinson (1971) Prison adjustment of alcoholic felons. *Q. J. Stud. Alcohol* **32,** 382–392.

[62]J. E. Overall (1973) MMPI personality patterns of alcoholics and narcotics addicts. *Q. J. Stud. Alcohol* **34,** 104–111.

[63]T. R. Holland, M. Levi, and C. G. Watson (1981) MMPI basic scales vs. two point codes in the discrimination of psychopathological groups. *J. Clin. Psychol.* **37,** 394–396.

[64]R. K. Blashfield (1985) Meta-analysis on MMPI studies of alcoholics. *Bull. Soc. Psychol. Addict. Behav.* **4,** 29–40.

[65]S. G. Goldstein and J. D. Linden (1969) Multivariate classification of alcoholics by means of the MMPI. *J. Abnorm. Psychol.* **6,** 661–669.

[66]D. M. Donovan, E. F. Chaney, and M. R. O'Leary (1978) Alcoholic MMPI subtypes. *J. Nerv. Mentl. Dis.* **166,** 553–561.

[67]T. Loberg (1981) MMPI-based personality subtypes of alcoholics: Relationships to drinking history, psychometrics, and neuropsychological deficits. *J. Stud. Alcohol* **42,** 766–782.

[68]V. J. Nerviano, D. McCarty, and S. M. McCarty (1980) MMPI profile patterns of men alcoholics in two contrasting settings. *J. Stud. Alcohol* **41,** 1143–1152.

[69]J. R. Graham (1987) *The MMPI: A Practical Guide.* Oxford University, New York.

[70]R. L. Greene (1980) *The MMPI: An Interpretative Manual.* Grune and Stratton, New York.

[71]H. Gilberstadt and J. Duker (1965) *A Handbook for Clinical and Actuarial MMPI Interpretation.* Saunders, Philadelphia, PA.

[72]P. A. Marks, W. Seeman, and D. L. Haller (1974) *The Actuarial Use of the MMPI with Adolescents and Adults.* Williams and Wilkins, Baltimore, MD.

[73]S. Svanum and C. L. Dallas (1981) Alcoholic MMPI types and their relationship to patient characteristics, polydrug abuse, and abstinence following treatment. *J. Pers. Assess.* **45,** 278–287.

[74]W. J. Filstead, D. A. Drachman, J. J. Rossi, and S. H. Getsinger (1983) The relationship of MMPI subtype membership to demographic variables and treatment outcome among substance misusers. *J. Stud. Alcohol* **44,** 917–922.

[75]K. S. Pfost, J. T. Kunce, and M. J. Stevens (1984) The relationship of MacAndrew Alcoholism scale scores to MMPI profile type and degree of elevation. *J. Clin. Psychol.* **40,** 852–857.

[76]J. J. Conley and L. A. Prioleau (1983) Personality typology of men and women alcoholics in relation to etiology and prognosis. *J. Stud. Alcohol* **44,** 996–1010.

[77]J. J. Conley (1981) An MMPI typology of male alcoholics: admission, discharge, and outcome comparisons. *J. Pers. Assess.* **45,** 33–39.

[78]C. MacAndrew (1981) What the MAC scale tells us about alcoholics: an interpretative review. *J. Stud. Alcohol* **42,** 604–625.

[79]P. B. Sutker and R. P. Archer (1979) MMPI characteristics of opiate addicts, alcoholics, and other drug abusers, in *MMPI Clinical and Research Trends.* C. E. Newmark, ed., Praeger, New York, pp. 105–148.

[80]D. Lachar, W. Berman, J. L. Grisell, and K. Schoot (1979) The MacAndrew Alcoholism Scale as a general measure of substance misuse. *J. Stud. Alcohol* **37,** 1609–1615.

[81]P. B. Sutker, R. P. Archer, P. Brantly, and D. Kilpatrick (1979) Alcoholics and opiate addicts: Comparison of personality characteristics. *J. Stud. Alcohol* **40,** 635–644.

[82]G. D. Walters, R. Greene, T. B. Jeffrey, D. J. Kruzich, and J. J. Haskin (1983) Racial variations on the MacAndrew Alcoholism Scale of the MMPI. *J. Consult. Clin. Psychol.* **51,** 947–948.

[83]K. W. Preng and J. R. Clopton (1986) Application of the MacAndrew Alcoholism Scale to alcoholics with psychiatric diagnoses. *J. Pers. Assess.* **50,** 113–122.

[84]C. MacAndrew (1979) On the possibility of the psychometric detection of persons who are prone to the abuse of alcohol and other substances. *Addict. Behav.* **4,** 11–20.

[85]P. M. O'Neil, J. P. Giacinto, S. R. Waid, J. C. Roitzsch, W. C. Miller, and D. G. Kilpatrick (1983) Behavioral psychological, and historical correlated of MacAndrew scale scores among male alcoholics. *J. Behav. Assess.* **5,** 261–273.

[86]Z. Z. Cernovsky (1985) Detection of false positives. *Psychol. Rep.* **57,** 191–194.

[87]Z. Z. Cernovsky (1987) A failure to detect MAC's false positives in female alcohol and drug addicts. *Addict. Behav.* **12,** 367–369.

[88]J. P. Allen, V. Faden, R. Rawlings, and A. Miller (1990) Subtypes of substance abusers: Personality differences associated with MacAndrew scores. *Psychol. Rep.* **66,** 691–698.

[89]C. MacAndrew (1986) Similarities in self-depictions of female alcoholics and psychiatric outpatients: An examination of Eysenck's dimension of emotionality in women. *J. Stud. Alcohol* **47,** 478–484.

[90]C. MacAndrew (1987) Differences in the self-depictions of female alcoholics and psychiatric outpatients: Towards a depiction of the modal female alcoholic. *J. Stud. Alcohol* **49,** 71–77.

[91]D. G. Jansen and H. Hoffmann (1973) Demographic and MMPI characteristics of male and female state hospital alcoholic patients. *Psychol. Rep.* **33,** 561–562.

[92]J. Curlee (1970) A comparison of male and female patients at an alcoholism treatment center. *J. Psychol* **74,** 239–247.

[93]M. F. Schwartz and J. R. Graham (1979) Construct validity of the MacAndrew Alcoholism scale. *J. Consult. Clin. Psychol.* **47,** 1090–1095.

[94]S. Svanum and R. G. Hoffman (1982) The factor structure of the MacAndrew Alcoholism scale. *Addict. Behav.* **7,** 195–198.

[95]R. J. Craig (1979) Personality characteristics of heroin addicts: A review of the empirical literature with critique-part II. *Int. J. Addict.* **14**, 607–626.

[96]A. W. Astin (1959) A factor study of the MMPI Psychopathic Deviate scale. *J. Consult. Psychol.* **23**, 550–554.

[97]R. W. Olson (1964) MMPI sex differences in narcotic addicts. *J. Gen. Psychol.* **71**, 257–266.

[98]J. I. Berzins, W. F. Ross, and J. J. Monroe (1974) Subgroups among opiate addicts: A typological investigation. *J. Abnorm. Psychol.* **83**, 65–73.

[99]P. B. Sutker and C. Moan (1972) Personality characteristics of socially deviant women: Incarcerated heroin addicts, street addicts, and nonaddict prisoners, in *Drug Addiction: Clinical and Socio-Legal Aspects.* J. M. Singh, L. Miller, and H. Lal, eds., Futura, Mount Kisco, NY, pp. 107–114.

[100]W. Parr, W. Woodward, R. Robinowitz, and W. Penk (1981) Cross-validation of a Heroin Addiction (HE) scale in a treatment setting. *Int. J. Addict.* **16**, 549–553.

[101]L. D. Zager and E. I. Megargee (1981) Some MMPI alcohol and drug abuse scales: An empirical investigation of their interrelationships, convergent and discriminate validity and degree of racial bias. *J. Pers. Soc. Psychol.* **40**, 532–544.

[102]R. J. Craig (1984) MMPI substance abuse scales on drug addicts with and without concurrent alcoholism. *J. Pers. Assess.* **48**, 495–499

[103]H. A. Collins, G. K. Burger, and G. A. Taylor (1976) An empirical typology of heroin abusers. *J. Clin. Psychol.* **32**, 473–476.

[104]D. T. Marsh, S. A. Stile, N. L. Stoughton, and B. L. Trout-Landen (1988) Psychopathology of opiate addiction: Comparative data from the MMPI and MCMI. *Am. J. Drug Alcohol Abuse* **14**, 17–27.

[105]R. J. Craig (1988) Psychological functioning of cocaine free-basers derived from objective psychological tests. *J. Clin. Psychol.* **44**, 599–606.

[106]S. Walfish, R. Massey, and A. Krone (1990) MMPI profiles of cocaine-addicted individuals in residential treatment: Implications for practical treatment planning. *J. Subst. Abuse Treatment* **7**, 151–154.

[107]J. M. Rothauzer (1980) A typological study of substance abusers using the MMPI. *J. Clin. Psychol* **36**, 1019–1021.

[108]W. P. Rohan, R. L. Tatro, and S. R. Rotman (1969) MMPI changes in alcoholics during hospitalization. *Q. J. Stud. Alcohol* **30**, 389–400.

[109]W. P. Rohan (1972) MMPI changes in hospitalized alcoholics; a second study. *Q. J. Stud. Alcohol* **33**, 65–76.

[110]A. E. Wilkinson, W. M. Prado, W. O. Williams, and F. W. Schnadt (1971) Psychological test characteristics and length of stay in treatment. *Q. J. Stud. Alcohol* **32**, 60–65.

[111]A. F. Chang, A. B. Calwell, and T. Moss (1973) Stability of personality traits in alcoholics during and after treatment as measured by the MMPI: A one year follow-up study. *Proc. Am. Psychol. Assoc.* **81**, 387–388.

[112]N. A. Huber and S. Danahy (1975) Use of the MMPI in predicting completion and evaluating changes in a long-term alcoholism treatment program. *J. Stud. Alcohol* **36**, 1230–1237.

[113]H. Hoffmann, R. G. Loper, and M. L. Kammeier, (1974) Identifying future alcoholics with MMPI alcoholism scales. *Q. J. Stud. Alcohol* **35**, 490–498.

[114]R. J. Craig, J. S. Verinis, and S. Wexler (1985) Personality characteristics of drug addicts and alcoholics on the Millon Clinical Multiaxial Inventory. *J. Pers. Assess.* **49**, 156–160.

[115]R. J. Craig and R. E. Olson (1990) MCMI comparisons of cocaine abusers and heroin addicts. *J. Clin. Psychol.* **46,** 230–237.

[116]T. Millon (1987) *Manual for the MCMI-I* (2nd ed.) National Computer Systems Inc., Minneapolis, MN.

[117]D. A. Calsyn and A. J. Saxon (1990) Personality disorder subtypes among cocaine and opioid addicts using the Millon Clinical Multiaxial Inventory. *Int. J. Addict.* **25,** 1037–1049.

[118]J. R. Corbisiero and M. Reznikoff (1991) The relationship between personality type and style of alcohol use. *J. Clin Psychol.* **47,** 291–298.

[119]P. F. Flynn and R. C. McMahon (1984) An examination of the drug abuse scale of the Millon Clinical Multiaxial Inventory. *Int. J. Addict.* **19,** 459–468.

[120]D. A. Calsyn, A. J. Saxon, and F. Daisy (1990) Validity of the MCMI drug abuse scale with drug abusing and psychiatric samples. *J. Clin. Psychol.* **46,** 244–246.

[121]D. A. Calsyn and A. J. Saxon (1991) Validity of the MCMI drug abuse scale as a function of drug of choice, race, and Axis II subtypes. *Am. J. Drug Alcohol Abuse* **17,** 153–159.

[122]D. L. Haller and S. H. Schnoll (1992) Rates of MCMI drug abuse detection. Unpublished data from NIDA study. Supported by NIDA Grant #DA06094.

[123]N. De Palma and H. D. Clayton (1958) Scores of alcoholics on the Sixteen Personality Factor Questionnaire. *J. Clin. Psychol.* **14,** 390–392.

[124]R. B. Cattell, H. W. Eber, and M. M. Tatsouka (1970) *Handbook for the Sixteen Personality Factor Questionnaire (16PF)*. Institute for Personality and Ability Testing, Champaign, IL.

[125]W. F. Gross and L. L. Carpenter (1971) Alcoholic personality; reality or fiction? *Psychol. Rep.* **28,** 375–378.

[126]C. F. J. Ross (1971) Comparison of hospital and prison alcoholics. *Br. J. Psychiatry* **118,** 75–78.

[127]P. V. Ciotola and J. F. Peterson (1976) Personality characteristics of alcoholics and drug addicts in a merged treatment program. *J. Stud. Alcohol* **37,** 1229–1235.

[128]E. M. Jellinek (1960) *The Disease Concept of Alcoholism*. Hillhouse, Highland Park, NJ.

[129]H. J. Walton (1968) Personality as a determinant of the form of alcoholism. *Br. J. Psychiatry* **114,** 761–766.

[130]G. F. Lawlis and S. E. Rubin (1971) 16-PF study of personality patterns in alcoholics. *Q. J. Stud. Alcohol* **32,** 318–327.

[131]V. J. Nerviano and W. F. Gross (1973) A multivariate delineation of two alcoholic profile types on the 16 PF. *J. Clin. Psychol.* **29,** 371–374.

[132]V. J. Nerviano and W. F. Gross (1983) Personality types of alcoholics on objective inventories. *J. Stud. Alcohol* **44,** 837–851.

[133]W. H. Replogle and J. F. Hair Jr. (1977) A multivariate approach to profiling alcoholic typologies. *Multivariate Exp. Clin. Res.* **3,** 157–164.

[134]R. M. Hoy (1969) The personality of inpatient alcoholics in relation to group psychotherapy, as measured by the 16 PF. *Q. J. Stud. Alcohol* **30,** 401–407.

[135]W. F. White (1965) Personality and cognitive learning among alcoholics with different intervals of sobriety. *Psychol. Rep.* **516,** 1125–1140.

[136]R. K. Brooner, P. T. Costa, L. T. Felch, E. E. Rousar, G. E. Bigelow, and C. W. Schmidt (1991) The personality dimensions of male and female drug abusers with and without antisocial personality disorder, in *NIDA Research Monograph Series, vol. 119,*

Problems of Drug Dependence 1991: Proceedings of the 53rd Annual Scientific Meeting. College on Problems of Drug Dependence, U.S. Government Printing Office, 1992b, Washington, DC., pp. 232.

[137]D. L. Knoblaugh (1988) A psychological component of women's alcoholism. *Alcohol. Treatment Q.* **5,** 219–229.

[138]S. J. Nixon and O. A. Parsons (1990) Application of the tridimensional personality questionnaire to a population of alcoholics and other substance abusers. *Alcohol. Clin. Exp. Res.* **14,** 513–517.

[139]R. G. Knight and C. T. Prout (1951) A study of results in hospital treatment of drug addictions. *Am. J. Psychiatry* **108,** 303–308.

[140]P. Zimmerling, J. Tollan, R. Safrin, and S. Wortis (1952) Drug addiction in relation to problems of adolescence. *Am. J. Psychiatry* **109,** 272–278.

[141]J. E. Bleckner (1974) Psychological characteristics of the "Haight" junkies. *J. Psychedelic Drugs* **6,** 21–28.

[142]D. L. Gerard and C. Kornetsky (1955) Adolescent opiate addiction: A study of control and addict subjects. *Psychiatr. Q.* **29,** 457–486.

[143]L. H. Silverman and D. Silverman (1960) Womb fantasies in heroin addiction: A psychological study. *J. Projective Techniques* **24,** 52–63.

[144]S. J. Blatt and W. H. Berman (1990) Differentiation of personality types among opiate addicts. *J. Pers. Assess.* **54,** 87–104.

[145]J. N. Butcher (1990) *MMPI-2 in Psychological Treatment.* Oxford University, New York.

[146]J. R. Graham (1990) *MMPI-2 in Assessing Personality and Psychopathology.* Oxford University, New York.

[147]J. T. Webb (1971) Regional and sex differences in MMPI scale high-point frequencies of psychiatric patients. *J. Clin. Psychol.* **27,** 483–486.

Why Women Smoke

Cynthia S. Pomerleau, Barbara A. Berman, Ellen R. Gritz, Judith L. Marks, and Susan Goeters

Smoking as a Public Health Problem for Women

The "Feminization" of Tobacco Use in the United States

Although tobacco use by both men and women has been documented throughout history,[1–3] two technological developments in the 19th century radically and irreversibly changed societal patterns of nicotine use. First, the introduction of flue-curing yielded a product with a lower pH and milder smoke that could be readily inhaled through the lungs, producing a rapid rise of nicotine in plasma that appears to contribute to the reinforcing and addictive properties of nicotine by partially overcoming tolerance,[4] and delivering nicotine via a process that maximizes exposure to carcinogens. Second, the invention by a Virginian named James Bonsack of a cigaret-rolling machine, which could turn out as many cigarets as could 40 workers rolling manually,[5] made that product widely and cheaply available. With these innovations, tobacco use was fairly quickly transformed from a somewhat distasteful and unhealthful habit, alternately lauded and reviled, to what is arguably the most critical public health problem we face today. Certainly, in terms of morbidity and mortality, as well as of fetal loss, cigaret-smoking is a far more devastating form of drug abuse than the substances on which we

From: *Drug and Alcohol Abuse Reviews, Vol. 5: Addictive Behaviors in Women*
Ed.: R. R. Watson ©1994 Humana Press Inc., Totowa, NJ

regularly wage war and to which we are frequently exhorted to "just say no."
(In 1989, cocaine and heroin combined accounted for about 6000 deaths in the
United States; smoking accounted for more than 60 times that number.[6,7])

During the early decades of the 20th century, tobacco use was primarily a male behavior.[8,9] Smoking by males exceeded 50% by 1925 and reached
70% in the 1940s and 1950s.[10] In 1964, when Luther Terry's landmark *Surgeon General's Report* documenting the health hazards of smoking was
issued, a downturn in smoking by men had already begun, going from around
50% in the mid-1960s to the current rate of approx 28.4%.[11,12]

The history of smoking in women is not coterminous with that for
men; not only is there a phase lag of 25–30 yr, there are also differences in
the patterns of initiation, maintenance, and cessation. Reflecting existing
and changing social norms and roles, smoking in women began to accelerate in the 1940s and 1950s,[2,10,13,14] increasing from approx 18% in 1935 to a
peak of 33.4% in 1965. It remained at about that level until 1977, then
began to decrease gradually to the current rate of 22.8%.[2] Although more
men than women now smoke, current rates of decline suggest that smoking
prevalence could be at parity by 1995, and female smokers could outnumber male smokers by the year 2000.[15,16] Recent downward trends in smoking initiation among 20- to 24-yr-old women, the only group for whom
prevalence was increasing before 1985, however, offer a ray of hope that
convergence is not inevitable.[17]

Patterns in Smoking Initiation and Nicotine Use

Nearly all smoking initiation occurs during the early teen years.[18–21]
The mean age of initiation is declining, particularly for young women, and
is currently between 12 and 13 yr of age. For boys and girls, about 25% of
those who smoke start by the age of 12, 50% by age 13–14, and 90% by the
age of 20. For the high school class of 1990, 19% had their first cigaret in
elementary school, 32% in grades 7–9, and 14% in grades 10–12.[22] Some
groups of young people are at particularly high risk for initiation,[23] including vocational students, students with chronic educational and other problems, children who are substance abusers, and children from single-parent
families.[24] "Latchkey children" are almost twice as likely to begin smoking
as other children, regardless of socioeconomic status.[25] Although there has
been a decline in smoking initiation across all educational groups, it is particularly noticeable among college-bound young people;[1,26] 19% of those with
only a high school education smoke half-a-pack a day or more, compared
with 8% of those who are college-bound.[22] That is not to imply that college
students are at no risk for smoking; among college students, 23% report
smoking in the past month, and one in seven (13.8%) report smoking daily.

Since 1977, smoking prevalence has been consistently higher for female high school seniors than males. Currently, these rates are approx 18.6% for males and 19.3% for females. To be sure, these figures may give a distorted picture of gender differences in nicotine use, as during the 1970s and 1980s the use of smokeless tobacco increased dramatically among young males in the United States.[1] Except for young Native American females, who are as likely as males to use these products,[27] regular use of smokeless tobacco has so far been limited among females in this country.[27,28] Substantial numbers of adolescent women report having tried smokeless tobacco at least once, however, pointing to the need for careful attention to possible changes in female use patterns.[27]

Interestingly, smoking prevalence among women does not appear to be affected by employment status.[29] Moreover, occupational differences are less predictive of smoking for women than for men; to the extent that occupational differences in prevalence are noted, they seem to be linked to socioeconomic status.[30] Fewer White than Black women smoke (although Black women are lighter smokers), and fewer Hispanic than non-Hispanic women. Neither race/ethnicity nor occupation accounts for as much of the variation in smoking prevalence as education (a marker of socioeconomic status); for both men and women, those with less education are most likely to smoke.[1,15–17]

Health Consequences of Smoking

All smokers are at significant health risk from tobacco use. Simply put, tobacco use remains the single major preventable cause of death and disease, and, despite the decline in prevalence, disease implications are likely to increase in coming decades, particularly for women.[31,32] Smoking is responsible for one of every five deaths, or about 435,000 total deaths each year in this nation and approx 2.5 million deaths worldwide.[33] Of the 3000 young people who begin to smoke each day in the United States, 750 will be killed by a smoking-related disease.[16,26] Five hundred million people in the world today will die from use of tobacco, half in their middle years, with an average loss of 20 yr of life. The cost to the nation in health expenses or time lost from work have been estimated at over 50 billion dollars annually.

Tobacco use has been implicated in cancers of the mouth, pharynx, larynx, esophagus, pancreas, uterine cervix, bladder, and kidney. It accounts for about 30% of all cancer deaths and over 85% of all lung cancer deaths.[11] The dramatic increase in lung cancer among women, to the point where lung cancer surpassed breast cancer as the leading cause of cancer death in the United States in 1986, is directly attributable to the adoption of cigaret smoking in this population.[34–36] Smoking is also a major cause of other cancers, heart disease, stroke, chronic obstructive pulmonary disease, and lung disease, and is linked to conditions ranging from chronic bronchitis, emphysema, and cerebrovascular disease to colds and gastric ulcers. Tobacco has a synergistic effect with other substances; industrial workers are especially susceptible to lung disease as a result of the combined effect of cigaret smoking and exposure to certain toxic industrial substances, such as fumes from rubber and chlorine and dust from cotton and coal. Exposure to asbestos in combination with cigaret smoking increases an individual's lung cancer risk nearly 60 times.[33]

Tobacco use is also harmful to nonsmokers.[11] Sidestream smoke poses risks for children and for nonsmoking adults who live or work with smokers. Environmental tobacco smoke (ETS) causes an estimated 53,000 deaths annually in this country, including about two-thirds from heart disease and about 4000 from lung cancer.[33] Passive smoking can aggravate asthmatic conditions and impaired blood circulation. Children living with smokers experience increased rates of lower respiratory tract infections, bronchitis, and other childhood illnesses.[33] Surveys indicate that between half and three-quarters of the homes in this nation contain at least one smoker, and that children of lower socioeconomic status are most likely to live in such circumstances.[37] Between 8.7 and 12.4 million American children under age 5 are exposed to cigaret smoke in their homes.[33]

Females are at risk for all of the aforementioned conditions. In addition, there are special risks among women. An association has been found between smoking and reduced fertility. Smoking during pregnancy has been associated with increased risk of tubal pregnancy, spontaneous abortion, perinatal mortality, stillbirth, preterm delivery, low birthweight babies, intrauterine growth retardation, the sudden infant death syndrome, oral clefting, a depressed or low 1- and 5-min Apgar score, and lower respiratory tract illness during the first 5 yr of life.[11,33,39–56] Despite widespread public health efforts, approx 25% of US women smoke throughout pregnancy, with higher proportions in unmarried women and women with less education.[57,58] A substantial proportion of women report having quit after becoming pregnant (16–41%), with estimates of those resuming smoking while still pregnant ranging from 20–35%.[58] About 80% of women who quit during pregnancy relapse following delivery, although there is some evidence that women who quit early in pregnancy are more likely to stay quit.[45,57,59,60]

Other health consequences among women throughout the life cycle have also been established. Smokers who use oral contraceptives face an increased risk of stroke.[11] An increased risk of cervical neoplasia is associated with active cigaret smoking.[61] Female smokers have higher rates of osteoporosis and experience earlier menopause than do other women.

Increased risks of threefold or greater for vertebral and twofold for hip fracture have been reported, although negative findings exist regarding the risk
of hip fracture.[62] Smoking increases central adiposity,[63] so that the body fat
distribution in women smokers tends to become more like the male pattern
of body fat distribution, which is associated with increased risk of diabetes,
cardiovascular disease, hypertension, stroke, and ischemic heart disease.[64]
Smoking appears to be more detrimental in its effects on lung function in
women than in men.[65] The mechanism underlying at least some of the
increased risks listed above is probably the apparent antiestrogenic and mas-
culinizing effect of smoking in women,[66,67] which compromises some of the
protection that estrogen confers on women during the premenopausal years
against cardiovascular disease, osteoporosis, and other conditions. Smoking may counteract the protective effect of oral estrogen replacement against
osteoporotic hip[62] and other fractures in women.

Exposure to tobacco from sources other than cigarets—e.g., smokeless tobacco, snuff, or chewing tobacco—is implicated in oral cancer and
noncancerous oral pathology (leukoplakia and erythroplakia).[28,33] Oral cancer occurs several times more frequently among snuff dippers than among
nontobacco users, and the excess risk of cancer of the cheek and gum may
reach nearly 50-fold among long-term snuff users. In nations where there is
extensive use of smokeless tobacco (e.g., India), oral cancer is the most
common cancer.[68] Although noncigaret tobacco use is not currently an important female health issue in this country, such products are widely used by
women in other cultures and societies.

Why Women Smoke

Experimentation and Initiation of Smoking

Environmental and Heredity Factors

Although extensive demographic data have been collected, much
remains to be learned about smoking initiation. Experimentation rates are
high, with an ever-use rate of over 60% cutting across educational aspirations, parents' educational level, population density, region, and gender.[22]
Experimentation is seen as particularly likely during times of social transition (i.e., movement from elementary to junior high school),[69] and over 50%
of smokers report having smoked their first cigaret with a friend. Gender-
specific social influences have also been reported. For young girls, for example, the desire to gain approval from opposite-sex peers seems to be a more
potent factor in smoking initiation that for their male counterparts.[70] Such
observations have been used to underscore the role of peer pressure in smok-

ing initiation, and undoubtedly it is an important factor in the process. Nevertheless, not all of those who experiment go on to become regular smokers. Very little is known about individual differences in vulnerability to nicotine use that might underlie the sorting process—particularly with respect to the relative contributions of hereditary and environmental influences. Adolescent girls, for example, are five times as likely to smoke if one or both parents or an older sibling in the household smokes.[71] It may be that parental/sibling smoking encourages initiation by establishing a socially acceptable climate for experimentation and making materials needed for experimentation available. On the other hand, considerable evidence has been amassed from twin studies and related investigations demonstrating a heritability of 53% for smoking—higher than for alcohol or caffeine use/abuse.[72,73] Furthermore, a number of investigations have shown that smokers consistently score higher than nonsmokers on scales designed to measure the (presumably inherited) trait of novelty-seeking or sensation-seeking.[74,75] In line with these observations, young girls who start to smoke have been described as more socially aggressive, sexually precocious, self-confident, rebellious, and rejecting of authority than their male counterparts.[76] Recent evidence points to the possibility of greater constitutional sensitivity to nicotine in people destined to become smokers.[77,78] Unfortunately, the kind of controlled experimentation that would be required to assess sensitivity to the various pharmacological effects of nicotine prior to exposure, to determine its power to predict subsequent smoking initiation and development of nicotine dependence, and to explore possible interactive effects of gender is limited by both ethical and practical considerations. (Interestingly, female smokers seem to show greater physiological reactivity to smoking than do male smokers.[79])

Advertising

By providing social reinforcement of and support for a self-image that includes smoking behavior,[69] cigaret advertising may contribute to smoking initiation[80–82] as well as facilitate the shift from experimentation to habituation and regular smoking.[69] Although industry spokespersons insist that their efforts are designed to encourage brand-switching, antitobacco advocates point out that smoking has accelerated in direct correlation with intensified, targeted promotional activities, particularly among women. Tobacco advertising ties smoking to the dramatic changes that have occurred in female roles during the past half century[83] and underscores its social acceptability. The linking of tobacco products to female independence, sophistication, youth, health, and success has been a touchstone of expensive advertising campaigns, which include magazines, outdoor displays, sponsorship of special events, clothing promotions, and other strategies.[10,13,14,34,83–90] Tobacco companies get extra mileage for their investment: The economic dependence of magazines on tobacco advertising has been shown to have a "chilling effect" on editorial policy and on the content of published articles.[83,91,92]

There is also evidence of subtargeting in tobacco advertising. Specific campaigns have been designed to enlist women with less education and of diverse racial and ethnic backgrounds.[34,93,94] Perhaps most controversial have been advertisements that appeal to young children and adolescents.[18,82,95–97] An estimated 3.3% of all cigaret sales are to children under 18 yr of age, representing 947 million packs and 1.23 billion dollars annually.

Evidence supports the effectiveness of such advertising; there has been a dramatic increase in Camel cigarets' share of the children's cigaret market following the introduction of the "Joe Camel" cigaret advertisements,[82,98] for example, and 6-yr-olds are as capable of identifying this figure as they are of recognizing Mickey Mouse.[82,95] Such product recognition is seen as an important element in product marketing and in establishing the basis for future consumer behavior.[95]

Current low prevalence of tobacco use does not insulate any population from increasing enrollment in the ranks of smokers in the future; on the contrary, such populations represent unsaturated markets that may serve as particular targets of tailored advertising. One population at risk for recruitment because of current low prevalence is Hispanic women.[99] Looking beyond our borders, a decline in US consumption has already been accompanied by vigorous activity in international marketing, particularly in some Third World countries.[100–104] A concomitant increase in smoking-related morbidity and mortality is already emerging.[100,102,104,105] Marketing efforts include aid to tobacco companies in these nations, joint ventures, exporting tobacco products, and the like. In countries where prevalence among women is lower than among men (e.g., in Japan and China), it is among women that increased consumption is most likely to occur.

Weight Management

Starting at an early age, women are more likely to be concerned with weight than men. Survey data indicate that 33–40% of women are currently trying to lose weight, as opposed to 20–24% of men. For high school students the gender gap is even larger—44% of female students vs 15% of male students.[106] In a survey of college freshmen, 89.2% of normal-weight women expressed a wish to be thinner than they were, as opposed to 52.6% of normal-weight men.[107]

Smoking depresses body weight and therefore represents a potential tool for weight management. On average, smokers weigh several pounds less than nonsmokers of the same age and gender;[108,109] on cessation, weight tends to increase until eventually smokers reach the weight they would have attained had they never smoked.[110] The mechanisms underlying this phenomenon are not entirely understood, but probably include effects on metabolic rate, food hedonics and intake (perhaps specifically of sweet-tasting foods), motor activity, and other factors.[111] Nicotine may even have greater efficacy as an anorectic in women than in men; Grunberg et al.[108] have presented animal data suggesting that females are more sensitive than males to the effects of nicotine on body weight and feeding during and after drug administration. In smokers who quit, mean weight gain is 3.8 kg in women and 2.8 kg in men.[110] Moreover, 13.4% of women, compared with 9.8% of men, experience major weight gain (more than 13 kg).[110]

Although a causal relationship is difficult to demonstrate conclusively, use of nicotine as a weight control strategy may be a factor in both in initiation and maintenance of smoking.[112] The belief that cigaret smoking is a means of weight control rises after age 12 and is more prevalent among smokers than nonsmokers.[113] This belief is fostered by the tobacco industry via advertising that not only links tobacco use to weight control, but also encourages tobacco use by contributing to societal preferences for thinness. For both sociocultural and biological reasons, as indicated earlier, women may be more susceptible than men to the allure of nicotine use as a weight control strategy. Overweight females, for example, are more likely than other groups to report desire to control weight as a motivating factor in initiation.[114] Moreover, women smokers are consistently more likely than men smokers to state that fear of weight gain reduces motivation to quit.[115]

Maintenance of Smoking Behavior
Nicotine Dependence

The 1988 *Surgeon General's Report* explored the characteristics of tobacco use that can make cessation so difficult for male and female smokers of all ages. That document clearly established that cigarets and other forms of tobacco are addicting, that nicotine is the drug in tobacco that causes addiction, and that the pharmacological and behavioral processes that determine tobacco addiction are similar to those that determine addiction to drugs such as heroin and cocaine.

Whether there are gender differences in vulnerability to the addictive properties of nicotine is not known. Interestingly, however, women smokers trying to quit are more likely to describe themselves as "hooked" than are their male counterparts.[116] Benowitz and Jacob[117] reported that male smokers metabolize and excrete nicotine from the body more rapidly than female smokers, raising the possibility that a given dose of nicotine has more pronounced effects in women than in men.

Affect Regulation

Investigation of situations that cue smoking[118,119] and retrospective examination of factors associated with craving[120] indicate that environmental stimuli can reliably increase the probability of smoking and decrease intercigaret interval. Analysis of the circumstances surrounding recidivism strengthen this inference,[121,122] as do studies involving the use of a variety of laboratory stressors.[123–126]

Nicotine can produce both stimulant and sedative effects in humans, depending on dose, initial state of arousal, and perhaps other factors, such as degree of addiction;[127] individual differences in susceptibility to anxiety may determine which effect, stimulation or sedation, is primary in a given smoker.[128] It has been suggested that women may be particularly susceptible to the anxiety-reducing properties of nicotine—for example, that women are more likely to smoke in situations of high anxiety than of low anxiety, to smoke when experiencing "negative affect," and to smoke at times of high job stress.[129–131] Russell et al.,[132] in their compilation of smoking motives, noted that women scored significantly lower in "sensorimotor smoking" and significantly higher in "sedative" (reduction of arousal) smoking than did men. Pomerleau et al.[74] found that female but not male smokers were somewhat more likely to score high in the harm–avoidance trait (thought to reflect a predisposition to anxiety). There is also evidence that for women, more than for men, degree of dependence is associated with the harm–avoidance trait[74] and with desire to smoke in stress-inducing circumstances.[133] A more speculative possibility is that women are more sensitive to external stimuli than men and may therefore find the distraction-filtering effects of nicotine more "useful" than do men.[134]

Endocrinological Influences

It is tempting to speculate that the more than 200 physical, psychological, and behavioral changes associated with the ovarian cycle[135] have an impact on smoking behavior in regularly cycling smokers. Unfortunately, the few attempts to investigate this question have produced conflicting and unconvincing results, with smoking variously reported to be highest during the menses,[136] midcycle,[137] and the late luteal phase.[138] It remains possible, however, that women smokers with Late Luteal Phase Dysphoric Disorder, or women smokers studied under stressful conditions, will be found to manifest more dramatic phase-related changes in smoking behavior.

Depression and Anxiety Disorders

Results from several studies have suggested that there is a relationship between smoking and Major Depressive Disorder[139–141] or depressive symptoms.[142,143] A relationship has also been suggested between smoking and panic disorder.[144] Even in the absence of any evidence of gender specificity, these relationships may be of particular importance to women, as the incidence of both depressive[145,146] and anxiety disorders[147] in women is twice that seen in men.

The percentage of smokers in an unselected adult population is approx 25%; this percentage is dramatically increased in samples of people with a current or past history of depression. Hughes et al.,[148] for example, found that 49% of a group of psychiatric outpatients with Major Depressive Disorder were smokers. Carney et al.[149] reported that 89% of depressed cardiac patients were smokers, compared with 54% of nondepressed patients.

Glassman et al.[139] studied the effectiveness of clonidine, an α-2-noradrenergic agonist, in relieving withdrawal symptoms associated with smoking cessation. Although subjects with a current diagnosis of depression were not entered into their protocol, the authors found not only that 61% of their subjects had a history of definite major depression, but also that this history had an impact on smoking cessation success rates, which were significantly lower in those subjects with a history of depression. Clonidine increased the success rate of smoking cessation in both the group with a history of depression and the group without such a history, but this effect was limited to women. The authors speculated that a higher dose of clonidine might have produced similar effects in men, since the same dose (50 μg) was administered regardless of gender or weight.

Frerichs et al.[142] assessed depressive symptoms in a Los Angeles community sample using the Center for Epidemiologic Studies Depression Scale (CES-D)[150] and found that both male and female smokers had significantly higher depression scores than nonsmokers. Similarly, Anda et al.[143] analyzed cross-sectional data collected in the National Health and Nutrition Examination Survey (NHANES I) and follow-up data from the NHANES I Epidemiologic Follow-up Study (NHEFS) to explore the relationship between depression and smoking. They found that the percentage of smokers increased significantly as depression (measured by CES-D score) increased—a relationship that held for both men and women. In addition, analysis of the follow-up data demonstrated that people who were depressed, regardless of gender, had the lowest incidence of quitting.

Glassman et al.[140] also looked at the relationship between smoking and depression in a community sample utilizing data from the St. Louis site of the Epidemiologic Catchment Area Program. The Diagnostic Interview Schedule[151] was used to collect data concerning smoking and depression in this sample. The lifetime prevalence of major depressive disorder in the entire sample was 5.1%; prevalence for never-smokers was 2.9%, compared to 6.6% among those who had ever smoked daily for at least 1 mo. The relationship between depression and smoking in this study was independent of sex, education, marital status, and race. Further analysis of the associations among gender, smoking status, and diagnostic status revealed that males without major depressive disorder and males with no psychiatric diagnosis were more likely than their female counterparts to have ever smoked and to have been successful in their attempts to quit smoking. These gender differences disappeared among the depressed group. The authors concluded that as smoking rate in the general population declines in response to changes in social attitudes and public policy, both the pools of people who start and those who cannot stop will increasingly consist of individuals vulnerable to depression. Since major depression is more common in women, an increase in the proportion of female smokers can be expected—a prediction that already seems to be borne out among young smokers.[140]

The data supporting an association between smoking and anxiety disorders or panic disorder are less conclusive. Anda et al.[143] and Glassman et al.[140] failed to detect such a relationship, but Breslau et al.,[141] studying a sample of 1007 young adults, recently reported a functional relationship between rate of anxiety disorders and severity of nicotine dependence using DSM-III-R criteria. Brodsky[144] reported clinical observations suggesting that patients with panic disorder may use nicotine to control panic symptoms, triggering the suggestion[152] that nicotine polacrilex could be used to diminish panic attacks. Debate ensued,[152–154] but the question of the efficacy of nicotine replacement in alleviating panic attacks remains open. In smokers with phobic anxiety, Fleming and Lombardo[155] found no effect of smoking on either self-reported anxiety in the presence of the phobic object or motoric anxiety (distance traversed toward the phobic object and average approach rate).

Associations with Alcohol and Other Drug Use

Smoking often occurs as part of a pattern of polydrug use/abuse. Smokers of both sexes tend to use more drugs than nonsmokers, including caffeine and alcohol.[10] Women smokers have been shown to use more prescription drugs of all types than do their nonsmoking counterparts.[156] Since many drugs are cleared more rapidly in smokers than in nonsmokers because of enzyme induction by nicotine in the liver, these findings are perhaps not altogether surprising. It seems unlikely that metabolic factors alone account for the observed differences, however.

Tobacco has been identified as a "gateway drug"[21]—that is, a drug that is often the first drug to which a young person is exposed, paving the way for subsequent involvement with other legal and illegal drugs. The other important "gateway drug" in our culture is alcohol in the form of wine or beer. Yamaguchi and Kandel[157] have noted gender differences in patterns of drug progression, with cigarets being more important for women than for men in the total progression; indeed, women who do not experiment with cigarets (i.e., smoke at least 10 cigarets) seldom proceed to other illicit drugs, whereas for men, alcohol use is more likely to be a critical step in the sequence. The existence of such stages does not necessarily imply causation; but it is noteworthy that for many women who use multiple drugs, nicotine is likely to be the "index" drug, the initial experience of a psychoactive substance.

Habitual users of alcohol, cocaine, and heroin are likely to be smokers.[6] A particularly strong relationship of alcohol use and alcoholism with cigaret smoking has frequently been noted.[158] Alcohol availability induces smoking in both men[159] and women.[138] Dreher and Fraser[160] found a smoking prevalence of 93% for males and 91% for females in an outpatient sample of alcoholics; similar percentages were reported by Ashley et al.[161] and Gritz et al.[162] Alcoholism manifests itself somewhat differently in men than in women.[163] Women (and some men) tend to exhibit "loss-of-control" drinking—that is, they can abstain for long periods of time but once started are unable to terminate binges; the "inability to abstain" pattern, with persistent drink-seeking behavior often associated with fighting and public intoxication, is limited almost exclusively to men. The prevalence of alcoholism in males is five times that in females. Those women who do meet criteria for alcohol dependence, however, are more likely to have concomitant psychiatric diagnoses (65%) than are male alcoholics (44%)—largely because women alcoholics, like women nonalcoholics, are more likely than men to meet criteria for depression and phobia.[164] Whether nicotine use in alcoholics represents an effort to counteract or enhance the effects of alcohol, whether both represent "self-medication" of an underlying psychiatric disorder, or whether both are manifestations of a nonspecific vulnerability to drug dependence remains to be determined. Regardless of the answer, the above observations suggest that efforts to dissect the relationship between alcohol use and smoking will have to take into account the likely differences between men and women in the mechanisms underlying alcohol abuse.

Solutions to the Problem

Attempts to develop cigarets that eliminate or minimize the negative health effects of tobacco products have not been successful. Evidence does not support the effectiveness of filters, low tar cigarets, and so forth. Avoidance of initiation and, once initiated, smoking cessation, are the only known effective public health strategies.

Prevention of Smoking Initiation in Young Women

For the most part, the decline that has occurred in smoking prevalence nationwide has resulted from a decrease in initiation among young people, rather than as a result of cessation among tobacco users. Daily cigaret smoking declined from 26.9 to 19.9% between 1975 and 1990 for high school seniors; smoking half-a-pack or more per day declined from 17.9 to 11.3% during the same period. Nonetheless, substantial uptake continues to occur.[22] In fact, between 1980 and 1987, after several years of dramatic decline, the rate of smoking initiation among high school seniors seems to have leveled off;[22,26] about a million new smokers are recruited to the ranks of regular smokers each year.[16] Nearly five million teenagers 12–17 yr of age smoke, as do over half a million 8- to 11-yr-olds. These trends are in contrast to the declining drug use seen in young people for marijuana, LSD, and virtually all other substances besides alcohol. Cigarets are the class of substance most frequently used on a daily basis by high school students.

Since almost all initiation begins in the adolescent or preadolescent period, considerable prevention/education resources have been allocated to school-based programs. Despite difficulties in assessing and evaluating such programs,[69] there is evidence that they can delay smoking onset, which in turn may reduce the likelihood that regular smoking will occur, result in a lower smoking rate in adulthood, and make smoking cessation more likely among those who start.[26,165] Less experimentation and regular smoking have occurred in schools where programs are in place than where such programs are absent. Although results have sometimes been modest, the potential for reaching large numbers of children somewhat offsets the weakness of the intervention.

Despite gender differences in initiation, school-based preventive/education programs virtually never distinguish between male and female adolescents and preadolescents. Although an in-depth survey of the relative effectiveness of the various techniques that have been tried is outside the scope of this chapter, it would seem evident that just as treatment-matching has been lauded as a way of increasing efficacy, "prevention-matching" might also be profitably applied to the problem of maximizing outcome. For example, young women may be particularly responsive to social inoculation and life-skill approaches, including:

1. Strategies that emphasize social skills, competencies in decision making, self-awareness, coping, goal-setting, and assertiveness;[166–168]
2. Participation in small groups offering opportunities for social support, self-assessment, and role-playing; and
3. Establishment of buddy system or peer counseling capacities.

Health-related information has not been proven effective as the central component of school-based programs, but other types of information addressing the specific concerns of young women may be more helpful—e.g., information correcting misconceptions about prevalence and social acceptance, and short-term reasons for not smoking such as decreased athletic ability and the unpleasant smells, tastes, and yellow teeth that accompany the behavior.[69] Focusing on the weight concerns of young women and teaching alternative strategies of weight management may also be helpful.

Given the average age of initiation, it is already too late for prevention for many high school women. To date, smoking cessation programming is not as well established as smoking prevention/education in the school setting.[23] Distinct elements for experimenters and those already habituated need to be included, so that young women at varied stages on the initiation continuum, from anticipation/preparation through regular smoking, are reached.[23]

In addition to traditional school-based programs, innovative approaches to education and prevention in such contexts as extracurricular activities (e.g., sports, music, and the like), vocational and alternative schools, substance abuse treatment programs, and family service programs are needed to reach young women at high risk of initiation. Finally, attention is needed to the development of more effective antitobacco programming to counteract the messages purveyed by the tobacco industry. An unfortunate byproduct of the women's movement and other forces of social change in this country is that sanctions against smoking in women have been lifted and women are now much freer to adopt practices whose devastating effects were previously confined largely to men. The tobacco industry has been highly responsive to and indeed instrumental in this transformation, finding numerous clever and insidious ways of telling young women, "You've come a long way, baby." Although billboards, magazines, newspapers, radio, and television reach a vast audience, antitobacco programming is enormously expensive, and there is a lack of a powerful positive image of the nonsmoker to match the image of the attractive, sexy, successful, and slim woman smoker.

Approaches to Smoking Cessation in Women

The risk of dying within the next 15 yr is halved in smokers who quit before the age of 50, as compared with continuing smokers. The risk of lung cancer drops to 30–50% that of smokers within 10 yr of quitting. The risk of coronary heart disease is comparable to that of never-smokers after 15 yr of abstinence; the risk of stroke diminishes to that of never-smokers as soon as 5 yr after quitting. These and numerous other health benefits of cessation have been extensively documented elsewhere.[57]

Although the majority of smokers indicate that they would like to stop smoking, cessation remains difficult to achieve, and sustained abstinence a particularly elusive goal. A quarter to a third of all adult smokers—approx 17 million men and women—attempt to quit each year; fewer than 10% of them succeed. Over 80% of adults who try to quit fail on the first attempt (i.e., relapse within 1 yr) and over 50% fail on their second attempt.[4]

Whether there are gender differences in ability to quit and stay quit has been the subject of some controversy. The 1980 *Surgeon General's Report* stated unequivocally that "women have more difficulty giving up smoking than men, both at the end of treatment and at long-term points of measurement" (p. 307).[10] Data from formal treatment programs would seem to support this contention[169]—and women are more likely than men to enroll in such programs.[170] Among unaided quitters, however—who comprise 85–95% of smokers wishing to quit[11,170–172]—fewer gender differences have been found.[173] Although the quit ratio (proportion of ever-smokers who have become ex-smokers) is smaller for women (39.8% in 1985) than for men (45.8%), it is increasing in both genders at an equal rate.[16] Regarding relapse, a higher percentage of males than females report that they were able to sustain abstinence for more than 6 mo, but data over longer periods of time do not suggest significant gender differences in relapse rate.[174] Such findings have led some to argue that not only cessation behavior, but the ability to remain quit, have become more alike for men and women.[175]

Regardless of how one interprets the data on differences in quitting and relapse, considerable evidence has been amassed to suggest that the process of quitting differs between men and women. Women—at least those who participate in smoking cessation programs—may be more tentative and less committed to quitting.[169] Although overall withdrawal symptomatology does not differ markedly between men and women, women report wanting to eat more following quitting and greater weight gain, as well as much more concern about that weight gain.[176] Weight concerns may not actually hinder cessation efforts,[177] once the commitment is made, but they do deter women smokers from making quit attempts.[178] (Several studies, however, have demonstrated that weight gain during cessation is positively associated with continued abstinence,[179,180] indicating that weight gain does not necessarily lead to relapse—although those smokers who cannot tolerate postcessation weight gain may not persist in their efforts long enough to be included in such statistics.) Despite the absence of clearcut menstrual phase effects on smoking behavior and nicotine intake, menstruating women may experience more severe withdrawal symptomatology during the luteal phase than during the follicular phase of their cycle,[137,181] suggesting that women may need extra support in their efforts at that time of the month. Social support may be particularly important for women.[10,182-185] As described below, gender interactions have been observed for various pharmacological interventions. These facts argue that greater attention to the specific needs of women and treatment-matching that takes gender into account, in the context of public education campaigns as well as in formal cessation clinics, would be worthwhile and could potentially lead to higher quit rates for women.

In the wake of the first *Surgeon General's Report* documenting the health hazards of smoking,[186] many optimistically believed that once people recognized the health risks associated with smoking, large numbers of smokers would quit. The resulting public information campaigns have resulted in dramatic increases in public knowledge of the health consequences of smoking and passive smoking. Many smokers, however, remain unaware of or willing to accept these risks.[11,187] Moreover, there is evidence to suggest that the level of knowledge varies in the population, and is lower among older age groups, women, those with less education, and current smokers.[187] Although information campaigns in and of themselves have failed to produce extensive cessation in the absence of additional support components,[188,189] small percentages can add up to substantial numbers of quitters if large segments of the population are reached. Even in the absence of direct success, such campaigns clearly lay the groundwork for future quit attempts; and when nested in a more extensive or multicomponent community effort, the effectiveness of educational campaigns using the media can be enhanced. Thus, efforts to increase awareness, knowledge, and motivation, particularly among neglected populations, are worth pursuing.[188]

Health encounters are particularly appealing as sites for minimal contact, ideally supported by self-help interventions. The strategy is to use circumstances (i.e., doctors' appointments, clinic visits, and so on) where access to smokers is established for purposes other than the smoking cessation goal. The value of utilizing such settings is well supported.[28,190-198] Physicians and other health providers need to learn that their patients welcome such intervention,[199] that their patients report receiving such messages far less frequently than physicians report giving such advice[197] and that specific steps at institutionalizing the delivery of anti-tobacco messages have been identified.[198] Younger smokers, minorities, and those without cigaret-related diseases are currently less likely than others to receive such counseling[197] and could profitably be targeted for special attention.

Although all such encounters are potentially productive, some circumstances may constitute a particularly appropriate "teachable moment." For example, new mothers may be motivated to make lifestyle changes, and the pediatrician has an important "window of opportunity" through which to intervene.[38,199] Physicians may play an especially important role in cessation among older female smokers.[200] Health visits during pregnancy have received particular attention as opportunities for smoking cessation counseling. Interventions delivered at such times, including in the context of programs targeting multiethnic populations attending public health clinics, have been found to be effective in improving cessation rates.[58] Even minimal interventions involving generalizable and relatively inexpensive self-help materials tailored to pregnant women in a single brief session have proved successful.[45,201–205] Ways to assist women in remaining abstinent postpartum need to be developed.[45] Some assumptions about circumstances that have not been thought conducive to smoking interventions now need to be reconsidered; for example, the belief that those enrolled in alcohol or other substance abuse treatment programs were not good candidates for smoking cessation has been disconfirmed.[206,207]

In addition to physician advice, specific skills and steps are needed to facilitate cessation. To this end, voluntary and government agencies, researchers, and for-profit and professional organizations have developed programs that usually include written (and illustrated) self-help materials as a central component. Serialized delivery, materials adjusted to readiness-to-change stage, and additional supports (hotlines, letters) have been included. (A minimal level of motivation seems to be required for such programs to be efficacious, however; a serialized, six-booklet intervention mailed to nonvolunteer women smokers did not appear to promote quitting.[208]) Content has been tailored to particular groups such as specific race/ethnic groups, populations with limited literacy, smokers at specific ages and life stages, individuals with smoking-related diseases, women, and others.[11,200,202,208–211] Subtargeting has also been attempted (i.e., women in specific occupations, pregnant women, and so forth), although more needs to be done to ensure that elements of such tailored programs reflect the particular concerns and needs of high-risk populations.[209,212] Specific skills are introduced and practiced, including commitment to a quit date, coping with smoking triggers, avoiding weight gain, utilizing support, developing alternative rewards, and dealing with withdrawal symptoms. These programs provide ways in which smokers can: reduce the reinforcing value of smoking, self-monitor, deal with the addiction, cope with slips, and recycle back into the program as needed.

Formal programs are used by fewer than 10% of those who smoke. Cost, access, and other barriers have been noted with regard to group programs, and success rates within such programs have until recently (with the introduction of nicotine replacement strategies) been discouragingly low. Despite these shortcomings, such programs should not be dismissed as valueless. Indeed, they may represent the best hope for the "hard core" of smokers who are unable to quit on their own.[170] A wide range of individualized approaches (i.e., behavioral techniques, psychotherapy, hypnosis, acupuncture, and so on) is available, although evaluation is not always available or uniform, and claims of for-profit organizations cannot always be substantiated.

The most exciting recent advance in smoking treatment has been the development of pharmacological adjuncts available by prescription. The best known and most widely tested have been nicotine replacement products: nicotine polacrilex (Nicorette), introduced in the 1980s, and more recently, the transdermal nicotine patch; both have proven effective when prescribed and used correctly, in the context of a behavioral change program.[6,11,213–220] A nicotine nasal spray that mimics the fast rise-time of plasma nicotine from smoking has shown promising initial results and may be particularly beneficial in heavy smokers.[221]

Other pharmacological strategies that have been tested with varying degrees of success include nicotinic cholinergic receptor blockade (mecamylamine), α-adrenergic agonists (clonidine), antidepressants (buspirone and tricyclics), serotonin agonists or precursors (*d*-fenfluramine, fluoxetine, L-tryptophan), sympathomimetics (phenylpropanolamine), and miscellaneous other drugs (e.g., depot ACTH).[10,139,222–228] Although the transdermal patch has had a great impact on the treatment of smoking, drugs in other categories are likely to assume increasing importance in treating special populations— that is, women for whom nicotine replacement may be contraindicated (e.g., pregnant women), as supplements to treat specific withdrawal symptoms during time-limited portions of the cessation process, or as treatments for psychiatric conditions that might be unmasked by cessation (e.g., depression). Although some forms of nicotine replacement, for example, have been found by some (although not all) investigators to be helpful in controlling postcessation weight gain,[221,229,230] particularly in heavy smokers,[231] serotonergic agents (e.g., fluoxetine, *d*-fenfluramine) are likewise effective for this purpose[224–226] and have the added potential advantage of providing a temporal separation between the emergence of weight gain and the other nicotine withdrawal symptoms. Although these agents have so far produced disappointing results as a cessation treatment, it is possible that they could play an important role in the context of a program specifically designed for women with fear of weight gain.

It should be noted that a number of drugs used for other purposes (e.g., antidepressants, antipsychotics) are known or suspected to have gender-specific effects or side effects,[232] and the drugs used to promote smoking cessation may likewise have differential effects in women. Killen et al.[233] found nicotine polacrilex to be more effective in men than in women; Glassman et al.[139] found the opposite for clonidine. Inclusion in treatment trials of adequate numbers of both men and women to test for gender inter-actions will be needed to ensure detection of such differences and facilitate treatment-matching.

Conclusion

In light of the trend toward feminization of tobacco use, it would seem particularly important that smoking be accorded a prominent place on the agenda of agencies and organizations concerned with research initiatives on women's health issues. An encouraging start has been made, partly as a result of several decades of programmatic efforts targeting research, legis-lation, education/prevention, and cessation interventions. Maintaining and building on these gains will require a serious commitment to research as well as to public health programs. Imaginative new approaches to assess-ment of nicotine dependence and nicotine pharmacology in women will be needed if further elucidation of the biological mechanisms underlying smok-ing behavior is to be anticipated.

Unfortunately, support for such efforts is not a foregone conclusion, nor is the discouragement of tobacco use an established health priority. Indeed, the seriousness of our commitment as a society to dealing effec-tively with this problem is open to question. Although the government funds research and intervention efforts, tobacco sales remain an important source of revenue, spurring government trade and price policies that support tobacco production and encourage export to other nations. Tobacco is a legal sub-stance (although not for young people). Messages provided in the class-room and elsewhere discouraging tobacco use compete with messages from adult role models and with implicit messages communicated by school poli-cies that sanction tobacco use.[234] Drugs associated with violence or whose use disrupts ongoing behavior claim a disproportionate share of public inter-est and produce clarion calls for action, even though their actual cost to society may be far less. Alcohol is associated with incapacitating cognitive and motor dysfunction, heroin results in sedation, and cocaine use can lead to psychotic symptoms. Smoking, by contrast, does not produce a dramatic intoxication; it may even enhance attention and reduce fatigue, thereby improving performance requiring cognitive and motor skills.[6] Only several decades later do cancer and other smoking-related diseases emerge. All of these considerations tend to perpetuate our time-honored ambivalence toward this drug and undermine perception of smoking as the public health disaster that it is. (At the 1992 meeting of the College on Problems of Drug Depen-dence, for example, at a symposium devoted to the consequences of prena-tal exposure to drugs, tobacco remarkably received no mention until the question period following the formal presentations.) Continued vigilance

and lobbying will clearly be needed to ensure that the single most important cause of preventable morbidity and mortality in women remains in the
forefront of public awareness.

Acknowledgment

Preparation of this chapter was supported by Grants CA 42730, CA
43461, and CA 41616 from the National Cancer Institute and Grant DA
06529 from the National Institute on Drug Abuse.

References

[1]M. C. Fiore (1992) Trends in cigarette smoking in the United States. The epidemiology of tobacco use. *Med. Clin. N. Am.* **76,** 289–303.
[2]E. R. Gritz (1980) Problems related to the use of tobacco by women, in *Advances in
Alcohol and Drug Problems in Women*. O. Kalant, ed. Plenum, New York, pp. 487–
544.
[3]J. Wilbert (1975) Magico-religious use of tobacco among Southern American Indians, in *Cannabis and Culture*. V. Rubin, ed. Mouton, The Hague, pp. 439–461.
[4]U.S. Department of Health and Human Services (1988) *The Health Consequences
of Smoking: Nicotine Addiction. A report of the Surgeon General, 1988*. U.S. Department of Health and Human Services, Public Health Service, Centers for Disease Control, Center for Health Promotion and Education, Office on Smoking and Health. DHHS
Publication No. (CDC) 88-8406, Rockville, MD.
[5]P. Taylor (1985) *The Smoke Ring: Tobacco, Money and Multinational Politics*, 2nd
ed. Mentor, New York.
[6]M. E. Jarvik and N. G. Schneider (1992) Nicotine, in *Substance Abuse: A Comprehensive Textbook*. J. H. Lowinson, P. Ruiz, R. B. Millman, and J. G. Langrod, eds.
Williams and Wilkins, Baltimore, MD, pp. 334–356.
[7]Centers for Disease Control (1991) Smoking-attributable mortality and years of
potential life lost—United States, 1988. *Morbidity Mortality Weekly Rep.* **40,** 62–71.
[8]R. K. Heimann (1960) *Tobacco and Americans*. McGraw-Hill, New York.
[9]J. C. Robert (1952) *The Story of Tobacco in America*. Knopf, New York.
[10]U.S. Department of Health and Human Services (1980) *The Health Consequences
of Smoking for Women. A Report of the Surgeon General*. U.S. Department of Health
and Human Services, Public Health Service, Office of the Assistant Secretary for Health,
Office on Smoking and Health, Rockville, MD.
[11]U.S. Department of Health and Human Services (1989) *Reducing the Health Consequences of Smoking: 25 Years of Progress. A Report of the Surgeon General*. U.S.
Department of Health and Human Services, Public Health Service, Centers for Disease
Control, Center for Chronic Disease Prevention and Health Promotion, Office on Smoking and Health. DHHS Publication No. (CDC) 89-8411, Rockville, MD.
[12]Centers for Disease Control (1992) Cigarette smoking among adults—United States,
1990. *Morbidity Mortality Weekly Rep.* **41,** 354–362.
[13]V. L. Ernster (1985) Mixed messages for women: A social history of cigarette
smoking and advertising. *NY State J. Med.* **85,** 335–340.

[14]H. Howe (1984) An historical review of women, smoking, and advertising. *Health Educ.* **15**, 3–8.

[15]J. P. Pierce, M. C. Fiore, T. E. Novotny, E. J. Hatziandreu, and R. M. Davis (1989) Trends in cigarette smoking in the United States. Projections to the year 2000. *JAMA* **261**, 61–65.

[16]M. C. Fiore, T. E. Novotny, J. P. Pierce, E. J. Hatziandreu, K. M. Patel, and R. M. Davis (1989) Trends in cigarette smoking in the United States—the changing influence of gender and race. *JAMA* **261**, 49–55.

[17]J. P. Pierce, M. C. Fiore, T. E. Novotny, E. J. Hatziandreu, and R. M. Davis (1989) Trends in cigarette smoking in the United States. Educational differences are increasing. *JAMA* **261**, 56–60.

[18]J. R. DiFranza and J. B. Tye (1990) Who profits from tobacco sales to children? *JAMA* **263**, 2784–2787.

[19]U.S. Department of Health and Human Services (1986) *Smoking and Health: A National Status Report. Report to Congress.* U.S. Department of Health and Human Services, Public Health Services, Centers for Disease Control, Center for Health Promotion and Education, Office on Smoking and Health. DHHS Publication No. (CDC) 87-8396, Rockville, MD.

[20]L. G. Escobedo, R. F. Anda, P. F. Smith, P. L. Remington, and E. E. Mast (1990) Sociodemographic characteristics of cigarette smoking initiation in the United States. Implications for smoking prevention policy. *JAMA* **264**, 1550–1555.

[21]D. B. Kandel and J. A. Logan (1984) Patterns of drug use from adolescence to young adulthood I: Periods of risk for initiation, continued use, and discontinuation. *Am. J. Public Health* **74**, 660–666.

[22]L. D. Johnston, P. M. O'Malley, and J. G. Bachman (1991) Drug use among American high school seniors, college students and young adults, 1975–1990. Rockville, MD: U.S. Department of Health and Human Services, Public Health Service, Alcohol, Drug Abuse, and Mental Health Administration, National Institute on Drug Abuse. *Vol. 1: High School Seniors*, pp. 91–115.

[23]T. J. Glynn, D. M. Anderson, and L. Schwarz (1991) Tobacco-use reduction among high-risk youth: Recommendations of a National Cancer Institute Expert Advisory Panel. *Prev. Med.* **20**, 279–291.

[24]L. S. Covey and D. Tam (1990) Depressive mood, the single-parent home, and adolescent cigarette smoking. *Am. J. Public Health* **80**, 1330–1333.

[25]J. L. Richardson, K. Dwyer, K. McGuigan, W. B. Hansen, C. Dent, C. A. Johnson, S. Y. Sussman, B. Brannon, and B. Flay (1989) Substance use among eighth-grade students who take care of themselves after school. *Pediatrics* **84**, 556–566.

[26]T. J. Glynn (1990) *School Programs to Prevent Smoking: The National Cancer Institute Guide to Strategies that Succeed.* U.S. Department of Health and Human Services, National Institutes of Health, Bethesda, MD.

[27]G. M. Boyd and E. D. Glover (1989) Smokeless tobacco use by youth in the U.S. *J. School Health* **59**, 189–194.

[28]U.S. Department of Health and Human Services (1986) *Clinical Opportunities for Smoking Intervention. A Guide for the Busy Physician.* Public Health Service, National Institutes of Health Publication No. 82178, Bethesda, MD.

[29]I. Waldron and D. Lye (1989) Employment, unemployment, occupation, and smoking. *Am. J. Prev. Med.* **5**, 142–149.

[30]S. D. Stellman, P. Boffetta, and L. Garfinkel (1988) Smoking habits of 800,000 American men and women in relation to their occupations. *Am. J. Ind. Med.* **13,** 43–58.

[31]J. P. DeVesa, W. J. Blot, and J. F. Fraumeni (1989) Declining lung cancer rates among young men and women in the United States: A cohort analysis. *J. Natl. Cancer Inst.* **81,** 1568–1571.

[32]T. E. Novotny, M. C. Fiore, E. J. Hatziandreu, G. A. Giovino, S. L. Mills, and J. P. Pierce (1990) Trends in smoking by age and sex, United States, 1974–1987: The implications for disease impact. *Prev. Med.* **19,** 552–561.

[33]American Cancer Society (1992) *Cancer Facts and Figures.* American Cancer Society, New York.

[34]R. M. Davis (1990) Women and smoking in the United States: How lung cancer became an "equal opportunity" disease. Paper presented at the Seventh World Conference on Tobacco and Health. Perth, Australia.

[35]L. Garfinkel and S. D. Stellman (1988) Smoking and lung cancer in women: Findings in a prospective study. *Cancer Res.* **48,** 6951–6955.

[36]S. D. Stellman and L. Garfinkel (1989) Proportions of cancer deaths attributable to cigarette smoking in women, 1988. *Women Health* **15,** 19–28.

[37]W. J. Miller and L. Hunter (1990) The relationship between socioeconomic status and household smoking patterns in Canada. *Am. J. Health Promotion* **5,** 36–42.

[38]P. J. Landrigan (1986) Involuntary smoking—A hazard to children. *Pediatrics* **77,** 755–757.

[39]E. L. Abel (1980) Smoking during pregnancy. *Hum. Biol.* **52,** 593–625.

[40]B. A. Berman and E. R. Gritz (1988) Smoking and pregnancy: Present and future challenges. *Wellness Perspect.* **4,** 19–26.

[41]S. Cnattingius (1989) Smoking habits in early pregnancy. *Addict. Behav.* **14,** 453–457.

[42]S. M. Garn, M. Jonston, S. A. Ridella, and A. S. Petzold (1981) Effects of maternal cigarette smoking on Apgar Scores. *Am. J. Dis. Child* **135,** 503–506.

[43]S. Kramer, E. Ward, A. T. Meadows, and K. E. Malone (1987) Medical and drug risk factors associated with neuroblastoma: a case-control study. *J. Natl. Cancer Inst.* **78,** 797–804.

[44]M. J. Khoury, A. Weinstein, S. Panny, N. A. Holtzman, P. K. Lindsay, K. Farrel, and M. Eisenberg (1987) Maternal cigarette smoking and oral clefts: A population-based study. *Am. J. Public Health* **77,** 623–625.

[45]P. D. Mullen, V. P. Quinn, and D. H. Ershoff (1990) Maintenance of nonsmoking by women who stopped smoking during pregnancy. *Am. J. Public Health* **80,** 992–994.

[46]D. R. Peterson (1981) The sudden infant death syndrome—reassessment of growth retardation in relation to maternal smoking and the hypoxia hypothesis. *Am. J. Epidemiol.* **113,** 583–589.

[47]B. Taylor and J. Wadsworth (1987) Maternal smoking during pregnancy and lower respiratory tract illness in early life. *Arch. Dis. Child.* **62,** 786–791.

[48]R. L. Naeye and E. C. Peters (1984) Mental development of children whose mothers smoked during pregnancy. *Obstet. Gynecol.* **64,** 601–607.

[49]J. D. Buckley, W. L. Hobbie, K. Ruccione, H. N. Sather, W. G. Woods, and G. D. Hammond (1986) Maternal smoking during pregnancy and the risk of childhood cancer [Letter]. *Lancet* **76,** 520.

[50]M. Stjernfeldt, K. Berglund, J. Lindsten, and J. Ludvigsson (1986) Maternal smoking during pregnancy and risk of childhood cancer. *Lancet* **i,** 1350–1352.

[51]P. Rantakallio (1983) A follow-up study to the age of 14 of children whose mothers smoked during pregnancy. *Acta Paediatr. Scand.* **72**, 747–753.

[52]J. C. Byrd, R. S. Shapiro, and D. L. Schiedermayer (1989) Passive smoking: A review of medical and legal issues. *Am. J. Public Health* **79**, 209–215.

[53]P. Correa, L. Pickle, G. Fontham, Y. Lin, and W. Haenszell (1983) Passive smoking and lung cancer. *Lancet* **2**, 595–597.

[54]N. Butler and H. Goldstein (1973) Smoking in pregnancy and subsequent child development. *Br. Med. J.* **4**, 573–575.

[55]H. A. Pattinson, P. J. Taylor, and M. H. Pattinson (1991) The effect of cigarette smoking on ovarian function and early pregnancy outcome of in vitro fertilization treatment. *Fertil. Steril.* **55**, 780–783.

[56]A. Stergachis, D. Scholes, J. R. Daling, N. S. Weiss, and J. Chu (1991) Maternal cigarette smoking and the risk of tubal pregnancy. *Am. J. Epidemiol.* **133**, 332–337.

[57]U.S. Department of Health and Human Services (1990) *The Health Benefits of Smoking Cessation. A Report of the Surgeon General.* U.S. Department of Health and Human Services, Public Health Service, Centers for Disease Control, Center for Chronic Disease Prevention and Health Promotion, Office on Smoking and Health. DHHS Publication No. (CDC) 90-8416, Rockville, MD.

[58]P. D. Mullen (1990) Smoking cessation counseling in prenatal care, in *New Perspectives on Prenatal Care.* I. R. Merkatz and J. E. Thompson, eds. Elsevier, New York, pp. 161–176.

[59]J. C. Kleinman and A. Kopstein (1987) Smoking during pregnancy, 1967–1980. *Am. J. Public Health* **77**, 823–825.

[60]L. A. Fingerhut, J. C. Kleinman, and J. S. Kendrick (1990) Smoking before, during, and after pregnancy. *Am. J. Public Health* **8**, 541–544.

[61]A. L. Coker, A. J. Rosenberg, M. F. McCann, and B. S. Hulka (1992) Active and passive cigarette smoke exposure and cervical intraepithelial neoplasia. *Can. Epidemiol. Biomarkers Prev.* **7**, 349–356.

[62]D. P. Kiel, J. A. Baron, J. J. Anderson, M. T. Hannan, and D. T. Felson (1992) Smoking eliminates the protective effect of oral estrogens on the risk for hip fracture among women. *Ann. Intern. Med.* **116**, 716–721.

[63]E. Barrett-Connor and K. T. Khaw (1989) Cigarette smoking and increased central adiposity. *Ann. Intern. Med.* **11**, 783–787.

[64]R. J. Troisi, J. W. Heinold, P. S. Vokonas, and S. T. Weiss (1991) Cigarette smoking, dietary intake, and physical activity: Effects on body fat distribution—the Normative Aging Study. *Am. J. Clin. Nutr.* **53**, 1104–1111.

[65]Y. Chen, S. A. Horne, and J. A. Dosman (1991) Increased susceptibility to lung dysfunction in female smokers. *Am. Rev. Resp. Dis.* **143**, 1224–1230.

[66]J. A. Baron, C. La Vecchia, and F. Levi (1990) The antiestrogenic effect of cigarette smoking in women. *Am. J. Obstet. Gynecol.* **162**, 502–514.

[67]J. J. Michnovicz, R. J. Hershcopf, H. Naganuma, H. L. Bradlow, and J. Fishman (1986) Increased 2-hydroxylation of estradiol as a possible mechanism for the antiestrogenic effect of cigarette smoking. *N. Engl. J. Med.* **315**, 1305–1309.

[68]R. C. Brownson, T. M. DiLorenzo, M. V. Tuinen, and W. W. Finger (1990) Patterns of cigarette and smokeless tobacco use among children and adolescents. *Prev. Med.* **19**, 170–180.

[69]B. R. Flay, J. R. d'Avernas, J. A. Best, M. W. Kersell, and K. B. Ryan (1983) Cigarette smoking: Why young people do it and ways of preventing it, in *Pediatric and*

Adolescent Behavioral Medicine: Treatment Issues. P. McGrath and P. Firestone, eds. Springer, New York, pp. 132–160.

[70]Skelly, White, and Yankelovich, Inc. (1977) *A Study of Cigarette Smoking Among Teen-age Girls and Young Women. Summary of Findings.* DHEW Publication No. NIH 77-1203, Department of Health, Education and Welfare, Public Health Service, National Institutes of Health, National Cancer Institute, Bethesda, MD.

[71]L. Chassin, C. C. Presson, and S. J. Sherman (1984) Cognitive and social influence factors in adolescent smoking cessation. *Addict. Behav.* **9,** 383–390.

[72]G. E. Swan, D. Carmelli, R. H. Rosenman, R. R. Fabsitz, and J. C. Christian (1990) Smoking and alcohol consumption in adult male twins: Genetic heritability and shared environmental influences. *J. Subst. Abuse* **2,** 39–50.

[73]J. R. Hughes (1986) Genetics of smoking: A brief review. *Behav. Ther.* **17,** 335–345.

[74]C. S. Pomerleau, O. F. Pomerleau, K. A. Flessland, and S. M. Basson (1992) Relationship of Tridimensional Personality Questionnaire scores and smoking variables in female and male smokers. *J. Subst. Abuse* **4,** 143–154.

[75]M. Zuckerman, S. Ball, and J. Black (1990) Influences of sensation seeking, gender, risk appraisal, and situational motivation on smoking. *Addict. Behav.* **15,** 209–220.

[76]L. D. Gilchrist, S. P. Schinke, and P. Nurius (1989) Reducing onset of habitual smoking among women. *Prev. Med.* **18,** 235–248.

[77]O. F. Pomerleau, A. C. Collins, S. Shiffman, and C. S. Pomerleau (in press) Differences between smokers and never-smokers in sensitivity to nicotine: A preliminary report. *J. Clin. Consult. Psychol.*

[78]M. A. H. Russell (1989) Subjective and behavioural effects of nicotine in humans: Some sources of individual variation, in *Progress in Brain Research*, vol. 79. A. Nordberg, K. Fuxe, B. Holmstedt, and A. Sundwall, eds. Elsevier Science Publishers, Amsterdam, pp. 289–302.

[79]S. Stone, M. Dembroski, P. Costa Jr., and J. MacDougall (1990) Gender differences in cardiovascular reactivity. *J. Behav. Med.* **13,**137–156.

[80]S. Broder (1992) Cigarette advertising and corporate responsibility. *JAMA* **268,** 782–873.

[81]J. R. DiFranza, J. W. Richards, P. M. Paulman, N. Wolf-Gillespie, C. Fletcher, R. D. Jaffe, and D. Murray (1991) RJR Nabisco's cartoon camel promotes Camel cigarettes to children. *JAMA* **266,** 3149–3154.

[82]J. P. Pierce, E. Gilpin, D. M. Burns, E. Whalen, B. Rosbrook, D. Shopland, and M. Johnson (1991) Does tobacco advertising target young people to start smoking? *JAMA* **266,** 3154–3159.

[83]R. Roemer (1990) Fighting the smoking epidemic: Legislative and economic weapons. *Arctic Med. Res.* **49,** 69–77.

[84]R. M. Davis (1987) Current trends in cigarette advertising and marketing. *N. Engl. J. Med.* **316,** 725–732.

[85]V. L. Ernster (1986) Women, smoking, cigarette advertising and cancer. *Women Health* **11,** 217–235.

[86]A. O. Goldstein, P. M. Fischer, J. W. Richards Jr., and D. Creten (1987) Relationship between high school student smoking and recognition of cigarette advertisements. *J. Pediatr.* **110,** 488–491.

[87]C. L. Albright, D. G. Altman, M. D. Slater, and N. Maccoby (1988) Cigarette advertisements in magazines: Evidence for a differential focus on women's and youth magazines. *Health Educ. Q.* **15,** 223–233.

[88]E. R. Gritz (1984) Cigarette smoking by adolescent females: Implications for health and behavior. *Women Health* **9,** 103–115.

[89]N. E. Grunberg, S. E. Winders, and M. E. Wewers (1991) Gender differences in tobacco use. *Health. Psychol.* **10,** 143–153.

[90]B. A. Berman and E. R. Gritz (1991) Women and smoking: Current trends and issues for the 1990s. *J. Subst. Abuse* **3,** 221–238.

[91]K. E. Warner (1985) Cigarette advertising and media coverage of-smoking and health. *N. Engl. J. Med.* **312,** 384–388.

[92]L. White and E. M. Whelan (1986) How well do American magazines cover the health hazards of smoking? The 1986 survey. *ACSH News Views* **7,** 7–10.

[93]A. M. O'Keefe (1990) Targeted marketing: selling cigarettes to women. Paper presented at the 118th Annual Meeting of the American Public Health Association, New York.

[94]T. R. Isbell and R. C. Klesges (1992) Cigarette advertising and smoking rates in women and minorities. Poster presented at the Society of Behavioral Medicine 13th Annual Scientific Sessions, March 25–28, New York.

[95]P. M. Fischer, M. P. Schwartz, J. W. Richards, A. O. Goldstein, and T. H. Rojas (1991) Brand logo recognition by children aged 3 to 6 years. *JAMA* **266,** 3145–3149.

[96]H. Waxman (1991) Editorial: Tobacco marketing: Profiteering from children. *JAMA* **266,** 3185.

[97]R. M. Davis (1991) Editorial: Reducing youth access to tobacco. *JAMA* **266,** 3186.

[98]J. R. DiFranza (1992) Preventing teenage tobacco addiction. *J. Fam. Pract.* **34,** 753–756.

[99]M. A. Greenberg, C. L. Wiggins, D. M. Kutvirt, and J. M. Samet (1987) Cigarette use among Hispanic and non-Hispanic white school children, Albuquerque, New Mexico. *Am. J. Public Health* **77,** 621–622.

[100]J. J. Yu, M. E. Mattson, G. M. Boyd, M. D. Mueller, D. R. Shopland, T. F. Pechacek, and J. W. Cullen (1990) A comparison of smoking patterns in the People's Republic of China with the United States: An impending health catastrophe in the Middle Kingdom. *JAMA* **264,** 1575–1579.

[101]N. E. Grunberg, S. E. Winders, and M. E. Wewers (1991) Gender differences in tobacco use. *Health Psychol.* **10,** 143–153.

[102]K. E. Warner and G. N. Connolly (1991) Viewpoint. The global metastasis of the Marlboro man. *Am. J. Health Promotion* **5,** 325–327.

[103]J. W. Cullen, J. W. McKenna, and M. M. Massey (1986) International control of smoking and the U.S. experience. *Chest* **89(suppl.),** 206S–217S.

[104]J. Crofton (1990) Tobacco and the third world. *Thorax* **45,** 164–169.

[105]W. V. Chandler (1988) Smoking epidemic widens. *World Watch* **3(article #81),** 39–40.

[106]NIH Technology Assessment Conference Panel (1992) Methods for voluntary weight loss and control. *Ann. Intern. Med.* **116,** 942–949.

[107]A. Drewnowski and D. K. Yee (1987) Men and body image: Are males satisfied with their body weight? *Psychosom. Med.* **49,** 626–634.

[108]N. E. Grunberg (1986) Nicotine as a psychoactive drug: appetite regulation. *Psycopharmacol. Bull.* **22**, 875–881.

[109]R. C. Klesges, A. W. Meyers, L. M. Klesges, and M. E. LaVasque (1989) Smoking, body weight, and their effects on smoking behavior: a comprehensive review of the literature. *Psychol. Bull.* **106**, 204–230.

[110]D. F. Williamson, J. Madans, R. F. Anda, J. C. Kleinman, G. A. Giovino, and T. Byers (1991) Smoking cessation and severity of weight gain in a national cohort. *N. Engl. J. Med.* **324**, 739–745.

[111]R. C. Klesges and S. A. Shumaker (1992) Understanding the relations between smoking and body weight and their importance to smoking cessation and relapse. *Health Psychol.* **11(suppl.)**, 1–3.

[112]E. R. Gritz, S. T. St. Jeor, G. Bennett, L. Biener, S. N. Blair, D. J. Bowen, R. L. Brunner, A. Deltorn, J. P. Foreyt, D. Haire-Joshu, S. M. Hall, D. R. Hill, J. Jensen, J. Kristeller, B. H. Marcus, M. Nides, P. L. Pirie, L. J. Solomon, F. Stillman, J. Ernst, and C. Z. Mealer (1992) Task Force 3: Implications with respect to intervention and prevention. *Health Psychol.* **11(suppl.)**, 17–25.

[113]E. R. Gritz (1986) Gender and the teenage smoker. *NIDA Res. Monogr.* **65**, 70–79.

[114]R. C. Klesges and L. M. Klesges (1988) Cigarette smoking as a dietary strategy in a university population. *Int. J. Eating Disord.* **7**, 413–417.

[115]E. R. Gritz, R. C. Klesges, and A. W. Meyers (1989) The smoking and body weight relationship: Implications for intervention and postcessation weight control. *Ann. Behav. Med.* **11**, 144–153.

[116]J. R. Eiser and J. van der Pligt (1986) "Sick" or "hooked": Smoker's perceptions of their addiction. *Addict. Behav.* **11**, 11–15.

[117]N. L. Benowitz, F. Kuyt, and P. Jacob (1984) Influence of nicotine on cardiovascular and hormonal effects of cigarette smoking. *Clin. Pharmacol. Ther.* **36**, 74–81.

[118]J. A. Best and A. R. Hakstian (1978) A situation-specific model for smoking behavior. *Addict. Behav.* **3**, 79–92.

[119]L. Epstein and F. Collins (1977) The measurement of situational influences of smoking. *Addict. Behav.* **2**, 47–54.

[120]A. L. Myrsten, A. Elgerot, and B. Edgren (1977) Effects of abstinence from tobacco smoking on physiological and psychological arousal levels in habitual smokers. *Psychosom. Med.* **39**, 25–38.

[121]O. F. Pomerleau, D. Adkins, and M. Pertschuk (1978) Predictors of outcome and recidivism in smoking cessation treatment. *Addict. Behav.* **3**, 65–70.

[122]S. Shiffman (1982) Relapse following smoking cessation: A situational analysis. *J. Consult. Clin. Psychol.* **50**, 71–86.

[123]S. D. Dobbs, D. P. Strickler, and W. E. Maxwell (1981) The effects of stress and relaxation in the presence of stress on urinary pH and smoking behavior. *Addict. Behav.* **6**, 345–353.

[124]J. F. Golding and G. L. Managan (1982) Effects of cigarette smoking on measures of arousal, response suppression, and excitation/inhibition balance. *Int. J. Addict.* **17**, 793–804.

[125]C. S. Pomerleau and O. F. Pomerleau (1987) The effects of a psychological stressor on cigarette smoking and subsequent and physiological responses. *Psychophysiology* **24**, 278–285.

[126]J. E. Rose, S. Ananda, and M. E. Jarvik (1983) Cigarette smoking during anxiety-provoking and monotonous tasks. *Addict. Behav.* **8,** 353–359.

[127]O. F. Pomerleau and C. S. Pomerleau (1984) Neuroregulators and the reinforcement of smoking: Towards a biobehavioral explanation. *Neurosci. Biobehav. Rev.* **8,** 503–513.

[128]A. L. Myrsten, K. Andersson, M. Frankenhauser, and A. Elgerot (1975) Immediate effects of cigarette smoking as related to different smoking habits. *Percept. Motor Skills* **40,** 515–523.

[129]C. D. Frith (1971) Smoking behaviour and its relation to the smoker's immediate experience. *Br. J. Soc. Clin. Psychol.* **10,** 73–78.

[130]F. F. Ikard and S. Tomkins (1973) The experience of affect as a determinant of smoking behavior: a series of validity studies. *J. Abnorm. Psychol.* **81,** 172–181.

[131]R. Karasek, B. Gardell, and J. Lindell (1987) Work and non-work correlates of illness and behavior in male and female Swedish white collar workers. *J. Occup. Behav.* **8,** 187–207.

[132]M. A. Russell, E. Armstrong, and U. A. Patel (1976) Temporal contiguity in electric aversion therapy for cigarette smoking. *Behav. Res. Ther.* **14,** 103–123.

[133]A. Elgerot (1976) Note on selective effects of short-term tobacco-abstinence on complex versus simple mental tasks. *Percept. Motor Skills* **42,** 413–414.

[134]L. Biener (1987) Gender differences in the use of substances for coping, in *Gender and Stress.* R. C. Barnett, L. Beiner, and G. K. Baruch, eds. Free, New York, pp. 330–349.

[135]A. L. Magos (1988) Effects and analysis of the menstrual cycle. *J. Biomed. Eng.* **10,** 105–109.

[136]J. L. Steinberg and D. R. Cherek (1989) Menstrual cycle and cigarette smoking behavior. *Addict. Behav.* **14,** 173–179.

[137]C. S. Pomerleau, A. W. Garcia, O. F. Pomerleau, and O. G. Cameron (1992) The effects of menstrual phase and nicotine abstinence on nicotine intake and on biochemical and subjective measures in women smokers: A preliminary report. *Psychoneuroendocrinology,* **17,** 627–638.

[138]N. K. Mello, J. H. Mendelson, and S. L. Palmieri (1987) Cigarette smoking by women: interactions with alcohol use. *Psychopharmacology (Berlin)* **93,** 8–15.

[139]A. H. Glassman, F. Stetner, B. T. Walsh, P. S. Raizman, J. L. Fleiss, T. B. Cooper, and L. S. Covey (1988) Heavy smokers, smoking cessation, and clonidine. *JAMA* **259,** 2863–2866.

[140]A. H. Glassman, J. E. Helzer, L. S. Covey, L. B. Cottler, F. Stetner, J. E. Tipp, and J. Johnson (1990) Smoking, smoking cessation, and major depression. *JAMA* **264,** 1546–1549.

[141]N. Breslau, M. M. Kilbey, and P. Andreski (1991) Nicotine dependence, major depression, and anxiety in young adults. *Arch. Gen. Psychiatry* **48,** 1069–1074.

[142]R. R. Frerichs, C. S. Aneshensel, V. A. Clark, and P. Yokopenic (1981) Smoking and depression: a community survey. *Am. J. Public Health* **71,** 637–640.

[143]R. F. Anda, D. F. Williamson, L. G. Escobedo, E. E. Mast, G. A. Giovino, and P. L. Remington (1990) Depression and the dynamics of smoking. A national perspective [see comments]. *JAMA* **264,** 1541–1545.

[144]L. Brodsky (1985) Can nicotine control panic attacks? [Letter]. *Am. J. Psychiatry* **142,** 524.

[145]M. M. Weissman and G. L. Klerman (1977) Sex differences in the epidemiology of depression. *Arch. Gen. Psychiatry* **34,** 98–111.

[146]M. M. Weissman, M. L. Bruce, P. J. Leaf, L. P. Florio, and C. Holzer III (1991) Affective disorders, in *Psychiatric Disorders in America: The Epidemiologic Catchment Area Study.* L. N. Robins and D. A. Regier, eds. Free Press, New York, pp. 53–80.

[147]W. W. Eaton, A. Dryman, and M. M. Weissman (1991) Panic and phobia, in *Psychiatric Disorders in America: The Epidemiologic Catchment Area Study.* L. N. Robins and D. A. Regier, eds. Free, New York, pp. 155–179.

[148]J. R. Hughes, D. K. Hatsukami, J. E. Mitchell, and L. A. Dahlgren (1986) Prevalence of smoking among psychiatric outpatients. *Am. J. Psychiatry* **143,** 993–997.

[149]R. M. Carney, M. W. Rich, A. TeVelde, J. Saini, K. Clark, and A. S. Jaffe (1987) Major Depressive Disorder in coronary artery disease. *Am, J. Cardiol.* **60,** 1273–1275.

[150]L. S. Radloff (1977) The CES-D scale: A self-report depression scale for research in the general population. *Appl. Psychol. Measurement* **1,** 385–401.

[151]L. N. Robins, J. E. Helzer, and J. Croughan, et al. (1979) *The NIMH Diagnostic Interview Schedule.* National Institute of Mental Health, Rockville, MD.

[152]J. R. Hughes (1986) Nicotine gum to treat panic attacks? [Letter]. *Am. J. Psychiatry* **143,** 271.

[153]L. Brodsky (1986) Can nicotine control panic attacks? [Reply]. *Am. J. Psychiatry* **143,** 271.

[154]I. Maany, G. Woody, and E. Foulks (1987) Nicotine and panic attacks [letter]. *Am. J. Psychiatry* **144,** 255.

[155]S. E. Fleming and T. W. Lombardo (1987) Effects of cigarette smoking on phobic anxiety. *Addict. Behav.* **12,** 195–198.

[156]C. C. Seltzer, G. D. Friedman, and A. B. Siegelaub (1974) Smoking and drug consumption in white, black, and oriental men and women. *Am. J. Public Health* **64,** 466–473.

[157]K. Yamaguchi and D. B. Kandel (1984) Patterns of drug use from adolescence to young adulthood: II. Sequences of progression. *Am. J. Public Health* **74,** 668–672.

[158]J. Istvan and J. D. Matarazzo (1984) Tobacco, alcohol, and caffeine use: A review of their interrelationships. *Psychol. Bull.* **95,** 301–326.

[159]R. R. Griffiths, G. E. Bigelow, and I. Liebson (1976) Facilitation of human tobacco self-administration by ethanol: a behavioral analysis. *J. Exp. Anal. Behav.* **25,** 279–292.

[160]K. F. Dreher and J. G. Fraser (1967) Smoking habits of alcoholic outpatients I. *Int. J. Addict.* **3,** 65–80.

[161]M. J. Ashley, J. S. Olin, W. H. leRiche, A. Kornaczewski, W. Schmidt, and J. G. Rankin (1981) Morbidity patterns in hazardous drinkers: Relevance of demographic sociologic, drinking, and drug use characteristics. *Int. J. Addict.* **16,** 593–625.

[162]E. R. Gritz, J. M. Stapleton, M. A. Hill, and M. E. Jarvik (1985) Prevalence of cigarette smoking in VC medical and psychiatric hospitals. *Bull. Soc. Psychol. Addict. Behav.* **4,** 151–165.

[163]C. R. Cloninger (1987) Neurogenetic adaptive mechanisms in alcoholism. *Science* **236,** 410–416.

[164]J. E. Helzer, A. Burnam, and L. T. McEvoy (1991) Alcohol abuse and dependence, in *Psychiatric Disorders in America: The Epidemiologic Catchment Area Study.* L. N. Robins and D. A. Regier, eds. Free, New York, pp. 81–115.

[165]E. Taioli and E. L. Wynder (1991) Effect of the age at which smoking begins on frequency of smoking in adulthood [letter]. *N. Engl. J. Med.* **325,** 968–969.

[166]L. D. Gilchrist and S. P. Schinke (1985) Improving smoking prevention programs. *J. Psychosoc. Oncol.* **3**, 67–78.

[167]University of Southern California Institute for Health Promotion and Disease Prevention (1989) *Tobacco/Drug Abuse Prevention Recommendations to the United States Senate.* Los Angeles, CA.

[168]B. F. Flay (1985) Psychosocial approaches to smoking prevention: A review of the findings. *Health Psychol.* **4**, 449–488.

[169]S. M. Blake, K. I. Klepp, T. F. Pechacek, A. R. Folsom, R. V. Luepker, D. R. Jacobs, and M. B. Mittelmark (1989) Differences in smoking cessation strategies between men and women. *Addict. Behav.* **14**, 409–418.

[170]M. C. Fiore, T. E. Novotny, J. P. Pierce, G. A. Giovino, E. J. Hatziandreu, P. A. Newcomb, T. S. Surawicz, and R. M. Davis (1990) Methods used to quit smoking in the United States. Do cessation programs help?. *JAMA* **263**, 2760–2765.

[171]J. K. Ockene (1984) Toward a smoke-free society [editorial]. *Am. J. Public Health* **74**, 1198–1200.

[172]S. J. Schneider, A. Benya, and H. Singer (1984) Computerized direct mail to treat smokers who avoid treatment. *Comput. Biomed. Res.* **17**, 409–418.

[173]S. Cohen, E. Lichtenstein, J. O. Prochaska, J. S. Rossi, E. R. Gritz, C. R. Carr, C. T. Orleans, V. J. Schoenbach, L. Biener, D. Abrams, C. DiClemente, S. Curry, G. A. Marlatt, K. M. Cummings, S. L. Emont, G. Giovino, and D. Ossip-Klein (1989) Debunking myths about self-quitting. Evidence from 10 prospective studies of persons who attempt to quit smoking by themselves. *Am. Psychol.* **44**, 1355–1365.

[174]M. A. Orlandi (1986) Gender differences in smoking cessation. *Women Health* **11**, 237–251.

[175]E. J. Hatziandreu, J. P. Pierce, M. Lefkopoulou, M. C. Fiore, S. L. Mills, T. E. Novotny, G. A. Giovino, and R. M. Davis (1990) Quitting smoking in the United States in 1986. *J. Natl. Cancer Inst.* **82**, 1402–1406.

[176]P. L. Pirie, D. M. Murray, and R. V. Luepker (1991) Gender differences in cigarette smoking and quitting in a cohort of young adults. *Am. J. Public Health* **81**, 324–327.

[177]S. A. French, R. W. Jerrery, P. L. Pirie, and C. M. McBride (1992) Do weight concerns hinder smoking cessation efforts? *Addict. Behav.* **17**, 219–226.

[178]C. K. Weekley, R. C. Klesges, and G. Reylea (1992) Smoking as a weight-control strategy and its relationship to smoking status. *Addict. Behav.* **17**, 259–271.

[179]E. R. Gritz, B. A. Berman, L. L. Read, A. C. Marcus, and J. Siau (1990) Weight change among registered nurses in a self-help smoking cessation program. *Am. J. Health Promotion* **5**, 115–121.

[180]S. M. Hall, D. Ginsberg, and R. T. Jones (1986) Smoking cessation and weight gain. *J. Consult. Clin. Psychol.* **54**, 342–346.

[181]P. O'Hara, S. A. Portser, and B. P. Anderson (1989) The influence of menstrual cycle changes on the tobacco withdrawal syndrome in women. *Addict. Behav.* **14**, 595–600.

[182]H. C. Coppotelli and C. T. Orleans (1985) Partner support and other determinants of smoking cessation maintenance among women. *J. Consult. Clin. Psychol.* **53**, 455–460.

[183]E. B. Fisher Jr., D. B. Bishop, J. Goldmuntz, and A. Jacobs (1988) Implications for the practicing physician of the psychosocial dimensions of smoking. *Chest* **93**, 69S–78S.

[184]R. Mermelstein, S. Cohen, E. Lichtenstein, J. S. Baer, and D. Kamarck (1986) Social support and smoking cessation and maintenance. *J. Consult. Clin. Psychol.* **54**, 447–453.

[185]R. Mermelstein, E. Lichtenstein, and K. McIntyre (1983) Partner support and relapse in smoking-cessation programs. *J. Consult. Clin. Psychol.* **51**, 465–466.

[186]U.S. Public Health Service (1964) *Smoking and Health. Report of the Advisory Committee to the Surgeon General of the Public Health Service.* U.S. Department of Health, Education, and Welfare, Public Health Service, Center for Disease Control. PHS Publication No. 1103, Washington, DC.

[187]R. C. Brownson, J. Jackson-Thompson, J. C. Wilderson, J. R. Davis, N. W. Owens, and E. B. Fisher (1992) Demographic and socioeconomic differences in beliefs about the health effects of smoking. *Am. J. Public Health* **82**, 99–103.

[188]B. R. Flay (1987) Mass media and smoking cessation: A critical review. *Am. J. Public Health* **77**, 153–160.

[189]U.S. Department of Health and Human Services (1991) *Strategies to Control Tobacco Use in the United States: A Blueprint for Public Health Action in the 1990's.* DHHS Publication No. 92-3316, U.S. Government Printing Office, Washington, DC.

[190]T. J. Glynn and M. W. Manley (1989) *How to Help Your Patients Stop Smoking: A National Cancer Institute Manual for Physicians.* National Institutes of Health Publication 89-3064, U.S. Department of Health and Human Services, Bethesda, MD.

[191]E. R. Gritz, C. R. Carr, and A. C. Marcus (1988) Unaided smoking cessation. Great American Smokeout and New Year's Day quitters. *J. Psychosoc. Oncol.* **6**, 41–63.

[192]T. E. Kottke, R. N. Battista, G. H. DeFriese, and M. L. Brekke (1988) Attributes of successful smoking cessation interventions in medical practice: A meta-analysis of 39 controlled trials. *JAMA* **259**, 2883–2889.

[193]T. E. Kottke, H. Blackburn, M. L. Brekke, and L. T. Solberg (1987) The systematic practice of preventive cardiology. *Am. J. Cardiol.* **59**, 690–694.

[194]D. H. Longsdon, C. M. Lazaro, and R. V. Meier (1989) The feasibility of behavioral risk reduction in primary medical care. *Am. J. Prev. Med.* **5**, 249–256.

[195]R. E. Mecklenburg (1990) The National Cancer Institute's invitation to dental professionals in smoking cessation. *J. Am. Dent. Assoc.* **(January suppl.)**, 40S–41S.

[196]L. I. Solberg (1988) Implementing a tobacco cessation program in clinical practice. *Med. Times* **116**, 119–124.

[197]E. Frank, M. A. Winkleby, D. G. Altman, B. Rockhill, and S. P. Fortmann (1991) Predictors of physicians' smoking cessation advice. *JAMA* **266**, 3139–3145.

[198]M. Manley, R. P. Epps, C. Huston, T. Glynn, and D. Shopland (1991) Clinical interventions in tobacco control. *JAMA* **266**, 3172–3174.

[199]R. P. Epps and M. W. Manley (1992) The clinician's role in preventing smoking initiation. *Med. Clin. N. Am.* **76**, 439–449.

[200]C. T. Orleans, B. K. Rimer, S. Cristinzio, M. K. Keintz, and L. Fleisher (1991) A national survey of older smokers: Treatment needs of a growing population. *Health Psychol.* **10**, 343–351.

[201]N. K. Aaronson, D. H. Ershoff, and B. G. Danaher (1985) Smoking cessation in pregnancy: A self-help approach. *Addict. Behav.* **10**, 103–108.

[202]D. H. Ershoff, P. D. Mullen, and V. P. Quinn (1989) A randomized trial of a serialized self-help smoking cessation program for pregnant women in an HMO. *Am. J. Public Health* **79**, 182–187.

[203]J. P. Mayer, B. Hawkins, and R. Todd (1990) A randomized evaluation of smoking cessation interventions for pregnant women at a WIC clinic. *Am. J. Public Health* **80**, 76–78.

[204]M. Sexton and J. R. Hebel (1984) A clinical trial of change in maternal smoking and its effect on birth weight. *JAMA* **251,** 911–915.

[205]R. A. Windsor, G. Cutter, J. Morris, Y. Reese, B. Manzella, E. E. Bartlett, C. Samuelson, and D. Spanos (1985) The effectiveness of smoking cessation methods for smokers in public health maternity clinics: A randomized trial. *Am. J. Public Health* **75,** 1389–1392.

[206]C. T. Orleans, J. Martin, J. Slade, L. C. Sobell, and L. T. Kozlowski (1992) Understanding and treating nicotine addiction in smokers with other chemical dependencies. Paper presented at the Annual Meeting of the Society for Behavioral Medicine, March 25–28, New York.

[207]A. M. Joseph, K. L. Nichol, M. L. Wallenbring, J. E. Korn, and L. S. Lysaght (1990) Beneficial effects of treatment of nicotine dependence during an inpatient substance abuse treatment program. *JAMA* **263,** 3043–3046.

[208]E. R. Gritz, B. A. Berman, R. Bastani, and M. Wu (1992) A randomized trial of a self-help smoking cessation intervention in a non-volunteer female population: Testing the limits of the public health model. *Health Psychol.* **11,** 280–289.

[209]E. R. Gritz, A. C. Marcus, B. A. Berman, L. L. Read, L. E. Kanim, and S. J. Reeder (1988) Evaluation of a worksite self-help smoking cessation program for registered nurses. *Am. J. Health Promotion* **3,** 26–35.

[210]E. R. Gritz, C. R. Carr, D. A. Rapkin, C. Chang, J. Beumer, and P. H. Ward (1991) A smoking cessation intervention for head and neck cancer patients: Trial design, patient accrual and characteristics. *Can. Epidemiol. Biomarkers Prev.* **1,** 67–73.

[211]American Cancer Society (1988) *Special Delivery: Smoke Free*, 88-1C-No. 2422.01-.06-LE. American Cancer Society, New York.

[212]C. Manfredi, L. Lacey, R. Warnecke, and M. Buis (1992) Smoking-related behavior, beliefs and social environment of young black women in subsidized public housing in Chicago. *Am. J. Public Health* **82,** 267–271.

[213]D. P. L. Sachs (1990) Smoking cessation strategies: What works, what doesn't. *J. Am. Dent. Assoc.* **(January suppl.),** 13S–19S.

[214]D. P. L. Sachs (1991) Advances in smoking cessation treatment. *Curr. Pulmonology* **12,** 139.

[215]J. Rose, E. D. Levin, F. M. Behm, C. Adivi, and C. Schur (1990) Transdermal nicotine facilitates smoking cessation. *Clin. Pharmacol. Ther.* **47,** 323–330.

[216]P. Tonnesen, J. Norregaard, K. Simonson, and U. Sawe (1991) A double-blind trial of a 16-hour transdermal nicotine patch in smoking cessation. *N. Engl. J. Med.* **325,** 311–315.

[217]Omaha, Nebraska Transdermal Nicotine Study Group (1991) Transdermal nicotine for smoking cessation. *JAMA* **266,** 3133–3139.

[218]N. L. Benowitz (1991) Pharmacodynamics of nicotine: Implications for rational treatment of nicotine addiction. *Br. J. Addict.* **86,** 495–499.

[219]R. D. Hurt, G. G. Lauger, K. P. Offord, T. E. Kottke, and L. C. Dale (1990) Nicotine-replacement therapy with use of a transdermal nicotine patch—a randomized double-blind placebo controlled trial. *Mayo Clin. Proc.* **65,** 1529–1537.

[220]J. A. Peters (1990) Editorial: Nicotine-related therapy in cessation of smoking. *Mayo Clin. Proc.* **65,** 1619–1623.

[221]G. Sutherland, J. A. Stapelton, M. A. H. Russell, M. J. Jarvis, P. Hajek, M. Belcher, and C. Feyerabend (1992) Randomized controlled trial of nasal nicotine spray in smoking cessation. *Lancet* **340,** 324–329.

[222]F. S. Tennant Jr., A. L. Tarver, and R. A. Rawson (1984) Clinical evaluation of mecamylamine for withdrawal from nicotine dependence. *NIDA Res. Monogr.* **49,** 239–246.

[223]A. H. Glassman, W. K. Jackson, B. T. Walsh, and S. P. Roose (1984) Cigarette craving, smoking withdrawal, and clonidine. *Science* **226,** 864–866.

[224]B. Spring, J. Wurtman, R. Gleason, R. Wurtman, and K. Kessler (1991) Weight gain and withdrawal symptoms after smoking cessation: a preventative intervention using *d*-fenfluramine. *Health Psychol.* **10,** 216–223.

[225]O. F. Pomerleau, C. S. Pomerleau, E. M. Morrell, and J. M. Lowenbergh (1991) Effects of fluoxetine on weight gain and food intake in smokers who reduce nicotine intake. *Psychoneuroendocrinology* **16,** 433–440.

[226]D. J. Bowen, B. Spring, and E. Pox (1991) Tryptophan and high-carbohydrate diets as adjuncts to smoking cessation therapy. *J. Behav. Med.* **14,** 97–110.

[227]R. C. Klesges, L. M. Klesges, A. W. Meyers, M. L. Klem, and T. Isbell (1990) The effects of phenylpropanolamine on dietary intake, physical activity, and body weight after smoking cessation. *Clin. Pharmacol. Ther.* **47,** 747–754.

[228]S. Bourne (1985) Treatment of cigarette smoking with short-term high-dosage corticotrophin therapy: Preliminary communication. *J. Roy. Soc. Med.* **78,** 649–650.

[229]J. Gross, M. L. Stitzer, and J. Maldonado (1989) Nicotine replacement: Effects on postcessation weight gain. *J. Consult. Clin. Psychol.* **57,** 87–92.

[230]P. Hajek, P. Jackson, and M. Belcher (1988) Long-term use of nicotine chewing gum occurrence, determinants, and effect on weight gain. *JAMA* **260,** 1593–1596.

[231]S. L. Emont and K. M. Cummings (1987) Weight gain following smoking cessation: a possible role for nicotine replacement in weight management. *Addict. Behav.* **12,** 151–155.

[232]J. A. Hamilton (1986) An overview of the clinical rationale for advancing gender-related psychopharmacology and drug abuse research. *NIDA Res. Monogr.* **65,** 14–20.

[233]J. D. Killen, S. P. Fortmann, B. Newman, and A. Varady (1990) Evaluation of a treatment approach combining nicotine gum with self-guided behavioral treatments for smoking relapse prevention. *J. Consult. Clin. Psychol.* **58,** 85–92.

[234]S. G. Brink, D. G. Simons-Morton, C. M. Harvey, G. S. Parcel, and K. M. Tiernau (1988) Developing comprehensive smoking control programs in school. *J. School Health* **58,** 177–180.

Drugs, Alcohol, and the Dysfunctional Family

Male/Female Differences

Barbara C. Wallace

Introduction

Any discussion of drugs, alcohol, and the dysfunctional family, which pays special attention to male and female differences, should aspire to prepare the clinician or counselor to work more effectively with the large female population of chemically dependent clients. The crack cocaine epidemic of the 1980s permitted women to demonstrate their equality in access to an inexpensive, potent, and chic ready-to-smoke cocaine product, as well as equal access to the path of addiction. Society and its media readily projected on these women of all colors and classes a negative image of being a criminal, with nothing being more disdainful than to continue the use of illicit chemicals once pregnant and carrying a vulnerable fetus. The incarceration of women so convicted for drug distribution and drug possession, as well as the incarceration and punishment of women who have either given birth to infants testing positive for cocaine, or abused and neglected their children because of addiction, means that the therapeutic and treatment challenge is considerable.

From: *Drug and Alcohol Abuse Reviews, Vol. 5: Addictive Behaviors in Women*
Ed.: R. R. Watson ©1994 Humana Press Inc., Totowa, NJ

As we navigate the 1990s, we find fewer new adolescent initiates into crack cocaine smoking, but a cohort of crack smokers continue their varying and diverse habits, ranging from some probable recreational use, to abuse and chemical dependence. We also observe a purer and cheaper heroin product readily available in the drug culture today, so that intranasal snorting remains a viable route of self-administration, reducing the risk of injected drug use spreading HIV/AIDS, and perhaps foreboding the fulfillment of the prophecy that a sedative epidemic follows a stimulant epidemic. Meanwhile, the cocaine and crack epidemic of the 1980s led us toward recognition that polydrug-use patterns involving alcohol and other innovative chemical cocktails are the prevailing reality today. Our contemporary chemical dependency treatment umbrella therefore encompasses the array of chemical-use patterns to be found.

In this era, those treating the new and large population of chemically dependent women in their childbearing years observe how this population brings with them the baggage of past histories of trauma. This trauma involves three eras that include:

1. Trauma sustained in childhood when growing up within a dysfunctional family;
2. The typical trauma of experiencing some form of abuse in adolescent and adult relationships; and
3. The trauma of violence in the streets and drug culture. This drug culture violence also overlaps with the trauma of hitting rock bottom.[1]

A clear implication is that the training and knowledge base of the clinicians and counselors working with this population must include some adequate appreciation of the role of trauma in the etiology and maintenance of addiction, the role of trauma in the manifestations of psychopathology, and common patterns of symptom substitution observable in clients who are pursuing abstinence. A consideration of problems of poor self-regulation[2] permits grounding treatment professionals and paraprofessionals in that requisite knowledge base.

An additional dimension of this complex treatment challenge involves the reality that cocaine's aphrodisiac effects promoted promiscuity and group sexual experimentation in the drug culture—in particular among freebase cocaine smokers and smokers of crack cocaine who developed the highest states of intoxication and most severe states of chemical dependence. Whether it involves sexual partners experiencing extended sexual sessions with the assistance of cocaine, the exchange of sex for drugs, or engagement in more outright forms of prostitution, the painful reality is that our cohort of chemically dependent women in their childbearing years, who were a part of the cocaine and crack culture, are wondering if they are HIV-positive and in danger of contracting AIDS; this nagging question remains even if these women are hopeful about avoiding relapse and staying drug- and alcohol-free.

Hence, clinicians and counselors find themselves faced with the painful reality that chemical dependency treatment not only involves trauma resolution at some point, but also necessitates health education on HIV/ AIDS, as well as counseling on death, dying, and the grieving process, since these women have already had lovers and loved ones die from AIDS, violence, and/or addiction. How does one acquire expertise in bereavement counseling as a subspecialty within chemical dependency treatment? How does one avoid it? In this day and age, no one can; and all treatment professionals are obligated to face the difficult look of denial in the eyes of clients who have canceled HIV tests and repeatedly not shown up for results, while admitting to some continuing sexual contacts without regular condom use. The active and persuasive health educator must emerge from within the clinician or counselor at such times, because once the wall of denial is cracked, the bereavement counselor must emerge from within, and be there for the torrential outpouring of pain and grief over the lover or loved one for whom they have never as yet grieved and are terrified of following unto death.

Since women in our society are largely exposed to treatment facilities developed for men, and are still subject to unique socialization forces and societal dynamics as women, certainly there is something different from the male experience in light of complex issues that impact women in a certain fashion. Consider the following:

1. A young mother who is incarcerated for drug distribution or drug possession, and thereby separated from her children;
2. A mother who loses custody of her infant at its birth, as well as of her other children;
3. A mother who has to seek out treatment in order to regain custody of her children in a society that has lacked adequate treatment slots for pregnant women, still has fewer treatment slots for women in programs that were specifically designed and structured for male heroin addicts, and typically asks women to separate from their infants and children in order to pursue 1 or 2 yr of residential therapeutic community treatment for their addiction in that male-structured program; and
4. A woman in receipt of chemical dependency treatment within a program that typically advises separation from a drug-dealing spouse or partner who may have been violent and abusive at times; however, the program typically fails to appreciate the woman's need for more innovative and culturally sensitive counseling and family outreach components that appreciate the ties a woman has to her children's father.

Do many residential therapeutic communities find themselves ever so subtly permeated with subtle dynamics that convey the notion that women have some lower status within these programs, just as they do in the larger society? Have the criminal justice system and our treatment programs been guilty of failing to appreciate the not so subtle pressure on women who are chemically dependent, but also concerned about the children from whom they are typically separated during incarceration, inpatient, and residential treatment, whereas male-structured programs indoctrinate women to keep the focus on themselves if they are to recover? How much sensitivity to the relationships women have with their children and with the father of their children prevails? And, when no simple solution exists, but a woman's spouse clearly needs chemical dependency treatment, job training and placement, and they both need couple's counseling and professional psychotherapy, can clinicians and counselors handle at present this complex task of family mental health promotion while striving toward the goal of family reunification? Although clear and consistent answers to these questions may not exist, a complex treatment challenge can clearly be seen as the context for this chapter's discussion.

This chapter will provide clinicians and counselors, attempting to improve their treatment efficacy with the new and large population of chemically dependent women, with the knowledge base needed in order to appreciate how drugs, alcohol, and dysfunctional families represent factors that intersect and blend to create today's complex treatment challenge. In particular, some discussion and elaboration of the issues touched on in this introduction will highlight important differences in male and female chemically dependent populations that significantly impact the treatment challenge. Specifically, this chapter will:

1. Present and discuss evidence that the chemically dependent are adult children of dysfunctional families and survivors of several eras of trauma that creates significant psychopathology, which must be remediated as a form of relapse prevention;
2. Consider the implications of HIV/AIDS and death, dying, and bereavement counseling emerging as components of chemical dependency treatment; and
3. Recommend ways in which treatment programs must become more sensitized to the task of recovery when one is a woman, a mother, and has children by a man who was her drug partner and drug dealer.

Female Addicts, Alcoholics, and Dysfunctional Family Background

Whether we are considering the female alcoholic or addict, we are in effect discussing that large population of chemically dependent women who are using novel polydrug combinations, such as alcohol, pills, and cigarets, combining alcohol with cocaine or crack, using heroin and marijuana, combining intranasal heroin use with crack smoking, or are dependent on some other innovative and idiosyncratic chemical combination. The bottom line is that the commonly encountered chemically dependent female client will, on assessment, produce disturbing and compelling tales as she pours forth her family history. Quite often, it is only within the context of a clinical interview, in which the clinician or counselor tries to gather the woman's psychosocial history, that it becomes apparent that some significant trauma has occurred.

The Importance of a Thorough Individualized Assessment

Clearly, only a thorough individualized assessment that asks standard questions, such as the following, can begin to document the nexus between chemical dependency and dysfunctional family experiences: What was it like growing up as a child? Did anything traumatic, shocking, or hurtful ever happen to you? Were your parents alcoholic? Did any alcohol or drug use change your parents' personalities? What kind of problems did your parents have when you were growing up? Were you ever sexually abused or molested? Although not a comprehensive listing of the kinds of questions that comprise a thorough, individualized assessment obtained in the course of a clinical interview,[3] these sample assessment questions begin to illustrate the importance of ascertaining a history of what may begin to constitute the experience of trauma.

The common history of some significant childhood or developmental trauma sustained within a dysfunctional family, which is to be found in female chemically dependent clients, will emerge via this kind of clinical interview. In some cases, clients need to receive some brief psychoeducation about what constitutes parental alcoholism, physical abuse, fondling, molestation, or sexual abuse. Therefore, clinicians aspire both to collect sufficient data on a client's psychosocial history, and also to end all clinical interviews with a technique that maximizes the clinician's therapeutic impact.

The clinician's therapeutic impact is maximized when the client emerges from the interview with some new understanding of how, for example, her mother's behavior did constitute alcoholism, physical abuse, and verbal abuse, which the client survived in a difficult childhood. The metaphoric pieces of a client's life-story might also be therapeutically put in place so that a tentative puzzle is formed, which is utilized to assist the client. A client might, for example, come to understand that because of her mother's alcoholism, and her subsequent experience of physical abuse and verbal abuse, the client was left with a tendency to get depressed sometimes as an adolescent and adult, and the client's own alcoholic drinking emerged as a way to cope with feelings of depression.[3] Perhaps even more common is to find that such a client utilizes some other chemical in vogue, such as crack cocaine, with which to cope with those intermittent periods of depression remaining as the legacy of some childhood trauma of physical and verbal abuse delivered by an alcoholic mother in a dysfunctional family.

The point is that those clinicians and counselors who have come to accept the reality of a drug, alcohol, and dysfunctional family nexus have arrived at that view because of countless experiences of merely performing a mandatory psychosocial history and assessment, but in the process having the experience of hearing horrendous tales of abuse that put the client's chemical dependency in a fresh perspective. Typically, that fresh perspective was a growing appreciation of probable etiological factors—among a host of multiple interacting variables recognized within biopsychosocial approaches—involving significant childhood trauma sustained within dysfunctional families.

A Definition of Trauma and Dysfunctional Family

At this time, it seems necessary to offer definitions of trauma and a dysfunctional family. Trauma can be defined as resulting from any experience of violence—the delivery of physical force, displays of power, delivery of misinformation/myths—which constitutes an assault against one's physical body, self-concept, identity, cognitions, affects, and consciousness. Typically, the experience of personal trauma involves witnessing or experiencing domestic violence, incest, child sexual abuse, physical abuse, or being the victim of some street or school violence, or of taunts and verbal abuse. In this chapter, the focus is primarily on the traumatic violence that has been sustained within one's very own family environment. A second part of the definition of trauma considers trauma as involving any moment when the ego is overwhelmed, cannot integrate or make sense out of an experience based on its wealth of knowledge, or experiences a state of overstimulation.

In terms of a definition of a dysfunctional family, consider the following: A dysfunctional family involves a setting in which parental figures responsible for the care of children engage in behavioral patterns characterized by inconsistency and unpredictability. The overall family environment may also, at times, appear to be chaotic, particularly at times when some form of violence—the use of physical force, displays of power, and the spreading of misinformation/myths—is transpiring in the form of domestic violence, physical abuse, sexual abuse, or verbal abuse. The concept of a dysfunctional family permits one to characterize the setting in which trauma has been sustained by children and adolescents who were somehow left vulnerable and susceptible to the development of chemical dependency.

Having made explicit the definition of trauma and dysfunctional family, it can be seen even more clearly that the kinds of horrendous tales clinicians have heard women share regarding their lives have in their simplest terms been tales about trauma sustained as they survived within dysfunctional families. Beyond what is heard within clinical interviews during the performance of thorough, individualized assessments, a growing body of supportive literature and data speaks more directly to the existence of a chemical dependency and dysfunctional family nexus.

Support for the Chemical Dependency/Dysfunctional Family Nexus

Support for the view that there is this nexus between chemical dependency and having experienced some trauma within a dysfunctional family while growing up as a child or adolescent rests in the literature. Schiffer, in his work with mostly White cocaine-dependent clients, treated first on an inpatient unit and then subsequently seen by the same therapist on a protracted basis in individual psychotherapy, has identified the way in which all of his clients had in common the experience of some trauma.[4] Wallace has conceptualized this trauma through a content analysis of psychosocial histories and assessments ($n = 245$), documenting that background trauma in her crack cocaine-dependent clients involved the following kinds of experiences within dysfunctional families: 51% are adult children of alcoholics, whereas others were exposed to domestic violence (20%), parental abandonment (22%), parental separation (20%), physical abuse (14%), emotional abuse (7%), and sexual abuse (7%).[3] A full 91% of this rather large sample were from one kind of dysfunctional family or another.

Voluntary reporting of trauma without specific and systematic questioning about sexual abuse experiences may have contributed to Wallace's low rates of reported sexual abuse in childhood.[3] Others assert that rates of sexual abuse among the female chemically dependent range from 20–75%.[5]

Walker reported on a residential therapeutic community sample where 70% of residents came from a home where one or both parents were alcoholic or had a drug problem; over two-fifths had either been battered, sexually molested, or raped as children.[6] Rohsenow et al. argued that actual rates of molestation during childhood for the chemically dependent are actually much higher.[7] They found that before they began to specifically ask about the problem, only 4% of men and 20% of women disclosed sexual abuse in childhood. Most interestingly, according to Rohsenow et al., after routine inquiries began, 42% of teenage boys, 75% of adult women, and 71–90% of teenage girls reported having been sexually abused as children.[7]

These figures strongly indicate that for both men and women the chemically dependent tend to possess striking rates of childhood sexual abuse. However, a clear male/female difference involves the higher rates of sexual abuse among women, fueling speculation on a probable etiological role for the trauma of sexual abuse, and underscoring the importance of this chapter's focus.

A critically needed advance in the field of chemical dependency, which would illustrate a sensitivity to male/female differences and the importance of special trauma resolution treatment components for women in particular, is to do the following: Clinicians and researchers need to pay explicit attention to the variable of the experience of trauma within a dysfunctional family in one's childhood. It is important to pay attention to this variable—which is really a set of variables once the age of trauma, duration, and severity of trauma are considered and explored—as it may distinguish categories of clients who can be matched to a much needed trauma resolution component providing professional psychotherapy (even if in a cost-effective group modality) and remediation of clients' psychopathology and other symptoms rooted within past trauma. Ultimately, client-to-intervention matching strategies within diverse treatment settings could lie in those thorough, individualized assessment findings gathered, perhaps ideally through a clinical interview, which reveal traumatic histories of incest, sexual abuse, physical abuse, domestic violence, and verbal abuse. This needed advance to more sophisticated matching strategies would address a prime criticism of the field, i.e., that clients are treated as though they are a monolithic group. Clearly, the presence of a trauma history distinguishes an entire subset of the chemically dependent population, and the male/female difference of yet higher rates of sexual abuse among women call for special women's groups for trauma resolution.[8]

Other compelling pieces in the literature underscore the importance of appreciating that this is a special issue for chemically dependent women, which if left unaddressed by male-structured and male-dominated treatment programs can lead to relapse in recovering women. Young focused on the experiences of women alcoholics and spelled out in some detail the way in which newly sober women may experience the re-emergence of memories of sexual abuse and may readily relapse, resorting once again to chemical management of symptoms rooted in their sexual abuse.[5] Quite often these symptoms in the newly abstinent chemically dependent female actually meet criteria for posttraumatic stress disorder.[9]

Wanck has documented the way in which a higher risk of relapse does seem to exist for adult children of alcoholics being treated for their own alcoholism.[10] Thus, the legacy of some adult child of a dysfunctional family status, in general, may translate not only into some susceptibility or vulnerability to the development of chemical dependency, but perhaps also to a greater risk of relapse.

In this regard, Bollerud urged the establishment of specialized treatment components for the resolution of trauma in women in light of the reported high rates of sexual abuse and incest in this population, as well as other sources of trauma within dysfunctional families.[11] Rohsenow et al. would concur that if histories of trauma within dysfunctional families are a major contributing factor to the development of addiction and are not addressed in treatment programs, then this factor may contribute to early relapse.[7]

The Nature of Psychopathology in Chemically Dependent Women

The work of Meyer[12] forces the reader to recognize that it is ever so difficult to answer the questions, What came first, the chicken or the egg? or, What came first, the addiction or the psychopathology? Does psychopathology, as that resulting from the experience of childhood trauma within a dysfunctional family, precede and perhaps contribute to the development of the addiction? or, Does the experience of addiction lead to the development and manifestation of some psychopathology? As a result of these kinds of questions, and without adequate longitudinal studies of children growing up within dysfunctional families who do and do not end up chemically dependent, it is not yet understood what percent of the variance in research exploring the role of biological, psychological, and social/environmental/cultural factors is accounted for by childhood development and the experience of some trauma within dysfunctional families.

Regression and Trauma from Chemical Dependence

Bean-Bayog[1] and Levin[13] argued for the view that some trauma and psychopathology follows from the experience of alcoholism or addiction. For her part, Bean-Bayog explained how there is the trauma of addiction, partly understandable as we consider the trauma of hitting rock bottom.[1] On the other hand, Levin drew on psychoanalytic concepts to explain how a predominance of narcissism in the newly abstinent chemically dependent reflects either a regression to a fixation point (perhaps from a childhood trauma), or a common regression observable in the newly abstinent to a narcissism that temporarily predominates.[13]

Wallace argued that, in her inpatient sample of crack cocaine-dependent patients ($n = 245$), sufficient evidence exists that the trauma of addiction and hitting rock bottom—as documented in the loss of infant custody, child custody, housing, spouses, employment, and family support—really added insult to pre-existing injury.[3] In this view, Wallace argued that the temporary regression, as in a regression to a predominance of narcissism, also involves a regression to those fixation points her clients possess from histories of significant childhood trauma sustained within dysfunctional families.[3] Therefore, in the chemically dependent, one can observe a population suffering from the influence of an era of childhood trauma preserved in fixation points, as well as the influence of an era of addiction in a drug culture characterized by the trauma of hitting rock bottom.

A Regression on Seven Lines of Development

Meanwhile, this author also observes in the chemically dependent a regression on each one of seven different lines of development as a consequence of the trauma of addiction. The seven areas negatively impacted by chemical dependency and upon which clients have regressed are as follows and involve:

1. Poor self-care;
2. Poor regulation of impulses;
3. Poor regulation of affects;
4. Poor regulation of self-esteem;
5. Poor regulation of interpersonal behavior;
6. Increased alienation from and decreased integration into family, cultural, and community life; and
7. Decreased spirituality.

To conceptualize seven lines of development and therefore seven lines on which the chemically dependent regress is to expand on the assertion of Khantzian[2] and Khantzian et al.,[14] which states that the chemically dependent poorly self-regulate their affects, impulses, self-esteem, interpersonal behavior, and engage in poor self-care.

The value of considering the resulting seven expanded areas of regression and lines of development, and of ordering them in this particular sequence, involves the implication for treatment of the chemically dependent. The main implication is that treatment programs need to systematically foster the addict's or alcoholic's progressive movement and growth on each of these seven lines or areas of development in order to reduce the risk of relapse and symptom substitution as the period of abstinence lengthens.

Implications of the Seven Lines for Treatment

The concept of poor self-regulation permits one to go beyond any one diagnostic category and to appreciate that the concrete task of remediating psychopathology involves the fulfillment of some concrete therapeutic goals (*see* ref. 15 for further discussion). For example, consider the following prioritizing of treatment program goals and objectives for the chemically dependent:

1. Clients are guided toward adequate self-care ranging from hygiene, job skills training, employment, and maintaining one's own housing;
2. Clients learn to follow program rules of no sexual or aggressive acting out, learning enhanced control of impulses, and internalizing external limits;
3. Clients learn how to identify, label, and process a range of feelings or affects so that enhanced self-regulation of affects results;
4. Clients improve self-esteem regulation by learning how to identify and stop the internal, automatic delivery of negative self-statements (I'm no good, I'm a failure) via the cognitive–behavioral technique of thought-stopping, and to replace them with the delivery of positive self-statements or positive affirmations;
5. Individual and group psychotherapy and counseling permits clients to improve their regulation of interpersonal behavior, opening up opportunities for productive love and work relationships;
6. Clients become less alienated and more integrated into family, cultural, and community life so that the ethnic/racial self-concept is raised;
7. Clients experience an increased spirituality through 12-step program involvement, connection with one's higher power, and a continuing progressive spiritual growth as a relationship develops and expands with one's higher power—however so conceived by the individual.

The Challenge of Remediating Subtle and Well-Hidden Psychopathology

The work of Wurmser helps one to appreciate that the nature of compulsive drug use is such that some of the psychopathology to be found in the chemically dependent involves the existence of well-hidden inhibitions and phobias.[16] Their presence complicates the realization of any individual practitioner's or treatment program's goals and objectives, however prioritized. The much more complex reality is that where a well-hidden inhibition of sexual impulses exists because of molestation, more work must go into the task of improving the regulation of sexual impulses. Similarly, where there is a well-hidden phobia, on the part of the ego, then the client may be terrified of his/her own feelings of anger and aggressive impulses, leading to a difficult constriction of angry affect and inhibition of aggressive impulses. Generalization of a conditioned anxiety or fear response[15] that is conditioned at the moment of trauma can occur in such a way that a client was not only raped by a father she now fears, but also has a well-hidden phobia of men in general, perhaps barring realization of optimal intimacy goals. Thus, some professional psychotherapy or clinical intervention needs to be delivered by one adequately trained to detect and remediate this kind of well-hidden and subtle psychopathology.

Whether preceding the addiction, following from the trauma of the addiction, or, most likely, involving some reality that the two work in tandem, such psychopathology can be effectively therapeutically addressed. Cost-effective models for the remediation of psychopathology in the chemically dependent have been described in the literature.[8,14] One model designed specifically for women and, in light of the kinds of trauma and dysfunctional family dynamics to which women have been exposed, attempts to improve client self-regulation of affects, impulses, self-esteem, and interpersonal behavior, while providing for the working through and integration of trauma.[8] Meanwhile, within Wallace's model of group psychotherapy, key elements of the residential therapeutic community program itself promote enhanced self-care, including the fostering of goals involving receipt of jobs skills, employment, and housing.[8] The residential therapeutic community also fosters considerable progressive growth in the regulation of affects, impulses, and self-esteem through community living and program interventions, and involvement with 12-step groups while in the therapeutic community serves to promote an enhanced spirituality. The area of promoting increased integration into family, cultural, and community life begins with active and constructive involvement with the therapeutic community "family," and extends to include visits from and with family members. As may be true of most treatment programs, yet more can be done by way of training staff in family therapy and counseling to enhance realization of the goal of enhanced integration into family/cultural/community life,[17] along with the raising of an ethnic or racial self-concept.[18]

In this way, one can begin to tackle the difficult task of not only efficaciously treating the chemically dependent, but also designing adequate treatment program structure by considering how one must substantially foster progressive growth and development on seven lines of development in chemically dependent clients. However, in light of some significant, subtle, but well-hidden psychopathology being present in the chemically dependent because of the childhood trauma of some abuse within a dysfunctional family—and perhaps because of the trauma of addiction and hitting rock bottom—the provision of some professional psychotherapy even within cost-effective group modalities may be essential. Whether the cost-effective group psychotherapy model described by Khantzian et al.[14] or that of Wallace,[8] a significant body of literature suggests that the chemically dependent have experienced significant trauma typically within dysfunctional families in childhood, necessitating the adequate working through and resolution of this trauma in order to avoid relapse and symptom substitution.

The Risk of Relapse and Symptom Substitution in Recovery

Some reference has been made in this chapter to both the risk of relapse and symptom substitution; however, yet even more explicit points need to be made in this regard. It has been asserted that not only adult children of alcoholics who are now themselves recovering from alcoholism experience a higher risk of relapse, but also the chemically dependent in general who are from dysfunctional families. Yet, it has also been asserted that there is this chemical dependency and dysfunctional family nexus. It therefore follows that the vast majority of the chemically dependent are from dysfunctional families of one kind or another in which some significant trauma was sustained. It may be said that the majority of the chemically dependent, therefore, possess a high risk of relapse and symptom substitution. Perhaps we sum up the lack of methodologically rigorous, and sufficiently lengthy, outcome evaluation studies focusing on subtle, well-hidden, but significant psychopathology and the possible emergence of compulsive behavioral symptoms (anorexia, bulimia, compulsive overeating, compulsive sexuality, gambling, workaholism, shopaholism, compulsive exercise) as recovery proceeds.

Future quality outcome evaluation research will have to examine the ages, severity, and duration of the experience of trauma—in both childhood and in later eras, including the trauma of addiction itself and hitting rock bottom. And, even in sufficiently rigorous longitudinal studies, only a small percentage of the variance will be accounted for by the severity and duration of trauma if a range of "biopsycho–social" factors are examined. But, in relation to the risk of relapse and symptom substitution, for a subset of more difficult chemically dependent clients there appears to be some critical role that past trauma within dysfunctional families plays in creating psychopathology and therefore a continuing risk of relapse and symptom substitution; as the psychopathology creates the need for yet newer and more elaborate defensive strategies involving new, or re-emergent symptoms.

But, the age, severity, and duration of the experience of trauma are likely to emerge in future research as key variables in explaining any greater risk of relapse. As seen earlier, dysfunctional family experiences are really about the variable of trauma; and trauma is really about some remaining psychopathology that can be manifested in well-hidden and subtle symptoms.

Chemical Dependency as a Symptom
of Underlying Psychopathology

Chemical dependency may, therefore, represent just one symptom of some remaining psychopathology that is the legacy of the experience of trauma within a dysfunctional family. One could define chemical dependency as just one developmental, and often protracted and recurrent, symptom of an individual coping with the legacy of psychopathology remaining from the experience of some significant trauma that likely transpired during childhood development within a dysfunctional family. The addiction potential of the chemical chosen for use, as well as a host of other biological, psychological, and social/environmental/cultural factors also play a role in the manifestation of the symptom of chemical dependency.

If chemical dependency is just one symptom of an underlying psychopathology (in a client in desperate need of remediation of their psychopathology) because of the experience of trauma, then yet other symptoms may manifest when chemicals are not being used. And, as a symptom, chemical dependency may be drawn on yet again in the future as a symptom of convenience if the client's underlying psychopathology has not as yet been remediated. With the receipt of efficacious chemical dependency treatment and the remediation of psychopathology through professional psychotherapy, clients learn and practice alternative coping strategies, and new skills and tools that must be firmly internalized by the client—thereby removing the need to rely once again on a chemical for any defensive or self-regulatory strategy in the face of one's personal psychopathology.

Quite often, when a history of the client's drug use dating back to adolescence or childhood is heard, the initiation of chemical use served as a kind of defense against the chronic states of tension felt within a chaotic and violent household, or as escape from overwhelming, spontaneously emerging dysphoric states of pain and depression. In this way, chemical use seems to begin to serve a kind of defensive function, assisting a youth in self-regulating affects, self-esteem, impulses, or interpersonal behavior. Chemicals are experienced as extra-reinforcing when they assist the user in achieving a kind of self-regulation that the client would be unable to sustain all by themselves without the use of chemicals).[3] As a consequence of the extra-reinforcing nature of chemical use for those receiving the additional benefit of enhanced self-regulation, such individuals are more likely to advance through the stages of chemical use from experimental use, to recreational use, abuse, and dependence.[3]

An analysis of insurance industry data on first hospital admissions for a chemical-use problem by older adolescents and young adults who are still dependents on their parents' insurance policies supports this thesis. This data shows that when comparing the adolescents of alcoholics to those of nonalcoholic parents, those adolescents from alcoholic homes tended to receive a diagnosis of dependence, whereas those without an alcoholic parent tended to receive a diagnosis of abuse on their first admission for some chemical-use problem.[19] For these adolescents and young adults who likely experienced some trauma and moments of overstimulation within their alcoholic dysfunctional families, chemical use likely was experienced as extra-reinforcing, supporting more rapid advancement to a more extreme state of addiction or dependence.

Chemical Use as Replacement of Rigid and Overused Defenses

Data also supports that children of alcoholics suffer higher rates of broken bones, stomach complaints, headaches, as well as other behavioral, psychosomatic, and social problems.[19] Whether reflecting the experience of states of overstimulation as their ego's observed the delivery on some human object within the family of physical blows, displays of force, and the spreading of misinformation or myths—essentially, some violence served to produce chronic moments of overstimulation and trauma. In this way, the critical role of the specificity of this chapter's definition of a dysfunctional family becomes more apparent. To experience inconsistent behavior by parents within a family setting, where one needs care from parental figures, can be quite traumatic for a child needing some reasonable consistency. Many experience the following parental behavioral changes throughout childhood and adolescence: Parents are intoxicated, then sober; depressed, then manic; loving, then violent; sober, then intoxicated again; good judgment and parental supervision prevail, then infantile/primitive cognitive functioning in the parent predominates with either lax or overcontrolling parenting. Something as subtle as parental behavior being inconsistent might be overlooked, but can be seen as creating many moments of overstimulation to which a child's ego might adapt with defensive maneuvers.

Similarly, this chapter's definition of a dysfunctional family highlights the role of attempting to develop within a setting where parental behavior and events can be quite unpredictable, and family life can be quite chaotic—as intoxicated, manic, temporarily psychotic, or depressed parents engaged in domestic violence, incest, sexual abuse, physical abuse, and verbal abuse. Childhoods so tainted with one form or another of violence produce many moments when egos stood in states of overstimulation—

overwhelmed and unable to explain parental sex in the living room, or a bloody stabbing of a parent on a Saturday night, or witnessing a sibling's rape and torture, or experiencing one's own rape and torture, or verbal and physical abuse. During these moments, it can be said that the young egos of children—even as they try to engage in some repression—may fall back on splitting as a defense;[20] thereby suggesting how young, overstimulated, and overwhelmed egos witnessing trauma utilized defensive activity to survive. This involved some successful repression of trauma, or the discovery of the survival-permitting use of the defense of dissociation during the very act of sustaining a trauma of sexual or physical abuse.

In essence, young egos discovered the necessity of the use of some form of regular defensive activity. This resulted in adolescent and young adult egos finding that years of overreliance on defensive functions has produced some rigidity, proneness to compulsive behaviors, or depression, procrastination, inertia, lack of motivation, or fatigue. The very feelings needed for outward, progressive, and increasing social growth outside the immediate family circle may be blocked—as a healthy form of an aggressive drive—because of a longstanding overreliance on a defense against one's inner feelings of anger and the aggressive drive attached to that "well" of anger. Stimulant chemicals might be experienced as extra-reinforcing for this particular kind of symptom, as well as for the classic attendant low self-esteem. Alcohol would serve disinhibition functions, releasing the flow of feelings as well as of sexual and aggressive drives, regardless of the consequences. This means that alcohol would be extra-reinforcing for that experimental user from a dysfunctional family background who uses alcohol in childhood, adolescence, or adulthood, and discovers that it provides tremendous relief from a baseline state of rigid, defensive inhibition of affect and impulses. Also, others have suffered chronic states of tension, rage, or fear because of extreme and chronic trauma, which means that a sedating or calming effect from heroin, marijuana, or alcohol produces a state of relief that is highly extra-reinforcing.

In sum, chemical use can come to replace the rigid, defensive use of various ego maneuvers that serve to keep at bay either the visual image, smell, feeling, or impulse associated with the experience of some past trauma. When chemicals replace a childhood and adolescence full of an overreliance on ego defenses—and that ego is actually in possession of all sorts of well-hidden phobias and inhibitions involving generalization to all sorts of feelings and human objects—then chemicals begin to serve a defensive function. The development of chemical dependency translates into a symptom. This symptom of chemical dependency serves notice for all who may also want to trace the etiology of the addiction that there was once a trauma sustained by a frightened, or angry, or sad, or shocked little girl or boy who saw or experienced unspeakable forms of violence. Even though a significant amount of the variance must certainly be taken up by multiple biological, psychological, and social/environmental/cultural factors, a role is also played by the primary caretakers who may be responsible for inconsistent, unpredictable parenting in settings where abuse was unleashed during chaotic and violent episodes. If this is sufficiently identified as a probable etiological factor, then prevention, early intervention, and treatment strategies may emerge, justifying a focus on how the chemical dependency and dysfunctional family nexus operates.

The Many Layers
of the Chemical Dependency Onion

As each clinician and counselor approaches the female chemically dependent client, and if they continue to work with that client long enough and come to know something of their inner experience, well-hidden inhibitions and phobias, and past history of personal trauma, they will soon discover that there are many layers to this complex woman. Metaphorically, it is discovered that those clients who seem to be just in one stage or another of recovery are actually in the process of peeling away the chemical dependency layer of a metaphoric onion—providing proof that it was just one layer of symptom that may readily give way to another layer of symptom; or reveal that ego that quickly resorts to a rigid, defensive style of some sort, or to the performance of some compulsive behavior.

To no one's surprise, one can now talk about the way in which the recovering chemically dependent client may, anywhere from 1, to 3, to 6, to 9 mo in recovery, reveal yet another symptom. Typically, in women this symptom may be some degree of anorexia, bulimia, compulsive overeating, compulsive sexual acting out, or gambling. Meanwhile, those who consider themselves more "normal" may find few differences between a more commonly accepted and reinforced workaholism or shopaholism, which may also emerge in their clients. A classic observation is how chemical dependency is typically followed in recovery by workaholism. To learn how to play and relax without chemicals, perhaps a luxury not afforded to one's childhood, becomes a critical goal, which is far from the typically rigid ego functioning and reliance on defenses that characterizes early phases of recovery.

How does the ego go about the process of instituting a defense, or a defensive maneuver, that is elaborate enough to replace the ritual of chemical dependency that has been surrendered? An important principle that begins to explain this process involves the classic Freudian thinking that the ego receives the signal of anxiety. Think of it this way: When the ego receives the signal of anxiety, it indicates that something is about to emerge into conscious awareness, or something defended against threatens to emerge anew. This could be a feeling, an impulse, an image, a memory that is about to emerge. At this time, the ego either executes the use of a defense, or in the active chemically dependent the ego seeks out the use of some chemical, or in the recovering and abstinent client this signal to the ego leads the ego into the performance of some, literally any, compulsive behavior. This compulsive behavior can be something as immediately distracting as nail biting, nail cleaning, or something as elaborate as compulsive sexuality, compulsive overeating, anorexia, bulimia, or compulsively cleaning one's apartment. This new compulsive behavior represents a new symptom replacing the former symptom of chemical dependency. Just as it has been suggested that adolescent or adult chemical use can replace, in a defensive capacity, the former defenses utilized since childhood, the performance of any compulsive behavior—even compulsive nail cleaning—can serve to replace the former defensive dependence on chemicals as a symptom.

Matching Clients to Interventions
for Remediation of Psychopathology

Thus, women in recovery must receive treatment from clinicians who understand the chemical dependency and dysfunctional family nexus, and who appreciate that the key treatment task is to not only promote progressive growth on all seven lines of development mentioned earlier, but also involves a very specific task for the professional psychotherapist or counselor aspiring to be most efficacious. This very specific task is to be the kind of empathic, perceptive, consistent, and keenly observant therapist who can: engage in the kind of psychoeducation and use of cognitive–behavioral techniques that strengthens the ego; and permit that strengthened ego to undergo a regression with the therapist's own keenly observant and supportive ego, so that a regression to the level of trauma occurs and sufficient working through and integration of trauma transpires (see ref. 15 for further discussion). The remediation of psychopathology does involve the use of a multifaceted clinical technique, combining the use of psychoeducation, metaphor as a major psychoeducational tool and integrative clinical technique, as well as the use of cognitive–behavioral, and psychoanalytic/psychodynamic interventions.[3] In any event, it becomes absolutely essential that shorter-term forms of cost-effective group psychotherapy (3, 6, 9 mo) be implemented and evaluated),[8] as the remediation of psychopathology and working through and integration of trauma seem to be key elements of effective relapse prevention.

In sum, this discussion of the chemical dependency nexus, as it most intimately impacts a large percentage of female clients, forms an appreciation of how the experience of early trauma within dysfunctional families calls on young egos to become early and prematurely overreliant on defenses; also, the overreliance on defenses may result in the manifestation of many childhood psychosomatic complaints and symptoms of psychopathology resulting from their trauma and captured in the very state of overreliance on defensive strategies. As a consequence of this overreliance on defensive strategies and psychopathology, the child or adolescent possesses poor self-regulation of affects, impulses, self-esteem, and interpersonal behavior, which leaves them vulnerable to experience chemicals as extra-reinforcing—if any experimental use of chemicals seemingly just happens to occur with one's peer group. Chemicals experienced as extra-reinforcing permit advancement through stages of chemical use so that the more severe state of addiction or dependence is reached. Chemicals so used because they enhance the individual's capacity for self-regulation—a capacity that is deficient because of past childhood trauma within a dysfunctional family, a resulting overreliance on defenses, and the existence of subtle, well-hidden psychopathology—are not only extra-reinforcing, but lead to the development of dependence on the chemical coming to serve a defensive purpose.

In this way, relapse can, in some instances, represent the failure of treatment programs and recovering persons to remediate subtle and well-hidden psychopathology. When treatment programs do not provide chemically dependent women with special treatment components for adequate trauma resolution and remediation of their psychopathology, then as they enter into recovery clinicians and counselors will be able to observe both relapse and symptom substitution as women become anorexic and bulimic, and sexually act out, for example. Without adequate professional psychotherapy, female clients are left to negotiate early phases of recovery with only rigid egos that demonstrate once again in early sobriety their historical overreliance on defensive strategies. Eventually, that client may come upon a sufficiently difficult situation or really hard test in reality, outside the therapeutic milieu, which calls for an adequate level of self-regulation.

If treatment has not promoted a chemically dependent client's systematic and progressive growth on the seven lines of development identified earlier in this chapter, then the most critical self-regulation of affects, impulses, self-esteem, and interpersonal behavior remains typically poor and inadequate for the hardest tests in recovery occurring within the first 3–6 mo of abstinence. Hence, in the face of interpersonal stress, extreme emotional upset, and the mobilization of powerful aggressive drives, clients may readily relapse.[3,21]

Perhaps it is difficult to fully realize the magnitude of the loss that clients experience as they surrender their chemical dependency and have reason to grieve the loss of their addiction.[22] It is as though, upon detoxification, clients have merely experienced the removal of an elaborate defensive structure that served as some relief from a historical, prechemical use, baseline personality functioning, which is rooted in childhood and adolescent personality development, that had as its hallmark an overreliance on ego defenses. Left without chemical self-regulation, clients not only negotiate a new daily life without chemicals, but fall back on rigid ego defenses, which have not even been recently utilized. Ego functioning is therefore even more rigid and defenses of denial and temporary narcissistic inflation are barely adequate for purposes of sufficient defense against a range of affects and impulses arising and being felt without the defense of chemical intoxication for the first time in months and years.

Therefore, if clinicians and counselors move beyond their own denial and narcissism, they may permit themselves to see that there are going to be many moments for their clients when the return of the repressed, split-off, and otherwise defended-against impulse, affect, image, or memory of trauma creates considerable pain and suffering in their clients. Through adequate training, clinicians and counselors must aspire to be able to strengthen their clients egos as rapidly as possible, improve self-regulation as expeditiously as possible, and increase their client's capacity to begin to pass the hard tests in reality, calling for some basic ability to especially self-regulate one's affects, impulses, self-esteem, and interpersonal behavior. When relapse occurs, clinicians and counselors must bring this understanding and some empathy to the task of engaging in a microanalysis of a relapse episode,[3] so that they can identify new, idiosyncratic triggers or determinants of relapse and plan for more effective relapse prevention. Frequently, this relapse prevention-calls for matching clients to more intensive and comprehensive treatment;[3] and as emphasized throughout this chapter, at the very least this involves matching women clients to a cost-effective professional group psychotherapy modality that is designed to strengthen client's egos rather quickly, facilitate the surrender of an overreliance on ego defenses, remediate psychopathology, improve self-regulation, and resolve and work through trauma.[8]

And, clinicians and counselors must not permit their own denial and narcissism from preventing them from recommending that clients with lives exemplifying the chemical dependency and dysfunctional family nexus— with all its complex of intertwined factors involving trauma, psychopathology, and symptom manifestation—be matched, ideally within programs, to professional psychotherapy provided by adequately trained clinicians and counselors who can detect and remediate subtle, well-hidden psychopathology. Only if such referrals are made and we embrace the absolute necessity of this kind of client-to-intervention matching strategy do female chemically dependent clients have a chance of avoiding relapse and symptom substitution with other destructive and compulsive behaviors.

Final Comments on Other Key Male/Female Differences

Although many different dimensions of the chemical dependency and dysfunctional family nexus have been explored, yet one remaining issue that highlights other key male/female differences involves women's characteristic experience of yet other eras of trauma. Typically, survivors of trauma within dysfunctional families have an uncanny ability to select partners with whom they can reenact classic behavioral dramas, such as those that transpired within their own homes as children. In this way, women who witnessed or experienced parental alcoholism, domestic violence, or their own childhood physical abuse may very well have ended up with a man, lover, or partner with whom violence was unleashed in their adult relationship. The nature of interpersonal behavioral dramas, which reflect the basic role behavior unconsciously internalized during moments of trauma, assist[15] treatment professionals in understanding how so many women report a second era of trauma. This second era of trauma involved late adolescent and adult battering by partners, lovers, and spouses during domestic violence, which may have repeated in certain basic elements the woman's childhood physical abuse.

Unfortunately, yet a third era of trauma is tied into experiences within the drug culture, and the crack cocaine culture in particular, wherein women may have engaged in the exchange of sex for drugs or outright prostitution in order to support high-dose and high-frequency drug habits. Typically this kind of behavioral pattern translates into late night and early morning walks in the street so that rapes, beatings by "Johns," and exposure to crack culture violence easily occurs. Women who inhabit this violent and sexually explicit crack culture are much more vulnerable than men to rapes and violent beatings; women have found themselves forced into prostitution, exhibitionistic group sex, and drug dealing by the very husbands, boyfriends, and lovers that they had once trusted.

HIV/AIDS and Death and Dying Issues Among Women

Because of this explicit sexual behavior within the crack and drug culture, many of these women have engaged in promiscuous, unprotected sex with multiple partners. Moreover, those who have been tested know they are HIV positive, know their T-cell count, and know about good self-care to prevent AIDS. Others actually live with AIDS. Unfortunately, the majority are in a state of denial and have not been tested, perhaps feeling that, with just 3 or 5 mo in recovery, they are still not emotionally strong enough to handle any bad news without raising the risk of an immediate relapse. And, among those in a state of fear, hesitancy, or denial many do still engage in unprotected sex on occasion. Clinicians and counselors must educate themselves and prepare to be active health educators who can ever so gently break through walls of denial with facts and basic health education on HIV/AIDS and human sexuality.

In addition to walls of denial, however, clients often have much more intimate knowledge of the reality of HIV/AIDS than perhaps treatment professionals do, since they have already nursed AIDS-stricken lovers and loved ones unto that death they fear for themselves. Whether or not grieving was felt to be part of chemical-dependency treatment, the task before clinicians and counselors is to permit female clients to undergo a grieving process within the safe confines of therapeutic milieus—especially long-term residential therapeutic communities. Clinicians and counselors have to face the task of being with clients in an empathic, supportive, and real manner as they allow them to talk about issues of death and dying, and go through a period of bereavement counseling over past lovers and loved ones lost to AIDS or violence.

Toward Culturally Sensitive Counseling and Family Outreach

Another issue involves the extent to which professionals may need to receive continuing education training in crosscultural counseling and the use of a culturally sensitive empathy,[15] which permits them to work effectively across ethnic, class, and racial lines despite any differences. This training may overlap with growing efforts to recognize that it is unwise to work with a female chemically dependent client all alone, and merely advise her to discontinue relationships with former drug dealing and violent partners and spouses who are still the father of one or more of their children.[23] Dropout rates and poor program retention speaks to the difficulty of this approach and how it fails to appreciate a basic reality: One cannot merely recommend and facilitate the dissolution of the family—especially African-American, Latino, and other poor and already besieged minority family structures.

A greater cultural sensitivity is desperately needed and might show that treatment professionals can be found guilty of having possessed and projected a societal stereotype that all Black or minority men of color are criminal; within this view, clinicians and counselors do their very best in freeing chemically dependent women from their men's drug dealing and violent clutches. But, at this very moment, the clinicians and counselors fail in providing adequate services for that female client; for, her engagement in basic reasoning may make her distrust and reject the treatment program: What does it say about the potential the treatment program staff holds, envisions, and projects on her as a Black woman, or on her Black infant son, or on her 10-yr-old male child, if some subtle organizational dynamic explicitly conveys negative feelings and negative assumptions held about Black men?"

At the very least, mandatory training in crosscultural counseling and in the psychology of differences should be set in place. This may permit all treatment professionals to learn how to avoid the projection of negative and low expectations and stereotypes on people of color, or those who are different from themselves, while freeing treatment professionals to retract any projections put forth, in the past, on others. It also frees treatment professionals to see each other as human beings capable of reaching their own potential. If adequate family outreach components can be structured, then treatment professionals can learn and demonstrate effective ways to reach out to women's partners, how to engage them in chemical dependency treatment, and foster their acquisition of jobs skills training and placement, and constructive employment. All, while working toward the goal of family reunification, as clinicians and counselors trained in family counseling[17] foster the communication of partners and the strengthening of family systems.

Fewer women will eventually succumb to relapse if it is recognized from the outset that her partner possesses the same potential for recovery, employment, and independent living as does she, and that unless treatment professionals assist him in recovery and healing, along with his loved ones and family, then women may relapse when that intoxicated man merely arrives for a childcare visit. Without preparation or planning, recovering chemically dependent women may—despite recommendations to cut all ties with this former drug partner and drug dealer—immediately relapse, to the treatment professional's apparent dismay. Perhaps this brief discussion on this sensitive issue removes the option of reacting with dismay when such women do relapse, since the mandate for crosscultural counseling training and ending any collusion in projecting low, negative, and criminal expectations on male partners of color has been offered.

Conclusion

This chapter has examined drugs, alcohol, and the dysfunctional family, paying close attention to male/female differences, while aspiring to prepare clinicians and counselors for challenging work with the large chemically dependent female population. The author has emphasized a chemical dependency-dysfunctional family nexus in which close intertwining issues involve the legacy of some trauma sustained within a dysfunctional family in childhood, the emergence of defensive strategies and psychopathology as a consequence of trauma, and chemical dependency, as well as other compulsive behaviors representing symptoms of a subtle and well-hidden psychopathology. Specifically, this chapter has presented and discussed evidence that the chemically dependent are adult children of dysfunctional families and survivors of several eras of trauma that creates significant psychopathology, which must be remediated as a form of relapse prevention. In addition, we have briefly considered the implications of HIV/AIDS and death, dying, and bereavement counseling emerging as components of chemical dependency treatment. This chapter has also offered some general recommendations for ways in which treatment programs must become more sensitized to the task of recovery when the client is a woman, a mother, and has children by a man who was her drug partner and drug dealer.

What emerges from this chapter's discussion is the reality that treatment of chemically dependent women requires clinicians and counselors to develop several areas of expertise, and to permit themselves by necessity to go beyond a previous identity, as one with an expertise in chemical dependency. Adequate relapse prevention for clients only begins when clinicians and counselors emerge with an expertise in dysfunctional families and how they impact development, as well as expertise in trauma resolution. Moreover, they must also become active educators, with a particular expertise in health education on HIV/AIDS and even on some related aspects of human sexuality. And not to be forgotten is the challenge of acquiring even more expertise in working with those resolving issues of death, dying, and the need to undergo a period of bereavement for one's own health, or a husband, lover, or loved one who has died from AIDS or violence.

A major limitation of this chapter is that research data has yet to document adequately the extent to which trauma in dysfunctional families plays a etiological role in the development and maintenance of chemical dependency, nor the efficacy of the recommended cost-effective group modalities with this population. However, key variables involving the age, duration, and severity of trauma have been identified as worthy of investigation in future longitudinal research. Also, psychological variables are likely to account for only a small percentage of the variance in investigations examining a host of biopsycho-social/environmental/cultural variables.

In light of the large population of chemically dependent women in need of treatment—as are their spouses, children, and families—clinicians and counselors need to expand their understanding of the issues these women bring with them into treatment. Toward this end, and in anticipation that the reader will seek out additional sources of training in line with this author's recommendations, this chapter has aspired to improve clinicians' and counselors' preparation for a complex treatment challenge.

References

[1]M. Bean-Bayog (1986) Psychopathology produced by alcoholism, in *Psychopathology and Addictive Disorders*, R. E. Meyers, ed., Guilford, New York.

[2]E. J. Khantzian (1985) On the psychological predisposition for opiate and stimulant dependence. *Psychiatry Lett.* **3**, 1.

[3]B. C. Wallace (1991) *Crack Cocaine: A Practical Treatment Approach for the Chemically Dependent*. Brunner/Mazel, New York.

[4]F. Schiffer (1988) Psychotherapy of nine successfully treated cocaine abusers: Techniques and dynamics. *J. Subst. Abuse Treatment* **5**, 131–137.

[5]E. B. Young (1990) The role of incest issues in relapse. *J. Psychoactive Drugs* **22**, 249–258.

[6]B. Walker (1988) Odyssey House Inc. of New York. *J. Subst. Abuse Treatment* **5**, 113–115.

[7]D. J. Rohsenow, R. Corbett, and D. Devine (1988) Molested as children: A hidden contribution to substance abuse? *J. Subst. Abuse Treatment* **5**, 13–18.

[8]B. C. Wallace (1992 The therapeutic community as a treatment modality and the role of the professional consultant: spotlight on Damon house, in *The Chemically Dependent: Phases of Treatment and Recovery,* B. C. Wallace, ed., Brunner/Mazel, New York.

[9]M. Fullilove (1991) Personal communication. New York.

[10]B. Wanck (1985) Treatment of adult children of alcoholics. *Carrier Found. Lett.* **109,** 6.

[11]K. Bollerud (1990) A model for the treatment of trauma-related syndromes among chemically dependent inpatient women. *J. Subst. Abuse Treatment* **7**, 83–87.

[12]R. E. Meyer (ed.) (1986) *Psychopathology and Addictive Disorders*. Guilford, New York.

[13]J. D. Levin (1987) *Treatment of Alcoholism and Other Addictions: A Self-Psychology Approach*. Aronson, Norwood, NJ.

[14]E. J. Khantzian, K. S. Halliday, and W. E. McAuliffe (1990) *Addiction and the Vulnerable Self: Modified Dynamic Group Therapy for Substance Abusers*. Guilford, New York.

[15]B. C. Wallace (in progress). *Adult Children of Dysfunctional Families: Prevention, Intervention, and Treatment For Mental Health Promotion*, Praeger, New York.

[16]L. Wurmser (1992) Psychology of compulsive drug use, in *The Chemically Dependent: Phases of Treatment and Recovery,* B. C. Wallace, ed., Brunner/Mazel, New York.

[17]A. A. Weidman (1992) Family therapy and the TC: The chemically dependent adolescent, in *The Chemically Dependent: Phases of Treatment and Recovery,* B. C. Wallace, ed., Brunner/Mazel, New York.

[18]R. Harris-Offutt (1992) Cultural factors in the assessment and treatment of African-American addicts: Africentric considerations, in *The Chemically Dependent: Phases of Treatment and Recovery,* B. C. Wallace, ed., Brunner/Mazel, New York.

[19]Children of Alcoholics Foundation (1990) *A Report Analyzing Insurance Industry Data Comparing Children of Alcoholics To Children of Non-Alcoholic Parents.* Children of Alcoholics Foundation, New York.

[20]O. Kernberg (1976) *Object Relations Theory and Clinical Psychoanalysis,* Aronson, New York.

[21]B. C. Wallace (1989) Psychological and environmental determinants of relapse in crack cocaine smokers. *J. Subst. Abuse Treatment* **6,** 95–106.

[22]D. Rothschild (1992) Treating the substance abuser: Psychotherapy throughout the recovery process, in *The Chemically Dependent: Phases of Treatment and Recovery,* B. C. Wallace, ed., Brunner/Mazel, New York.

[23]H. D. Weiner, M. C. Wallen, G. L. Zankowski (1990) Culture and social class as intervening variables in relapse prevention with chemically dependent women. *J. Psychoactive Drugs* **22,** 239–248.

Alcohol's Role in Sexual Assault

Antonia Abbey, Lisa Thomson Ross, and Donna McDuffie

Introduction

A young woman who participated in one of our studies told of how she agreed to go back to her date's house after a party, "We played quarter bounce (a drinking game). I got sick drunk; I was slumped over a toilet vomiting. He grabbed me and dragged me into his room and raped me. I had been a virgin and felt it was all my fault for going back to his house when no one else was home." Another woman wrote, "He planned it. I believe he slipped something into my drink. I only had one drink but I was severely intoxicated. He started to rape me. I was scared, I froze, I cried, I begged him to stop."

The role of alcohol in sexual assault has also been described to us by male study participants. One man wrote, "Under alcohol, a few times I've noticed I've become more persistent and perhaps more annoying in approaching women. I'm more aggressive in my attitude." Another young man who forced sex on a female friend felt that, "Alcohol loosened us up and the situation occurred by accident. If no alcohol was consumed, I would never have crossed that line."

Alcohol and other drug use have been consistently linked to sexual assault. There are two main purposes of this chapter. The first is to review the empirical data that documents the relationship between sexual assault and substance use. The second is to provide some explanations for this rela-

From: *Drug and Alcohol Abuse Reviews, Vol. 5: Addictive Behaviors in Women*
Ed.: R. R. Watson ©1994 Humana Press Inc., Totowa, NJ

nship. Before reviewing the literature, some terms need to be defined in order to clarify the focus and limits of this chapter.

Definitions and Terminology

One difficulty associated with doing research in the area of sexual assault concerns the varying definitions and labels used by the legal system, researchers, laypeople, and individuals who have experienced or perpetrated sexual assault. Definitions "set the parameters of research and influence the results and conclusions" (p. 23),[1] so it is necessary to describe the way various terms will be used before a substantive discussion of the issues is presented.

The Federal Bureau of Investigation (FBI) defines rape as "carnal knowledge of a female forcibly and against her will."[2] This definition assumes that men cannot be raped, and it limits behavior to penile-vaginal intercourse. A broader federal rape law, which applies to acts committed on government property, defines rape as "nonconsensual penetration of an adolescent or adult obtained by physical force, by threat of bodily harm, or where the victim is incapable of giving consent by virtue of mental illness, mental retardation, or intoxication" (p. 62).[3] Here sexual penetration is defined as any intrusion, however slight, of any person's body, as well as oral-genital sexual contact.

Most rapes in the United States are prosecuted at the state level, rather than the federal level, and each state has its own criminal code. There is a great deal of variation across the states in the types of acts that constitute rape or sexual assault. For example, in Alabama, rape is limited to vaginal penetration. In contrast, there are four degrees of criminal sexual assault according to Michigan law, depending on the age, mental, and physical status of the victim; the relationship between the victim and offender; the degree of sexual contact; the absence or presence of a weapon; and whether the offense was committed in conjunction with a felony.[4] Whether or not spousal rape is a punishable offense also varies across the states. As of 1990, in seven states marital rape was not considered a crime unless the couple was legally separated or had filed for a divorce.[5]

For the purposes of this chapter, sexual assault is thought of as a continuum that includes all levels of nonconsensual sexual contact. The term sexual assault will be used to describe the full range of forced sexual acts including forced touching or kissing as well as vaginal, oral, and anal penetration. Following standard convention, the term rape will be reserved for sexual behaviors that involve some type of penetration by force or threat of force, a lack of consent, or inability to give consent due to age, intoxication, or mental status.[1]

Throughout this chapter the assumption will be made that men are the perpetrators of sexual assault and women are the victims of these experiences. Although this is true for the vast majority of instances, men are sometimes the victims of sexual assault. The Bureau of Justice estimated that <10% of rape victims are male.[6] Other authors have found that about 5–10% of the rape victims treated at rape crisis clinics are male (*see* ref. 7 for a review of this literature). Men are even more reluctant than women to report being a victim of sexual assault, so it is difficult to determine the accuracy of these statistics. Men are almost always raped by another man.[8] Both heterosexual and homosexual men have been victims of male assailants.[9]

This chapter will focus primarily on adolescent and adult experiences. Although incest and child molestation are disturbing and serious social problems, they are better explained by different psychosocial models of behavior.[10,11]

The Incidence and Prevalence of Sexual Assault

Estimates of the incidence and prevalence of sexual assault vary dramatically. This is partially because different sources use different definitions, and partially because of victims' reluctance to report rape to the police. Several estimates will be provided in this section of the chapter to give the reader a sense of the scope of sexual assault.

Estimates Based on Criminal Justice Data

The FBI provides an annual estimate of the number of rapes committed in the United States, using the definition described in the last section. In 1990, 102,555 rapes were reported by the FBI.[2] This represents a victimization rate of .8/1000 women. The FBI acknowledges that the vast majority of rapes are not reported to legal authorities and that this is a significant underestimate of the severity of the problem. The FBI estimated in 1990 that one rape is committed every 5 min in the United States. The Bureau of Justice Statistics (BJS) conducts the National Crime Survey (NCS). Although this survey includes rapes not reported to the police and includes male victims, the question-phrasing and context of the interview encourages underreporting.[3] Using the 1989 NCS data, 1.2 women/1000 were victims of rape and .1 men/1000 were victims of rape.[6]

Estimates Based on General Surveys

Several nongovernmental researchers have also conducted studies designed to estimate the incidence and prevalence of sexual assault. Russell conducted a survey of 930 randomly selected women in San Francisco.[12]

During the year prior to the interview, 25 women experienced a rape that met the FBI definition; this is an incidence rate of 26.88/1000 women. Twenty-four percent of these women had experienced rape at some point in their life; this is a prevalence rate of 239.77/1000 women. Fifteen percent of the women who had ever been married reported being physically forced to have intercourse with their husband.

Kilpatrick et al. interviewed 2004 randomly selected women in Charleston, South Carolina.[13] Sexual assault had been experienced by 14.5% of these women at least once in their lives; 9% had been the victims of rape using the FBI definition. There was an annual incidence rate of rape of 7.2/1000 women.

Estimates Based on College Surveys

Many researchers have examined the prevalence of sexual assault among college students. Sexual assault is most common in late adolescence and early adulthood,[2,6] so college students are at high risk. It is estimated that 15–30% of college women have experienced rape, usually perpetrated by a fellow student. The first research on this topic was conducted by Kanin and his colleagues in the 1950s. Kirkpatrick and Kanin surveyed 291 college women from 22 different university classes.[14] Twenty-eight percent of these women had experienced rape or attempted rape on a date during the academic year.

Koss et al. surveyed 3187 women students from 32 colleges across the country selected to represent the higher education enrollment in the United States.[15] Since the age of 14, 27.5% of the women had experienced an act that met the legal definition of rape (including attempted rapes). Seventeen percent had experienced rape or attempted rape in the previous year. This is an annual incidence rate of 166 rapes/1000 college women. Only 27% of the women who experienced an act that met the legal definition of rape labeled what occurred as rape and only 42% had told anyone about it. Because many women do not acknowledge the severity of what has happened to themselves or others, Koss and her colleagues have called acquaintance rape a "hidden crime."[15]

Not all college women who experience sexual assault are raped (using the standard legal definitions described earlier). In the Koss et al. sample, 53.4% of the women had experienced some form of forced sex.[15] The most serious level of sexual assault experienced by 14.4% of the women was forced sexual contact (kissing, petting, and other sex acts that do not involve penetration). Another 11.9% experienced sexual coercion (verbal pressure to engage in sexual intercourse), whereas the remaining women experienced physically forced attempted (12.1%) or completed (15.4%) acts of penetration.

College men acknowledge committing acts that meet the legal definition of rape, although at lower rates than these acts are reported by women. Depending on the study and the definitions used, 7–26% of college men have indicated that they perpetrated acquaintance rape. Kanin obtained a random sample of 381 college men from one university.[16] He reported that 26% of these men acknowledged forcing sexual intercourse on a date since entering college. Rapaport and Burkhart collected data from 190 college men from undergraduate psychology classes.[17] Fifteen percent of these men reported forcing intercourse on a woman at least once. Koss et al. found that 7.7% of the 2972 college men whom they surveyed reported committing an act that met the legal definition of rape.[15] Abbey and Thomson found that 10% of the 814 male undergraduates in their survey had perpetrated completed or attempted rape.[18]

Alcohol and Sexual Assault

Alcohol use by the perpetrator, the victim, or both is frequently associated with sexual assault. As is the case for statistics on the prevalence of sexual assault, each investigator finds somewhat different percentages. On average, however, at least 50% of rapes are found to be associated with alcohol use.[19,20] These findings are reviewed in this section of the chapter. It is important to keep in mind that the co-occurrence of sexual assault and alcohol use does not establish the causal connection between these variables. Cognitive impairments associated with alcohol consumption might make sexual assault more likely, or alcohol might be used as a post hoc justification for sexual assault, or their co-occurrence may be explained by other variables, such as an impulsive personality style. Possible explanations for the relationship between sexual assault and alcohol use are described in later sections of the chapter.

Criminal Justice Data

Some authors have collected data from incarcerated rapists. The majority of rapists are not imprisoned, so the generalizability of results from these studies to all sexual assaults is unclear. An advantage to these studies is that incarcerated rapists may be more honest about some topics because fear of prosecution is not typically an issue of concern for them. Rada collected data from 77 imprisoned rapists in California.[20] Fifty percent of these men had been drinking alcohol at the time of the rape and

35% were alcoholics. Scully described interviews conducted with 80 incarcerated rapists.[21] About three-quarters of them consumed alcohol or other drugs prior to the rape.

Vinogradov et al. studied 63 incarcerated adolescent rapists in California.[22] Seventy-two percent of these young men reported being under the influence of alcohol or another drug at the time of the rape; 15% had taken a drug <15 min prior to the rape. Alcohol and marijuana were the most frequently mentioned substances. Only 12% of the victims had used alcohol or marijuana prior to the rape.

Several authors have examined police records to estimate the association of alcohol consumption and rape. Amir reviewed all forcible rape cases in the Philadelphia police department records for 1958 and 1960.[23] He found that in 24% of these 646 cases, alcohol had been used by the perpetrator; in 31% of these cases, alcohol had been used by the victim. Rapes that involved alcohol were associated with sexual humiliation.

Johnson et al. examined the police records on rapes reported in Winnipeg, Canada from 1966 through 1975.[24] Alcohol was involved in 72.4% of the rapes. In 24.4% of the incidents only the assailant was drinking, in 9.2% only the victim was drinking, and in the remainder, both of them were drinking alcohol. Rapes in which the victim was physically injured were more likely to involve alcohol than those in which she was not physically injured.

Maldonado et al. examined 150 cases of sexual assault in Spain.[25] Forty-eight percent of the offenders had consumed alcohol; in 13% of these cases they also consumed an illicit drug. Twelve percent of the victims had consumed alcohol. Rapes that involved multiple perpetrators and those that caused injury to the victim were more likely to involve alcohol or other drug use than those that involved single perpetrators and no injuries.

Goodyear-Smith examined the information obtained as part of the medical examination of 81 adult women who were raped in New Zealand.[26] Approximately one-third of these women were under the influence of alcohol at the time of the assault. Information on perpetrators' alcohol consumption was not collected.

Survey Data

Koss, in her national representative sample of college students, found that 74% of the perpetrators and 55% of the victims had been drinking alcohol prior to the incident.[19] Furthermore, alcohol consumption was associated with the severity of the sexual assault. When alcohol was involved, acts that met the legal definition of rape were more likely to occur. In further analyses of this dataset, Koss and Dinero found that alcohol use at the time of the attack was one of the four strongest predictors of the likelihood of college women being raped.[27]

Muelenhard and Linton found that 55% of the college men in their sample who acknowledged committing forced sex were under the influence of alcohol or other drugs at the time of the assault.[28] In a parallel manner, 53% of the women in the Muelenhard and Linton study, who reported that they had been sexually assaulted on a date, also reported being under the influence of alcohol or drugs at the time of the incident.[28] Furthermore, dates in which sexual assault occurred were more likely to involve "heavy" alcohol or other drug use than these students' typical dates.

Abbey and Thomson surveyed 1160 college women and 814 college men from 94 different classes at an urban public university.[18] They found that 30% of the men who reported physically forcing a woman to engage in sexual intercourse had been drinking alcohol at the time of the incident. In this same study, 29% of the women forced by a man to engage in sexual intercourse reported drinking alcohol prior to the assault.

Russell interviewed women who had experienced marital rape.[12] About 25% of the perpetrators had consumed alcohol prior to the rape. In several instances, the rape occurred when the woman was too drunk to give consent.

Substance Abuse Treatment Data

Wilsnack reviewed several studies that collected data on the sexual assault history of women receiving treatment for alcohol abuse.[29] Across these studies, 30–75% of the female alcoholics interviewed had a history of incest and/or adult sexual assault. For example, Hammond et al. (1979; reviewed in ref. 29) interviewed 44 female alcoholic outpatients. Forty percent of these women reported a history of incest, and 39% reported being raped. Covington (1982; reviewed in ref. 29) compared the experiences of 35 alcoholic women in the early stages of sobriety and 35 nonalcoholic controls. Seventy-four percent of the alcoholic women had a history of incest or sexual assault as compared to 50% of the controls.

Two studies looked at the co-occurrence of substance abuse and sexual assault in settings other than substance abuse treatment clinics. Swett et al. surveyed 189 female psychiatric outpatients.[30] They found that patients with a history of sexual assault had higher scores on the Michigan Alcoholism Screening Test than did patients without a sexual assault history.

Kilpatrick completed telephone interviews with a random sample of 4009 adult women.[31] Twenty-three percent of these women had been victims of sexual assault at some point in their lives. Sexual assault victims (and victims of other types of crimes) were more likely to have a substance abuse disorder than were noncrime victims.

Although most studies that have examined the relationship between substance use and sexual assault have focused on alcohol use, reports of marijuana and cocaine use prior to sexual assault have also been made.[15,22,25,28] Goldstein et al. conducted qualitative interviews with drug users in Manhattan.[32] Women who used large quantities of cocaine were more likely to be the victims of sexual assault than were nonusers and light users of cocaine. Because of the paucity of empirical literature on the role of illicit drug use in sexual assault, this chapter will focus on alcohol consumption.

Psychosocial Explanations of the Relationship Between Alcohol Consumption and Sexual Assault

Past research consistently documents the relationship between alcohol use and sexual assault, however, it does not provide a theoretical framework for describing why this relationship exists. In this section of the chapter, some psychosocial explanations will be presented to help explain the co-occurrence of alcohol use and sexual assault. First, several caveats must be made about the scope of the model. The focus of this theoretical model is on how preexisting gender differences in beliefs about sexuality, dating, and alcohol interact with aspects of the immediate situation to increase the likelihood that sexual assault will occur among acquaintances. It is not our goal to thoroughly review all known correlates or predictors of sexual assault. Excellent reviews of early family influences, perpetrator and victim personality characteristics, peer group influences, and exposure to sexually violent media depictions of heterosexual relations are available for the interested reader.[15,21,33–38]

At many places in this chapter, factors are described that put women "at risk" or make them "vulnerable" to sexual assault. The identification of factors that put women at risk for being victimized is not intended to imply that women should be blamed or held responsible for being sexually assaulted (for a discussion of the different meanings of the terms *risk factors*, *blame*, and *responsibility*, *see* refs. 39 and 40). Perpetrators of sexual assault are responsible for their own behavior, as are perpetrators of other crimes. However, just as we can describe actions that potential robbery or mugging victims can take to reduce the likelihood of becoming a victim, without implying that they are responsible if a theft occurs (e.g., carry your purse close to your body, do not display your money in public), we can also describe actions that potential victims of sexual assault can take to minimize the likelihood of sexual assault occurring. By providing information about ways to reduce the likelihood of being sexually assaulted, women are provided a sense of personal control and empowerment, rather than powerlessness.[41]

Predisposing Belief Systems

Women and men bring a variety of different beliefs to their interactions with one another. Figure 1 displays the theoretical model that is described in this section of the chapter. As can be seen in Fig. 1, men's and women's beliefs about gender roles, alcohol's effects on behavior, and stereotypes about women who drink alcohol can increase the likelihood that an interaction between a woman and a man will end with sexual assault. The role of each of these predisposing beliefs is described in the following section.

Gender Role Norms
About Dating and Sexual Behavior

Several explanations for sexual assault focus on American society's gender role norms. These arguments are reviewed here, and then alcohol's role in this process is described. Gender role norms provide implicit and explicit rules about how males and females in a particular society or culture should act. Boys and girls grow up learning what is expected from them by virtue of their gender. Little boys are encouraged to be competitive, to win, to feel comfortable exerting power, to be task-oriented, and to avoid crying or other emotional displays of "weakness."[42,43] Little girls are encouraged to play nice, be nice, to take care of others, to make people happy, and to avoid conflict or "making waves."[42,43]

Within the dating and sexual arena, adolescent girls are taught strategies to attract boys' attention (i.e., to flirt), whereas adolescent boys are taught to pursue girls in the same task-oriented, competitive way in which they pursue other achievements.[44] Women learn that they should not appear too interested in engaging in sexual activities. In order to maintain their image, women are expected to initially resist men's sexual advances even when they find them desirable and plan on reciprocating.[44] Women are expected to set the limits on sexual activities and are they held responsible when men overstep them.[45,46] In a complementary manner, men have traditionally been socialized to initiate sexual encounters and to believe that women prefer lovers who are forceful, aggressive, and dominant. Also, men are led to believe they should ignore a woman's initial sexual resistance or refusal,

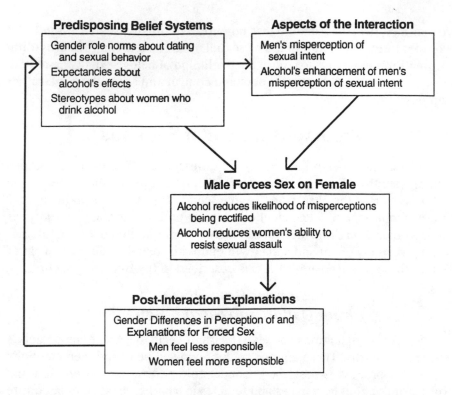

Fig. 1. Psychosocial explanations of alcohol's role in sexual assault.

otherwise they may not appear sufficiently masculine.[47] These gender role messages create in some men a sense of sexual entitlement and superiority over women.[48]

Beliefs About Forced Sex

Young men and women also internalize the message that forced sex is sometimes acceptable. Kikuchi (1988, reported in ref. 41) asked more than 1500 middle school youths if it was ever acceptable for a man to force sex on a woman. More than half of the youths viewed forced sex as acceptable if the woman was wearing "seductive" clothing or if the couple had been dating more than 6 mo. More than one-third said that forced sex was acceptable if the boy had spent "a lot" of money on the girl (a lot of money was defined as $10 by these youths).

Goodchilds and Zellman found similar results with high school youths.[49] They reported that more than half the young men and more than a quarter of the young women they interviewed believed that forced sex was acceptable if she "led him on," if she first said "yes" and then changed her mind, or if he was so excited he could not stop.

Individual Differences in Gender Role Beliefs

The theory and data previously described suggests that men with a strong belief in traditional gender roles would be more prone to perpetrate sexual assault. Data from several studies support this hypothesis. College men who acknowledge committing sexual assault have been found to believe strongly that men and women are sexual adversaries, to accept interpersonal violence as being appropriate, to believe traditional rape myths, to be hostile toward women, and to be sexually aroused in response to aggression.[50,51]

In contrast, women's gender role beliefs have not been consistently linked to the likelihood of experiencing sexual assault. For example, Koss and Dinero found that femininity was not associated with the likelihood of being sexually victimized.[27]

Alcohol's Effects on How Gender Role Norms Are Enacted

Alcohol has an impact on how the gender role norms about dating and sexuality previously described are expressed in heterosexual interactions. A man's alcohol consumption is likely to increase the persistence he uses to reach his sexual goals and his ability to ignore cues that suggest that his partner does not want to engage in sexual activities. Alcohol consumption makes it more difficult to communicate accurately across the gulf induced by gender differences. Alcohol reduces people's capacity to interpret ambiguous cues,[52,53] and many verbal and nonverbal aspects of dating behavior are ambiguous. If a young man suggests to his date that they go for a drive, he could mean exactly that—going for a drive. He could also mean let's park, kiss, and have sex. Although sexual messages are usually vague, it is even more difficult for people to communicate and send cues about their sexual desires and preferences if they are under the influence of alcohol. The role of alcohol in sexual miscommunication is described in greater detail in a later section of this chapter.

Expectancies about Alcohol's Effects on Behavior

In order to understand the role that alcohol has in sexual assault, one needs to consider the expectancies that most people have about alcohol's effects on sexual and aggressive behavior. Many of the effects of alcohol are psychological rather than pharmacological in nature. Meta-analyses by Steele and Southwick demonstrated similar mean effect sizes for people who believed that they had consumed alcohol, but had not actually done so, and for people who had consumed alcohol.[54] People's expectancies regarding alcohol greatly influence the effects that alcohol has on them.[55]

Men, as compared to women, expect to feel more powerful, sexual, and aggressive and less inhibited after drinking alcohol.[56–60] These expectancies may be stronger among men who themselves are more hostile.[61] Men who think they have been drinking alcohol feel sexually aroused and are more responsive to erotic stimuli, including rape scenarios.[62,63]

Research on women's alcohol expectancies has produced mixed results. Leigh reported that women, as compared to men, expected alcohol to make them feel more friendly and romantic.[58] Some authors have found sociability to be more associated with women's than men's alcohol consumption.[56,59] In contrast, Rohsenow found that as compared to men, women expected less social and physical pleasure, less relaxation, and more cognitive and motor impairment from drinking alcohol.[60] Other research has shown that alcohol increased women's anxiety in heterosexual situations but decreased men's anxiety in these situations.[64–66] Leigh described a study in which college students were asked to list positive and negative aspects of drinking alcohol.[67] Fourteen percent of the male college sample mentioned sexuality as a positive aspect of drinking alcohol, whereas only 5% of women did. In contrast, 18% of the women and 13% of the men viewed sexuality as a negative aspect of alcohol consumption. The "female vulnerability" hypothesis suggests that the costs of alcohol consumption are higher for women than for men, so women have good reason to be cautious when consuming alcohol.[68] Female drinkers are more often stigmatized than are male drinkers and they are also at greater risk for victimization.[69]

Because American society is in a period of transition regarding attitudes about appropriate roles and behaviors for women, it is easy to see why the alcohol expectancy literature produces mixed results for women. Some women have internalized traditional beliefs about women's alcohol consumption and are more likely to feel that alcohol consumption has negative consequences (the vulnerability hypothesis). Other women have not internalized these traditional attitudes about women's alcohol consumption, and instead they have adopted positive alcohol expectancies similar to those that most men hold (the convergence hypothesis).

Expectancies frequently become self-fulfilling prophecies.[70] When people consume alcohol, they think and behave in ways that make it likely that the effects they experience will correspond to their initial expectancies. If a woman believes that alcohol makes people more friendly and romantic, then she is likely to act friendly and romantic, even if she is not interested in having sexual intercourse with her companion. If a man believes that alcohol makes people more sexual and aggressive, then he is likely to act sexual and aggressive. He may be more willing to physically force sexual intercourse on a reluctant companion because of alcohol-induced feelings of power.

Expectancies About Illicit Drugs

Much less research has been conducted regarding people's expectancies about the effects of illicit drugs on human behavior. Several authors have found that marijuana and cocaine are perceived by drug users as aphrodisiacs.[71-73] These drugs are reported to enhance the enjoyment of sexual activity, increase sexual desire, and reduce sexual inhibitions. Although more research is needed, it is likely that these expectancies also serve as self-fulfilling prophecies and can contribute to sexual assault.

Stereotypes About Women Who Drink Alcohol

Women who drink alcohol are frequently perceived as being sexually available. George et al. asked college undergraduates to read a brief story about a young couple on a date.[69] The man in the story always drank alcohol. The woman in the story either drank alcohol or a soft drink. Both male and female college students viewed the woman who had a few drinks of alcohol as being more willing to be seduced, more favorably disposed to a sexual advance, and more willing to engage in sexual intercourse. Drinking just a few beers made her appear sexually loose. Similarly, Corcoran and Thomas reported that a woman (as well as a man) who consumed alcohol on a first date was perceived to be more likely to initiate intercourse on that date.[74] In this study, alcohol was linked to perceptions of women's sexual availability and sexual assertiveness. As described earlier, expectancies can become self-fulfilling. Consequently, if a man believes that his date's alcohol consumption is a sign of her willingness to have sex with him, then he is likely to act in ways (possibly including the use of force) which help insure that sex will occur.

Forty percent of the high school males interviewed by Goodchilds and Zellman thought it was acceptable to force sex on a drunk date.[49] Fifty-four percent of the college date rapists interviewed by Kanin thought that their reputation would be improved if they forced sex on a woman they picked up in a bar.[75] Koss et al. found that college women were more likely to be raped when incapacitated as a result of heavy alcohol consumption than to be raped through the use of physical force.[15] Thus, drinking women are perceived as fair game for sexual assault. As a college man who participated in one of our surveys of sexual assault wrote in justification of his behavior, "she was the sleazy type ... a typical bar slut."

Aspects of the Interaction

There are a number of aspects of heterosexual interactions that contribute to the likelihood that sexual assault will occur. This chapter focuses on misperception of friendliness as sexual interest. As can be seen in Fig. 1, the dating and alcohol beliefs described in the last section of the chapter increase the likelihood that friendly cues will be misperceived as sexual cues, and all these factors independently enhance the likelihood of sexual assault.

Misperception of Friendly Cues as a Sign of Sexual Interest

Several authors have found that cues that are intended to convey platonic friendliness are frequently perceived by the recipient as a sign of sexual interest. Abbey surveyed 598 (Study I) college undergraduates and found that two-thirds of them had their friendliness misperceived as sexual interest at least once.[76] Significantly more women (72%) than men (60%) reported that their friendliness had been misperceived by someone of the other sex as a sign of sexual attraction. Koss and Oros found that 70% percent of the women and 53% of the men in their college sample had a member of the other sex misinterpret the level of sexual intimacy that they desired.[77]

A large number of studies have demonstrated that men are more likely than women to interpret a variety of verbal and nonverbal cues as evidence that a woman is interested in having sex with a man. Goodchilds and Zellman asked high school students to rate the likelihood that various cues that might occur on a date would reflect one's willingness to have sex.[49] They found that male adolescents rated revealing clothing worn by either the male or the female, the male's prior reputation, secluded date locations, drinking alcohol, complimenting a date, and tickling a date to be more indicative of one's desire to have sexual intercourse with one's date than did adolescent females.

Abbey and her colleagues have repeatedly found that college men perceive college women as being more seductive and promiscuous and more interested in having sex than college women do. Irrespective of the amount of eye contact, physical closeness, type of touching that has occurred, and type of clothing worn, men perceive women to be more seductive and promiscuous and sexually available than do women.[78-81] Abbey argued that these results suggest that men view the world in a more sexualized manner than women do, and consequently, are more likely than women to interpret ambiguous cues as evidence of sexual intent.[82]

The traditional American gender roles and dating norms, which were described in an earlier section, also make misperception between men and women seem inevitable. Given men's traditional responsibility for initiating dates and sexual behavior, it is not surprising that they would carefully search their female partner's verbal and nonverbal cues for signs of their interest in engaging in sex. When an ambiguous cue is encountered, such as a pat on the arm, the man must decide if he should escalate, perhaps by kissing his date. If the man is interested in having sex, then he is likely to escalate because this is the response most likely to help him achieve his goal.

Alcohol's Role in Men's Misperceptions of Friendliness as Sexual Intent

A man who is drinking alcohol is more likely than a man who is not drinking alcohol to misperceive friendly cues as a sexual come-on, and to ignore his female companion's attempts to rectify his misperception of her. Alcohol consumption reduces people's capacity to analyze complex stimuli.[52–54,83] Intoxicated people are less able to simultaneously attend to multiple stimuli, integrate different sources of information, and engage in complex problem-solving.[84,85] People under the influence of alcohol, consequently, are likely to focus on the most salient, obvious aspects of the situation. Thus, ambiguous cues, such as a friendly date, are likely to be interpreted in a way that fits one's initial hypothesis. For many men, this initial hypothesis is that sex will occur.[86] Alcohol can cause a man to interpret any friendly cue from the woman as a sign of her desire to have sex with him. This may partially explain why the rate of acquaintance rape reported by women is consistently higher than that reported by men.[15] A man may view what happened as seduction, whereas his date views it as sexual coercion.

Men who simultaneously feel sexually aroused and aggressive may find it easy to force sex on their female companions. Their alcohol expectancies fuel their misperceptions and make force seem justifiable. Several authors have found that alcohol consumption causes men to ignore implicit cues inhibiting violence.[53,85] A college male who participated in a focus group conducted to provide background information for this chapter stated that:

> [When drinking alcohol] it's more acceptable to be aggressive. In one situation, I was hanging out with some guys. Some girl was bugging one of the guys, and the guy just slapped the girl, and everybody laughed about it. But I'll tell you one thing, if none of the people were drunk, it would have been a different situation. If they were sober and that happened, they'd all gang up on him.

Alcohol's Effect on Women's Ability to Rectify Misperceptions of Sexual Intent

The cognitive processing limitations associated with alcohol consumption may cause women to miss or ignore cues that suggest they have been misperceived. Alcohol can produce a narrowing of attention and a reduction in inferential processing,[52,83] which may keep a woman from realizing that her friendly behavior is being perceived as seduction.

Research suggests that misperceptions of friendliness for sexual interest are usually rectified before any forced sex occurs. Abbey asked more than 700 college students to describe their most recent experience of misperception of sexual intent.[76] Misperceptions most commonly occurred at parties where both the woman, the man, and their friends were drinking alcohol. Being touched or kissed, suggestive remarks, and extreme attentiveness served as signals to these students that they were being misperceived. Students were fairly evenly split in their use of direct (e.g., tell the other person you are not interested in them in that way) and indirect (e.g., make an excuse to get away, try to ignore it) strategies. The fact that almost half of these students responded to being misperceived by acting as if nothing had happened helps to explain how simple misperceptions can escalate into forced sexual experiences. Norms of politeness and indirectness regarding one's sexual intent may be so strong, that even when they are aware of being misperceived, some women may feel uncomfortable directly discussing it. Consequently, the misperceiver continues to interpret ambiguous words and actions as evidence of sexual interest. The longer the misperception lasts, the more likely it is that the misperceiver will feel justified in expecting sexual intercourse to occur.[49] Sexual provocation, whether intentional or not, is not a legal justification for rape. As described earlier, however, many men and women feel that sexual "teases" deserve forced sex.[49]

Alcohol's Effects on Women's Ability to Resist Sexual Assault

The physical effects of alcohol can make it difficult for a woman to either verbally or physically resist a man's efforts to force sex on her. Several studies have shown that women who successfully escape rape attempts engage in prompt verbal and physical resistance,[27,87] and that women who resist experience less severe levels of sexual assault.[88] The effects of alcohol on cognitive and motor functioning are likely to produce a slow and ineffective response to attack. Compared to women raped as a result of threat or force, women raped as a result of alcohol or drug intoxication were less likely to report physically struggling or running away.[89]

Kanin interviewed 71 college men who acknowledged committing date rape.[75] Three-quarters of these men had gotten a woman high on alcohol or marijuana in order to have sex with her. Kanin described these men as sexually predatory and as willing to use any available strategy to obtain sex (e.g., falsely professing love, threatening to terminate the relationship). These date rapists viewed dating as a "no-holds-barred contest" (p. 223). Similarly, Mosher and Anderson found that 66% of the college men they surveyed used alcohol and 42% used illegal drugs to obtain sex with a female partner (some used both, so percentages total to more than 100%).[90] In this study, using alcohol or other drugs to obtain sex was associated with traditional gender role beliefs and negative sexual attitudes about women.[90] Fifty-five percent of the college men surveyed by Bowker reported that they had used drugs at least once to make their dating partners more willing to have sex.[91]

In summary, alcohol exacerbates the effects of misperception in a variety of ways. Alcohol enhances the likelihood that misperceptions will occur, that they will not be quickly and easily rectified, that a man will feel comfortable forcing sex on a woman whose sexual intentions he misperceived, and that the woman will be unable to successfully resist his attack.

Postinteraction Factors

Both predisposing factors and aspects of the interaction influence how men and women perceive sexual assault after it has happened. Research suggests that alcohol consumption tends to decrease men's sense of responsibility and increase women's sense of responsibility for sexual assault.

Alcohol as a Justification
for Men's Sexual Aggression

Historically, alcohol has been used in American society as a justification for men's socially inappropriate behavior.[92,93] Several empirical laboratory studies have found drunken men to be held less responsible than sober men for a variety of crimes including vandalism, robbery, assault, spouse abuse, and rape.[94–97] For example, Barbaree and Seto (1991; reported in ref. 98) found that college undergraduates held a male perpetrator of date rape less responsible for his behavior if he was intoxicated at the time of the assault. There is also evidence from reviews of court records and interviews with convicted rapists that intoxication is used to justify criminal behavior.[99,100] Based on their crosscultural research, MacAndrew and Edgerton concluded that in many cultures, drunkenness represents a "time-out" during which men are not held to the usual behavioral limits.[93]

Either consciously or unconsciously, some men may choose to drink alcohol in order to facilitate their attempts to have sex with their partner.[100] Alcohol consumption reduces some men's sense of responsibility for their sexual behaviors, making forced sex seem excusable. One of the incarcerated rapists interviewed by Scully stated that "Straight, I don't have the guts to rape. I could fight a man but not that" (p. 124).[21] Twenty-one percent of the date rapists interviewed by Kanin said that the rape would not have happened if they had not been drinking alcohol.[101] An additional 41% of these men felt that their alcohol consumption was partially responsible for the rape because it led them to misperceive their partner's sexual interest and feel comfortable using force. Many male college students report drinking alcohol in order to experience the sense of disinhibition, power, and sexuality that they have come to associate with drinking.[102] Then some of them jokingly brag the next day about their socially unacceptable exploits including vandalism, fist fights, vomiting, memory loss, and forced sex.

When intoxicated, the violation of personal or social norms can easily be attributed to alcohol.[103] The alcohol provides a convenient external factor to blame. Thus, a perpetrator of acquaintance rape need not consider painful internal attributions such as "Am I a violent person?" If men are not held responsible, by themselves or society, for rapes committed while intoxicated, then this encourages future rape and societal norms tolerant of rape.

Alcohol as a Factor That Increases Women's Sense of Responsibility

Paradoxically, whereas alcohol consumption makes some men feel less responsible for sexual aggression, it makes some women feel more responsible for what happened. Men are more likely than women to report using alcohol to excuse socially inappropriate behavior.[104,105] Berglas argued that because society does not view intoxication as acceptable for women, drunkenness cannot be used by women to excuse errors of judgment.[104]

Women who were under the influence of alcohol when sexually assaulted are often viewed by others as partially responsible for what happened.[97,106] Many convicted rapists use their victim's intoxication to discredit their testimony and make the victim appear more responsible for what happened.[21] Even after being convicted, many of the men interviewed by Scully denied that rape occurred and said that alcohol or other drugs had sexually aroused their victims.[21]

Sexually assaulted women who have traditional gender role beliefs are likely to feel that they failed in their gatekeeper role. This sense of failure can cause women to feel partially responsible for the sexual assault.[107] As one woman who participated in our research wrote, "For years I believed it was my fault for being too drunk. I never called it 'rape' until much more recently, even though I repeatedly told him 'no.' "

Women who were under the influence of alcohol when sexually assaulted are likely to feel even more responsible because they may feel that their drunkenness caused the attack. Interviews with date rapists, however, suggest that it is more likely that the perpetrator purposely got the victim drunk in order to facilitate the forced sex.[75]

Richardson and Campbell asked college students to read a brief story about a college woman raped by one of the guests at the end of a party.[97] Some students read a version of the story in which the victim was drunk, whereas the other students read a version of the story in which the attacker was drunk. Both female and male students rated the male attacker as less responsible for the rape when he was intoxicated rather than sober. In contrast, both female and male students rated the female victim as more responsible when she was intoxicated rather than sober. She was also liked less and perceived as less moral when she was drunk. These findings demonstrate that many college students hold the traditional negative view of women who drink alcohol, and tend to denigrate women when they experience any negative consequences. Whereas men are allowed to "let loose," women who "let their hair down" do so at the risk of being judged harshly. This double standard regarding men's and women's responsibility for their behavior when intoxicated strengthens societal norms that tolerate and support rape.[108]

Substance Abuse as a Consequence of Childhood Sexual Assault

Several authors have found that childhood sexual assault is significantly related to experiencing sexual assault as an adult.[11,27,30,109] In an attempt to explain this relationship, Harney and Muehlenhard observed that victims of childhood sexual assault are significantly more likely than nonvictims to experience depression and substance abuse.[110] They suggested that substance abuse may be an intervening variable that explains the relationship between childhood and adult sexual assault experiences. Some victims of childhood sexual assault turn to substances as a strategy for coping with the depression they experience. Women who experienced incest frequently report feeling less sexually attractive, less positive about sex, and more guilty about sex than other women (Hammond et al., 1979; reviewed in ref. 29). Hammond et al. (1979; reviewed in ref. 29) also found that incest history was negatively correlated with the experience of sexual satisfaction when sober but not when intoxicated. Thus, some incest victims may begin abusing alcohol in an attempt to have more positive sexual experiences. Wilsnack suggested that "alcohol helped sedate these women against the negative feelings they associated with sexual activity" (p. 215).[29]

As described earlier, intoxication puts women at risk for sexual assault both because men may view them as an appropriate target and because they may be less able to fight off an attack. Thus a woman who uses substances to cope with the trauma associated with childhood sexual assault is vulnerable to additional sexual assaults.

Conclusions and Suggestions for Future Research

This chapter has focused on the role of alcohol in sexual assault. To summarize the main points of this chapter, alcohol is thought to increase the likelihood that sexual assault will occur by:

1. Encouraging the expression of traditional gender role beliefs about sexual behavior;
2. Triggering alcohol expectancies associated with male sexuality and aggression;
3. Engaging stereotypes about the sexual availability of women who drink alcohol;
4. Increasing the likelihood that men will misperceive women's friendly cues as a sign of sexual interest;
5. Limiting women's ability to rectify misperceptions of sexual intent;
6. Decreasing women's capacity to resist sexual assault;
7. Providing justification for men to commit sexual assault; and
8. Making women feel responsible for sexual assault.

Literature has been cited to support each of these points. However, most of these studies were not designed specifically to test these relationships, consequently the evidence must be viewed as supportive rather than conclusive. Research is needed to examine directly the role of the factors previously described in sexual assault.

Although it is easy to point to the need for further research, it is more difficult to specify the precise methods that should be used. Because exposure to sexual assault or alcohol use in potentially assaultive situations cannot be experimentally manipulated, questions about causality are difficult to address. Space limitations preclude a full discussion of research design issues, however, we want to encourage the use of a variety of different methods. There is a need for experimental analog studies, which systematically vary factors such as alcohol consumption or a female confederate's behavior and measure outcomes such as men's physiological sexual arousal and self-reported hypothetical likelihood of raping.[111-113]

There is also a need for studies that interview perpetrators and victims of sexual assault to obtain their perceptions of the role of alcohol and other drugs in their experiences. Scully's interviews with incarcerated rapists provide a wealth of qualitative information.[21] Similar interviews are needed with perpetrators of unreported sexual assaults. Prospective epidemiological designs can also be used to examine precursors of sexual assault, including substance abuse. If studies using a variety of different methods produce similar results, this provides greater confidence in their conclusions.

Prevention and Treatment Implications

One practical implication of the literature reviewed in this chapter is the need to coordinate sexual assault and substance abuse prevention and treatment services. The frequent co-occurrence of these two problems makes it essential that service providers in both fields are crosstrained. Individuals who work in substance abuse treatment must systematically assess previous sexual assault experiences in male and female clients. Male substance abusers may have a history of perpetration and/or victimization. Individuals who work with perpetrators and victims of sexual assault must systematically assess their level of substance use. Although substance abuse does not provide moral or legal justification for perpetrating sexual assault, it does require treatment. Similarly, although substance use does not make a woman responsible for being sexually assaulted, a substance abuse treatment referral should be made if necessary. Women need to know that even a few drinks of alcohol can make them more vulnerable to sexual assault, both because some men will interpret their alcohol consumption as a sign of sexual availability[69] and because they may be less effective in resisting an attempted sexual assault.[89] This conclusion is not meant to imply that women should not drink alcohol, but that they should be aware of its effects on themselves and others.

The gender role stereotypes and alcohol expectancies described in this chapter are an integral part of American culture. These beliefs develop in early childhood and are reinforced throughout people's lives.[108,114] Beliefs about alcohol and sexuality will be altered only if parental, peer, and media messages are changed. The mass media plays a large role in promoting these images,[115] and its portrayal of appropriate alcohol use must be altered if youths' impression of responsible decision making about alcohol use is to change.

There is no single cause of sexual assault and there is no single solution to this problem. Future research that clarifies the link between alcohol use and sexual assault will aid the development of more effective prevention and treatment programs.

Acknowledgments

This chapter was funded by grants from the U.S. Department of Education's Fund for the Improvement of Secondary Education and the National Institute on Alcohol Abuse and Alcoholism to the first author. We would like to thank Alan Berkowitz, Teresa Herzog, and Mary P. Koss for their thought-provoking comments on an earlier version of this chapter.

References

[1]C. L. Muehlenhard, I. G. Powch, J. L. Phelps, and L. M. Giusti (1992) Definitions of rape: Scientific and political implications. *J. Soc. Issues* **48,** 23–44.

[2]Federal Bureau of Investigation (1991) *Uniform Crime Reports.* U.S. Department of Justice, Washington, DC.

[3]M. P. Koss (1992) The underdetection of rape: Methodological choices influence incidence estimates. *J. Soc. Issues* **48,** 61–76.

[4]P. Searles and R. J. Berger (1987) The current status of rape reform legislation: An examination of state statutes. *Women's Rights Law Reporter* **10,** 25–43.

[5]D. E. H. Russell (1991) Wife rape, in *Acquaintance Rape: The Hidden Crime.* A. Parrot and L. Bechhofer, eds. Wiley, New York, pp. 129–139.

[6]Bureau of Justice Statistics (1991) *Criminal Victimization in the United States.* U.S. Department of Justice, Washington, DC.

[7]C. Struckman-Johnson (1991) Male victims of acquaintance rape, in *Acquaintance Rape: The Hidden Crime.* A. Parrot and L. Bechhofer, eds. Wiley, New York, pp. 192–213.

[8]G. Mezey and M. King (1989) The effects of sexual assault on men: A survey of 22 victims. *Psychological Med.* **19,** 205–209.

[9]A. N. Groth and A. W. Burgess (1980) Male rape: Offenders and victims. *Am. J. Psychiatry* **137,** 806–810.

[10]A. Browne and D. Finkelhor (1986) Impact of child sexual abuse: A review of the research. *Psychological Bull.* **99,** 66–77.

[11]D. E. H. Russell (1986) *The Secret Trauma: Incest in the Lives of Girls and Women.* Basic, New York.

[12]D. E. H. Russell (1982) The prevalence and incidence of rape and attempted rape of females. *Victimology* **7,** 81–93.

[13]D. G. Kilpatrick, L. J. Veronen, and C. L. Best (1984) Factors predicting psychological distress among rape victims, in *Trauma and Its Wake: The Study and Treatment of Post-Traumatic Stress Disorder.* C. R. Figley, ed. Brunner Mazel, New York, pp. 113–141.

[14]C. Kirkpatrick and E. J. Kanin (1957) Male sex aggression on a university campus. *Am. Sociol. Rev.* **22,** 52–58.

[15]M. P. Koss, C. A. Gidycz, and N. Wisniewski (1987) The scope of rape: Incidence and prevalence of sexual aggression and victimization in a national sample of higher education students. *J. Consult. Clin. Psychol.* **55,** 162–170.

[16]E. J. Kanin (1969) Selected dyadic aspects of males' sex aggression. *J. Sex Res.* **5,** 12–28.

[17]K. Rapaport and B. R. Burkhart (1984) Personality and attitudinal characteristics of sexually coercive college males. *J. Abnorm. Psychol.* **93,** 216–221.

[18]A. Abbey and L. I. Thomson (1992, June) Role of Alcohol Beliefs and Gender Beliefs in the Perpetration of Sexual Assault. Paper presented at the annual meeting of the American Psychological Society, San Diego.

[19]M. P. Koss (1988) Hidden rape: Sexual aggression and victimization in a national sample of students in higher education, in *Rape and Sexual Assault*, vol. 2. A. W. Burgess, ed. Garland, New York, pp. 3–25.

[20]R. T. Rada (1975) Alcoholism and forcible rape. *Am. J. Psychiatry* **132,** 444–446.

[21]D. Scully (1991) *Understanding Sexual Violence: A Study of Convicted Rapists.* Unwin Hyman, Boston, MA.

[22]S. Vinogradov, N. I. Dishotsky, A. K. Doty, and J. R. Tinklenberg (1988) Patterns of behavior in adolescent rape. *Am. J. Orthopsychiatry* **58,** 179–187.

[23]M. Amir (1971) *Patterns in Forcible Rape.* University of Chicago, Chicago, IL.

[24]S. D. Johnson, L. Gibson, and R. Linden (1978) Alcohol and rape in Winnipeg, 1966–1975. *J. Stud. Alcohol* **39,** 1887–1894.

[25]A. L. Maldonado, F. Martinez, E. Osuna, and R. Garcia-Ferrer (1988) Alcohol consumption and crimes against sexual freedom. *Med. Law* **7,** 81–86.

[26]A. Goodyear-Smith (1989) Medical evaluation of sexual assault findings in the Auckland region. *NZ Med. J.* **102,** 493–495.

[27]M. P. Koss and T. E. Dinero (1989) Discriminant analysis of risk factors for sexual victimization among a national sample of college women. *J. Consult. Clin. Psychol.* **57,** 242–250.

[28]C. L. Muehlenhard and M. A. Linton (1987) Date rape and sexual aggression in dating situations: Incidence and risk factors. *J. Counseling Psychol.* **34,** 186–196.

[29]S. C. Wilsnack (1984) Drinking, sexuality, and sexual dysfunction in women, in *Alcohol Problems in Women.* S.C. Wilsnack and L. J. Beckman, eds. Guilford, New York, pp. 189–227.

[30]C. Swett, C. Cohen, J. Surrey, A. Compaine, and R. Chavez (1991) High rates of alcohol use and history of physical and sexual abuse among women outpatients. *Am. J. Alcohol Abuse* **17,** 49–60.

[31]D. G. Kilpatrick (1990, August) Violence as a Precursor of Women's Substance Abuse: The Rest of the Drugs-Violence Story. Paper presented at the annual meeting of the American Psychological Association, Boston.

[32]P. J. Goldstein, P. A. Bellucci, B. J. Spunt, and T. Miller (1991) Volume of cocaine use and violence: A comparison between men and women. *J. Drug Issues* **21,** 345–367.

[33]S. S. Ageton (1983) *Sexual Assault Among Adolescents.* Lexington, Lexington, MA.

[34]A. Berkowitz (1992) College men as perpetrators of acquaintance rape and sexual assault: A review of recent research. *J. Am. Coll. Health* **40,** 175–181.

[35]E. R. Hall and P. J. Flannery (1984) Prevalence and correlates of sexual assault experiences in adolescents. *Victimology Int. J.* **9,** 398–406.

[36]J. W. White and M. P. Koss (1991) Courtship violence: Incidents in a national sample of higher education students. *Violence Victims* **6,** 247–256.

[37]N. M. Malamuth and J. Briere (1986) Sexual violence in the media: Indirect effects on aggression against women. *J. Soc. Issues* **42,** 75–92.

[38]N. M. Malamuth, R. J. Sockloskie, M. P. Koss, and J. S. Tanaka (1991) Characteristics of aggressors against women: Testing a model using a national sample of college students. *J. Consult. Clin. Psychol.* **59,** 670–681.

[39]A. Abbey (1987) Perceptions of personal avoidability versus responsibility: How do they differ? *Basic Appl. Soc. Psychol.* **8**, 3–20.

[40]K. G. Shaver (1987) *The Attribution of Blame.* Springer-Verlag, New York.

[41]L. Bechhofer and A. Parrot (1991) What is acquaintance rape?, in *Acquaintance Rape: The Hidden Crime.* A. Parrot and L. Bechhofer, eds. Wiley, New York, pp. 9–25.

[42]J. T. Spence and L. L. Sawin (1985) Images of masculinity and femininity: A reconceptualization, in *Women, Gender and Social Psychology.* V. E. O'Leary, R. K. Unger, and B. S. Wallerston, eds. Erlbaum, Hillsdale, NJ, pp. 35–66.

[43]P. D. Werner and G. W. LaRussa (1985) Persistence and change in sex role stereotypes. *Sex Roles* **12**, 1089–1100.

[44]R. J. Berger, P. Searles, R. G. Salem, and B. A. Pierce (1986) Sexual assault in a college community. *Sociol. Focus* **19**, 1–26.

[45]E. Grauerholz and R. T. Serpe (1985) Initiation and response: The dynamics of sexual interaction. *Sex Roles* **12**, 1041–1059.

[46]M. N. LaPlante, N. McCormick, and G. G. Brannigan (1980) Living the sexual script: College students' views of influence in sexual encounters. *J. Sex Res.* **16**, 338–355.

[47]C. L. Muehlenhard (1988) "Nice women" don't say yes and "real men" don't say no: How miscommunication and the double standard can cause sexual problems. *Women Ther.* **7**, 95–108.

[48]R. Warshaw and A. Parrot (1991) The contribution of sex-role socialization to acquaintance rape, in *Acquaintance Rape: The Hidden Crime.* A. Parrot and L. Bechhofer, eds. Wiley, New York, pp. 73–82.

[49]J. D. Goodchilds and G. L. Zellman (1984) Sexual signaling and sexual aggression in adolescent relationships, in *Pornography and Sexual Aggression.* N. M. Malamuth and E. Donnerstein, eds. Academic, Orlando, FL, pp. 233–243.

[50]N. M. Malamuth (1986) Predictors of naturalistic sexual aggression. *J. Pers. Soc. Psychol.* **50**, 953–962.

[51]K. R. Rapaport and C. D. Posey (1991) Sexually coercive college males, in *Acquaintance Rape: The Hidden Crime.* A. Parrot and L. Bechhofer, eds. Wiley, New York, pp. 217–228.

[52]R. Berkow (1982) *Merck Manual of Diagnosis and Therapy*, 14th ed. Merck, Rahway, NJ.

[53]K. E. Leonard (1989) The impact of explicit aggressive and implicit nonaggressive cues on aggression in intoxicated and sober males. *Pers. Soc. Psychol. Bull.* **15**, 390–400.

[54]C. M. Steele and L. Southwick (1985) Alcohol and social behavior I: The psychology of drunken excess. *J. Pers. Soc. Psychol.* **48**, 18–34.

[55]G. A. Marlatt and D. J. Rohsenow (1980) Cognitive processes in alcohol use, in *Advances in Substance Abuse: Behavioral and Biological Research.* N. K. Mello, ed. JAI, Greenwich, CT, pp. 159–199.

[56]S. A. Brown, M. S. Goldman, A. Inn, and L. R. Anderson (1980) Expectations of reinforcement from alcohol: Their domain and relation to drinking patterns. *J. Consult. Clin. Psychol.* **48**, 419–426.

[57]A. Crawford (1984) Alcohol and expectancy—I. Perceived sex differences in the effects of drinking. *Alcohol Alcohol.* **19**, 63–69.

[58]B. C. Leigh (1987) Beliefs about the effects of alcohol on self and others. *J. Stud. Alcohol* **48**, 467–475.

[59]K. G. Ratliff and B. R. Burkhart (1984) Sex differences in motivations for and effects of drinking among college students. *J. Stud. Alcohol* **45**, 26–32.

[60]D. J. Rohsenow (1983) Drinking habits and expectancies about alcohol's effects for self versus others. *J. Consult. Clin. Psychol.* **51,** 752–756.

[61]K. E. Leonard and H. T. Blane (1988) Alcohol expectancies and personality characteristics in young men. *Addict. Behav.* **13,** 353–357.

[62]J. A. Carpenter and N. P. Armenti (1972) Some effects of ethanol on human sexual and aggressive behavior, in *The Biology of Alcoholism*, vol. 2. B. Kissin and H. Begleiter, eds. Plenum, New York, pp. 509–543.

[63]G. T. Wilson and D. M. Lawson (1976) Expectancies, alcohol and sexual arousal in male social drinkers. *J. Abnorm. Psychol.* **85,** 587–594.

[64]D. B. Abrams and G. T. Wilson (1979) Effects of alcohol on social anxiety in women. *J. Abnorm. Psychol.* **88,** 161–173.

[65]M. Konovsky and S. C. Wilsnack (1982) Social drinking and self-esteem in married couples. *J. Stud. Alcohol* **43,** 319–333.

[66]G. T. Wilson and D. B. Abrams (1977) Effects of alcohol on social anxiety and physiological arousal: Cognitive versus pharmacological processes. *Cognitive Ther. Res.* **1,** 195–210.

[67]B. C. Leigh (1990) The relationship of sex-related alcohol expectancies to alcohol consumption and sexual behavior. *Br. J. Addict.* **85,** 919–928.

[68]C. Robbins (1989) Sex differences in psychosocial consequences of alcohol and drug use. *J. Health Soc. Behav.* **30,** 117–130.

[69]W. H. George, S. J. Gournic, and M. P. McAffee (1988) Perceptions of post drinking female sexuality: Effects of gender, beverage choice, and drink payment. *J. Appl. Soc. Psychol.* **18,** 1295–1317.

[70]J. M. Darley and R. H. Fazio (1980) Expectancy confirmation processes arising in the social interaction sequence. *Am. Psychol.* **35,** 867–881.

[71]R. H. Blum (1970) *Students and Drugs*. Jossey Bass, New York.

[72]G. R. Gay, J. A. Newmeyer, M. Perry, G. Johnson, and M. Kurland (1982) Love and Haight: The sensuous hippie revisited. Drug/sex practices in San Francisco, 1980–81. *J. Psychoactive Drugs* **14,** 111–123.

[73]W. C. Koff (1974) Marijuana and sexual activity. *J. Sex Res.* **10,** 194–204.

[74]K. J. Corcoran and L. R. Thomas (1991) The influence of observed alcohol consumption on perceptions of initiation of sexual activity in a college dating situation. *J. Appl. Soc. Psychol.* **21,** 500–507.

[75]E. J. Kanin (1985) Date rapists: Differential sexual socialization and relative deprivation. *Arch. Sex. Behav.* **14,** 219–231.

[76]A. Abbey (1987) Misperceptions of friendly behavior as sexual interest: A survey of naturally occurring incidents. *Psychol. Women Q.* **11,** 173–194.

[77]M. P. Koss and C. L. Oros (1982) Sexual experiences survey: A research instrument investigating sexual aggression and victimization. *J. Consult. Clin. Psychol.* **50,** 455–457.

[78]A. Abbey (1982) Sex differences in attributions for friendly behavior: Do males misperceive females' friendliness? *J. Pers. Soc. Psychol.* **42,** 830–838.

[79]A. Abbey, C. Cozzarelli, K. McLaughlin, and R. J. Harnish (1987) The effects of clothing and dyad sex composition on perceptions of sexual intent: Do women and men evaluate these cues differently? *J. Appl. Soc. Psychol.* **17,** 108–126.

[80]A. Abbey and C. Melby (1986) The effects of nonverbal cues on gender differences in perceptions of sexual intent. *Sex Roles* **15,** 283–298.

[81]R. J. Harnish, A. Abbey, and K. G. DeBono (1990) Toward an understanding of "the sex game." *J. Appl. Soc. Psychol.* **20,** 1333–1344.

[82]A. Abbey (1991) Misperception as an antecedent of acquaintance rape: A consequence of ambiguity in communication between women and men, in *Acquaintance Rape: The Hidden Crime*. A. Parrot and L. Bechhofer, eds. Wiley, New York, pp. 96–111.

[83]C. Ryan and N. Butters (1983) Cognitive deficits in alcoholics, in *The Pathogenesis of Alcoholism: Biological Factors*, vol. 7. B. Kissin and H. Begleiter, eds. Plenum, New York, pp. 485–538.

[84]J. G. Hull and R. R. Van Treuren (1986) Experimental social psychology and the causes and effects of alcohol consumption, in *Research Advances in Alcohol and Drug Problems*. H. D. Cappell, ed. Plenum, New York, pp. 211–244.

[85]S. P. Taylor and K. E. Leonard (1983) Alcohol and human physical aggression, in *Aggression: Theoretical and Empirical Reviews*, vol. 2. R. G. Green and E. I. Donnerstein, eds. Academic, New York, pp. 77–101.

[86]A. E. Gross (1978) The male role and heterosexual behavior. *J. Soc. Issues* **34**, 87–107.

[87]J. M. Seigal, S. B. Sorenson, J. M. Golding, M. A. Burnam, and J. A. Stein (1989) Resistance to sexual assault: Who resists and what happens? *Am. J. Public Health* **79**, 27–31.

[88]S. E. Ullman and R. A. Knight (1991) A multivariate model for predicting rape and physical injury outcomes during sexual assaults. *J. Consult. Clin. Psychol.* **59**, 724–731.

[89]B. K. Hawks and C. D. Welch (1991, August) Alcohol and the Experience of Rape. Paper presented at the meeting of the American Psychological Association, San Francisco.

[90]D. L. Mosher and R. D. Anderson (1986) Macho personality, sexual aggression, and reactions to guided imagery of realistic rape. *J. Res. Pers.* **20**, 77–94.

[91]L. H. Bowker (1978) The relationship between sex, drugs, and sexual behavior on a college campus. *Drug Forum* **7**, 69–80.

[92]B. Critchlow (1983) Blaming the booze: The attribution of responsibility for drunken behavior. *Pers. Soc. Psychol. Bull.* **9**, 451–473.

[93]C. MacAndrew and R. B. Edgerton (1969) *Drunken Comportment: A Social Explanation*. Aldine, Chicago.

[94]B. J. Carducci and J. A. McNeely (1981, August) Attribution of Blame for Wife Abuse by Alcoholics and Nonalcoholics. Paper presented at the annual meeting of the American Psychological Association, Los Angeles.

[95]B. Critchlow (1985) The blame in the bottle: Attributions about drunken behavior. *Pers. Soc. Psychol. Bull.* **11**, 258–274.

[96]D. R. Richardson and G. S. Hammock (1991) Alcohol and acquaintance rape, in *Acquaintance Rape: The Hidden Crime*. A. Parrot and L. Bechhofer, eds. Wiley, New York, pp. 83–95.

[97]D. Richardson and J. L. Campbell, (1982) Alcohol and rape: The effect of alcohol on attributions of blame for rape. *Pers. Soc. Psychol. Bull.* **8**, 468–476.

[98]H. E. Barbaree and W. L. Marshall (1991) The role of male sexual arousal in rape: Six models. *J. Consult. Clin. Psychol.* **59**, 621–630.

[99]W. A. Harrell (1981) The effects of alcohol use and offender remorsefulness on sentencing decisions. *J. Appl. Soc. Psychol.* **11**, 83–91.

[100]D. Scully and J. Marolla (1984) Convicted rapists' vocabulary of motive: Excuses and justifications. *Soc. Problems* **31**, 530–544.

[101]E. J. Kanin (1984) Date rape: Unofficial criminals and victims. *Victimology* **9**, 95–108.

[102]A. D. Berkowitz and H. W. Perkins (1987) Recent research on gender differences in collegiate alcohol use. *J. Am. Coll. Health* **36**, 123–129.

[103]G. T. Wilson (1981) The effects of alcohol on human sexual behavior, in *Advances in Substance Abuse*, vol. 2. M. Mello, ed. JAI, Greenwich, CT, pp. 1–40.

[104]S. Berglas (1987) Self-handicapping model, in *Psychological Theories of Drinking and Alcoholism*. H. T. Blane and K. E. Leonard, eds. Guilford, New York, pp. 305–345.

[105]R. M. Schwartz, B. R. Burkhart, and S. B. Green (1982) Sensation seeking and anxiety as factors in social drinking by men. *J. Stud. Alcohol* **43**, 1108–1114.

[106]B. Aramburu and B. C. Leigh (1991) For better or for worse: Attributions about drunken aggression toward male and female victims. *Violence Victims* **6**, 31–41.

[107]R. Warshaw (1988) *I Never Called it Rape*. Harper and Row, New York.

[108]M. R. Burt (1991) Rape myths and acquaintance rape, in *Acquaintance Rape: The Hidden Crime*. A. Parrot and L. Bechhofer, eds. Wiley, New York, pp. 26–40.

[109]D. L. Hurley (1991) Women, alcohol and incest: An analytical review. *J. Stud. Alcohol* **52**, 253–268.

[110]P. A. Harney and C. L. Muehlenhard (1991) Factors that increase the likelihood of victimization, in *Acquaintance Rape: The Hidden Crime*. A. Parrot and L. Bechhofer, eds. Wiley, New York, pp. 159–175.

[111]W. H. George and G. A. Marlatt (1986) The effects of alcohol and anger on interest in violence, erotica, and deviance. *J. Abnorm. Psychol.* **95**, 150–158.

[112]A. Lang, J. Searles, R. Lauerman, and V. Adesso (1980). Expectancy, alcohol and sex guilt as determinants of interest in and reaction to sexual stimuli. *J. Abnorm. Psychol.* **89**, 644–653.

[113]N. M. Malamuth (1988) Predicting laboratory aggression against female and male targets: Implications for sexual aggression. *J. Res. Pers.* **22**, 474–495.

[114]D. L. Spiegler (1983) Children's attitudes toward alcohol. *J. Stud. Alcohol* **44**, 542–552.

[115]E. Goffman (1976) *Gender Advertisements*. Harper and Row, New York.

Gender Differences in Biological Markers of Alcohol Use

Linda S. LaGrange

Introduction

In spite of the fact that much of the research data gathered on alcohol use and alcoholism has been elicited from a male population, it is clear that there are gender differences associated with almost all dimensions of human alcohol consumption. As more research is undertaken with female participants, examples of alcohol-related gender differences become more numerous and clear cut. For instance, there are indications that female alcoholics are more likely than male alcoholics to be polydrug users, displaying a preference for prescription CNS depressants.[1] As well, women have higher blood-alcohol levels and a lower volume of distribution (V_d) of alcohol than do males after an equivalent amount of acute alcohol consumption, a difference thought by some investigators to be attributable to the relatively higher levels of body fat in women;[2] or as other researchers assert, the result of a decreased first-pass metabolism by gastric alcohol dehydrogenase.[3] It also appears that there are differences in the effects of alcohol on both the morphological features[4] and cognitive functions[5] of the brain. It was noted some time ago that females seemed to suffer greater liver damage over a shorter period of drinking history than males.[6,7] This temporal foreshortening effect (referred to as telescoping) has not only been associated with severity of liver damage, but apparently applies to most of the adverse consequences

From: *Drug and Alcohol Abuse Reviews, Vol. 5: Addictive Behaviors in Women*
Ed.: R. R. Watson ©1994 Humana Press Inc., Totowa, NJ

of alcohol abuse.[8] In addition, some of the events leading to excessive drinking and the subsequent emotional and social problems appear to vary according to gender.[9-11] It seems logical, and in fact is the case, that because there are gender differences in endocrine function apart from alcohol consumption, the effects of alcohol on those different functions would also be quite distinct.[12,13] Finally, and certainly gender-related, the effects of continued abuse of alcohol throughout pregnancy may result in irrevocable damage to the developing fetus.[14]

Regardless of gender, alcoholism is an emotionally and physically costly disease. Because it is preventable, given appropriate treatment intervention, its early, unequivocal diagnosis is a primary goal of health care personnel. Currently, the assessment of alcohol use, whether by interview, questionnaire, or biomarker, is unacceptably inaccurate. With regard specifically to females and the use of interviews and questionnaires as assessment instruments, Ernhart et al.,[15] in retrospective interviews of women who 5 yr earlier had participated in a study of self-reported levels of alcohol consumption during pregnancy, found that 41% of the women recalled significantly more prenatal and in-pregnancy alcohol use than they had originally reported. A similar trend was observed by Robles and Day:[16] Retest responses indicated higher levels of in-pregnancy drinking than initial test reports. In a subsequent study, Morrow-Tlucak et al.[17] noted that women with the most severe alcohol problems were the most likely to underreport their alcohol consumption during pregnancy. They also noted that although the Michigan Alcoholism Screening Test (MAST) seemed to be a better indicator than self-report, it too was inadequate. The tendency to conceal the true extent of alcohol use is not confined to pregnant females. It appears to be particularly pronounced among many young females who abuse alcohol;[18,19] a population extremely vulnerable to the adverse consequences of alcohol abuse and urgently in need of early diagnosis.[20,21]

The diagnosis of alcoholism or assessment of alcohol abuse through the use of biomarkers is also somewhat unreliable, characterized by both a lack of sensitivity and specificity. Because the correlations between alcohol consumption and many of the better known biological laboratory tests are inconsistent and often weak,[22] these currently used biomarkers of alcohol consumption may be more a measure of tissue and organ damage or metabolic changes than alcohol consumption *per se*. Young females who are abusing alcohol might not be identified by current laboratory tests because the early stages of alcohol abuse do not usually manifest the pathological and metabolic changes detected by these tests.[23,24] Obviously, too, either the sensitivity or specificity of such biomarkers for alcohol-induced changes is limited in that similar tissue and organ damage or metabolic changes can be caused by factors other than alcohol consumption. Among females, the usefulness of biomarkers is further compromised by the fact that certain metabolic changes that mimic those caused by excessive alcohol consumption may actually be caused by hormonal fluctuations associated with the menstrual cycle or with pregnancy. The criteria for a useful biomarker of excessive alcohol consumption must accommodate gender-specific constraints, such that the biomarker itself is gender-specific or is unaffected by gender differences.

General considerations that have thus far governed the use and development of biomarkers of alcohol consumption have included the following:

1. The assessment of pattern of consumption; for instance, is the individual binging, or drinking heavily on a daily basis?
2. Is the heavy consumption chronic or short term?
3. Is the biomarker useful in detecting relapse or compliance with abstinence programs?
4. Can the biomarker be used to detect underlying alcohol-induced pathology?
5. Is the biomarker unaffected by disease states and the intake of drugs other than alcohol?
6. Is the biomarker of equivalent utility for both genders?
7. Will the efficacy of the biomarker be maintained throughout pregnancy?
8. Is the biomarker relatively accessible to sampling procedures?
9. Can the presence of the biomarker be detected by a relatively inexpensive and standardized assay?

It is likely that no single biomarker can meet all of the aforementioned criteria, in which case the alternative is to establish the simplest and most effective combination of biomarkers specific to the assessment of each criterion. The following review of biomarkers will describe each biomarker, note the type of assay required to detect the marker, discuss the overall research findings, provide some information about the possible mechanisms that alter the biochemical substance to the extent that it can be considered a marker, examine other nonalcohol-related factors that may influence the biomarker, and identify any gender differences that might have an influence on the efficacy of the biomarker to accurately reflect the abuse of alcohol.

Review of Biomarkers

Serum and/or Urinary Lipids

Urinary Dolichol

Dolichols are long chain 2,3-dihydropolyprenols that function as lipid carriers in the synthesis of glycoproteins. They can be found in biological fluids and tissue in the form of esters of fatty acids, phosphate esters, and free alcohols.[25] Levels of urinary dolichol can be determined by high-performance liquid chromatography (HPLC) after extraction on a reversed-phase sorbent.[26]

A number of studies have revealed that urinary dolichol is elevated in alcoholics.[27–29] It also appears that although acute heavy consumption lasting more than 1 d by nonalcoholics can cause urinary dolichol levels to increase,[27,30] moderate alcohol consumption does not affect dolichol levels. Reports of the sensitivity of this biomarker encompass an enormous range: 19–68%,[28,31] with specificity ranging from 64–94%.[31,32]

Because dolichols are thought to be oxidized by alcohol dehydrogenase, the mechanism by which urinary dolichol levels may increase in response to heavy alcohol consumption is via competitive oxidation of alcohol by alcohol dehydrogenase.[33] Another possible influence is that of enhanced dolichol formation from a saturated precursor as a result of the increased NADH/NAD ratio formed during alcohol metabolism.[34] Raised levels do not seem to be a consequence of liver damage.[28]

Other factors that appear to cause either tissue or urinary dolichol levels to increase include: Alzheimer's disease,[35] neuronal ceroid-lipofuscinosis,[36] Hermansky-Pudlak syndrome,[37] metastatic cancer,[38] advanced age,[39] pregnancy and bacterial infections,[40] strenuous physical exercise,[41] aspirin, and heat stress.[42] Excluding pregnant females, gender does not seem to be associated with increased or decreased dolichol levels.[28]

Clearly, if pregnancy is indeed associated with an increase in dolichol levels, the utility of urinary dolichol as a biomarker of alcohol consumption in females is severely limited. Why pregnancy is associated with elevated dolichol levels is not yet known. It is also not clear if the instance of alcohol consumption during pregnancy would drive urinary dolichol levels even higher than either pregnancy or alcohol consumption alone.

With the exception of the study on pregnant females,[40] the overwhelming majority of alcoholic participants in previous studies were male. If there were gender differences, it is possible the number of female participants was considered too low to report separately. A review of the studies conducted on the association of urinary dolichol levels with alcohol consumption reveals an approx 3:1 ratio of male to female participants. If only those participants who were alcoholics are considered, the ratio increases to approx 7:1.

Serum Dolichol

The effect of alcohol on serum dolichol has not been extensively studied, however there were some noteworthy observations made in a 1989 study of serum dolichol levels by Roine et al.[43] Dolichol levels were analyzed using HPLC after extraction on a reversed-phase sorbent with UV detection at 210 nm.

Briefly, serum dolichol levels were higher in alcoholics than in nonalcoholics, however group differences were not as pronounced as those found when using urinary dolichol as the marker. Heavy drinking by nonalcoholics for a period of more than 1 d did not raise serum dolichol levels. Finally, in alcoholics, elevated serum dolichol levels decreased more slowly than urinary dolichol levels during periods of abstinence. Reasons for the change in serum dolichol levels with alcohol consumption have not been elucidated. There is some speculation that the increase may be associated with the alcohol-induced increase in high-density lipoprotein (HDL).[43] With regard to other possible causes of elevated serum dolichol levels, it was thought that age may have been a factor,[44] however, this has not been confirmed in other studies.[45,46] Although there were female participants in the Roine et al.[43] study, no gender differences were noted in any of the other serum dolichol studies.

Plasma High-Density Lipoprotein Cholesterol (HDLC)

It has been demonstrated that HDL, at least in part, forms in plasma as a catabolic product of triglyceride-rich lipoproteins and lipoprotein lipase.[47] Because increased levels of HDL and HDLC are associated with a reduction in coronary heart disease[48] and atherosclerosis,[49] it is thought that HDL and HDLC act as carriers for cholesterol, removing it from arterial tissue. HDL protein can be determined by electroimmunoassay,[50] HDLC can be separated by precipitation, and the cholesterol on the supernatant can be measured enzymatically.[51]

As with many biomarkers, the sensitivity of HDLC as an indication of alcohol abuse varies from study to study. Barboriak et al.[52] found that HDLC levels were elevated in 20% of male alcoholics and 57% of female alcoholics. Yet, in an earlier study by Danielsson et al.,[53] 66% of the male alcoholics had elevated HDLC levels. A possible mechanism by which alcohol consumption causes an increase in HDLC is via its inhibitory effect on hepatic endothelial lipase (HL), an enzyme involved in the metabolism of HDL.[54]

In addition to the association between increased levels of HDLC and alcoholism,[52,55] elevated HDLC levels can also result from, or are associated with, exercise,[56] Black racial groups, estrogen treatment, certain families,[57] and ingesting particular classes of drugs.[58] HDLC can be decreased as a result of severe alcoholic liver disease,[59] thus limiting its use as a marker in individuals with impaired liver function. It is also negatively correlated with tobacco smoking and body weight.[60]

There are reports of gender differences in HDLC levels. Females, overall, have higher levels than males.[61,62] It also appears that HDLC as a marker of alcohol consumption is generally more sensitive when used among females.[52] Although, after a 3-wk 35 g/d alcohol intake, the levels of HDLC in both physically active and inactive females remained unchanged,[62] whereas a similar protocol induced an increase in HDLC in inactive males.[61] This would seem to indicate that, at least among females, elevated HDLC levels are more indicative of chronic alcohol abuse than isolated acute drinking bouts. As with all biomarkers, the data on females and HDLC is not as extensive as that collected on males.

Serum Apolipoprotein A-I and A-II (Apo A-I; A-II)

Apo A-I and A-II account for 80–85% of the apolipoprotein content of HDL.[63] They also act as cofactors in lipoprotein metabolism.[64] As with HDL, high levels of Apo-I and Apo-II are associated with a reduced risk of coronary heart disease.[65] There is evidence that concentrations of A-II are determined genetically.[66] Quantitation of A-I and A-II can be accomplished by electroimmunoassay.[67]

Heavy alcohol consumption results in increased Apo A-I in males.[65] However, in the Hartung et al. study, female levels of Apo A-I did not increase in response to 3 wk of sustained alcohol consumption.[62] It was speculated that this difference could be attributed to the higher baseline levels of Apo A-I found in females.[66] Because males are reported to have higher baseline levels of Apo A-II than females,[66] it would be interesting to determine if A-II levels would remain unchanged in males after a similar 3-wk alcohol challenge. In a separate study of both males and females, data reflected increased levels of Apo A-I and A-II in those participants known to abuse alcohol,[68] however results were not analyzed separately by gender. The sensitivity of Apo A-II as a marker of alcohol use in the Puchois et al. study was 42%. Pileire et al. found that Apo A-II was positively associated with alcohol consumption as assessed by the CAGE questionnaire, and was the only marker that could be used to distinguish between moderate and excessive levels of consumption.[69] Why alcohol consumption causes Apo A-I and A-II levels to increase is not known. Apo A-II was also found to be a sensitive marker of resumption or reduction of alcohol intake in alcohol-abusing males.[70]

Some data indicate seasonal variations in the concentrations of Apo A-I and A-II.[71] There has, however, been no mention of whether or not seasonal variation could interfere with the use of Apo A-I and A-II as biomarkers of alcohol consumption. Research on the association of APO A-I and A-II levels with alcohol use has not been that extensive, therefore additional gender differences may exist that simply have not been detected because of the relatively small number of studies.

Enzymes

There are a number of enzymes measurable in serum that have been examined as possible biomarkers of alcohol use. Most of them share many of the same advantages and disadvantages. Those less promising enzymatic markers will be listed and briefly commented on, whereas the more reliable or newer enzymatic biomarkers will be described in more depth.

Gamma Glutamyl-Transpeptidase (GGTP)

This membrane-bound enzyme is responsible for the transfer of gamma glutamyl groups between peptides and the transport of amino acids through outer membrane structures.[72] GGTP activity can be assessed by a relatively simple photometric technique.[73]

GGTP is perhaps the most well-studied of the biomarkers. General findings indicate that GGTP, although generally elevated in heavy drinkers,[74,75] displays considerable variability in sensitivity, ranging from 31%[76] to 53%.[24] The sensitivity improves to >80% if there is overt liver damage.[77] In a study of just females ($n = 100$), 42% of the alcoholics had elevated GGTP activity.[18] The mechanism underlying alcohol-associated elevations of GGTP is thought to be an induction of the enzyme in the endoplasmic reticulum.[78] However, in recent studies it has been noted that changes in GGTP may also be the result of alcohol-induced liver injury.[79] Indeed, Moussavian et al. observed that GGTP was elevated in only 22% of chronic alcoholics who had no detectable symptoms of liver disease.

Much of the difficulty in using GGTP as a biomarker of alcohol abuse stems from the fact that numerous factors other than alcohol can affect its activity. GGTP activity is frequently elevated when there is liver pathology.[80] Other disease states such as intracranial tumors,[81] pancreatitis,[82] and myocardial infarction,[83] are associated with increased GGTP activity. Harada et al. observed that 50% of elevated GGTP values in a hospital population were attributable to factors other than alcohol consumption.[84]

A number of gender differences have been observed in connection with the use of GGTP as a biomarker of alcohol abuse. Rosalki[77] found evidence that estrogens inhibit GGTP, which may be why GGTP and age are positively correlated in some females.[75] It should be mentioned, however, that this positive GGTP/age correlation in females was not observed in a later study by Persson et al.[85] It has also been noted that the use of oral contraceptives may cause up to a 20% increase in GGTP activity.[86] In general, GGTP does not appear to be as sensitive a marker among females as compared to males,[87] although there are exceptions. For example, Cushman et al.[24] found no gender difference in the efficacy of GGTP as a biomarker of alcohol abuse.

GGTP activity during pregnancy has been assessed in two separate studies. In the first study, the sensitivity of GGTP as a marker of excessive alcohol use was only 25%.[88] More recently, Ylikorkal et al.[89] found that pregnancy appeared not to affect GGTP activity, and that GGTP was elevated in 59.1% of the 29 pregnant alcoholics in their sample, indicating that

GGTP may be of some value as a biomarker of alcohol use during pregnancy. There does seem to be fairly unequivocal evidence for a gender difference in the baseline levels of GGTP wherein female enzyme activity is less than that of males.[90,91] Specifically, for the 40- to 50-yr age group, GGTP activity was 75% higher in males than in females.[92] It was also observed, in this same study, that there was a positive association between weight and serum GGTP in males that was not evident in females.

Serum Aspartate Transaminase (s-ASAT)

Serum ASAT is a soluble form of cytoplasmic enzyme distinct from the mitochondrial enzyme (m-ASAT).[93] As with most of the serum enzyme assays, s-ASAT can be determined by standard autoanalyzer techniques.[94]

Elevated s-ASAT is frequently associated with alcoholism, as has been established by a number of studies.[95–97] However, it is likely that the increased s-ASAT is the result of tissue or organ damage caused by alcohol consumption and not a direct action by alcohol on the enzyme. Because elevation is an indirect effect of alcohol, increased s-ASAT may also be attributable to nonalcohol-related disease states or the ingestion of other substances.[98] Its value as a biomarker of alcoholism is somewhat limited because the elevated activity is frequently a consequence of liver damage.[99] Sensitivity ranged from 38%[100] to 76% in a group of alcoholics known to have mild liver damage.[96] In a study of female alcoholics ($n = 100$), sensitivity was 18% and there was no correlation of s-ASAT with level of alcohol consumption.[18] ASAT increases with age and is a bit decreased in heavy smokers.[101] Whitfield et al. found that alcohol intake among females did not result in an increase of s-ASAT whereas there was a positive association of alcohol consumption and s-ASAT in males.[87] The Whitfield group suggested that s-ASAT is a less sensitive biomarker of alcohol abuse when used among females.

Ratio of Mitochondrial Aspartate Aminotransferase to Total Aspartate Aminotransferase (m-ASAT/t-ASAT)

The total ASAT activity in serum is comprised of two isoenzymes: one soluble (s-ASAT) and the other mitochondrial (m-ASAT).[102] Normally only a small portion of t-ASAT is accounted for by m-ASAT. It is the proportion of m-ASAT to t-ASAT that, when elevated, appears indicative of excessive alcohol use. An increased ratio of m-ASAT:t-ASAT has been found in chronic alcoholics with a sensitivity of up to 80%.[103,104] The ratio does not appear to be modified by acute alcohol consumption.[104] When studies are conducted on unselected populations, however, the sensitivity drops to 29%,[105] indicating that the m-ASAT:t-ASAT ratio is not suitable as a biomarker among those persons in the early stages of alcoholic disease. Speculation regarding the mechanism underlying the increased ratio include, first, the possibility that free fatty acids generated as a result of alcohol intake cause the mitochondria to swell, increasing the fragility of the membrane,[106] and, second, alcohol-induced m-ASAT synthesis.[107] The m-ASAT:t-ASAT ratio does not differentiate between alcoholics and patients with nonalcoholic steatohepatitis,[108] but is a relatively sensitive biomarker for alcoholics with liver damage.

In a study examining the efficacy of some of the newer biomarkers,[109] the authors concluded that although sensitivity of the m-ASAT:t-ASAT ratio among males was poor, among females it seemed almost nonexistent. The m-ASAT:t-ASAT normal cutoff points cited in the Nilssen et al. study reflect a slightly lower ratio for females. If there are additional gender differences, they have not yet been described.

Serum and Urinary Beta-Hexosaminidase (Hex-B)

The lysosomal enzyme Hex-B is one of a complex group of glycoprotein isoenzymes.[110] Blood serum contains a number of forms of hexosaminidase that can be separated and identified by isoelectric focusing.[110] Hex-B can be measured via a simple spectrophotometric method[111] or by immunoassay.[112]

Hex-B increases slightly with age.[113] It is also known to be elevated in patients with hyperthyroidism, Crohn's disease, myocardial infarction,[113,114] cholestasis,[115] and diabetes.[116] Hex-B has a biological half-life of 2–4 d.[117] The cause of Hex-B elevation in alcoholics may be the result of a decreased capacity of the nonparenchymal cells in the liver to clear the enzyme.[118]

It was noted in the Hultberg et al. study that Hex-B was a more sensitive marker of alcohol abuse than GGTP and ASAT.[117] Hultberg et al. speculated that since levels of Hex-B in control participants increased so little in response to acute alcohol challenge, the cause of the elevated Hex-B in alcoholics could be attributed to alcohol-associated liver damage, wherein the capacity of the nonparenchymal cells to clear the enzyme is decreased.[117]

Kärkkäinen compared urinary Hex (UHex) levels to serum Hex (SHex) levels and found UHex to be a more sensitive marker, in part because it remained elevated longer after initiation of abstinence.[119] In the all-male sample, UHex sensitivity was 81.3%, and SHex was 68.8%. When SHex, UHex, and GGTP values were combined, sensitivity rose to 93% and remained at 93% 7 d after admission to an inpatient treatment program. SHex, in another study of just males, seemed to be optimally responsive to recent alcohol consumption at moderate levels.[120]

During pregnancy, there is an increase in total Hex activity, with the peak increase occurring in the intermediate and Hex-B enzymes.[121,122] A possible cause for the increased activity may be, as mentioned earlier, a reduced function of the hepatic reticulo-endothelial system (RES), such that the nonparenchymal liver cells do not appropriately clear the enzymes from the serum.[123] Another possible reason for the elevation found during pregnancy is that of increased steroid levels that in turn trigger the release of the Hex enzymes.[124] The serum from females taking oral contraceptives reflects higher than normal Hex activity, similar to that observed during pregnancy.[125,126] As with dolichol levels, the variation in Hex-B associated with pregnancy limits its utility as a biomarker of alcohol abuse among women.

Other Enzyme Biomarkers

Alanine aminotransferase (ALAT), another of the hepatic enzymes, is frequently elevated in the serum of alcoholics.[32] It enters the bloodstream when hepatocyte damage contributes to liver cell membrane fragility,[127] thus its elevation can usually be attributed to liver damage. Babor et al.[128] found ALAT activity to be lower in both alcoholic and nonalcoholic females than in control group males. ALAT is sometimes used in conjunction with ASAT to form a ratio (ALAT:ASAT), which is computed to determine whether or not hepatic dysfunction is a consequence of alcohol abuse. If the ALAT:ASAT ratio is more than two, the indication is that alcohol-induced damage is likely.[22] Another enzyme marker, alkaline phosphatase (AFOS), is also located in the liver and measured in serum. It is elevated in alcoholics but does not respond to acute alcohol challenge.[129] Nonalcoholic liver disease can cause AFOS activity to increase, thus limiting its usefulness as an indication of excessive alcohol consumption. AFOS is also used in conjunction with GGTP activity to form the ratio GGTP:AFOS. As with the ALAT:ASAT ratio, this ratio is used to determine if liver damage is the result of alcohol abuse. A ratio of more than 1:4 is believed to be such an indication.[129] Also present in the liver, glutamate dehydrogenase (GDH) is a mitochondrial enzyme that, when elevated, indicates alcoholic liver cell necrosis;[130] although this association with necrosis was not replicated by Mills et al.[131] GDH does not seem to respond significantly to acute alcohol consumption.[132] Activity of GDH quickly returns to normal after initiation of abstinence.[133] Yet another enzyme, ornithine carbamoyl transferase (OCT), was elevated in 56% of the male alcoholic participants in a Konttinen et al. study;[134] an elevation thought to be the consequence of liver damage.[135] Finally, an enzyme associated with alcohol-induced myopathy, lactate dehydrogenase (LDH), is composed of several isoenzymes. The reactive levels of these isoenzymes change as a result of heavy alcohol consumption. Those isoenzymes most likely to change are LDH-1, LDH-2, and LDH-5 fractions.[136]

Typically, the normal limits of these enzymatic biomarkers are not broken down into gender-defined ranges, whereas GGTP norms usually are. This could be taken to indicate that, with the exception of GGTP, there are no significant gender differences in the activity of many of the hepatic enzymes. Or, it may simply reflect a lack of information.

Hematological Alterations

Mean Corpuscular Volume (MCV)

Mean corpuscular volume (MCV) is an indication of erythrocyte size. When MCV values are abnormally high, the condition is labeled macrocytosis.[137] The assessment of MCV is done by Coulter counter.

Even among alcoholics, MCV values are usually normal if there is no liver damage.[138] Yet, it appears that alcohol-related increased MCV is caused by an alcohol-induced aberration in the maturation of red blood cells in marrow.[139] Some research has indicated that MCV values increase concurrent with alcohol consumption, even at normal social levels of alcohol consumption.[140] However, these increases do not exceed the normal range of MCV values. Elevated MCV values are also associated with vitamin B12 and folic acid deficiency,[141] smoking,[142] and iron therapy.[143]

Barrison et al. observed that, in females, MCV seemed to be a more sensitive marker than among males, and that it correlated positively with GGTP, liver size, and previous levels of alcohol consumption.[144] In the Bhattacharya and Rake study,[138] MCV values were elevated in 90% of the female alcoholics with liver damage compared to a 65% elevation in male alcoholics with liver damage. In contrast to the Barrison et al. study,[144] Cushman et al.,[24] noted that although MCV was increased in 54% of their male alcoholic participants, only 27% of the female alcoholics had higher than normal values. In another study using female participants it was found that 48% of the female alcoholics had higher than normal values of MCV.[18] MCV values in females taking oral contraceptives are positively associated with age,[142] an association not evident in males nor in females not taking oral contraceptives. Finally, Nyström et al. found that MCV values were not significantly different for males drinking varying quantities of alcohol, however they were significantly higher for the female heavy drinkers.[126] Although females have not constituted the majority of participants in MCV studies, there have been some investigations, as noted earlier, designed to assess the link between MCV values and alcohol consumption specifically in women.

Other Hematological Parameters

Seppä et al.[145] conducted a study in which the Technicon H-1 analyzer was used to measure hematological parameters in three groups of middle-aged males: social drinkers, heavy drinkers, and alcoholics. Because the H-1 is available in a number of laboratories, Seppä et al. sought to determine if any of the hematological measures it was designed to assess could add to the sensitivity and specificity of MCV in detecting alcohol abuse.

It was found that MCV correlated significantly and positively with white blood cells and red blood cell distribution width, and negatively with red blood cells, hemoglobin (Hb) distribution width, Hb concentration (cell by cell), and measured Hb distribution width. The battery of hematological measures was insufficiently sensitive to identify heavy drinkers, but was somewhat more sensitive within the alcoholic group. For example, red blood cell distribution width had a sensitivity of 40.6%, the ratio of MCV:measured distribution width 17.1%, and the ratio MCV:erythrocytes 19.8%. The specificity of these measures is compromised in patients with pernicious anemia and vitamin B12 and folate deficiency. The incidence of pernicious anemia increases with age, thus limiting the specificity of these parameters in older age groups.[139]

Because MCV, as noted in the above review of MCV, is a more sensitive marker among females, the use of the H-1 hematological parameters might be a valuable approach in the identification of female alcoholics. This remains to be determined, however, because the Seppä et al. study did not include females.[145]

Condensation Products and/or Metabolic Products

Hemoglobin A1 Fraction (HbA1ach)

All but approx 6% of human hemoglobin is identified as simply hemoglobin A. The remaining hemoglobins have been identified, using cationic exchange resins and HPLC, as a series of glycosylated hemoglobin A molecules generally labeled as A1a-c,[146] and collectively referred to as the A1 fraction or "fast hemoglobins." Acetaldehyde, the first pass metabolite of alcohol, appears to elute with two minor hemoglobin fractions. The more sensitive of the two fractions to acetaldehyde has been named HbA1ach,[147] and falls close to the A1c subfraction. It is this subfraction that appears to be elevated in individuals who abuse alcohol,[148,149] thus contributing to the elevation of the overall A1 fraction. An additional technique for the detection of acetaldehyde-associated hemoglobin utilizes the immunogenic properties of the hemoglobin adducts by measuring the degree of reaction to antibodies[150] as detected by an enzyme-linked immunoabsorbent assay (ELISA).

Because glucose reacts with hemoglobin to form HbA1c, the subsequent increase in HbA1c has been used to monitor hyperglycemia in diabetic patients.[151] It was thought that HbA1ach could be used similarly to monitor alcohol consumption. In a study of male heavy drinkers ($n = 72$), a ratio of the subfraction HbA1ach to the subfraction HbA1c was computed and examined as a possible marker of alcohol consumption. The sensitivity of this ratio as a marker was 33%, as compared to 40% for GGTP and 24% for MCV.[147] The HbA1ach component appeared more useful as a marker of the early stages of alcohol abuse because it was not reliable in differentiating between heavy drinkers and alcoholics,[147] but could be used to distinguish heavy drinkers and alcoholics from light drinkers. When an individual is abstaining from alcohol, the half-life of the elevated total A1 fraction is approx 11 d.[148]

Regarding gender differences, it appears that the total A1 differences between alcoholic females ($n = 6$) and nonalcoholic females ($n = 18$) were greater than those found when comparing all alcoholics with all healthy controls.[148] However, there were no gender differences in the total A1 levels within the control group. Niemelä et al. conducted a study using 19 pregnant alcoholics.[152] Those participants who delivered infants with fetal alcohol effects (FAE) also had the highest levels of HbA1ach. The investigators stated that the use of HbA1ach as a biomarker of alcohol abuse could be further extended to monitor abstinence compliance, particularly among pregnant alcoholics. Although not directly relevant to the topic of gender differences in biomarkers of alcohol abuse, the authors also suggested that acetaldehyde may be implicated in the alcohol-associated fetal damage.

Whole Blood-Associated Acetaldehyde (WBAA); Hemoglobin-Associated Acetaldehyde (HbAA)

As acetaldehyde, the first pass metabolite of alcohol, enters the bloodstream, it is bound primarily to red blood cells (RBC).[153] More specifically, this binding occurs on the free amino group of N-terminal residues of hemoglobin.[154] The hemoglobin binding sites display a high affinity for acetaldehyde, whereas a lower affinity, higher capacity site exists on the protein-free supernatant, and is associated with the presence of free cysteine.[153] In addition to the measurement of acetaldehyde-induced hemoglobin subfractions, it is also possible to simply measure the amount of acetaldehyde bound to red blood cells or hemoglobin. The degree of acetaldehyde binding to RBC can be assessed by equilibrium dialysis.[155] The determination of hemoglobin-associated acetaldehyde (HbAA) or whole blood-associated acetaldehyde (WBAA) can be accomplished by fluorigenic HPLC.[156]

Hernandez-Munoz et al. noted that binding of acetaldehyde to the protein-free supernatant of RBC was higher in alcoholics than in controls.[157] This elevation persisted for up to 2 wk of withdrawal. It has been noted, however, that the oxidation of alcohol is not the only source of WBAA. Baraona et al. have established that intestinal overgrowth can provide a significant source of endogenous acetaldehyde.[158] Other causes for altered levels of HbAA include the ingestion of salicylic acid and sickle cell disease.[159]

Plasma- and hemoglobin-associated acetaldehyde (HbAA) were measured after a low dose of alcohol in teetotalers and alcoholics.[160] It appeared that elevated plasma acetaldehyde (PA) was the better indicator of acute alcohol consumption, whereas HbAA levels, which remained elevated above teetotaler levels 28 d into abstinence, was a better marker of chronic abuse. In discussing the results of their 1990 study, Peterson et al. stated that although HbAA levels could be used to distinguish alcoholics from social drinkers and teetotalers, they were not effective in separating social drinkers from teetotallers.[161]

Nathan et al. examined acetylated hemoglobin in several populations and found that values for pregnant females were elevated 1.9%, and for alcoholics 2.7%.[159] In newborns, HbAA levels have been found to range from 10–15%.[162] In the Nathan et al. study, there was an enormous amount of individual variation such that some of the nonalcoholic females had levels as high as those found in the alcoholic participants.[159] Turpenein et al.[163] stated that the reason for the high proportions of HbAA found in some nonalcoholic females was not yet known. They also mentioned the need for more data to establish age and gender norms.

One additional gender difference was observed in a study of mice in which the levels of whole blood-associated acetaldehyde (WBAA) were measured after alcohol consumption, and the levels then compared by gender. Female mice, when consuming more alcohol than males in proportion to their weight, had lower WBAA than males.[164] Further, female WBAA levels returned to baseline levels even while the mice were still consuming alcohol, whereas male WBAA levels remained elevated. The investigators stressed that the implications of this gender difference found in mice should be considered when investigating the use of WBAA as a biomarker of alcohol abuse among human females.

Blood Acetate

Alcohol is oxidized in the liver, where its metabolite, acetaldehyde, is metabolized to acetate,[165] which then enters the bloodstream. In the blood, acetate is oxidized to water and carbon dioxide by peripheral tissues.[166] Blood acetate concentration can be measured with a commercially available enzymatic test kit.[167]

The concentration of blood acetate is independent of blood alcohol level.[168] Levels of alcohol-induced acetate are controlled, in part, by the rate at which alcohol is metabolized in the liver.[169] Because alcoholics have developed a certain degree of metabolic tolerance that is demonstrated by a faster rate of alcohol metabolism, their blood acetate levels are higher than those of nondrinking individuals during alcohol oxidation.[170] Although small amounts of acetate can be formed endogenously in the gastrointestinal tract by microflora,[171] these levels of acetate should not approach those induced by alcohol ingestion.

In the Korri et al. study, no gender differences were observed for either the control or alcoholic group.[168] Sensitivity for both genders combined was

65% for alcoholics. It should be noted that as a marker of alcohol abuse, blood acetate can be used only during those times when the liver is actually oxidizing alcohol.

Urinary Salsolinol

Salsolinol is a condensation product of acetaldehyde, which is the first pass metabolite of alcohol, and dopamine.[172] It can, however, be formed endogenously independent of alcohol ingestion, and is also present in many foods[173] and drinks, one of which is beer.[174] Salsolinol can be detected in urine using a single-isotope radioenzymatic assay.[173]

Salsolinol has been found to be elevated in males after long-term moderate levels of alcohol consumption.[175] It has also been observed to increase transiently following acute bouts of alcohol ingestion and is highly correlated with blood acetaldehyde levels.[176]

Some investigators have postulated that dopamine alkaloids, such as salsolinol, contribute to the development of alcohol addiction.[177] Indeed, rats given intracerebral injections of salsolinol seem to display an increased preference for alcohol in a free choice paradigm.[178] Some alcoholics, both chronic and abstinent, with low monoamine oxidase (MAO) activity also have high urinary levels of salsolinol.[173] Because MAO activity is thought to be, at least in part, genetically determined,[179] and low MAO activity is associated with alcoholism,[180] it is possible that elevated salsolinol levels may, for example, be present in children of alcoholics, and utilized as a marker for increased risk for the development of alcoholism.

In one of the few studies to include females,[181] levels of urinary salsolinol were higher in female social drinkers than in males 3 h after alcohol ingestion. This gender difference was not evident in the 90-min postingestion sample. The authors suggested that the difference may reflect the fact that identical quantities of salsolinol were ingested by both males and females via salsolinol-rich foods, however differences in body mass were not taken into account. Apart from this single study, no other significant gender differences have been noted with regard to salsolinol levels and alcohol abuse.

Beta-Carbolines

Beta-carbolines are naturally occurring compounds that can be found in plants, foods, wine, and beer.[182] They possess a number of neurochemical properties, such as the blockade of catecholamine uptake systems, the inhibition of serotonin, the inhibition of monoamine oxidase,[183] and the antagonism of benzodiazepine receptor binding.[182] Measurement of beta-carbolines can be carried out by HPLC with fluorescence detection.[184]

Beta-carbolines can be formed endogenously by a reaction between an indole ethylamine and either puruvic acid or acetaldehyde.[185] Because acetaldehyde is a metabolic product of alcohol oxidation, the possibility exists that acetaldehyde reacts with the indole, serotonin, to form beta-carboline. In a recent series of studies, it was demonstrated that alcoholics excrete higher amounts of the urinary beta-carboline, harmon, than nonalcholics.[186,187] Rommelspacher et al. noted an association between patients with elevated beta-carboline levels and first-time consumption of alcohol, as well as number of first-degree alcoholic relatives.[186] In another study involving ethanol-loading of nonalcoholic participants, it was found that harmon increased in erythrocytes after alcohol ingestion.[188] Further observations in a subsequent study seemed to indicate that the beta-carboline increase was not state-dependent on the presence of alcohol, but may be more the consequence of some chronic alcohol-induced metabolic changes.[189] Although many of the studies included female participants, no gender-specific data were provided.

Urinary Ethanol, Ethanol Conjugates, and Acetaldehyde Conjugates

Tang et al. speculated that if stable acetaldehyde-protein adducts are formed as a result of alcohol consumption, eventually these adducts would be excreted in urine.[190] Subsequently, it was found that this was indeed the case.[191,192] It was observed that urinary levels of free ethanol, ethanol conjugates, and acetaldehyde conjugates were higher in abstaining alcoholics than in controls. Sensitivity for correctly classifying alcoholics on d 1 of hospital admission was 100%, and subsequently dropped to 91% 14 d after onset of abstention.

Measuring free ethanol and acetaldehyde conjugates is accomplished by gas chromatographic chemical ionization mass spectrometric (GC/MS) method.[192] There are other factors, such as nutrition and smoking, that may influence levels of acetaldehyde in the body.[84] If there were gender differences noticed in any of the abovementioned studies, they were not mentioned.

2,3-Butanediol, 1,2-Propanediol

Butanediol and propanediol are short chain, low-mol-mass diols. There seems to be a relationship between diol formation and carbohydrate metabolism, as well as formation subsequent to the metabolization of acetone.[193,194] Both diols can be measured by gas-liquid chromatography–mass spectrometry.[195]

These diols are elevated in alcoholic cirrhosis,[196] although there have been conflicting reports regarding the effects of abstinence and the presence of liver disease.[195] It is speculated that the presence of these compounds in the serum of alcoholics is indicative of an alteration in the metabolic pathway in response to prolonged excessive alcohol consumption.[197] Diols are the substrates for liver alcohol dehydrogenase,[198] and it has been postulated that competition with alcohol for degradation by alcohol dehydrogenase contributes to the increased concentration of diols.[199] Sysfontes et al.[195] were the only investigators to indicate the use of female participants, however the data were not reported separately by gender.

Plasma Levels of Alpha-amino-n-butyric Acid (AANB)

AANB is an amino acid found in the bloodstream. Diabetic ketoacidosis and consumption of carbohydrate-poor diets can cause an increase in plasma AANB.[200,201] The assay is rather difficult in that it requires the use of an amino acid analyzer.[202]

Long-term alcohol abuse is associated with high plasma levels of AANB.[203] The use of the AANB:leucine ratio was proposed to take advantage of the fact that the concentrations of both substances are decreased as a result of protein deficiency, but only AANB is increased as the result of alcohol abuse.[204,205] However, Ellingboe et al. speculated that the ratio values were the consequence of liver damage that may or may not be related to excessive alcohol consumption, and therefore were not always indicative of alcohol abuse.[206] Shaw et al. found AANB, used in combination with GGTP, to be useful in detecting episodes of relapse drinking.[207] Very few studies have included female participants, therefore there is little knowledge regarding possible gender differences.

Glycoproteins

Carbohydrate Deficient Transferrin (CDT)

Transferrin is a heterogeneous glycoprotein that is synthesized and metabolized primarily in the liver.[208] It serves as a vehicle for the transport of iron to cells throughout the body and also regulates blood plasma iron concentration.[209] There are three genetic types of transferrin found in humans: B, C, and D.[208] Each of the three main forms and their subtypes can be identified by determination of their isoelectric point (pI). Type C is the most common form of transferrin, with a pI that ranges from 5.2–5.7. In alcoholics, a variant of the normal type C transferrin appears in a band with a pI of 5.7, which differs from the main transferrin component by a pH of 0.3.[210] This variant is characterized by a deficiency in the terminal trisaccharide, which contains N-acetylglucosamine, galactos, and sialic acid.[211] The variant is sometimes referred to as desialylated transferrin as well as carbohydrate deficient transferrin (CDT) The procedure for determining CDT involves the isocratic anion-exchange chromatography of serum at pH 5.65 and a subsequent transferrin radioimmune assay.[212]

The sensitivity of CDT as a biomarker of alcohol abuse ranges from 79–93% and its specificity is usually above 95%.[212-215] A minimum alcohol intake of 60–80 g/d seems to be necessary to cause an increase in CDT values.[216] As well, there are indications that CDT is more sensitive to binge drinking than steady moderate consumption.[217] Kwoh-Gain et al. observed that there was no correlation between CDT values and severity of liver disease.[215] Drugs, such as opiates, other analgesics, sedatives, antiepileptics, and hormones, do not appear to be associated with changes in CDT values.[216]

Nyström et al. examined the efficacy of CDT as a biomarker of alcohol abuse among young university students.[126] Previous findings that CDT values were significantly higher in females than in males were confirmed in the Nyström et al. study. In this same study, however, the sensitivity of CDT among female heavy drinkers ($n = 7$) was 0%. CDT sensitivity was also low for young male university students, at 21%. Although the researchers reported a significant positive correlation between alcohol consumption and serum CDT, they stated that the use of CDT could not be recommended as a biomarker for early stages of alcohol abuse among young females.

Females, in a study by Stibler et al., had significantly higher CDT values than males.[218] Amounts of CDT in females taking oral contraceptives ($n = 48$) were within the normal range,[218] as well as those CDT values from the five pregnant nonalcoholic participants. CDT was elevated in 83% of female alcoholics with a recent history of alcohol abuse in a Stibler et al. study.[219] This level of sensitivity exceeded that of GGTP (59%), ASAT (50%), and ALAT (47%); but not MCV (91%). The higher figure for MCV may have been a reflection of the high percentage of smokers among the female alcoholics. False positives can be caused by the presence of primary biliary cirrhosis[220] and uncommon genetic D-variants of transferrin.[221] In Kapur et al.[214] and Stibler et al.[212] a number of false positives were found in elderly women whose medical diagnoses and drug treatments were varied and unrelated.

The proportion of female participants in CDT-related alcohol research has been more commensurate with the need for reasonable representation. With reference to young females, it appears that although CDT levels are not increased by pregnancy, nor are they raised by the use of oral contraceptives, they are also unresponsive to the early stages of alcohol abuse.

Ferritin

Ferritin is a protein that is the source of intracellular iron, and is present in serum in proportion to the amount of iron stored in the body.[222] In addition to chronic alcohol consumption, hemochromatosis, liver disease, cancer, and inflammatory diseases are all associated with an increased concentration of serum ferritin.[223–225]

Serum ferritin exists in several forms, and this microheterogeneity appears to be associated with the presence of sialic acid residues.[225] The microheterogeneity of serum ferritin can be determined by isoelectric focusing in polyacrylamide gel cylinders.[226] Serum ferritin can be measured by an immunoradiometric assay.[227] Ferritin concanavalin A is glycosylated and is measured by incubation of serum with concanavalin A-sepharose 4B.[228]

In the 1991 Moirand et al. study, it was observed that total serum ferritin was elevated in chronic alcoholics.[227] The investigators tentatively attributed this increase to an increased secretion of glycosylated ferritin. The sensitivity of ferritin ranges from 40–70%.[74,224,227] Although ferritin is elevated in chronic alcoholics, Bliding et al. found no association between ferritin and actual quantity of alcohol consumption among the male participants.[23] Females were included in the Moirand et al. study, however data were not analyzed by gender.[227]

Combination Measures

It has been suggested that a combination of the various laboratory tests might improve both sensitivity and specificity. However, a shortcoming of all test combination protocols is that there will still be an overlap between alcoholic and nonalcoholic sampling distributions; such that if sensitivity levels are high, specificity is likely to be low, and if specificity is high, sensitivity suffers.[32] Nevertheless, numerous studies have been conducted assessing the efficacy of various combinations of biomarkers.

Using discriminant function analysis, Chalmers et al. found that of the eight original laboratory measures taken in their study, MCV, log10GGTP, and log10AFOS provided the best discrimination for alcohol abuse.[229] Sensitivity for females was 92%, and for males 80%. Specificity was 100% for both females and males.

In 1982, Ryback et al. ran a quadratic multiple discriminant analysis on 25 commonly used laboratory tests.[230] This discriminant approach was relatively accurate in that it correctly identified 98% of the alcoholism treatment program patients. There were no females in this study.

Seven hematological and 20 serum biochemical parameters were examined in a 1982 study by Beresford et al.[231] Seven variables were identified by linear discriminant analysis as criteria for separation of alcoholics from nonalcoholics. The seven variables included log10urea nitrogen, ASAT, log10LDH, log10uric acid, log10total bilirubin, MCV, and creatinine. The sensitivity of these measures was 79%, and specificity was 80%. Although the study included both females and males, no gender differences were mentioned.

Also in 1982, Bliding et al.[23] ran a linear discriminant analysis on seven commonly used laboratory tests: APO AI, asparagine, aminotransferase, ALAT, GGTP, and MCV. No single laboratory test reliably discriminated between light and heavy drinkers, however the discriminant approach improved sensitivity somewhat to 54%. There were no female participants in this study.

A subsequent study also employed seven markers: GGTP, MCV, HDLC, ASAT, BAL, serum glutamic pyruvic transaminase (SGPT), and AFOS, with a consequent sensitivity of 71% in females and 82% in males. If the combination tests were limited to just GGTP, ASAT, and MCV, sensitivity was 61% in females and 72% in males.[24] The single gender difference noted in this study was that MCV values were lower in females than in males.

In another combination study GGTP, ALAT, ASAT, MCV, and creatinine were combined in various ways to maximize both sensitivity and specificity.[32] When the results of two or more of an individual's tests were beyond the decision limit set for each biomarker, the individual was classified as alcoholic. The sensitivity of this method was 85% and the specificity, 64%. Only males participated in this study.

A survey of 7735 middle-aged men was conducted by Shaper et al.[232] Alcohol consumption was assessed by an alcohol consumption questionnaire and 25 biochemical and hematological measurements. Five variables (GGTP, HDLC, urate, mean corpuscular hemoglobin, and lead) were combined to provide a composite discriminant score that was the criterion for separation of light drinkers from heavy drinkers. Sensitivity using this criterion was 41%, and specificity was 97.5%.

Hillers et al. ran a quadratic discriminant analysis on selected combinations of 33 common blood chemistry tests.[233] Their intent was not only to distinguish between alcoholics and nonalcoholics, but also to discriminate between levels of alcohol consumption. After 27 d of abstinence, a quadratic discriminant analysis of 24 of the blood tests correctly classified 92% of the alcoholics. The study did not include females.

Using 31 common laboratory tests, Chan et al. found that a combination of urea nitrogen (UN), potassium, and MCV seemed to be the most significant variables in identifying abusers of alcohol.[234] Sensitivity was 89%, and specificity was 92%. The only gender differences noted were that UN and potassium levels were appreciably higher in males than in females.

In a study of only female participants, Hollstedt and Dahlgren observed that by combining MCV, thrombocyte, ASAT, GGTP, and albumin measures, 75% of the female alcoholics were correctly classified.[18] Urate and triglycerides did not add to the discriminant power of the other five variables. When each biomarker was considered individually, MCV was the most sensitive at 48%. This relatively high sensitivity may be a consequence of the sensitizing effect smoking has on alcohol-induced changes in MCV.[235] Using only three variables, MCV, GGTP, and albumin, sensitivity was 73%.

Vanclay et al. undertook a discriminant analysis of a range of biochemical and hematological tests taken by an extended Multiple Biochemical Analysis as well as weight, smoking status, and systolic blood pressure.[236] Sensitivity for this community sample was 78%, and specificity was 87.2%. This was a males-only study.

Finally, the Svalbard study included 310 males and 171 females.[109] The biomarkers examined were CDT, GGTP, and mAST. The mAST measure was judged unsuitable for general population assessment, whereas CDT seemed most discriminating at lower alcohol intake levels, and GGTP discriminated best at higher levels. CDT was slightly better at discriminating male heavy drinkers, particularly those drinkers falling in the 95th percentile for quantity consumed. The authors concluded that, overall, the three biomarkers appeared to be of limited value as screening techniques in females.

Conclusion

After an extensive review of the literature on biomarkers of alcohol abuse, it is evident that although numerous studies have included females, far more studies were conducted using only male participants. When data from both genders were collected, the investigators frequently did not analyze or report the results by gender. Two factors may have contributed to the decision not to analyze results separately: Female sample sizes were considered too small to analyze separately, and/or there were no observable gender differences, hence no reason to do separate analyses. Any attempt to describe the gender differences in biomarkers of alcohol abuse is constrained by the relative paucity of information available on females. It is this gender-related informational imbalance that may be the most compelling of the gender differences. Until this artifactual difference is addressed, the biological-based gender differences in alcohol abuse cannot be accurately assessed.

References

[1]S. Blume (1986) Women and alcohol. A review. *JAMA* **256,** 1460–1470.

[2]M. Arthur, A. Lee, and R. Wright (1984) Sex differences in the metabolism of ethanol and acetaldehyde in normal subjects. *Clin. Sci.* **67,** 397–401.

[3]M. Frezza, C. DiPadova, G. Pozzato, M. Terpin, E. Baraona, and C. Lieber (1990) High blood alcohol levels in women: The role of decreased gastric alcohol dehydrogenase activity and first-pass metabolism. *N. Engl. J. Med.* **322,** 95–99.

[4]C. Harper, N. Smith, and J. Kvil (1990) The effects of alcohol on the female brain: A neuropathological study. *Alcohol Alcohol.* **25,** 445–448.

[5]B. Ober and R. Stillman (1988) Memory in chronic alcoholics: effects of inconsistent versus consistent information. *Addict. Behav.* **13,** 11–15.

[6]B. Jones and M. Jones (1976) Alcohol effects in women during the menstrual cycle. *Ann. NY Acad. Science* **272,** 576–587.

[7]D. Van Thiel, and J. Gavaler (1988) Ethanol metabolism and hepatotoxicity: Does sex make a difference? in *Recent Developments in Alcoholism.* M. Galanter, ed. Plenum, New York, pp. 291–304.

[8]N. Piazza, J. Vrbka, and R. Yeager (1989) Telescoping of alcoholism in women alcoholics. *Int. J. Addict.* **24,** 19–28.

[9]E. Morrisey and M. Schuckit (1978) Stressful life events and alcohol problems among women seen at a detoxification center. *J. Stud. Alcohol* **39,** 1559–1576.

[10]G. Perodeau (1984) Married alcoholic women: A review. *J. Drug Issues* **14,** 703–719.

[11]M. Schuckit (1986) Genetic and clinical complications of alcoholism and affective disorder. *Am. J. Psych.* **143,** 140–147.

[12]J. Gavaler (1985) Effects of alcohol on endocrine function in postmenopausal women: A review. *J. Stud. Alcohol* **46,** 495–516.

[13]N. K. Mello (1988) Effects of alcohol abuse on reproductive function in women, in *Recent Developments in Alcoholism.* M. Galanter, ed. Plenum, New York, pp. 253–276.

[14]C. Ernhart, R. Sokol, S. Martier, P. Moron, D. Nadler, J. Ager, and A. Wolf (1987) Alcohol teratogenicity in the human: A detailed assessment of specificity, critical period, and threshold. *Am. J. Obstet. Gynecol.* **156,** 33–39.

[15]C. Ernhart, M. Morrow-Tlucak, R. Sokol, and D. Martier (1988) Underreporting of alcohol use during pregnancy. *Alcohol. Clin. Exp. Res.* **12,** 506–511.

[16]N. Robles and N. Day (1990) Recall of alcohol consumption during pregnancy. *J. Stud. Alcohol* **51,** 403–407.

[17]M. Morrow-Tlucak, C. Ernhart, R. Sokol, S. Martier, and J. Ager (1989) Underreporting of alcohol use in pregnancy: Relationship to alcohol problem history. *Alcohol. Clin. Exp. Res.* **13,** 399–401.

[18]C. Hollstedt and L. Dahlgren (1987) Peripheral markers in the female "hidden alcoholic." *Acta Psychiatr. Scand.* **75,** 591–596.

[19]C. Hollstedt, L. Dahlgren, and U. Ryberg (1983) Outcome of pregnancy in women treated in an alcoholic clinic. *Acta Psychiatr. Scand.* **67,** 236–248.

[20]M. Serdula, P. Williamson, J. Kendrick, R. Anda, and T. Byers (1991) Trends in alcohol consumption by pregnant women. *JAMA* **265,** 876–879.

[21]R. Sokol and S. Bottoms (1989) Practical screening for risk-drinking during pregnancy, in *Diagnosis of Alcohol Abuse.* R. R. Watson, ed. CRC, Boca Raton, FL, pp. 252–260.

[22]M. Salaspuro (1987) Use of enzymes for the diagnosis of alcohol related organ damage, *Enzyme* **37,** 87–107.

[23]G. Bliding, A. Bliding, G. Fex, and C. Tornqvist (1982) The appropriateness of laboratory tests in tracing young heavy drinkers. *Drug Alcohol Dependence* **10,** 153–158.

[24]P. Cushman, G. Jacobson, J. Barboriak, and A. Anderson (1984) Biochemical markers for alcoholism: Sensitivity problems. *Alcohol. Clin. Exp. Res.* **8,** 253–257.

[25]A. Parodi and L. Leloir (1979) The role of lipid intermediates in the glycosylation of proteins in the eucaryotic cell. *Biochim. Biophys. Acta* **559,** 1–37.

[26]U. Turpeinen (1986) Liquid-chromatographic determination of dolichols in urine. *Clin. Chem.* **32,** 2026–2029.

[27]R. Roine (1987) Effects of moderate drinking and alcohol abstinence on urinary dolichol levels. *Alcohol* **5,** 229–231.

[28]R. Roine, U. Turpeinen, R. Ylikahri, and M. Salaspuro (1987) Urinary dolichol— A new marker of alcoholism. *Alcohol. Clin. Exp. Res.* **11,** 525–527.

[29]M. Salaspuro, U. Korri, H. Nuutinen, and R. Roine (1987) Blood acetate and urinary dolichols—new markers of heavy drinking and alcoholism, in *Genetics and Alcoholism.* Int. Titisee Symposium, Liss, New York, pp. 231–240.

[30]R. Roine, R. Ylikahri, P. Koskinen, A. Suokas, J. Hamalainen, and M. Salaspuro (1987) Effect of heavy weekend drinking on urinary dolichol levels. *Alcohol* **4,** 509–511.

[31]F. Stetter, H. Gaertner, G. Wiatr, K. Mann, and U. Breyer-Pfaff (1991) Urinary dolichol—A doubtful marker of alcoholism. *Alcohol. Clin. Exp. Res.* **15,** 938–941.

[32]D. Stamm, E. Hansert, and W. Feuerlein (1984) Detection and exclusion of alcoholism in men on the basis of clinical laboratory findings. *J. Clin. Chem. Clin. Biochem.* **22,** 79–96.

[33]R. Pullarkat and S. Raguthu (1985) Elevated urinary dolichol levels in chronic alcoholics. *Alcohol. Clin. Exp. Res.* **9,** 28–30.

[34]T. Chojuacki and G. Dallner (1988) The biological role of dolichol. *Biochem. J.* **251,** 1–9.

[35]L. Wolfe, N. Ng Ying Kin, J. Palo, and M. Haltia (1982) Raised levels of cerebral cortex dolichols in Alzheimer's disease. *Lancet* **ii,** 99.

[36]N. Ng Ying Kin, J. Palo, M. Haltia, and L. Wolfe (1983) High levels of brain dolichols in neuronal ceroid-lipofuscinosis and senescence. *J. Neurochem.* **40,** 1465–1473.

[37]C. Witcop Jr., L. Wolfe, S. Cal, J. White, D. Townsend, and K. Keenan (1987) Elevated urinary dolichol excretions in the Hermansky-Pudlak syndrome. *Am. J. Med.* **82,** 463–470.

[38]R. Pullarkat, S. Raguthu, and S. Pachchagiri (1984) Dolichols in metastatic cancer. *Am. Soc. Neurochem.* **15,** 171.

[39]R. Pullarkat and H. Reha (1982) Accumulation of dolichols in brains of elderly. *J. Biol. Chem.* **257,** 5591–5593.

[40]R. Roine, K. Humaloja, J. Hamalainen, R. Nykanen, R. Ylikahri, and M. Salapuro (1989) Significant increases in urinary dolichol levels in bacterial infections, malignancies and pregnancy but not in other clinical conditions. *Ann. Med.* **21,** 13–16.

[41]L. Wolfe, J. Palo, P. Santavuori, F. Andermann, E. Andermann, J. Jacob, and E. Kolodny (1986) Urinary sediment dolichols in the diagnosis of neuronal ceroid-lipofuscinosis. *Ann. Neurol.* **19,** 270–274.

[42]R. Roine, T. Heinonen, K. Salmela, E. Hlikkonen, A. Suokas, O. Luurila, P. Koskinen, J. Palo, and M. Salaspuro (1991) Strenuous physical activity, aspirin and heat stress increase urinary dolichols. Evidence for lysosomal origin of urinary dolichols. *Clin. Chim. Acta* **204,** 13–22.

[43]R. Roine, I. Nykanen, R. Ylikahri, J. Heikkila, A. Suokas, and M. Salaspuro (1989) Effect of alcohol on blood dolichol concentration. *Alcohol. Clin. Exp. Res.* **13,** 519–522.

[44]G. Elmberger and P. Engfeldt (1985) Distribution of dolichol in human and rabbit blood. *Acta Chem. Scand. [B]* **39,** 323–325.

[45]G. Norris and R. Pullarkat (1987) A micromethod for the estimation of blood dolichol. *Lipids* **22,** 58–60.

[46]K. Yamada, H. Yokohama, S. Abe, K. Katayama, and T. Sato (1985) High performance liquid chromatographic method for the determination of dolichols in tissues and plasma. *Analyt. Biochem.* **150,** 26–31.

[47]E. Nikkila, T. Kuusi, and M. Taskinen (1982) Role of lipoprotein lipase and hepatic endothelial lipase in the metabolism of high density lipoproteins: A novel concept on cholesterol transport in HDL cycle, in *Metabolic Risk Factors in Ischemic CV Disease*. B. Pernow and C. Carlson, eds. Raven, New York, pp. 205–215.

[48]N. Miller, O. Forde, D. Thelle, and O. Mjos (1977) The Tromso Heart Study. High density lipoproteins and coronary heart disease. *Lancet* 1, 965–967.

[49]N. Miller, F. Hammet, S. Saltissi, S. Rao, H. Van Zeller, J. Colthart, and B. Lewis (1981) Relation of angiographically defined coronary artery disease to plasma lipoprotein subfractions and apolipoproteins. *Br. Med. J.* 282, 1741–1744.

[50]C. Laurell (1972) Composition and variation of the gel electrophoretic fractions of plasma, cerebrospinal fluid and urine. *Scand. J. Clin. Lab. Invest.* 29, 124.

[51]G. Warnick, J. Benderson, and J. Albers (1982) Quantification of high density subclasses after separation by dextran sulfate and Mg^{2+} precipitation. *Clin. Chem.* 28, 1574.

[52]J. Barboriak, G. Jacobson, P. Cushman, R. Herrington, R. Lipo, M. Daley, and A. Anderson (1980) Chronic alcohol abuse and high density lipoprotein cholesterol. *Alcohol. Clin. Exp. Res.* 4, 346–349.

[53]B. Danielsson, R. Ekman, G. Fex, G. Johansson, H. Kristensson, P. Nilsson-Ehle, and J. Wadstein (1978) Changes in plasma high density lipoproteins in chronic male alcoholics during and after abuse. *Scand. J. Clin. Lab. Invest.* 38, 113–119.

[54]J. Kuusi, P. Kinnumen, and E. Nikkila (1979) Hepatic endothelial lipase antiserum influences rat plasma low and high density lipoproteins in vivo. *FEBS Lett.* 104, 384–388.

[55]M. Valimaki, E. Nikkila, M. Taskinen, and R. Ylikahri (1986) Rapid decrease in high density lipoprotein subfractions and postheparin plasma lipase activities after cessation of chronic alcohol intake. *Atherosclerosis* 59, 147–153.

[56]P. Wood and W. Haskell (1979) The effects of exercise on plasma high density lipoproteins. *Lipid* 14, 417–422.

[57]C. Glueck, R. Fallat, F. Millet, and P. Garside (1975) Familial hyperalphalipoproteinemia: Studies in eighteen kindreds. *Metabolism* 24, 1243–1250.

[58]P. Durrington (1979) Effects of phenobarbitone on plasma apolipoprotein B and plasma high-density lipoprotein cholesterol in normal subjects. *Clin. Sci.* 56, 501–506.

[59]P. Devenyi, G. Robinson, B. Kapur, and D. Roncari (1981) High density lipoprotein cholesterol in male alcoholics with and without liver disease. *Am. J. Med.* 71, 589–594.

[60]H. Bell, J. Stromme, H. Steensland, and J. Bache-Wiig (1985) Plasma-HDL-cholesterol and estimated ethanol consumption in 104 patients with alcohol dependence syndrome. *Alcohol Alcohol.* 20, 35–40.

[61]G. Hartung, J. Foreyt, R. Mitchell, J. Mitchell, R. Reeves, and A. Gotto (1983) Effect of alcohol intake on high-density lipoprotein cholesterol levels in runners and inactive men. *JAMA* 249, 747–750.

[62]G. Hartung, R. Reeves, J. Foreyt, W. Patsch, and A. Gotto (1986) Effect of alcohol intake and exercise on plasma high-density lipoprotein cholesterol subfractions and apolipoprotein A-1 in women. *Am. J. Cardiol.* 58, 148–151.

[63]A. Suenram, W. McConathy, and P. Alaupovic (1978) Evidence for the lipoprotein heterogeneity of human plasma high density lipoproteins isolated by three different procedures. *Lipids* 15, 505–511.

[64]J. Fruchart, C. Fievet, and P. Puchois (1985) Apo-lipoproteins, in *Methods of Enzymatic Analysis*, vol. 8. H. Bergmeyer, J. Bergmeyer, and M. Grabl, eds. VCH, Weinheim, pp. 126–137.

[65]C. Camargo Jr., P. Williams, K. Vranizan, J. Albers, and P. Wood (1985) The effect of moderate alcohol intake on serum apolipoprotein A-I and A-II. *JAMA* **253,** 2854–2857.

[66]P. Sistonen and C. Ehnholm (1980) On the heritability of serum high density lipoprotein in twins. *Am. J. Hum. Genet.* **32,** 107.

[67]J. Fruchart, I. Kora, C. Cachera, V. Clavey, and Y. Moschetto (1982) Simultaneous measurement of plasma apolipoprotiens A-I and B by electroimmunoassay. *Clin. Chem.* **28,** 59–62.

[68]P. Puchois, M. Fontan, J. Gentilini, P. Gelez, and J. Fruchart (1984) Serum apolipoprotein A-II, a biochemical indicator of alcohol abuse. *Clin. Chim. Acta* **185,** 185–189.

[69]B. Pileire, J. Bredent-Bangou, and M. Valentino (1991) Comparison of questionnaire and biochemical markers to detect alcohol abuse in a West Indian population. *Alcohol Alcohol.* **26,** 353–358.

[70]I. Puddey, J. Masarei, R. Vandongen, and L. Berlin (1986) Serum apolipoprotein A-II as a marker of change in alcohol intake in heavy drinkers. *Alcohol Alcohol.* **21,** 375–383.

[71]C. Van Gent, A. Van Der Voort, and L. Hessl (1978) High density lipoprotein and cholesterol. Monthly variation and association with cardiovascular risk factors in 1,000 forty-year-old Dutch citizens. *Clin. Chim. Acta* **88,** 155–162.

[72]M. Nishimura and R. Teschke (1983) Alcohol and gamma-glutamyltransferase. *Klin. Wochenschr.* **61,** 265–275.

[73]H. Gjerde and J. Morland (1985) Determination of gamma glutamyl transferase in completely haemolyzed blood samples. *Scand. J. Clin. Lab. Invest.* **45,** 661–664.

[74]J. Chick, J. Pikkarainen, and M. Plant (1987) Serum ferritin as a marker of alcohol consumption in working men. *Alcohol Alcohol.* **22,** 75–77.

[75]L. Papoz, J. Warnet, G. Pequignot, E. Eschwege, J. Claude, and D. Schwartz (1981) Alcohol consumption in a healthy population: Relationship to gamma-glutamyl transferase activity and mean corpuscular volume. *JAMA* **245,** 1748–1751.

[76]H. Kristenson and E. Trell (1982) Indicators of alcohol consumption: Comparisons between a questionnaire (Mn-MAST), interviews and serum gamma-glutamyl transferase (GGT) in a health survey of middle-aged males. *Br. J. Addict.* **77,** 297–304.

[77]S. B. Rosalki (1984) Identifying the alcoholic, in *Clinical Biochemistry of Alcoholism.* S. B. Rosalki, ed. Churchill Livingston, New York, pp. 65–92.

[78]M. Nishimura, H. Stein, B. Wilhem, and R. Teschke (1981) Gamma-glutamyl transferase activity of liver plasma membrane: Induction following chronic alcohol consumption. *Biochem. Biophys. Res. Comm.* **99,** 142–148.

[79]S. Moussavian, R. Becker, J. Piepmeyer, E. Mezey, and R. Bozian (1985) Serum gamma-glutamyl transpeptidase and chronic alcoholism. *Dig. Dis. Sci.* **30,** 211–214.

[80]G. Lum and S. Gambino (1972) Serum gamma-glutamyl transpeptidase activity as an indicator of disease of liver, pancreas, or bone. *Clin. Chem.* **18,** 358–362.

[81]L. Ewen and J. Griffiths (1973) Gamma-glutamyl transpeptidase elevated activities in certain neurological diseases. *Am. J. Clin. Pathol.* **59,** 2–9.

[82]A. Rutenberg, J. Goldbarg, and E. Pineda (1963) Serum gamma-glutamyl transpeptidase activity in hepatobiliary pancreatic disease. *Gastroenterology* **45,** 43–45.

[83]K. Ravens, S. Gudbjarnson, C. Cowan, and R. Bing (1969) Gamma-glutamyl-transpeptidase in myocardial infarction. Clinical and experimental studies. *Circulation* **39,** 693–700.

[84]S. Harada, D. Agarwal, and H. Goedde (1989) Biochemical and hematological markers of alcoholism, in *Alcoholism.* S. Harada and D. Agarwal, eds. Pergamon, NY, pp. 238–254.

[85]J. Persson, P. Magnusson, and S. Borg (1990) Serum gamma-glutamyl transferase (GGT) in a group of organized teetotalers. *Alcohol* **6,** 87–89.

[86]E. Arnesen, N. Huseby, T. Bren, and K. Try. (1986) The Tromsø Heart Study: Distribution of, and determinants for, gamma glutamyltransferase in a free living population. *Scand. J. Clin. Lab. Invest.* **46,** 63–70.

[87]Whitfield, J., Hensley, W., Bryden, D., and Gallagher, H. (1978) Effects of age and sex on biochemical responses to drinking habits. *Med. J. Aust.* **22,** 629–632.

[88]G. Larsson, C. Ottenblad, L. Hagenfeldt, A. Larrson, and M. Forsgren (1983) Evaluation of serum gamma-glutamyl transferase as a screening method for excessive alcohol consumption during pregnancy. *Am. J. Obstet. Gynecol.* **147,** 654–657.

[89]O. Ylikorkala, U. Stenman, and E. Halmesmaki (1987) Gamma-glutamyl transferase and mean cell volume reveal maternal alcohol abuse and fetal alcohol effects. *Am. J. Obstet. Gynecol.* **157,** 344–348.

[90]E. Arnesen, N. Huseby, T. Brenn, and K. Try (1986) The Tromsø Heart Study: Distribution of, and determinants for, gamma glutamyltransferase in a free living population. *Scand. J. Clin. Lab. Invest.* **46,** 63–70.

[91]O. Nilssen, O. Forde, and T. Brenn (1990) The Tromso study: Distribution and population determinants of gamma-glutamyl transferase. *Am. J. Epidemiol.* **132,** 318–326.

[92]F. Schiele, A. Guilmin, H. Detienne, and G. Siest (1977) Gamma-glutamyltransferase activity in plasma: Statistical distributions, individual variations, and reference intervals. *Clin. Chem.* **23,** 1023–1028.

[93]H. Teranishi, H. Kagamiyama, K. Teranishi, H. Wada, T. Yamano, and Y. Morino (1978) Cystolic and mitochondrial isozymes of glutamate-oxaloacetic transaminase from human heart. *J. Biol. Chem.* **253,** 8842–8847.

[94]M. Devgun, J. Dunbar, J. Hagart, B. Martin, and S. Ogston (1985) Effects of acute and varying amounts of alcohol consumption on alkaline phosphatase, aspartate transaminase, and gamma-glutamyltransferase. *Alcohol. Clin. Exp. Res.* **9,** 235–237.

[95]H. Ishii, F. Okuno, Y. Shegeta, and M. Tsuchuja (1979) Enhanced serum glutamic oxalacetic transaminase activity of mitochondrial origin in chronic alcoholics, in *Currents in Alcoholism,* vol. 5. M. Galanter, ed. Grune and Stratton, New York, pp. 101–108.

[96]H. Orrego, H. Kalant, Y. Israel, J. Blake, A. Medline, J. Rankin, A. Armstrong, and B. Kapur (1979) Effects of short term therapy with propylthiouracil in patients with alcoholic liver disease. *Gastroenterology* **76,** 105–115.

[97]G. Skude and J. Wadstein (1977) Amylase, hepatic enzymes and bilirubin in serum of chronic alcoholics. *Acta Med. Scand.* **201,** 53–58.

[98]N. McIntyre and J. Heathcote (1974) The laboratory in the diagnosis and management of viral hepatitis. *Clin. Gastroenterol.* **3,** 317–336.

[99]S. Shaw, D. Korts, and B. Stimmel (1983) Abnormal liver function tests as biological markers for alcoholism in narcotic addicts. *Am. J. Drug Alcohol Abuse* **9,** 345–354.

[100]M. Bernadt, C. Taylor, J. Mumford, B. Smith, and R. Murray (1982) Comparison of questionnaire and laboratory tests in the detection of excessive drinking and alcoholism. *Lancet* **2,** 325–331.

[101]M. Chana Young, P. Ferriera, J. Frolich, M. Shulzer, and F. Tan (1981) The effects of age and smoking on routine laboratory tests. *Am. J. Clin. Pathol.* **75,** 320–326.

[102]R. Rej (1978) Aspartate aminotranferase activity and isoenzyme proportions in human liver tissues. *Clin. Chem.* **24,** 1971–1979.

[103]G. Alveyn, J. Beresford, F. Bull, and R. Wright (1987) Mitochondrial aspartate aminotransferase (mAST) as a marker for alcohol misuse in patients with liver disease and controls. *Gut* **28,** 1349.

[104]B. Nalpas, A. Vassault, S. Charpin, B. Lacour, and P. Berthelot (1986) Serum mitochondrial aspartate aminotransferase as a marker of chronic alcoholism: Diagnostic value and interpretation in a liver unit. *Hepatology* **6,** 608–614.

[105]B. Nalpas, R. Poupon, A. Vassault, P. Hauzmanneau, Y. Sage, F. Schellenberg, B. Lacour, and P. Berthelot (1989) Evaluation of mAST/tAST ratio as a marker of misuse in a non-selected population. *Alcohol Alcohol.* **24,** 415–419.

[106]D. Acosta and D. G. Wenzel (1974) Injury produced by free fatty acids to lysosomes and mitochondria in cultured heart muscle and endothelial cells. *Atherosclerosis* **20,** 417–426.

[107]W. J. Jenkins and T. J. Peters (1978) Mitochondrial enzyme activities in liver biopsies from patients with alcoholic liver disease. *Gut* **19,** 341–344.

[108]L. Fletcher, I. Kwoh-Gain, E. Powell, L. Powell, and J. Halliday (1991) Markers of chronic alcohol ingestion in patients with nonalcoholic steatohepatitis: An aid to diagnosis. *Hepatology* **13,** 455–459.

[109]O. Nilssen, N. Huseby, G. Hoyer, T. Brenn, H. Schirmer, and O. Forde (1992) New alcohol markers—How useful are they in population studies: The Svalbard study 1988–89. *Alcohol. Clin. Exp. Res.* **16,** 82–86.

[110]S. Nakagawa, S. Kumin, and H. Nitowsky (1977) Human hexosaminidase isozymes: chromatographic separation an aid to heterozygote identification. *Clin. Chim. Acta* **75,** 181–191.

[111]P. Kärkkäinen, P. Poikalainen, and M. Salaspuro (1990) Serum beta-hexosaminidase as a marker of heavy drinking. *Alcohol. Clin. Exp. Res.* **2,** 187–190.

[112]A. Isaksson and B. Hultberg (1989) Immunoassay of beta-hexosaminidase isoenzymes in serum in patients with varied total activities. *Clin. Chim. Acta* **183,** 155–162.

[113]Ö. Eriksson, B. Ginsburg, B. Hultburg, and P. Öckerman (1972) Influence of age and sex on plasma acid hydrolases. *Clin. Chim. Acta* **40,** 181–185.

[114]B. Hultberg, A. Isaksson, and G. Tiderström (1980) β-hexosaminidase, leucine aminopeptidase, cystidyl aminopeptidase, hepatic enzymes and bilirubin in serum of chronic alcoholics with acute ethanol intoxication. *Clin. Chim. Acta* **105,** 317–323.

[115]B. Hultberg, A. Isaksson, and L. Jansson (1981) Beta-hexosaminidase in serum from patients with cirrhosis and cholestasis. *Enzyme* **26,** 296–300.

[116]P. Poon, T. Davis, T. Dornan, and R. Turner (1983) Plasma N-acetyl, D-glucose-aminidase activities and glycaemia in diabetes mellitus. *Diabetologia* **24,** 433–436.

[117]B. Hultberg, A. Isaksson, M. Berglund, and A. Moberg (1991) Serum beta-hexosaminidase isoenzyme: A sensitive marker for alcohol abuse. *Alcohol. Clin. Exp. Res.* **15,** 549–552.

[118]A. Isaksson, B. Gustavii, B. Hultberg, and P. Masson (1984) Activity of lysosomal hydrolases in plasma at term and post partum. *Enzyme* **31,** 229–233.

[119]P. Kärrkäinen (1990) Serum and urinary B-hexosaminidase as markers of heavy drinking. *Alcohol Alcohol.* **25,** 365–369.

[120]P. Kärkkäinen, K. Jokelainen, R. Roine, A. Suokas, and M. Salaspuro (1990) The effects of moderate drinking and abstinence on serum and urinary beta-hexosaminidase levels. *Drug Alcohol Dependence* **25,** 35–38.

[121]J. Huddleston, R. Cefalo, G. Lee, and J. Robinson (1971) An investigation of the gestational increase in serum hexosaminidase. *Am. J. Obstet. Gynecol.* **111,** 804–807.

[122]J. Lowden (1979) Serum beta-hexosaminidase in pregnancy. *Clin. Chim. Acta* **93**, 409–417.

[123]B. Hultberg and A. Isaksson (1981) A possible explanation for the occurrence of increased beta-hexosaminidase activity in pregnancy serum. *Clin. Chim. Acta* **113**, 135–140.

[124]M. Briggs and M. Briggs (1975) Serum activity of lysosomal enzymes in relationship to contraceptive steroid doses. *Curr. Med. Res. Opinions* **3**, 203–205.

[125]H. Nitowsky, J. Davis, S. Nakagawa, and D. Fox (1979) Human hexosaminidase isoenzymes: effects of oral contraceptive steroids on serum hexosaminidase activity. *Am. J. Obstet. Gynecol.* **134**, 642–647.

[126]M. Nyström, J. Peräsalo, and M. Salaspuro (1992) Serum beta-hexosaminidase in young university students. *Alcohol. Clin. Exp. Res.* **15**, 877–880.

[127]E. Coodley (1971) Enzyme diagnosis in hepatic disease. *Am. J. Gastroent.* **56**, 413–419.

[128]T. Babor, H. Kranzler, and R. Lauerman (1989) Early detection of harmful alcohol consumption: Comparison of clinical, laboratory, and self-report screening procedures. *Addict. Behav.* **14**, 139–157.

[129]C. Lai, R. Ng, and A. Lok (1982) The diagnostic value of the ratio of serum gammaglutamyl transpeptidase to alkaline phosphatase in alcoholic liver disease. *Gastroenterol.* **17**, 41–47.

[130]L. van Waes and C. Lieber (1977) Glutamate dehydrogenase: A reliable marker of liver cell necrosis in the alcoholic. *Br. Med. J.* **ii**, 1508–1510.

[131]P. Mills, R. Spooner, R. Russell, P. Boyle, and R. MacSween (1981) Serum glutamate dehydrogenase as a marker of hepatocyte necrosis in alcoholic liver disease. *Br. Med. J.* **283**, 754–755.

[132]S. Holt, H. Skinner, and Y. Israel (1981) Early identification of alcohol abuse: 2: Clinical and laboratory indicators. *CMA J.* **124**, 1279–1284.

[133]T. Worner and C. Lieber (1980) Plasma glutamate dehydrogenase: A marker of alcoholic liver injury. *Pharmacol. Biochem. Behav.* **13**, 107–110.

[134]A. Konttinen, G. Hartel, and A. Louhija (1970) Multiple serum enzyme analyses in chronic alcoholics. *Acta Med. Scand.* **188**, 257–264.

[135]S. Takase, A. Takada, M. Tsutsumi, and Y. Matsuda (1985) Biochemical markers of chronic alcoholism. *Alcohol* **2**, 405–410.

[136]A. Nygren and L. Sunblad (1971) Lactate dehydrogenase isoenzyme patterns in serum and skeletal muscle in intoxicated alcoholics. *Acta Med. Scand.* **189**, 303–307.

[137]K. Seppä, P. Laippala, and M. Saarni (1991) Macrocytosis as a consequence of alcohol abuse among patients in general practice. *Alcohol. Clin. Exp. Res.* **15**, 871–876.

[138]D. Bhattacharya and M. Rake (1983) Correlation of alcohol consumption with liver damage in men and women. *Alcohol Alcohol.* **18**, 181–184.

[139]J. Chanarin (1982) Haemopoisis and alcohol. *Br. Med. J.* **38**, 81–86.

[140]R. Asker, J. Renwick, and A. Goldstone (1982) Erythrocyte volume as a crude indicator of ethanol consumption in pregnancy. *Clin. Lab. Haematol.* **4**, 326–329.

[141]R. Davidson and P. Hamilton (1978) High mean red cell volume: its incidence and significance in routine haematology. *J. Clin. Pathol.* **31**, 493–498.

[142]D. Chalmers, A. Levi, I. Chanarin, W. North, and T. Meade (1979) Mean cell volume in a working population: the effects of age, smoking, alcohol, and oral contraception. *Br. J. Haematol.* **43**, 631–636.

[143]D. Taylor and T. Lind (1976) Haematological changes during normal pregnancy: iron-induced macrocytosis. *Br. J. Obst. Gynaecol.* **83,** 760.

[144]I. Barrison, J. Ruzek, and I. Murray-Lyon (1987) Drinkwatchers—Description of subjects and evaluation of laboratory markers of heavy drinking. *Alcohol Alcohol.* **22,** 147–154.

[145]K. Seppä, P. Sillanaukee, and T. Koivula (1991) Abnormalities of hematologic parameters in heavy drinkers and alcoholics. *Alcohol. Clin. Exp. Res.* **16,** 117–121.

[146]M. McDonald, R. Shapiro, M. Bleichman, J. Solway, and H. Bunn (1978) Glycosylated minor components of human adult hemoglobin. Purification, identification and partial structural analysis. *J. Biol. Chem.* **253,** 2327.

[147]P. Sillanaukee, K. Seppä, and T. Koivula (1991) Effect of acetaldehyde on hemoglobin: HbA1$_{ach}$ as a potential marker of heavy drinking. *Alcohol* **8,** 377–381.

[148]H. Hoberman and S. Chiodo (1982) Elevation of the hemoglobin A1 fraction in alcoholism. *Alcohol. Clin. Exp. Res.* **6,** 260–266.

[149]V. Stevens, W. Fantl, C. Newman, R. Sims, A. Cerami, and C. Peterson (1981) Acetaldehyde adducts with hemoglobin. *J. Clin. Invest.* **67,** 361–369.

[150]O. Niemelä, Y. Israel, Y. Mizui, T. Fukunaga, and C. Eriksson (1990) Hemoglobin-acetaldehyde adducts in human volunteers following acute alcohol ingestion. *Alcohol. Clin. Exp. Res.* **14,** 838–841.

[151]R. Koenig, C. Peterson, C. Kelo, A. Cerami, and J. Williamson (1976) Hemoglobin A1c as an indicator of the degree of glucose intolerance in diabetes. *Diabetes* **25,** 230–232.

[152]O. Niemelä, E. Halmesmaki, and O. Ylikorkala (1991) Hemoglobin-acetaldehyde adducts are elevated in women carrying alcohol-damaged fetuses. *Alcohol. Clin. Exp. Res.* **15,** 1007–1010.

[153]E. Baraona, C. DiPadova, J. Tobasco, and C. Lieber (1987) Red blood cells: A new major modality for acetaldehyde transport from liver to other tissues. *Life Sci.* **40,** 253–258.

[154]R. San George and H. Hoberman (1986) Reaction of acetaldehyde with hemoglobin. *J. Biol. Chem.* **261,** 6811–6821.

[155]H. H. Stein (1965) Studies of binding by macromolecules. A new dialysis technique for obtaining quantitative data. *Analyt. Biochem.* **13,** 305–313.

[156]C. Peterson and C. Polizzi (1987) Improved method for acetaldehyde in plasma and hemoglobin-associated acetaldehyde: Results in teetotalers and alcoholics reporting for treatment. *Alcohol* **4,** 477–480.

[157]R. Hernandez-Munoz, E. Baraona, I. Blacksburg, and C. Lieber (1989) Characterization of the increased binding of acetaldehyde to red blood cells in alcoholics. *Alcohol. Clin. Exp. Res.* **13,** 654–659.

[158]E. Baraona, R. Julkunen, L. Tannenbaum, and C. Lieber (1986) Role of intestinal bacterial overgrowth in ethanol production and metabolism in rats. *Gastroenterology* **90,** 103–110.

[159]D. Nathan, T. Francis, and J. Palmer (1983) Effects of aspirin on determinations of glycosylated hemoglobin. *Clin. Chem.* **29,** 466–469.

[160]C. Peterson, L. Jovanovic-Peterson, and F. Schmid-Formby (1988) Rapid association of acetaldehyde with hemoglobin in human volunteers after low dose ethanol. *Alcohol* **5,** 371–374.

[161]C. Peterson, S. Ross, and B. K. Scott (1990) Correlation of self-administered alcoholism screening test with hemoglobin-associated acetaldehyde. *Alcohol* **7,** 289–293.

[162]E. Abraham, A. Abraham, and M. Stallings (1984) High-pressure liquid chromatographic separation of glycosylated and acetylated minor hemoglobins in newborn infants and in patients with sickle cell disease. *J. Lab. Clin. Med.* **104,** 1027–1034.

[163]U. Turpenin, U. Stenman, and R. Roine (1989) Liquid-chromatographic determination of acetylated hemoglobin. *Clin. Chem.* **35,** 33–36.

[164]C. Peterson, D. Scott, and S. McLaughlin (1991) Studies of whole blood associated acetaldehyde as a marker for alcohol intake: Effect of gender in mice. *Alcohol* **8,** 35–38.

[165]F. Lundquist (1960) The concentrate of acetate in blood during alcohol metabolism in man. *Acta Physiol. Scand.* **175(suppl.),** 97.

[166]N. Karlsson, E. Fellenius, and K.-H. Kiessling (1975) The metabolism of acetate in the perfused hindquarter of the rat. *Acta Physiol. Scand.* **12,** 400.

[167]H. Nuutinen, K. Lindros, P. Hekali, and M. Salaspuro (1985) Elevated blood acetate as indicator of fast ethanol elimination in chronic alcoholics. *Alcohol* **2,** 623–626.

[168]U. Korri, H. Nuutinen, and M. Salaspuro (1985) Increased blood acetate: A new laboratory marker of alcoholism and heavy drinking. *Alcohol. Clin. Exp. Res.* **9,** 468–471.

[169]F. Lundquist, N. Tygstrup, K. Winkler, K. Mellemgaard, and S. Munck-Peterson (1962) Ethanol metabolism and production of free acetate in the human liver. *J. Clin. Invest.* **41,** 955–961.

[170]M. Salaspuro and H. Nuutinen (1983) Increased blood acetate: a new laboratory marker of alcoholism. *Scand. J. Gastroenterol.* **18,** 877–880.

[171]B. Buckley and D. Williamson (1977) Origin of blood acetate in the rat. *Biochem. J.* **166,** 539–545.

[172]L. Lumeng (1986) New diagnostic markers of alcohol abuse. *Hepatology* **6,** 742–745.

[173]V. Camp, J. Lenton, T. Stammers, S. Lee, and B. Faraj (1986) Detection of significant excretion of salsolinol in urine of alcoholics by a specific radioenzymatic assay (Abstract) *Alcohol. Clin. Exp. Res.* **10,** 93.

[174]M. Duncan and G. Smythe (1982) Salsolinol and dopamine in alcoholic beverages. *Lancet* **1,** 904–905.

[175]K. Matsubara, S. Fukushima, A. Akane, K. Hama, and Y. Fukui (1986) Tetrahydrobeta-carbolines in human urine and rat brain—no evidence of formation by alcohol drinking. *Alcohol Alcohol.* **21,** 339–345.

[176]J. Adachi, Y. Mizoi, T. Fukunaga, M. Kogame, I. Ninomiya, and T. Naito (1986) Effect of acetaldehyde on urinary salsolinol in healthy men after ethanol intake. *Alcohol* **3,** 215–220.

[177]C. L. Melchior (1979) Interaction of salsolinol and tetrahydropapaveroline with ethanol and monoamines. *Alcohol. Clin. Exp. Res.* **3,** 364–367.

[178]C. Duncan and R. Dietrich (1980) A critical evaluation of tetrahydroisoquinoline-induced preference in rats. *Pharmacol. Biochem. Behav.* **13,** 265–281.

[179]G. Oxenstierna, G. Edman, L. Iselius, L. Oreland, S. Ross, and G. Sedvall (1986) Concentrations of monoamine metabolites in the CSF of twins and unrelated subjects. Agenentic study. *J. Psych. Res.* **20,** 19–29.

[180]B. Faraj, J. Lenton, M. Kutner, V. Camp, T. Stammers, S. Lee, P. Lolies, and D. Chandora (1987) Prevalence of low monoamine oxidase function in alcoholism. *Alcohol. Clin. Exp. Res.* **11,** 464–467.

[181]M. Hirst, D. Evans, C. Gowdey, and M. Adams (1985) The influences of ethanol and other factors on the excretion of urinary salsolinol in social drinkers. *Pharmacol. Biochem. Behav.* **22,** 993–1000.

[182]H. Rommelspacher, C. Nanz, H. Borbe, K. Fehske, W. Muller, and U. Wollert, (1981) Benzodiazepine antagonism by harmane and other beta carbolines in vitro and in vivo. *Eur. J. Pharmacol.* **70**, 409–416.

[183]N. Buckholtz and W. Boggan (1976) Effects of tetrahydro-beta-carbolines on monoamine oxidase and serotonin uptake in mouse brain. *Biochem. Pharmacol.* **25**, 2319–2321.

[184]T. Bosin (1988) Measurement of beta-carbolines by high-performance liquid chromatography with fluorescence detection. *J. Chromatog.* **428**, 229–236.

[185]H. Rommelspacher and H. Susilo (1985) Tetrahydroisoquinolines and beta-carbolines: putative natural substances in plants and mammals, in *Progress in Drug Research,* vol. 29. E. Ticker, ed. Birkhäuser Verlag, Basel, pp. 415–459.

[186]H. Rommelspacher, H. Damm, L. Schmidt, and G. Schmidt (1985) Increased excretion of harmon by alcoholics depends on events of their life history and the state of the liver. *Psychopharmacology* **87**, 64–68.

[187]H. Rommelspacher, S. Strauss, and J. Lindemann (1980) Excretion of tetrahydro-harmane and harmane in the urine of man and rat after a load with ethanol. *FEBS Lett.* **109**, 209–212.

[188]H. Rommelspacher, H. Damm, S. Lutter, L. Schmidt, M. Otto, N. Sachs-Ericsson, and G. Schmidt (1990) Harmon (1-methyl-beta-carboline) in blood plasma and erythrocytes of nonalcoholics following ethanol loading. *Alcohol* **7**, 27–31.

[189]H. Rommelspacher, L. Schmidt, and T. May (1991) Plasma norharmon (beta-carboline) levels are elevated in chronic alcoholics. *Alcohol. Clin. Exp. Res.* **15**, 553–559.

[190]B. Tang, P. Devenyi, D. Teller, and Y. Israel (1986) Detection of an alcohol specific product in urine of alcoholics. *Biochem. Biophys. Res. Commun.* **140**, 924–927.

[191]B. Tang (1987) Detection of ethanol in urine of abstaining alcoholics. *Can. J. Physiol. Pharmacol.* **65**, 1225–1227.

[192]B. Tang (1991) Urinary markers of chronic excessive ethanol consumption. *Alcohol. Clin. Exp. Res.* **15**, 881–885.

[193]J. Casazza, M. Felver, and K. Veech (1984) The metabolism of acetone in rat. *J. Biol. Chem.* **259**, 231–236.

[194]D. Lewis, W. Griffiths, and J. Tucci (1981) Detection of 2,3-butanediol in the serum of an abstinent alcohol abuser and its relationship to glucose metabolism. *Ann. Clin. Lab. Sci.* **11**, 468.

[195]L. Sysfontes, G. Nyborg, A. Jones, and R. Blomstrand (1986) Occurrence of short chain aliphatic diols in human blood: Identification by gas chromatography—mass spectrometry. *Clin. Chim. Acta* **155**, 115–122.

[196]J. Casazza, J. Frietas, D. Stambuck, M. Morgan, and R. Veech (1987) The measurement of 1,2-propanediol, D,L-2,3-butanediol and meso-2,3-butanediol in controls and alcoholic cirrhotics. *Alcohol Alcohol.* **1(suppl.)**, 607–609.

[197]D. Rutstein, R. Nickerson, A. Vernon, P. Kishore, R. Veech, M. Felver, L. Needham, and S. Thacker (1983) 2,3-Butanediol: An unusual metabolite in the serum of severely alcoholic men during acute intoxication. *Lancet* **ii**, 534–537.

[198]G. Munst, M. Ris-Steiger, R. Galeazzi, J. Von Wartburg, and J. Bircher (1981) The fate of the ethanol analogue 1,3-butanediol in the dog. *Biochem. Pharmacol.* **30**, 1987–1997.

[199]F. Poldrugo, O. Snead, and S. Barker (1985) Chronic alcohol administration produces an increase in liver 1,4-butanediol concentration. *Alcohol Alcohol.* **20**, 251–253.

[200]P. Felig, E. Marliss, J. Ohman, and J. Cahill (1970) Plasma amino acid levels in diabetic ketoacidosis. *Diabetes* **19**, 727–729.

[201]M. Swendseid, C. Yamada, E. Vinyard, W. Figuero, and E. Drenick (1967) Plasma amino acid levels in subjects fed isonitrogen diets containing different proportions of fat and carbohydrate. *Am. J. Clin. Nutr.* **20,** 52–55.

[202]R. Herrington, G. Jacobsen, M. Daley, R. Lipo, H. Biller, and C. Weissberger (1981) The use of plasma alpha-amino-*n*-butyric acid:leucine ratio to identify alcoholics. *J. Stud. Alcohol* **42,** 492–499.

[203]S. Shaw and C. Lieber (1976) Characteristic plasma amino acid abnormalities in the alcoholic; respective roles of alcoholism, nutrition, and liver injury (abstract) *Clin. Res.* **24,** 2914.

[204]J. Chick, M. Longstaff, N. Kreitman, M. Plant, D. Thatcher, and J. Waite (1982) Plasma alpha-amino-*n*-butyric acid: leucine ratio and alcoholic consumption in working men and in alcoholics. *J. Stud. Alcohol* **43,** 583–587.

[205]S. Shaw, B. Stimmel, and C. Lieber (1976) Plasma alpha amino-*n*-butyric acid to leucine ratio: an empirical biochemical marker of alcoholism. *Science* **194,** 1057–1058.

[206]J. Ellingboe, J. Mendelsohn, C. Varanelli, O. Neuberger, and W. Burysow (1978) Plasma alpha amino-*n*-butyric acid:leucine ratio: nonspecificity as a marker for alcoholism. *Gastroenterology* **75,** 561–565.

[207]S. Shaw, T. Worner, M. Borysow, R. Schmitz, and C. Lieber (1979) Detection of alcoholism relapse: comparative diagnostic value of MCV, GGTP, and AANB. *Alcohol. Clin. Exp. Res.* **3,** 297–301.

[208]H. Van Eijk, W. van Noort, M. Dubelaar, and C. van der Heul (1983) The microheterogeneity of human transferrin in biological fluids. *Clin. Chim. Acta* **132,** 167–171.

[209]S. Petren and O. Vesterberg (1989) Separation of different forms of transferrin by isoelectric focusing to detect effects on the liver caused by xenobiotics. *Electrophoresis* **10,** 600–604.

[210]H. Stibler and K. Kjellin (1979) Isoelectric focusing and electrophoresis of the CSF proteins in tremor of different origins. *J. Neurol. Sci.* **30,** 269–285.

[211]H. Stibler and S. Borg (1986) Carbohydrate composition of serum transferrin in alcoholic patients. *Alcohol. Clin. Exp. Res.* **10,** 61–63.

[212]H. Stibler, S. Borg, and M. Joustra (1986) Micro anion exchange chromatography of carbohydrate-deficient transferrin in serum in relation to alcohol consumption (Swedish patent 8400587-5) *Alcohol. Clin. Exp. Res.* **10,** 535–544.

[213]U. Behrens, T. Worner, and C. Lieber (1988) Changes in carbohydrate-deficient transferrin levels after alcohol withdrawal. *Alcohol. Clin. Exp. Res.* **12,** 539–544.

[214]A. Kapur, G. Wild, A. Milford-Ward, and D. Triger (1989) Carbohydrate deficient transferrin: a marker for alcohol abuse. *Br. Med. J.* **299,** 427–431.

[215]I. Kwoh-Gain, L. Fletcher, J. Price, L. Powell, and J. Halliday (1990) Desialylated transferrin and mitochondrial apsartate aminotransferase compared as laboratory markers of excessive alcohol consumption. *Clin. Chem.* **36,** 841–845.

[216]H. Stibler, S. Borg, M. Joustra, and R. Hultcrantz (1988) Carbohydrate-deficient transferrin (CDT) in serum as a marker of high alcohol consumption. *Adv. Biosci.* **71,** 353–357.

[217]F. Schellenberg, J. Benard, A. Le Goff, and J.Weill (1989) Evaluation of carbohydrate-deficient transferrin compared with Tf index and other markers of alcohol abuse. *Alcohol. Clin. Exp. Res.* **13,** 605–610.

[218]H. Stibler, S. Borg, and G. Beckman (1988) Transferrin phenotype and level of carbohydrate-deficient transferrin in healthy individuals. *Alcohol. Clin. Exp. Res.* **12,** 450–453.

[219]H. Stibler, L. Dahlgren, and S. Borg (1988) Carbohydrate-deficient transferrin (CDT) in serum in women with early alcohol addiction. *Alcohol* 5, 393–398.

[220]H. Stibler and R. Hultcrantz (1987) Carbohydrate-deficient tranferrin in serum in patients with liver diseases. *Alcohol. Clin. Exp. Res.* 11, 468–473

[221]J. Jaeken, E. Eggermont, and H. Stibler (1987) An apparent homozygous X-linked disorder carbohydrate-deficient serum glycoproteins. *Lancet* 2, 1398.

[222]M. Worwood (1979) Serum ferritin. CRC Critical Reviews. *Clin. Lab. Sci.* 10, 171–204.

[223]A. Jacobson, A. Norden, J. Qvist, and J. Wadstein (1978) Serum ferritin—a new marker for alcoholism? *Acta Soc. Med. Suec.* 87, 3314.

[224]H. Kristenson, G. Fex, and E. Trell (1986) Serum ferritin, gamma-glutamyltranspeptidase and alcohol consumption in healthy middle-aged men. *Drug Alcohol Dependence* 8, 43–50.

[225]M. Worwood, S. Cragg, M. Wagstaff, and A. Jacobs (1979) Binding of human serum ferritin to concanavalin A. *Clin. Sci.* 56, 83–87.

[226]M. Wagstaff, M. Worwood, and A. Jacobs (1978) Properties of human tissue isoferritins. *Biochem. J.* 173, 974–977.

[227]R. Moirand, G. Lescoat, D. Delamaire, L. Lauvin, J. Campion, Y. Dengnier, and P. Brissot (1991) Increase in glycosylated and nonglycosylated serum ferritin in chronic alcoholism and their evolution during alcohol withdrawal. *Alcohol. Clin. Exp. Res.* 15, 963–969.

[228]M. Worwood, D. Hourahane, and B. Jones (1984) Accumulation and release of isoferritins during incubation in vitro of human peripheral blood mononuclear cells. *Br. J. Haematol.* 56, 31–43.

[229]D. Chalmers, M. Rinsler, S. MacDermott, C. Spicer, and A. Levi (1981) Biochemical and haematological indicators of excessive alcohol consumption. *Gut* 22, 992–996.

[230]R. Ryback, M. Eckardt, B. Felsher, and R. Rawlings (1982) Biochemical and hematologic correlates of alcoholism and liver disease. *JAMA* 248, 2261–2265.

[231]T. Beresford, D. Low, R. Hall, R. Adduci, and F. Goggans (1982) A computerized biochemical profile for detection of alcoholism. *Psychosomatics* 23, 713–720.

[232]A. Shaper, S. Pocock, D. Ashby, M. Walker, and T. Whitehead (1985) Biochemical and haematological response to alcohol intake. *Ann. Clin. Biochem.* 22, 50–61.

[233]V. Hillers, J. Alldredge, and L. Massey (1986) Determination of habitual alcohol intake from a panel of blood chemistries. *Alcohol Alcohol.* 21, 199–205.

[234]A. Chan, J. Welte, and R. Whitney (1987) Identification of alcoholism in young adults by blood chemistries. *Alcohol* 4, 175–179.

[235]L. Dahlgren, C.-M. Ideström, and T. Bjerver (1982) The EWA project: Specialized treatment for female alcoholics. *Läkartidningen* 79, 1257–1258.

[236]F. Vanclay, B. Raphael, M. Dunne, J. Whitfield, T. Lewin, and B. Singh (1991) A community screening test for high alcohol consumption using biochemical and haematological measures. *Alcohol Alcohol.* 26, 337–346.

Peer Support Groups for Women in Treatment and Aftercare

Lisa Roth and Patricia James

Introduction

Substance abuse among women has traditionally received less attention and treatment dollars than chemical dependence among men. This is owing to the social stigma attached to women's drug abuse, the hidden nature of much female substance abuse, and the comparatively fewer numbers of female substance abusers. However, in the early 1970s recognition of the magnitude of the problem of substance abuse among women began to increase as the women's movement drew attention to women's unmet needs in many areas. Unfortunately, at the same time the number of chemically dependent women also began to rise. There is also evidence that the problems of chemically dependent women have increased in complexity and severity in the past 20 yr.[1] The pattern of drug usage by women also changed from licit drugs, primarily prescription medications and alcohol, to illicit "hard" drugs.[1] The epidemic of crack cocaine usage among urban women of childbearing age, which began in the late 1980s, is perhaps the most visible evidence of this trend.

Although the number of drug-dependent women has increased since 1970, women continue to seek out and enter treatment programs less often than men.[2] Furst and his colleagues found that even when actual utilization rates were corrected for prevalence, alcoholic men entered treatment 2.5

From: *Drug and Alcohol Abuse Reviews, Vol. 5: Addictive Behaviors in Women*
Ed.: R. R. Watson ©1994 Humana Press Inc., Totowa, NJ

times as frequently as did women.[3] Various psychosocial and environmental factors for this trend have been advanced, including: social expectations and pressures, different help-seeking behaviors, denial of addiction, lack of adequate treatment facilities for women, and lack of facilities for the children of women in treatment. In many cases, women seeking treatment must give up custody of their children to relatives or state-sponsored foster care[4] because most treatment models and services lack childcare facilities. The traditional assumption has been that men, and not women, are the population at risk.[5,6] As a result, it has been estimated that <20% of treatment programs offer childcare or other specialized services for women.[7]

At the same time that the numbers of drug-dependent women were increasing, a growing body of research suggested that female and male substance abusers differ markedly in their drug abuse histories, reasons for addiction, and service needs.[8-12] These studies, although not conclusive, suggested that new treatment approaches specifically designed for women might be more effective in drawing women into treatment and improving treatment outcomes. These are briefly described in the following.

One specific treatment modality, the self-help group, was popularized almost 50 yr ago by Alcoholics Anonymous (AA) as an informal alternative to formal treatment programs. AA continues to be one of the fastest-growing self-help organizations in the world, with the formation of other 12-step groups such as Narcotics Anonymous and Cocaine Anonymous.[13] Peer support, or self-help, groups became a major force in formal treatment programs in the 1970s.[14] Feminist self-help models have been developed for domestic violence programs, and, in the addictions field, by therapeutic communities and outpatient programs.

Feminist-oriented women's consciousness-raising (CR) groups developed in the late 1960s and continued for almost two decades. These groups had both personal growth and social change agendas and were informed by the slogan "The personal is political." The antirape and battered women's movements grew out of CR activities. For both political and economic reasons, rape crisis centers and battered women's shelters employed self-help models that promoted personal healing and empowerment. This included the sharing of information resources; developing coping skills; destigmatization about being a survivor of male violence; and organizing for fundamental social change. Despite their feminist origins, these groups had much in common with other self-help groups, including AA. The two issues— addictions and abuse in women's lives—have recently come together as researchers and service providers gain greater understanding of the role that physical and sexual violence against women plays in fostering addiction, and the role that healing from the effects of this violence must play in women's treatment and recovery. Recognizing the efficacy of self-help groups in women's healing from incest, rape and battering, and in improving self-esteem and a sense of control, researchers in addictions treatment began to suggest that self-help groups be included in female-oriented treatment programs.[5,10,14,15] Unfortunately, because of the lack of proportionate funding for research demonstration projects specifically designed for addicted women, few evaluative studies of treatment models for women that provide this new treatment technique have been published.

The purpose of this chapter is to provide a theoretical basis for the utilization of women-only peer support groups for the treatment of substance abuse. It will provide an overview of the literature on the needs of women in treatment, the uses of women-only peer support groups, and the efficacy of peer support groups in women's treatment and aftercare in formal settings. This chapter does not address the effectiveness of specific self-help groups as an informal treatment or aftercare method, such as Alcoholics or Narcotics Anonymous, Recovery Inc., or Women for Sobriety. There is a large body of literature demonstrating that these groups have helped many individuals to overcome their addiction, both with or without formal treatment.[16]

Needs of Women in Substance Abuse Treatment

The need of drug-dependent women for different types of treatment programs and services than those traditionally available to the male substance-abusing population is related to the unique characteristics of drug-dependent women.[9] First, addicted women are more likely than men to need emotional support, because they are more likely to be socially isolated. For example, a 1979 study comparing addicted and nonaddicted men and women concluded that addicted women were more likely to be separated from spouses, less likely to have friends in their neighborhood, and more likely to report feelings of loneliness than both nonaddicted women and addicted men from the same environment. When supportive relationships exist, they are more likely to be a source of practical rather than emotional support.[12] Lacking an emotionally supportive network, female addicts are also especially sensitive to the effects of life stressors, which leave them highly vulnerable to becoming addicted or relapsing after treatment.[17]

Addicted women are also more in need of social services and psychotherapeutic services than addicted men. They tend to have primary childcare responsibility, less vocational preparation, more health problems and concerns, and they tend to come from drug-dependent and/or dysfunctional families. They tend to have lower self-esteem. They are more likely to report symptoms of depression and anxiety, to have alcoholic or drug-abusing spouses, and to have been battered or sexually abused as children, than drug-dependent men.[5,9,11,12,18,19]

Third, drug-dependent women are more likely to benefit from women-only treatment than from programs that serve both men and women. Generally speaking, when men and women interact, men's language and interaction predominate, especially when women are substantially outnumbered by men, as they are in many drug treatment programs. The consequences of being outnumbered in a group are heightened visibility and stereotyping of those individuals who are outnumbered. These dynamics have been documented between men and women in small groups.[20] Therefore, woman-only treatment programs give recovering women more of an opportunity to fully participate in group discussions. Furthermore, drug-dependent women, who are more likely than other women to be victims of domestic and sexual violence, often need an exclusively female group in which they can feel completely free to discuss their experiences with abusive men.[21,22]

Thus, treatment programs that provide three components—social services, psychotherapeutic services, and an enhanced network of supportive women—would seem to be more attractive to drug-dependent women and better able to meet their needs. The specific components of female-oriented treatment programs and their rationale are discussed in more detail in the following section.

Substance Abuse
Treatment Models for Women

Based on the research conducted on the unique characteristics of female substance abusers, several authors have suggested treatment program components that could attract more women into treatment and improve program outcomes. Unfortunately, there are few published evaluations of such programs and their effectiveness remains unknown.

Broadly speaking, programs that offer female-oriented drug-dependence treatment services generally can be defined as those that:

1. Address women's treatment needs;
2. Reduce barriers to recovery from drug dependence that are likely to occur for women;
3. Are delivered in a context that is compatible with women's styles and orientations and is safe from exploitation; and
4. Take into account women's roles, socialization, and relative status within the larger culture.[5]

Program Components

Since women who abuse drugs and alcohol have a wider range of needs than men, any female-oriented treatment program should target a wide range of addicted women, provide a broader range of treatment goals, and provide a staff that is trained in a diverse range of treatment modalities and can offer a wide range of services.

Treatment Model

Program philosophy should be clearly articulated, with concrete goals for staff and clients,[10] and treatment interventions should build on women's strengths and help them develop relationships with other women.[23] The treatment of the woman's addiction should include a focus on her family and significant others, since women tend to be highly influenced by others in their use of drugs.[5]

Target Population

Because addicted women tend to abuse more than one substance, programs should not be restricted to women who abuse a particular type of substance. Programs should also include client and staff training on abuse of licit substances, such as prescription drugs and diet pills.[8,10]

Staff Composition

Staff, particularly leadership, should be predominantly or all female in order to serve as role models for program participants, and to help women feel comfortable in discussing their histories of domestic violence and childhood sexual abuse. It has also been suggested that an all-female staff is useful in avoiding sexual harassment and other sexist behavior by male staff members. If the program includes both male and female staff, frequent training sessions are necessary, focusing on the needs of women in treatment and the identification and correction of sexism in the staff.[10,23]

Outreach

Since women tend to be solitary drug users, traditional outreach (through the criminal justice system, physicians, and employee assistance programs) are not as effective with women as with men. Female-oriented programs should include a strong outreach component to identify women in the community who need treatment[10] by utilizing individuals who see women regularly, such as hairdressers, those who work with their children, or others who have some influence with women, such as clergy or family.[5] Staff should have strong links with the community agencies offering the ancillary services that women in treatment need in order to facilitate referrals for clients.[5]

Services

Ancillary services have been shown to be instrumental in attracting women into treatment,[8] an important consideration since women are less likely to seek out treatment than men. Because the majority of women in treatment bear primary responsibility for themselves and their children, on-site childcare, or assistance with an affordable, reliable source of childcare, is probably the single most important factor in increasing access to treatment for women.[5,7,10,23,24]

Other program services that are important in reducing environmental stressors on addicted women, and, thus, in improving the chances of long-term abstinence from drugs, are: vocational training and counseling; referrals to a regular source of healthcare and education on health and nutrition, especially for pregnant women; counseling on domestic violence, rape, and childhood sexual abuse; basic life-skills training; parenting training and education in child development; assertiveness training; medical and psychiatric treatment for children as necessary; socialization activities to replace drug-taking behaviors; counseling and psychotherapy for family and significant others; assistance with housing; aftercare planning and services; and, of course, women's support groups.[4,5,7,10]

In one of the few published studies of a treatment program sensitive to women, Stevens and colleagues described the results of measures taken to make a mixed-gender residential treatment program more oriented toward female clients. Women were permitted to bring their children into treatment if no other childcare arrangements were possible. This female-based treatment model included an expanded female staff; a women's support group; training on assertiveness, basic living skills, sexuality, and health; and referrals to vocational opportunities. A female counselor was also hired to conduct outreach and coordinate childcare, healthcare, education, and vocational opportunities with the women. As a result, the proportion of women in the program increased from 0.08 to 32% in 2 yr. The length of stay also increased for both men and women.[4]

These results illustrate how ancillary services that meet women's needs are useful in attracting women to treatment and increasing their length of stay. Unfortunately, very little research that evaluates the effectiveness of female-oriented treatment models, and specifically of women's support groups, has been published.

Peer Support Groups

Peer support, or self-help, in small groups is a process that has been widely researched since the 1940s, when "T-groups" (training groups developed around human relations problem-solving techniques) and group psychotherapy processes gained acceptance.[25] Researchers characterize self-help groups as those that are voluntarily formed by the members to meet needs not met by existing institutions. Members generally share a stigmatizing or handicapping circumstance that represents a departure from the normative ideal and is often socially isolating. Many self-help groups develop a specific language that promotes a unique ideology to which members adhere. Leadership and authority are shared by all members, and leadership by professionals is often discouraged. Self-help groups serve several critical functions in members' lives. Membership fosters a sense of personal responsibility and empowerment among participants. Often members "confess" their qualifications for membership, and experience catharsis and eventual self-acceptance and destigmatization. They meet others who have overcome or learned to live with the stigmatizing condition, and they learn skills and obtain needed resources to improve their own coping abilities. They develop social supports, networks, and a sense of community with other members. One of the most important functions of self-help is the sense of empowerment and personal worth experienced by members who help other members.[26–33]

The initial relationship between professional human service providers and self-help groups was often characterized by mutual suspicion, trivialization, ignorance, and, at best, skepticism about the other's ethics and efficacy. Balgopal noted that although "self-help groups are increasingly becoming an accepted part of our social fabric, the relationship between such groups and other professional helpers has been a tenuous one in many cases" (p. 124).[34] Alcoholics Anonymous (AA), founded in 1935, is the first contemporary self-help group movement. Originally, AA was widely criticized as antitherapeutic. Now, however, substance abuse treatment programs increasingly refer clients to AA and other 12-step programs as part of their recovery and aftercare planning. Similarly, the women's groups that developed during the late 1960s and 1970s had the reputation of being in the "radical fringe," especially among human service providers whose traditional treatment approaches to women were being questioned. Women-only self-help groups are often used in programs for battered women, rape victims, and incest survivors. Moreover, a number of 12-step programs offer women-only meetings. In fact, Al-Anon, the second 12-step program founded in 1949, was established by women for the wives and families of male alcoholics.[35]

Self-help groups are increasingly accepted by professional human service providers as research on self-help group processes demonstrates the efficacy of this model in physical and mental health promotion, and as the number of viable self-help groups continues to grow.[36,37] Nationally, there are over 126 organizations using 12-step models alone.[35] In 1988, the Surgeon General's

Workshop on Self-Help and Public Health presented a list of recommendations that included promotion of the use of self-help organizations and models
by professionals, support for collaborative research and demonstration
projects, systematic study of the self-help process, and an increase in federal, state, and local funding for self-help groups and activities.[38]

Women and Self-Help

Traditionally, women have often met informally in groups that fostered caring, support, and sharing of information.[35] Use of self-help models
is particularly appropriate for women given increasing levels of social isolation and the socialization of women to defer to men in groups.[39] Self-help
groups emphasize the ability of each to help the other. New members learn
hope from senior members who are examples that healing, recovery, and
growth are possible. Senior members gain self-esteem as they become role
models and increase their competence to help others.[40] Wedenoja and Reed
noted that early research on women's groups revealed an increase in members' self-awareness, self-respect, and self-esteem, and propose the use of
this technique in treatment of drug-dependent women.[15]

Women-only groups offer women the opportunity to discuss issues
such as survival of incest, rape, or battering in a supportive, nonthreatening
atmosphere. Peer models validate personal experience and responses that
may be treated as symptoms of individual pathology by professionals. Battered women, for example, are often labeled masochistic, borderline, paranoid, or even schizophrenic. Often the symptoms resolve themselves in peer
support environments, such as shelters and support groups.[41,42] Rape and
incest survivors may learn in groups that their experience of posttraumatic
stress is normal for these events, and in the context of peer support they
stop feeling "crazy," ashamed, and "dirty" and can begin to relearn trust.[43]
Because the low self-esteem, depression, anxiety, and isolation from experiences of incest, rape, and battering are often at the core of a woman's addiction, self-help groups in women's treatment and aftercare settings could be
an effective recovery strategy.

Peer Support in Treatment
and Aftercare of Addicted Women

Although most treatment programs employ group processes that promote peer support strategies, relatively little research has been done specifically on the role these processes play in treatment and aftercare. The
authors found less than a dozen articles that discuss peer support groups in
women's recovery, and apparently no research has been published evaluat-

ing self-help processes in women-only treatment and aftercare programs. Nor does there seem to be any published research on comparing treatment outcomes of women and men in mixed-gender self-help groups. Existing evaluative research on peer support in mixed-gender treatment settings, social networks, and self-help recovery models do not differentiate between outcomes for women and men.

Gordon and Zrull examined the social network influences on drinking behavior of alcoholics in their first year after completion of inpatient rehabilitation.[44] Their study cohort included 85 males and 71 females, and measured the role of support by nondrinking coworkers. Although previous research[12] suggests that male and female drug abusers differ significantly in the origin and pattern of their addiction and the nature of their support networks and need for services, the authors did not examine the effect of differences in gender on the influence of social networks on drinking behavior.

In another study, Humphreys et al.[45] followed 201 male (70.6%) and female (29.4%) substance abusers for 6 mo after entry into treatment in a publicly funded program. They found that Blacks and women were significantly more likely to attend self-help groups such as NA and AA. Measures of social stability did not predict attendance, but persons who attended the groups had significantly more severe problems in psychological, family/social, and substance abuse domains. The authors concluded that self-help groups appeal to Black and female substance abusers, contrary to the popular notion that self-help groups appeal more to the educated, White, male, middle class. Neither study explored whether women in mixed-gender self-help groups are inhibited from fully participating, and thus benefiting, in mixed-gender groups. Neither examined the role of barriers to attendance that are specific to women, such as childcare, transportation, and personal safety concerns for attending night meetings.

Most of the literature on self-help groups for addicted women is descriptive, rather than evaluative. For example, Wedenoja and Reed offered practical guidelines for establishing and maintaining all-women groups.[15] They noted that traditional male models of group work for substance abusers use confrontational, self-confessional methods that tend to exacerbate the effects of sexual and physical abuse experienced by many women, and reinforce women's depression and low self-esteem. In fact, they noted that in mixed-gender groups, "issues relevant to women are often neglected or avoided" (p. 65). Since most mixed-gender treatment groups have many more male than female members, women's behavior, opportunities, and influence are restricted by expectations and norms controlled by male members. Women are expected to conform to male-defined standards of feminine behavior, such as passivity and dependence, and male members and group leaders pathologize women who fail to conform.[15] Finally, traditional treatment models do not recognize the double standard inherent in assumptions about gender roles and substance abuse. "Getting high" does not call men's masculinity into question (as it probably should), but the same behavior puts women at risk of being considered unfeminine, showing evidence of poor moral judgment, of being a "bad" wife and mother, and of deserving sexual and/or physical abuse.

All-women groups are becoming a major mode of treatment for drug-dependent women. Some programs use groups as the exclusive form of treatment, other programs use groups in combination with individual therapy, and some in combination with mixed-gender groups and/or therapy. The feminist orientation of many groups promotes valuing women, examining the impact of sexism on women's lives, overcoming stereotypes that devalue women, and developing personal and social approaches to problem solving.

On the other hand, some women may be reluctant to participate in all-female support groups. This resistance often stems from the fact that greater value is placed on men by this culture, and many drug-dependent women have been socialized to play subservient roles to men and to depend on them for status, resources, identity, and sense of self-worth. All-women groups challenge women to learn new ways of interacting with others on an equal basis.[15]

There is some controversy about the appropriateness of the 12-step model for women. Covington noted that AA was built on male model of alcoholism, adding that "neither the understanding of alcoholism in a person's life, nor the meaning of recovery have been completely relevant for women" (p. 86).[35] She added that until other models are developed, "AA is a viable resource for women." Feminist criticism of AA has focused on the concept of a higher power, which is often misunderstood to be religious doctrine. Early AA publications frequently refer to a male God figure. The concept of powerlessness in 12-step programs is also questioned as counterproductive and reinforcing of patriarchal notions of female passivity. Covington took issue with this: "The paradox is that admitting where you are powerless in life actually empowers you. For example, a woman involved in an abusive relationship may admit to her powerlessness over drinking and, once sober, be able to identify areas in her life where she can make choices about how to think and how to behave with regard to her relationship."[35]

Other limitations of 12-step groups for women include insistence on individual pathology and individual change without discussions of the social and political context of addiction. According to Covington, "For women, it may be that the environment contributed to the drinking and the environment prevents recovery from occurring. Many of the problems women have with alcohol exist through systems of domination. ... AA does not provide a forum for discussion of structural and political issues that contribute to a woman's alcoholic drinking and may prohibit her recovery" (p. 90). Therefore, many support groups formed specifically for women use a feminist empowerment model instead of the original 12 steps developed by AA.

Self-Help Processes in Aftercare

Unfortunately, there is little published research on the utilization of female-oriented support groups as aftercare to prevent relapse by recovering women. "Relapse is the rule across all treatment approaches" (p. 1229), according to DeLeon, who added that aftercare activities can help maintain treatment gains and sustain the recovery process.[46] He suggested that the goals of aftercare should include "socialization, psychological improvement, recognition of the triggers or cues of relapse, and the development of new coping skills consistent and establishment of drug-free networks" (p. 1229). Absence of a strong posttreatment support network and lack of involvement in productive roles and leisure activities are among the significant predictors of relapse identified by Hawkins and Catalano.[47]

The only current research on the characteristics of drug-dependent women suggests that these relapse factors are exacerbated by problems specific to women, notably the prevalence of physical, sexual and emotional abuse in addicted women's lives and extreme stigmatization.[17,48,49] Meeting this wide range of needs is consistent with the purpose of many self-help groups. There is broad agreement that social networks play a key role in posttreatment recovery, and several researchers affirm the value of self-help groups in improving social networks and other aftercare strategies.[14,16,47,50–52]

Treatment alone does not prepare clients for the transition to community life. Aftercare can mitigate the stresses of adjusting to a new, and possibly indifferent, community and creating a new lifestyle.[14] Self-help groups are a primary component of most aftercare activities,[14] but DenHartog et al.[16] and Washton[51] both noted relatively low rates of referral to self-help by professional treatment programs, however. McAuliffe and Ch'ien suggested that self-help and professional models of aftercare combined may offer the most effective relapse-reduction strategies.[50] Their Recovery Training and Self-Help program, which featured a weekly recovery training session, a weekly self-help style meeting, weekend recreational and social activities, and a support network of long-term ex-addicts, significantly reduced the probability of relapse to illicit opiates for the entire 12-mo period of follow-up. Although 15% of their 144 subjects were female, they did not discuss the effect of gender on peer support group attendance and recovery. On the other hand, Havassy and colleagues examined links between social support and abstinence from cocaine in a sample of 104 persons completing treatment.[53] At follow-up 6 mo after treatment, they found that greater functional support and higher levels of perceived emotional support predicted a decreased risk of relapse to cocaine use across race and gender groups.[53]

More recently, Mumme' reviewed the general literature on the role of aftercare in women's recovery.[54] She found that, although there are small but consistent findings that aftercare greatly enhances treatment for both male and female substance abusers, there have been no formal, published studies carried out on women's needs in aftercare. The published formal studies concentrate, for the most part, on male populations, or do not examine differences in the aftercare needs of males and females. She suggested that self-help is one of the most important factors in recovery for women, as it is for men, and that aftercare for women should include peer support with other women as well as mixed groups, such as AA.

The authors of this chapter are currently conducting a 5-yr study on the effectiveness of a non-12-step peer support group in preventing relapse for formerly homeless women in recovery from substance abuse. This research/demonstration project, the Aftercare Project, compares outcomes over an 18-mo period for volunteers who are randomly assigned to control or experimental groups. Women in the control group receive intensive case management, whereas members of the experimental group receive intensive case management and participate in weekly peer support groups. Results remain preliminary in nature. To date, 63 women have been enrolled in the study. The majority of participants are African-American women in their late 20s. Data from intake interviews indicate that most of the women had a history of sexual and physical abuse and intimidation. Almost three-quarters (74%) reported at least one episode of physical abuse by a sexual partner. Almost half reported having been raped, and 30% were sexually abused as children. Half were raised by an alcoholic single mother. More than 25% have attempted suicide at least once. Cocaine (90%) was the most frequently reported drug of abuse, followed by marijuana (64%) and alcohol (44%). More than two-thirds are polydrug abusers.

Since the study is only in its second year, the sample size remains rather small. Thus far no significant differences in outcomes, or measures of self-esteem, presence of social supports, or depression have been observed between the control and experimental groups. However, the results of the participant observation study indicate that the peer support group has been very successful. Peer group meetings are convened by project staff who originally played an active role in facilitating meetings, using a meeting format based on empowerment models from the battered women's movement. Group members now display a high level of motivation to attend meetings, even though for most it involves transporting multiple preschoolers across town by public transportation. Strollers are provided by the project, and childcare is available free of charge during peer group meetings. Group members, their children, and aftercare staff share a lunch following meetings. Members even decided to meet on both Christmas and New Year's Eves. In many ways, this level of commitment contradicts traditional thinking that self-help groups are more important to middle class people who are not as overwhelmed with material needs as women who have just left homeless shelters and are trying to avoid relapse into drug abuse.

As the group has stabilized, members have begun to take greater responsibility for group tasks, maintenance, and facilitation. The group has developed its own rituals for opening and closing meetings. Members hold each other accountable for meeting personal goals set during group meetings. There are frequent reports of social contact between members outside the group. A second group has been formed during nonworking hours to meet the needs of original group members who have since found jobs or are enrolled in educational programs. Ethnographic data gathered by the participant observer at peer group meetings documents the members' need to have a safe place to discuss issues of childhood abuse, incest, battering by a recent or current sexual partner, and feelings of inadequacy as daughters, mothers, lovers, and workers. The women frequently mention their need for a woman-only group. Many have indicated that women-only 12-step groups do not always provide a setting in which these ancillary issues can be safely addressed because of the narrow focus of meetings on addiction and recovery, and because membership in 12-step groups is more open and transient. These observations, together with our survey data, point toward a strong need for aftercare programs that address the specific needs of women in recovery, and that employ self-help models that foster peer support and extended social networks.

Conclusion

There has been a substantial increase in the number of addicted women since the early 1970s. Research in the past 20 yr has demonstrated that addicted women differ from men in their sociodemographic characteristics and patterns of drug abuse, and, therefore, in the type of treatment and after-care that they need. However, there has been little growth in the number of programs for women and their families that address this need. Carefully controlled research studies that examine the role of different components of treatment, including women-only self-help groups, are crucial in validating these experimental treatment forms and in obtaining funding for badly needed new programs. More important, of course, is the elimination of the causes of addiction in women through the establishment of more programs that identify and intervene to prevent the effects of dysfunctional and substance-abusing families, poverty, and the physical, sexual, and emotional abuse of women and their children.

Acknowledgments

This research was supported by a grant from the National Institute on Drug Abuse. The authors wish to gratefully acknowledge the assistance of Rose A. Cheney, Kathleen Coughey, and Amanda Merwin, of the Philadelphia Health Management Corporation, in researching and editing this chapter.

References

[1]P. A. Harrison (1989) Women in treatment: Changing over time. *Int. J. Addict.* **24,** 655–673.

[2]S. Gutierres, R. Jonathan, and D. L. Rhoades (1981) Women and drugs: Use and abuse. Unpublished paper, CODAMA Services, Inc., Phoenix, AZ.

[3]C. J. Furst, L. J. Beckman, C. Y. Nakamura, and M. Weiss (1981) Utilization of Alcoholism Treatment Services. Report prepared for the State of California Department of Alcohol and Drug Programs, University of California at Los Angeles Alcohol Research Center.

[4]S. Stevens, N. Arbiter, and P. Glider (1989) Women residents: Expanding their role to increase treatment effectiveness in substance abuse programs. *Int. J. Addict.* **24,** 425–434.

[5]B. G. Reed (1987) Developing women-sensitive drug dependence treatment services: Why so difficult?. *J. Psychoactive Drugs* **19,** 151–164.

[6]C. Lubinski (1991) Advocacy: Prevention strategies and treatment services sensitive to women's needs, in *Alcohol and Drugs are Women's Issues*, vol. 1. P. Roth, ed. Women's Action Alliance and Scarecrow Press, Metuchen, NJ, pp. 178–182.

[7]L. J. Beckman and H. Amaro (1984/5) Patterns of women's use of alcohol treatment agencies. *Alcohol Health Res. World* **9,** 15–25.

[8]J.C. Marsh and N. A. Miller (1985) Female clients in substance abuse treatment. *Int. J. Addict.* **20,** 995–1019.

[9]P. B. Sutker (1982) Drug dependent women: An overview of the literature, in *Treatment Services for Drug Dependent Women*, vol. 1. G. M. Beschner, B. G. Reed, and J. Mondanaro, eds. National Institute on Drug Abuse, Rockville, MD, pp. 25–51.

[10]T. Doshan and C. Bursch (1982) Women and substance abuse: Critical issues in treatment. *J. Drug Educ.* **12,** 229–239.

[11]L. P. Finnegan (1980) Women in treatment, in *Handbook on Drug Abuse.* R. L. DuPont, A. Goldstein, and J. O'Donnell, eds. National Institute on Drug Abuse, Rockville, MD, pp. 121–131.

[12]M. B. Tucker (1979) A descriptive and comparative analysis of the social support structure of heroin-addicted women, in *Addicted Women: Family Dynamics, Self Perceptions, and Support Systems.* B. G. Reed, E. Leibson, and E. Donovan, eds. National Institute on Drug Abuse, Rockville, MD, pp. 37–76.

[13]L. F. Kurtz (1990) The self-help movement: review of the past decade of research. *Soc. Work Groups* **13,** 101–115.

[14]B. S. Brown and R. S. Ashery (1979) Aftercare in drug abuse programming, in *Handbook on Drug Abuse.* R. L. DuPont, A. Goldstein, and J. O'Donnell, eds. National Institute on Drug Abuse, Rockville, MD, pp. 165–173.

[15]M. Wedenoja and B. G. Reed (1982) Women's groups as a form of intervention for drug dependent women, in *Treatment Services for Drug Dependent Women,* vol. 2. B. G. Reed, G. M. Beschner, and J. Mondanaro, eds. National Institute on Drug Abuse, Rockville, MD, pp. 62–136.

[16]G. L. DenHartog, A. L. Homer, and R. B. Wilson (1986) *Cooperation: A Tradition in Action. Self-Help Involvement of Clients in Missouri Alcohol and Drug Abuse Treatment Programs.* Missouri Department of Mental Health, Jefferson City, MO.

[17]D. L. Rhoades (1983) A longitudinal study of life stress and social support among drug abusers. *Int. J. Addict.* **18,** 195–222.

[18]B. G. Reed (1982) Intervention strategies for drug dependent women: An introduction, in *Treatment Services for Drug Dependent Women,* vol. 1. G. M. Beschner, B. G. Reed, and J. Mondanaro, eds. National Institute on Drug Abuse, Rockville, MD, pp. 1–24.

[19]B. Haver (1987) Female alcoholics: IV. The relationship between family violence and outcome 3–10 years after treatment. *Acta Psychiatr. Scand.* **75,** 449–455.

[20]P. Y. Martin and K. A. Shanahan (1983) Transcending the effects of sex composition in small groups, in *Groupwork with Women/Groupwork with Men.* B. G. Reed and C. G. Garvin, eds. Haworth, New York, pp. 19–32.

[21]R. M. Kanter (1977a) *Men and Women of the Corporation.* Basic Books, New York.

[22]R. M. Kanter (1977b) Some effects of proportions in group life: Skewed sex ratios and responses to token women. *Am. J. Sociol.* **82,** 965–990.

[23]B. G. Reed and E. Leibson (1981) Women clients in special women's demonstration drug abuse treatment programs compared with women entering selected co-sex programs. *Int. J. Addict.* **16,** 1425–1466.

[24]N. Naierman, B. Savage, B. Haskins, J. Lear, H. Chase, K. Marvelle, and R. Lamothe (1979) *An Assessment of Sex Discrimination in the Delivery of Health Development services.* Final report to the Department of Health, Education, and Welfare, Office of Civil Rights (ABT Associates), Contract HEW-100-78--137.S.

[25]I. D. Yalom (1985) *The Theory and Practice of Group Psychotherapy.* Basic, New York, pp. 486–514.

[26]P. Antze (1979) Role of ideologies in peer psychotherapy groups, in *Self-Help Groups for Coping with Crisis.* M. A. Lieberman and L. D. Bordman, eds. Jossey-Bass, San Francisco, pp. 272–304.

[27]P. R. Balgopal and T. V. Vassil (1983) Group work: historical overview and current status. *Groups in Social Work—An Ecological Perspective*, pp. 1–18.

[28]A. H. Katz and E. I. Bender (1976) Self-help groups in western society: history and prospects. *J. Appl. Behav. Sci.* **12**, 265–282.

[29]M. Levine (1988) How self-help works. *Am. J. Community Psychol.* **16**, 167–183.

[30]M. A. Lieberman and G. R. Bond (1978) Self-help groups—problems in measuring outcome. *Small Group Behav.* **9**, 221–241.

[31]L. Maguire (1983) *Understanding Social Networks*. Sage, Beverly Hills, CA.

[32]P. Rosenberg (1984) Support groups—a special therapeutic entity. *Small Group Behav.* **15**, 173–186

[33]L. Shulman (1986) The dynamics of mutual aid. *Soc. Work Groups* **8**, 51–60.

[34]P. R. Balgopal, P. H. Ephross, and T. V. Vassil (1986) Self-help groups and professional helpers. *Small Group Behav.* **17**, 123–137.

[35]S. S. Covington (1991) Sororities of helping and healing: women and mutual help groups in *Alcohol and Drugs are Women's Issues,* vol. 1. P. Roth, ed. Women's Action Alliance and Scarecrow Press, Metuchen, NJ, pp. 85–92.

[36]L. F. Kurtz and T. J. Powell (1987) Three approaches to understanding self-help groups. *Soc. Work Groups* **10**, 69–80.

[37]G. S. Leventhal, K. I. Maton, and E. J. Madara (1988) Systemic organization support for self-help groups. *Am. J. Orthopsychiatry* **58**, 592–603.

[38]P. Petrakis (1988) Research report of the surgeon general's workshop on self-help and public health. *Soc. Policy* **11**, 36–38.

[39]B. Gottlieb (1983) Social networks and social support: an overview of research, practice and policy implications. *Health Educ. Q.* **12**, 5–22.

[40]S. Hartman (1983) A self-help group for women in abusive relationships. *Soc. Work Groups* **6**, 133–146.

[41]P. Cooper-White (1990) Peer vs clinical counseling—is there a place for both in the battered women's movement? *Response* **13**, 2–6.

[42]M. Habib and B. J. Landgraf (1977) Women helping women. *Soc. Work* **22**, 510–512.

[43]S. Xenarios (1988) Sounds of practice I: group work with rape survivors. *Soc. Work Groups* **11**, 95–101.

[44]A. J. Gordon and M. Zrull (1991) Social networks and recovery: one year after inpatient treatment. *J. Subst. Abuse Treatment* **8**, 143–152.

[45]K. Humphreys, B. Mavis, and B. Stofflemayr (1991) Factors predicting attendance at self-help groups after substance abuse treatment: preliminary findings. *J. Consult. Clin. Psychol.* **59**, 591–593.

[46]G. DeLeon (1991) Aftercare in therapeutic communities. *Int. J. Addict.* **25**, 1225–1237.

[47]R. F. Catalano and J. D. Hawkins (1985) Project skills: preliminary results from a theoretically based aftercare experiment. *Natl. Inst. Drug Abuse Res. Monogr. Ser.* **58**, 157–181.

[48]G. B. Ladwig and M. D. Andersen (1989) Substance abuse in women: Relationship between chemical dependency of women and past reports of physical and/or sexual abuse. *Int. J. Addict.* **24**, 739–754.

[49]B. L. Underhill (1986) Issues relevant to aftercare programs for women. *Alcohol Health Res. World* **11**, 46–47.

[50]W. E. McAuliffe and J. M. N. Ch'ien (1986) Recovery training and self help: a relapse-prevention program for treated opiate addicts. *J. Subst. Abuse Treatment* **3,** 9–20.

[51]A. M. Washton (1988) Preventing relapse to cocaine. *J. Clin. Psychiatry* **49,** 34–38.

[52]H. D. Weiner, M. C. Wallen, and G. L. Zankowski (1990) Culture and social class as intervening variables in relapse prevention with chemically dependent women. *J. Psychoactive Drugs* **22,** 239–248.

[53]B. E. Havassy, S. M. Hall, and D. M. Wasserman (1990) Relapse to cocaine use following treatment: Preliminary findings on the role of social support, in *Problems of Drug Dependence 1990: Proceedings of the 52nd Annual Scientific Meeting.* L. Harris, ed. National Institute on Drug Abuse, Rockville, MD, pp. 502–503.

[54]D. Mumme' (1991) Aftercare: Its role in primary and secondary recovery of women from alcohol and other drug dependence. *Int. J. Addict.* **26,** 549–564.

Dieting and Alcohol Use in Women

Dean D. Krahn, Blake Gosnell, and Candace Kurth

Introduction

The connection between dieting, which involves the restriction of caloric intake and especially the avoidance of the intake of "empty" calories, and alcohol consumption, which involves the intake of calories that are not nutritionally vital, is not intuitively obvious to many. Therefore, the reader of this chapter may benefit from a recounting of the way in which we came to study this problem. We recognize that this may be viewed as a rather egocentric approach by some, but in our experience with talking about this area of interest with colleagues, we have found that this type of review tends to be an understandable approach to this topic. The comorbidity of eating disorders and substance abuse have also been reviewed extensively elsewhere,[1,2] and more emphasis regarding family history and clinical implications are available in these sources.

Several years ago, one of the authors (Krahn) was given the task of establishing an eating disorders program on the same unit that housed the substance abuse program. It quickly became difficult to establish the clear lines of demarcation between the programs desired by staff, administrators, and third party payers, as many of the patients with eating disorders also met diagnostic criteria for alcohol and/or other substance abuse disorders, whereas many of the substance abuse patients reported unusual and/or for-

From: *Drug and Alcohol Abuse Reviews, Vol. 5: Addictive Behaviors in Women*
Ed.: R. R. Watson ©1994 Humana Press Inc., Totowa, NJ

mally disordered eating behaviors. Patients with eating disorders would demand that the staff confront patients admitted for substance abuse treatment about their abnormal eating behaviors, and substance abuse patients would chide the staff for failing to recognize the substance abuse problems of patients with eating disorders. The magnitude of this comorbidity of eating disorders and substance abuse was somewhat surprising to us at the time. However, the frequent co-occurrence of these two disorders is now well documented.[3-30] Crisp was one of the first to comment on the relationship between anorexia and alcoholism stating that "chronic patients who have progressed to a state of overeating and vomiting not infrequently appear to become dominated by oral behavior, and may sometimes present with alcoholism" (p. 372).[14] Others have found prevalences of alcoholism or alcohol abuse of 6.7–23% in anorexic populations, with those patients who also have problems with bulimia and/or kleptomania reporting far higher rates of alcohol problems.[3,4] Although these prevalences of alcohol problems are high, they are even higher when one considers that these diagnoses are found in samples of women in late adolescence and early adulthood. The fact that anorexics who have progressed to bulimic behaviors are also at highest risk of substance use disorders suggests that the mechanism by which an individual, after months or years of deprivation, becomes unable to control the use of one orally administered substance (e.g., palatable food) also involves the inability to control the use of other reinforcers, such as alcohol. This incidence of alcoholism is high, and it is even higher when one considers that the average age of this sample was 20 yr.

The frequency of alcohol and other drug abuse is even higher in studies of bulimic patients. Normal weight bulimics show frequencies of substance abuse ranging from 6–31%.[5,7,9,31,32] For example, Mitchell et al. reported that 49% of a large sample of 275 bulimia nervosa patients collected at a university-based clinic reported using alcohol several times per week or more, although not all of these were judged to be abusers or dependent.[8] Pyle et al. reported in their initial description of normal weight bulimia that 24% of their bulimic patients had significant chemical dependency problems.[9] At the time of evaluation, 41% were using alcohol at least several times per week and 18% were using it daily. In all, 21% reported intermittent amphetamine abuse, and 12% admitted to daily amphetamine use. Weiss and Ebert reported that significantly more bulimics than normal controls used marijuana, cocaine, amphetamines, and barbiturates, indicating that this relationship was not limited to alcohol, which contains calories, or amphetamines, which suppress appetite.[27] Conversely, cross-sectional studies have shown a high prevalence of eating disorders in female patients presenting with substance abuse.[30,33] Beary et al. compared 20 consecutive alcoholic women under age 40 with 20 age-matched patients with bulimia nervosa and 17 age-matched normal controls.[20] In all, 35% of alcoholics had a previous major eating disorder, and 50% of the bulimics either abused alcohol or used it to excess. Thus, eating disorders and alcohol and other drug abuse are found together whether one studies populations presented for treatment of eating disorders or alcoholism.

Hypothesis Generation

However, the simple recognition that these two disorders were also frequently co-occurring in other investigators' patient populations did little beyond reassuring us that our observations were not the result of an unusual selection of patients as a result of housing both units on one ward. These observations did not provide answers to the vexing questions of patients and professionals, such as: Am I addicted to food and drugs? Is this all one illness? Do I use both food and drugs to treat my depression? Do I need 12-step groups for both disorders? Is my drug use secondary to my eating disorder so that if I get over my eating disorder, then I won't have to deal with the drug problem? Can you treat both disorders with one treatment?. Answers to all of these questions remain elusive, but this area of research was not one in which we could formulate testable hypotheses as long as we lacked a reasonable theory regarding the relationship of the two disorders.

The two hypotheses extant several years ago regarding the nature of the relationship of these two disorders seemed unlikely to be proven correct. One hypothesis, which posited that the pathological use of food and drugs was related to an underlying addictive personality, seemed doubtful as little evidence had been marshaled that defined a personality type (other than the antisocial variant) as being specifically connected to alcoholism or other drug dependency.[34] We reasoned that it was unlikely that a hypothesis that had failed to explain one set of abnormal behaviors would be better at explaining two sets of abnormal behaviors. The other hypothesis, which posited that both alcohol abuse and pathological eating patterns were secondary to depression, also was of dubious validity. Although bulimic women are clearly frequently depressed and benefit to some degree from antidepressants,[31,32,35,36] insightful analyses by Strober and Katz as well as Hinz and Williamson clearly showed that bulimia was not simply a form of affective disorder.[37,38] Again, it seemed unlikely that an explanation that had failed to explain one disorder would prove better in explaining two disorders.

Unfortunately, at that time, we had no better explanation for this relationship. Then, quite by accident, we came across a body of literature showing that food deprivation is one of the most potent environmental stimulants of drug self-administration in animals.[39] Food deprivation increases the self-administration of drugs by both intravenous[35,41] and oral[42,43] routes, and this effect occurs in both rats and rhesus monkeys.[44,45] Alcohol,[46] barbiturates,[47] opiates,[41] stimulants,[48] hallucinogens,[44] and nicotine[51] are all self-administered in greater amounts by animals when they are deprived of food. Food restriction is part of standard paradigms for establishing drugs as reinforcers in animals.[52,53] Thus, food deprivation increases the likelihood of acquisition of the drug as a reinforcer as well as the consumption of drugs already established as reinforcers. Food deprivation also increases the rate of electrical intracranial self-stimulation.[54,55] Therefore, it is likely that food deprivation alters the function of the central reward mechanism rather than specifically altering drug intake. Given that patients with eating disorders are almost exclusively severe and chronic dieters and have a high frequency of alcohol and drug self-administration, we hypothesized that the food restriction practiced by these patients had the same effect on their response to the rewarding effects of alcohol and drugs as that which was previously documented in food-restricted animals.

There was little evidence that the stimulatory effect of food deprivation on alcohol and drug consumption was operative in humans. However, in a classic study, normal males who were placed on half their normal caloric intake for 6 mo dramatically increased their consumption of coffee and tobacco, which were the only drugs available to these laboratory-confined subjects.[56] Chewing of cocoa leaf increases during food deprivation and decreases when food is plentiful in Quechua Indians of Peru.[57]

Of note, a number of the men who were deprived of food in a laboratory setting experienced binge-eating episodes on sweet, high-fat foods in addition to the increase in drug intake.[56] Additional studies show that food deprivation increases the intake of saccharin (i.e., sweet substances)[58,59] and fat[60] in animals. Bulimic and anorectic women (groups with high incidences of alcohol and other drug use and abuse) have higher preferences for sweet tastes than do normals.[61] Thus, it seems likely that restricted food intake in humans, like animals, simultaneously increases the preference for and/or intake of highly palatable, "binge" foods and the preference for and/or intake of drugs. Increased intakes of alcohol, drugs, and sweet, high-fat foods resemble alcohol and drug use and binge-eating episodes seen in bulimics. Food deprivation may alter the dynamics of central reward mechanisms, increasing the consumption of reinforcing chemicals and palatable foods. It may be the case that the process by which anorexics or severe dieters switch to bulimia (an event which occurs in many chronic patients) carries with it not only a change in one's ability to control food intake, but also a change in the capacity to control alcohol and other drug intake. The converse hypothesis, that drug use significantly alters the regulation of food intake is not as well documented. Although the self-administration of some drugs with potent anorectic effects, such as cocaine, do affect patterns of food intake, alcohol drinking is compensated for by laboratory animals.[62]

Of course, some women use drugs as anorectic agents in order to help them in their pursuit of thinness. Data from the NIDA High School Senior Survey show that 1.9% of high school senior females use diet pills daily and 43% of high school senior females have used diet pills at some time.[63] These anorectic drugs could act as gateway drugs to more widespread or severe drug use. It has been hypothesized on the basis of animal studies, however, that women who deprive themselves of food and also use anorectic agents in that deprived state are using these agents at a point of increased sensitivity to their reinforcing effects and, therefore, are at increased risk for addiction to these agents.[64,65]

If food deprivation was an important potentiator of drug self-administration and preference for sweet, high-fat foods in humans as in animals, it provided a possible explanation for the relationship of eating disorders and alcoholism and other drug abuse. One could predict that those people who restricted food intake most severely and chronically would be more prone to frequent or pathological use of substances than those who restricted food intake moderately, who, in turn, would be more prone to use of substances than those who rarely or never food restricted. One could also predict that the onset of food deprivation behaviors (i.e., dieting) would precede frequent or pathological substance use. However, because all patients with eating disorders attempt to deprive themselves of food to a severe degree, studying a sample of eating disorders for the relationship of severity of dieting and frequency of alcohol and other drug consumption was pointless as there was too little variability in severity of food restriction. Therefore, we needed to compare the alcohol and drug use of populations with widely differing degrees of severity of dieting pathology to determine whether the severity of perceived food restriction was related to the frequency and intensity of alcohol and drug intake. Prior to formulating new studies of our own to address this point, we reviewed two sets of studies, one set that documented a possible relationship between increased alcohol/drug use and subclinical levels of eating disorder symptoms and the other set that documented the clinical impression that eating disorder symptoms precede frequent or pathological alcohol or drug use.

Relevant Previous Studies

Bulimic behaviors that did not meet diagnostic criteria also show a close relationship with alcohol and other substance use. Killen et al. reported that high school student subjects with either bulimia and bulimic behaviors reported higher usage rates than normal for cigarets and marijuana and more frequent episodes of drunkenness.[66] College freshman women who were smokers or drinkers reported higher prevalences of bulimic behaviors by Frank et al.[67] Bradstock et al. reported that women who reported dieting were more likely to be binge drinkers than those who did not report dieting.[68] A study at the University of Michigan examined the relationship of dieting behaviors and alcohol use in general psychiatric patients.[1] Our hypothesis was that those patients with histories of frequent dieting or bulimic behaviors would answer more questions positively (i.e., pathologically) on the CAGE screening questionnaire for alcoholism.[69] We reviewed the records of 243 consecutive female patients between ages 18 and 40 evaluated in clinics (other than the eating disorders clinic) who did not receive an eating disorders diagnosis in their evaluation. Each patient completed a questionnaire assessing dieting and bulimic behaviors as well as the CAGE questionnaire. Patients were classified as positive or negative for any history of pathological weight control efforts (i.e., purging or fasting behavior consistent with eating disorders). Results showed that 98 of the 236 patients reported a positive history for pathological weight control efforts. In the 98 patients with this positive history, 41.8% responded positively to two or more CAGE questions, and patients with a positive history were more than twice as likely to answer two or more CAGE questions positively as those with no history of pathological weight control efforts. ($\chi^2 = 16.01$, $p < .001$). In these 98 patients with positive history for pathological weight control efforts, 51% responded positively to one or more CAGE questions whereas only 29.7% of those with negative histories answered similarly ($\chi^2 = 10.99$, $p < .001$). From these data it was concluded that, at least in the general psychiatric population, bulimic behavior that does not meet diagnostic criteria for bulimia nervosa carries with it an increased risk of pathological use of alcohol. These data also suggest that a history of bulimic behaviors is associated with a risk of alcohol abuse over and above any increased risk conferred by being a psychiatric patient. Thus, there is some evidence that not only bulimia nervosa or anorexia nervosa but also bulimic behaviors are related to increased alcohol and/or drug abuse.

Several authors further noted that the development of eating disorders or problems usually antedate the onset of alcohol or other drug abuse. Jones et al. reviewed 27 cases in which the onset of an eating disorder antedated the onset of alcohol abuse.[20] Reflecting on more than two decades of clinical work with a stable population, the authors noted that "the most striking feature has been the reemergence of the same individuals with alcoholism who had suffered eating disorder in earlier years." Hatsukami et al. demonstrated that the frequency of use of alcohol by bulimic patients increased significantly after the onset of bulimic behavior.[70] In bulimic patients who were eventually diagnosed as substance abusers, daily alcohol use increased to 41.1% of patients after the onset of bulimia compared to 14.7% before the onset of bulimia. Mitchell et al. reported that 20% of a sample of 275 bulimic patients admitted to using alcohol several times a week or more prior to onset of bulimia and 49% reported this pattern of alcohol consumption after the onset of bulimia.[8] Beary et al. also noted that 35% of alcoholic subjects reported a previous major eating disorder and that 50% of bulimic subjects reported significant alcohol abuse following the onset of their eating disorders.[30] By age 35, 50% of bulimic patients use excessively or abuse alcohol.[70] The authors infer that ongoing eating-disordered behavior results in a gradual increase in alcohol use and that a history of previous eating disorder should alert physicians to the future diagnosis of alcoholism.

Thus, the available data suggested that the presence of eating disorders symptomatology might also be associated with increased use of alcohol and that eating disordered behaviors usually preceded problems with abuse of substances. However, no study had actually looked for the relationship between dieting severity over the entire continuum of dieting severity.

A Test of the Relationship of Dieting Severity and Alcohol and Other Drug Use

In order to clarify the relationship between substance use and dieting across a wide range of severity, we surveyed incoming freshman women at a major midwestern university. Results of this study are more completely presented elsewhere.[71] We hypothesized that dieting severity would be continuously related to the prevalence, frequency, and intensity of substance use in a graded manner, such that subjects who reported symptoms that fulfilled DSM-III-R criteria for bulimia nervosa would report the highest levels of substance use; those who reported subthreshold levels of dieting behaviors would report intermediate levels of substance use; and those who reported little or no dieting would report the lowest levels of substance use.

All females attending a freshman orientation at a major midwestern university were invited to participate. Subjects completed a self-administered questionnaire regarding weight, dieting, exercise, purging, weight-related attitudes, and substance use (cigarets, alcohol, and marijuana). Questions were obtained from earlier studies of dieting behavior by our group[72] and the Monitoring the Future Project (MTF), a national, ongoing assessment of substance use patterns in high school seniors and young adults.[73] Participation in the study was voluntary and anonymous. Questionnaires were completed by 1796 women, a 90% response rate.

Frequencies of alcohol, cigaret, and marijuana use over the last month, past year, and lifetime were assessed, along with two indicators of heavy drinking (i.e., the frequencies of having five or more drinks in a row [question from MTF] and of drinking enough alcohol to get "buzzed" [question modified from MTF]). Questions regarding dependence were not included.

Six mutually exclusive dieting severity categories were defined prior to data analyses according to rules described elsewhere.[71] The categories were based on DSM-III-R criteria for bulimia nervosa and results of previous studies.[72,74] In all, 1.6% of the sample was classified as bulimic dieters, 16.6% as at-risk dieters, 22.3% as severe dieters, 12.4% as intense dieters, 33.2% as casual dieters, and 13.8% as nondieters. This rate of bulimia in college women is very similar to that reported by similar previous studies.[74,75]

Prevalence of alcohol use was positively associated with dieting severity. The prevalence of drinking in the past month by dieting severity categories is presented in Table 1. The prevalence of alcohol use increased across the entire range of dieting severity from 43.9% for nondieters to approx 72% for at risk and bulimic dieters. Nondieters were significantly less likely than casual dieters to have consumed alcohol, whereas the severe and at-risk groups were significantly more likely to have used alcohol. The frequency of alcohol use was also positively related to dieting severity. As dieting severity increased, the reported number of occasions of alcohol consumption increased. The bulimic and at-risk groups were similar in their frequency of alcohol use, with >40% of the subjects using alcohol on an approximately weekly or more frequent basis. In contrast, <20% of the nondieters and <30% of casual dieters consumed alcohol at that frequency. Thus, dieting severity was related not only to the prevalence of alcohol use but also to the frequency of alcohol consumption.

The frequency of heavy drinking (consuming five or more drinks in a row) in the past 2 wk was positively related to dieting severity. As dieting severity increased, the reported number of occasions of heavy drinking increased. Almost 20% of the bulimic and at-risk subjects, compared to 5% nondieters, drank five or more drinks in a row on a weekly basis. Similarly, the frequency of drinking enough to alter their mental state was also positively related to dieting severity. Fifty to sixty percent of the subjects in the at-risk and bulimic groups achieved a change in mental state in most or all drinking occasions, compared to approximately half that percentage in the lower two dieting severity groups. Thus, dieting severity was positively related to the intensity of alcohol use.

Table 1
Prevalence of Drinking Alcohol and Bivariate Odds Ratios
and 95% Confidence Intervals for Past Month Drinking

Dieting severity categories	Prevalence of drinking, %	Bivariate odds ratio[a]	95% CI[b]
Bulimic	72.0	1.92	0.85–4.36
At Risk	71.7	1.85	1.37–2.50
Severe	65.0	1.33	1.02–1.73
Intense	61.8	1.18	0.86–1.63
Casual	57.7	—	—
Nondieting	43.9	0.56	0.43–0.78

Reproduced from ref. 71 with permission.
[a]Test for linear trend, $\chi^2 = 46.5$, $p < .0001$.
[b]Casual dieters used as reference group.

Prevalence of smoking was positively associated with dieting severity (test for linear trend = 25.1, $p < .001$). The prevalence of cigaret smoking in the past month for each dieting severity category are: nondieting, 4.9%; casual, 9.5%, intense, 15.7%; severe, 11.8%; at risk, 18.6%; and bulimic, 20.7%. The prevalence of smoking increased across the entire range of dieting severity. Nondieters were significantly less likely than casual dieters to have smoked whereas the intense and at-risk groups were significantly more likely to have smoked. The prevalence of marijuana use in the past month for each dieting severity category are: nondieting, 6.8%; casual, 5.4%; intense, 5.3%; severe, 7.2%; at risk, 9.7%; and bulimic, 14.8%. The at-risk and bulimic dieters were significantly more likely to have used marijuana ($p < .05$). It is important to note that virtually all smokers and marijuana users consumed alcohol, making it impossible to assess independent relationships with dieting severity.

These data show that the relationship between dieting behaviors and increased substance use is not limited to the categories of clinically diagnosable bulimia nervosa and alcoholism, but also extends across the wide range of less severe, but far more frequent levels of dieting and substance use observed in a large population of incoming college women. These results support the hypothesis that there is a positive, continuous relationship between dieting severity and the prevalence, frequency, and intensity of alcohol use. Hence, the most frequent and intense alcohol use was reported by the bulimic and at-risk dieting groups; an intermediate level of alcohol use was reported by the severe and intense groups; and the lowest alcohol use was reported by the nondieters. Furthermore, the prevalence of cigaret and marijuana use was also positively related to dieting severity.

As noted above, bulimics have a markedly increased prevalence of alcohol and other drug use problems. Considering that those subjects who were categorized as at-risk (16.6% of the sample) behaved similarly in their use of alcohol and other drugs to those subjects reporting behaviors and attitudes consistent with bulimia nervosa (1.6%), the at-risk group of dieters may also be at increased risk for the development of chemical dependency. It should be noted that the more severe dieting groups not only consumed alcohol frequently, but also got "buzzed" more often when drinking. In other words, the differences between dieting-severity groups in the qualitative use of alcohol as a mood-altering substance were even larger than indicated by the simple frequency of alcohol use. Intermediate levels of dieting, which we categorized as severe or intense, were also associated with increased substance use. Finally, this pattern occurred even in casual dieters, who used alcohol more than nondieters.

An Extension of the Hypothesis and Potential Implications of Our Findings

The finding that the relationships between dieting behaviors and alcohol and drug use extends to all levels of dieting behavior is consistent with our hypothesis that deprivation of calories or palatable foods is a stimulant of the use of other potential reinforcers, such as alcohol or drugs. It is important to note, however, that we did not measure actual food intake and that our dieting severity scale may measure a perception of deprivation as well as certain responses to deprivation, such as binging rather than actual caloric deficits. Therefore, the possibility remains that the emergence of the belief or feeling that one is deprived of food is sufficient to stimulate use of alcohol or drugs and that no caloric deficit is necessary. It is possible that the deprivation of an important reinforcer of any type has an important stimulatory effect on the subsequent self-administration of other reinforcers. This explanation of the food deprivation effect is bolstered by the fact that other types of deprivation, including water deprivation and sensory isolation, result in increases in drug self-administration in animals.[76,77] Carroll and Meisch concluded that "drug self-administration is controlled by the availability of a variety of reinforcing events in the environment" (p. 59).[78] It is also possible, however, that the deprivation of alcohol or other drugs in people who have become dependent on these substances results also in the use of or cravings for, not only the drugs they are deprived of, but also in the use of or cravings for other reinforcers, such as other drugs or highly palatable foods (*see* Fig. 1). Thus, just as a food-deprived (i.e., dieting) person may use more alcohol and drugs and even develop cravings for alcohol and drugs in addition to cravings for specific foods, an alcohol-dependent person deprived of alcohol may use more highly palatable foods and even develop cravings for foods in addition to cravings for alcohol.[79] Recovering alcoholics who have the longest periods of postdetoxification sobriety report markedly increased intake of sugar in beverages.[80] Sweet cravings are frequently reported by opiate addicts, and large intakes of sweet foods have been reported in this population.[81,82] Anorexic and bulimic patients have increased preferences for sweet-tasting substances[83,84] (although they typically deprive themselves of these foods) and increased rates of alcoholism and other substance abuse.[7,8,20,27,29] Thus, the interactions between preference for sweet substances and the preference for and intake of drugs may be important in both drug-abusing and eating-disordered populations.

The fact that food deprivation increases both sweet and fat preferences and alcohol and drug preferences raises questions about the relationship of preferences for palatable foods and alcohol and other drugs in nondeprived states. Our group has shown that rats selected for preference for a high-fat diet drink more alcohol than do rats selected for preference for a low-fat diet.[85] Likewise, rats that highly prefer saccharin drink more alcohol than rats that show low preference for saccharin.[86] Rats that prefer fat also are more likely to self-administer morphine.[21] Conversely, AA rats bred for high preference for alcohol have higher fat intakes than ANA rats which have low preferences for alcohol.[87] Finally, rats from the LC-Hi strain, which are bred for high rates of self-stimulation in the lateral hypothalamus (presumably evidence of differences in their "reward" systems), drink markedly more saccharin than the LC-Lo strain.[88] Therefore, differences in preferences for palatable qualities of food or fluids may indicate differences in preferences for alcohol and drugs. Whether or not these baseline vulnerabilities would be accentuated by deprivation is unknown.

Thus, the food deprivation practiced by so many people in our society may be just one visible type of deprivation state, which may affect one's vulnerability to frequent or pathological drug use. For years, Alcoholics Anonymous has been advising recovering alcoholics to avoid HALT, an acronym for hunger, anger, loneliness, and tiredness, if they wanted to avoid relapse.[89,90] Other groups are now telling dieters that they need to substitute alternative reinforcers when they deprive themselves of food.[89] Thus, this phenomenon of deprivation of one reinforcer leading to the increased and, possibly, pathological use of alternative reinforcers may be of clinical rel-

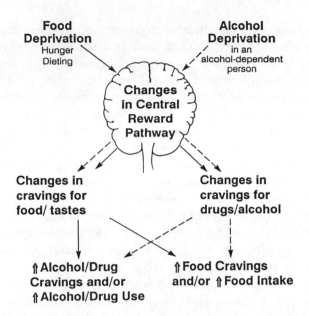

Fig. 1. The proposed reciprocal relationship between deprivation of preferred, palatable foods and increased intake of drugs as well as the deprivation of reinforcing drugs and increased intake of preferred, palatable foods. This relationship is presumably mediated by the central reward mechanisms, which involve dopaminergic and opioid pathways.

evance. However, many questions remain to be answered prior to being satisfied that these clinical recommendations are supported by evidence. These include:

1. Do alcoholics and other drug abusers report increased cravings for and use of alternative reinforcers such as highly palatable foods? If so, are there any important subgroups that seem to be especially prone to pathological use of these alternative reinforcers or should these alternative reinforcers be offered as a means to avoid relapse to use of alcohol or drugs?;
2. Does the relationship between dieting severity and alcohol and other drug use extend to other populations besides young college women?;
3. Does the relationship between dieting severity and alcohol and other drug use hold over time?; and
4. Do deprivations of other types of reinforcers also lead to increased drug and alcohol use?

All of these questions are currently foci of interest for our research group.

Other possible implications of this relationship between deprivation of food and the increased use of alcohol and drug reinforcers include:

1. If food deprivation or deprivation of preferred, highly palatable diets (a common dieting strategy) does trigger increases in drug use in certain populations, then specific prevention programs could be developed, which would focus on young women (as they diet frequently) and highlight the relationship of dieting, binge eating as a result of cravings for highly palatable foods, and alcohol and drug abuse;
2. The avoidance of dieting and the treatment of eating disordered behaviors in the recovery process of young women with alcoholism or other drug abuse problems should be emphasized;
3. Warning labels could be developed for diet pills and other diet products so that consumers would be informed of the increased risk of alcohol and drug abuse that is associated with dieting; and
4. Programs designed to reduce or prevent malnutrition in socioeconomically depressed populations may have the added benefit of reducing vulnerability to drug abuse.

References

[1]D. D. Krahn (1991) The relationship of eating disorders and substance abuse. *J. Subst. Abuse* **3,** 239–253.

[2]D. D. Krahn The relationship of eating disorders and substance abuse, in *Women and Substance Abuse.* E. Gomberg and T. Nirenberg, eds. Ablex, Norwood, NJ, 1993, in press.

[3]R. G. Laessle, H. U. Wittchen, M. M. Fitcher et al. (1989) The significance of subgroups of bulimia and anorexia nervosa: Lifetime frequency of psychiatric disorders. *Int. J. Eating Disorders* **8,** 569–574.

[4]E. D. Eckert, S. C. Goldberg, K. A. Halmi, R. C. Casper, and J. M. Davis (1982) Depression in anorexia nervosa. *Psychol. Med.* **12,** 115–122.

[5]D. K. Hatsukami, E. D. Eckert, J. E. Mitchell, and R. L. Pyle (1984) Affective disorder and substance abuse among women with bulimia. *Psychol. Med.* **14,** 701–704.

[6]D. Hatsukami, P. Owen, R. Pyle, and J. Mitchell (1982) Similarities and differences on the MMPI between women with bulimia and women with alcohol or drug abuse problems. *Addict. Behav.* **7,** 435–439.

[7]G. R. Leon, K. Carroll, B. Chemyk, and S. Finn (1985) Binge eating and associated habit patterns within college student and identified bulimic populations. *Int. J. Eating Disorders* **4,** 43–57.

[8]J. E. Mitchell, D. Hatsukami, E. D. Eckert, and R. L. Pyle (1985) Characteristics of 275 patients with bulimia. *Am. J. Psychiatry* **142,** 482–485.

[9]R. L. Pyle, J. E. Mitchell, and E. D. Eckert (1981) Bulimia: A report of 34 cases. *J. Clin. Psychiatry* **42,** 60–64.

[10]R. L. Pyle, J. E. Mitchell, E. D. Eckert, P. A. Halvorson, P. A. Neuman, and G. M. Goff (1983) The incidence of bulimia in freshmen college students. *Int. J. Eating Disorders* **2,** 75–85.

[11]B. T. Walsh, S. P. Roose, A. H. Glassman, M. Gladis, and C. Sadik (1985) Bulimia and depression. *Psychosom. Med.* **47,** 123–131.

[12]P. J. W. Beaumont, G. C. W. George, and D. E. Smart (1976) Dieters and vomiters and purgers in anorexia nervosa. *Psychol. Med.* **6,** 617–622.

[13]R. C. Casper, E. D. Eckert, K. A. Halmi, S. Goldberg, and J. Davis (1980) Bulimia: Its incidence and clinical importance in patients with anorexia nervosa. *Arch. Gen. Psychiatry* **37,** 1036–1040.

[14]A. H. Crisp (1968) Primary anorexia nervosa. *Gut* **9,** 370–372.

[15]P. E. Garfinkel and D. M. Garner (1982) *Anorexia Nervosa: A Multidimensional Perspective.* Brunner/Mazel, New York.

[16]P. E. Garfinkel, H. Moldofsky, and D. M. Garner (1980) The heterogeneity of anorexia nervosa. *Arch. Gen. Psychiatry* **37,** 1036–1040.

[17]D. M. Garner and P. E. Garfinkel (1980) Socio-cultural factors in the development of anorexia nervosa. *Psychol. Med.* **10,** 647–656.

[18]M. Strober (1981) The relationship of personality characteristics to body image disturbances in juvenile anorexia nervosa: A multivariate analysis. *Psychosom. Med.* **43,** 323–330.

[19]M. Strober (1982) Focus of control psychopathology, and weight gain in juvenile anorexia nervosa. *J. Abnorm. Child Psychol.* **10,** 97–106.

[20]D. A. Jones, N. Cheshire, and H. Moorhouse (1985) Anorexia nervosa, bulimia and alcoholism-association of eating disorder and alcohol. *J. Psychiat. Res.* **19,** 377–380.

[21]H. E. Gwirtsman, P. Roy-Bryne, J. Yager, and R. H. Gerner (1983) Neuroendocrine abnormalities in bulimia. *Am. J. Psychiatry* **140,** 559–563.

[22]J. I. Hudson, H. G. Pope, J. M. Jonas, and D. Yurgelun-Todd (1983) Family history study of anorexia nervosa and bulimia. *Br. J. Psychiatry* **142,** 133–138.

[23]M. Strober, B. Salkin, J. Burroughs, and W. Morrell (1982) Validity of the bulimia-restrictor distinction in anorexia nervosa. *J. Nerv. Ment. Dis.* **170,** 345–351.

[24]D. B. Herzog (1982) Bulimia in the adolescent. *Am. J. Dis. Child.* **136,** 985–989.

[25]J. Brisman and M. Siegel (1984) Bulimia and alcoholism: Two sides of the same coin? *J. Subst. Abuse Treatment* **1,** 113–118.

[26]S. C. Wooley and O. W. Wooley (1981) Overeating as substance abuse. *Adv. Subst. Abuse* **2,** 41–67.

[27]S. Weiss and M. Ebert (1983) Psychological and behavioral characteristics of normal-weight bulimics and normal-weight controls. *Psychosom. Med.* **45,** 293–303.

[28]K. Carroll and G. Leon (1981) The bulimic-vomiting disorder within a generalized substance abuse pattern. Paper presented at the annual meeting of the Association for the Advancement of Behavior Therapy, Toronto, Canada.

[29]J. M. Jonas, M. S. Gold, D. Sweeny, and A. L. C. Pottash (1987) Eating disorders and cocaine abuse: A survey of 259 cocaine abusers. *J. Clin. Psychiatry* **48,** 47–50.

[30]M. D. Beary, J. H. Lacey, and J. Merry (1986) Alcoholism and eating disorders in women of fertile age. *Br. J. Addict.* **81,** 685–689.

[31]J. I. Hudson, H. G. Pope, J. M. Jonas, and D. Yurgelun-Todd (1983) Family history study of anorexia nervosa and bulimia. *Br. J. Psychiatry* **142,** 133–138.

[32]J. I. Hudson, H. G. Pope Jr., J. M. Jonas, and D. Yurgelun-Todd (1983) Phenomenologic relationship of eating disorders to major affective disorder. *Psychiatry Res.* **9,** 345–354.

[33]R. N. Marcus and K. A. Halmi (1989) Eating disorders in substance abuse patients. Paper presented at the meeting of the American Psychiatric Association, San Francisco.

[34]G. E. Vaillant (1983) *The Natural History of Alcoholism Causes, Patterns, and Paths to Recovery.* Harvard University Press, Cambridge, MA.

[35]D. K. Hatsukami, J. E. Mitchell, and E. D. Eckert (1984) Eating disorders: A variant of mood disorders? *Psychiat. Clin. N. Am.* **7.**

[36]J. I. Hudson, H. G. Pope Jr., J. M. Jonas, and D. Yurgelun-Todd (1983) Phenomenologic relationship of eating disorders to major affective disorder. *Psychiatry Res.* **9,** 345–354.

[37]M. Strober and J. Katz (1987) Do eating disorders and affective disorders share a common etiology? A dissenting opinion. *Int. J. Eating Disorders* **6,** 171–180.

[38]L. D. Hinz and D. A. Williamson (1987) Bulimia and depression: A review of the affective variant hypothesis. *Psychol. Bull.* **102,** 150–158.

[39]M. E. Carroll and R. A. Meisch (1984) Increased drug-reinforced behavior due to food deprivation, in *Advances in Behavioral Pharmacology,* vol. 4. T. Thompson, J. E. Barrett, and P. B. Davis, eds. Academic, New York, pp. 47–88

[40]M. E. Carroll, C. P. France, and R. A. Meisch (1979) Food deprivation increases oral and intravenous drug intake in rats. *Science* **205,** 319–321.

[41]M. E. Carroll, C. P. France, and R. A. Meisch (1981) Intravenous self-administration of etonitazene, cocaine, and phencyclidine in rats during food deprivation and starvation. *J. Pharmacol. Exp. Ther.* **217,** 241–247.

[42]M. E. Carroll and R. A. Meisch (1979) Effects of food deprivation on etonitazene consumption in rats. *Pharmacol. Biochem. Behav.* **10,** 155–159.

[43]R. A. Meisch and D. J. Kliner (1979) Etonitazene as a reinforcer for rats: Increased etonitazene-reinforced behavior due to food deprivation. *Psychopharmacology* **63,** 97,98.

[44]M. E. Carroll and R. A. Meisch (1980) Oral phencyclidine (PCP) self-administration in rhesus monkeys: Effects of feeding conditions. *J. Pharmacology Exp. Ther.* **214,** 339–346.

[45]M. E. Carroll (1982) Rapid acquisition of oral phencyclidine self-administration in food-deprived and food-satiated rhesus monkeys: Concurrent phencyclidine and water choice. *Pharmacol. Biochem. Behav.* **17,** 341–346.

[46]R. A. Meisch and T. Thompson (1973) Ethanol as a reinforcer: Effects of fixed ratio size and food deprivation. *Psychopharmacologia* **28,** 171–183.

[47]M. E. Carroll, D. C. Stotz, D. J. Kliner, and R. A. Meisch (1984) Self-administration of orally-delivered methohexital in rhesus monkey with phencyclidine or pentobarbital histories: Effects of food deprivation and satiation. *Pharmacol. Biochem. Behav.* **20,** 145–151.

[48]D. J. Kliner and R. A. Meisch (1989) Oral pentobarbital intake in rhesus monkeys: Effects of drug concentration under conditions of food deprivation and satiation. *Pharmacol. Biochem. Behav.* **32,** 347–354.

[49]S. D. Glick, P. A. Hinds, and J. N. Carlson (1987) Food deprivation and stimulant self-administration in rats: Differences between cocaine and d-amphetamine. *Psychopharmacology (Berlin)* **91,** 372–374.

[50]R. N. Takahashi, G. Singer, and T. P. S. Oei (1978) Schedule-induced self-injection of d-amphetamine by naive animals. *Pharmacol. Biochem. Behav.* **9,** 857–861.

[51]T. P. S. Oei, G. Singer, D. Jeffreys, W. Lang, and A. Latiff (1978) Schedule induced self-injection of nicotine, heroin, and methadone by naive animals, in *Stimulus Properties of Drugs: Ten Years of Progress.* F. C. Colpaert and J. A. Rosecrans, eds. Elsevier, Amsterdam, North Holland, pp. 503–516.

[52]R. B. Stewart and L. A. Grupp (1984) A simplified procedure for producing ethanol self-selection in rats. *Pharmacol. Biochem. Behav.* **21,** 255–258.

[53]J. E. Henningfeld and R. A. Meisch (1975) Ethanol-reinforced responding and intake as a function of volume per reinforcement. *Pharmacol. Biochem. Behav.* **3,** 437–441.

[54]J. Olds (1958) Effects of hunger and male sex hormones on self-stimulation of the brain. *J. Comp. Physiol. Psychology* **51,** 320–324.

[55]J. R. Stellar and C. R. Gallistel (1975) Runway performance of rats for brain stimulation or food reward: Effects of hunger and priming. *J. Comp. Physiol. Psychology* **89,** 590–599.

[56]J. C. Franklin, B. C. Schiele, J. Brozek, and A. Keys (1948) Observations on human behavior in experimental semistarvation and rehabilitation. *J. Clin. Psychology* **4,** 28–45.

[57]J. M. Hanna and C. A. Hornick (1977) Use of coca leaf in southern Peru: Adaptation or addiction. *Bull. Narc.* **29,** 63–74.

[58]F. D. Sheffield and T. B. Roby (1950) Reward value of a nonnutritive sweet taste. *J. Comp. Physiol. Psychology* **43,** 471–481.

[59]S. R. Hursh and R. C. Beck (1971) Bitter and sweet saccharin preference as a function of food deprivation. *Psychol. Rep.* **29,** 419–422.

[60]D. R. Reed, R. J. Contreras, C. Maggio, M. R. C. Greenwood, and J. Rodin (1988) Weight cycling in female rats increases dietary fat selection and adiposity. *Physiol. Behav.* **42,** 389–395.

[61]A. Drewnowski, K. A. Halmi, B. Pierce, J. Gibbs, and G. P. Smith (1987) Taste and eating disorders. *Am. J. Clin. Nutrition* **46,** 442–450..

[62]C. P. Richter (1941) Alcohol as a food. *Q. J. Study Alcohol* **1,** 650–662.

[63]L. D. Johnston, P. M. O'Malley, and J. G. Bachman (1985) *Use of Licit and Illicit Drugs by America's High School Students, 1975–1984.* DHHS Publication No. (ADM) 85-1394, U.S. Government Printing Office, Washington, DC.

[64]E. R. Gritz (1986) Gender and the teenage smoker, in *Women and Drugs: A New Era for Research.* NIDA Research Monograph Series No. 65, U.S. Government Printing Office, Washington, DC, pp. 70–79.

[65]M. Papasava and G. Singer (1985) Self-administration of low-dose cocaine by rats at reduced and recovered body weight. *Psychopharmacology* **85,** 419–425.

[66]J. D. Killen, C. B. Taylor, M. J. Telch, T. N. Robinson, D. J. Maron, and K. E. Saylor (1987) Depressive symptoms and substance use among adolescent binge eaters and purgers: A defined population study. *Am. J. Public Health* **77,** 1539–1541.

[67]R. E. Frank, M. Serdula, and G. G. Abel (1987) Bulimic eating behaviors: Association with alcohol and tobacco. *Am. J. Public Health* **77,** 369,370.

[68]K. Bradstock, M. R. Forman, N. J. Binkin, E. M. Gentry, G. C. Hogelin, D. F. Williamson, and F. L. Trowbridge (1988) Alcohol use and health behavior lifestyles among U.S. women: The behavioral risk factor surveys. *Addict. Behav.* **13,** 61–71.

[69]J. A. Ewing (1987) Detecting alcoholism, the CAGE questionnaire. *JAMA* **252,** 111–121.

[70]D. Hatsukami, J. E. Mitchell, E. D. Eckert, and R. Pyle (1986) Characteristics of patients with bulimia only, bulimia with affective disorder, and bulimia with substance abuse problems. *Addict. Behav.* **11,** 399–406.

[71]D. D. Krahn, C. Kurth, M. Demitrack, and A. Drewnowski (1992) The relationship of dieting severity and bulimic behaviors to alcohol and other drug use in young women. *J. Subst. Abuse* **4,** 341–353.

[72]A. Drewnowski, D. K. Yee, and D. D. Krahn (1989) Dieting and bulimia: A continuum of behaviors. Paper presented at the meeting of the American Psychiatric Association, San Francisco, May, 1989.

[73]L. O. Johnston, P. M. O'Malley, and J. G. Buchman (1988/1989) Monitoring the Future (MTF). Institute for Social Research, The University of Michigan, Ann Arbor, MI.

[74]A. Drewnowski, D. K. Yee, and D. D. Krahn (1988) Bulimia in college women: Incidence and recovery rates. *Am. J. Psychiatry* **145**, 753–755.

[75]E. E. Schotte and A. J. Stunkard (1987) Bulimia vs. bulimic behaviors on a college campus. *JAMA* **258**, 1213–1215.

[76]M. E. Carroll and I. N. Boe (1984) Effect of dose on increased etonitazene self-administration by rats due to food deprivation. *Psychopharmacology* **82**, 151,152.

[77]C. W. Cole and G. S. Goldstein (1971) Consumption of ethanol as a function of sensory isolation. *Learning Motivation* **2**, 363–370.

[78]M. E. Carroll and R. A. Meisch (1984) Increased drug-reinforced behavior due to food deprivation, in *Advances in Behavioral Pharmacology*, vol. 4. T. Thompson, J. E. Barrett, and P. B. Davis, eds. Academic, New York, pp. 47–88.

[79]R. M. Gunther (1980) The effect of nutritional therapy on rehabilitation of alcoholics. PhD Thesis, University of Michigan.

[80]L. Yung, E. Gordis, and J. Holt (1983) Dietary choices and likelihood of abstinence among alcoholic patients in an outpatient clinic. *Drug Alcohol Dependency* **12**, 355–362.

[81]A. Morabia, J. Fabre, E. Chee, S. Zeger, E. Orsat, and A. Robert (1989) Diet and opiate addiction: A quantitative assessment of the diet of non-institutionalized opiate addicts. *Br. J. Addict.* **84**, 173–180.

[82]J. R. Tallman, M. Willenbring, G. Carlson, M. G. Boosalis, D. D. Krahn, A. S. Levine, and J. E. Morley (1984) Effect of chronic methadone use in humans on taste and dietary preference [abstract]. *Federal Proc.* **43**, 1057.

[83]A. Drewnowski, K. A. Halmi, and B. Pierce (1987) Taste and eating disorders. *Am. J. Clin. Nutrition* **46**, 442–450.

[84]A. Drewnowski, F. Bellisle, P. Aimez, and B. Remy (1987) Taste and bulimia. *Physiol. Behav.* **41**, 621–626.

[85]D. D. Krahn and B. Gosnell (1991) A. Fat-preferring rats consume more alcohol than carbohydrate-preferring rats. *Alcohol* **8**, 313–316.

[86]B. A. Gosnell and D. D. Krahn (1991) The relationship between saccharin and alcohol intake in rats. *Alcohol* **9**, 203–206.

[87]O. A. Forsander (1988) The interaction between voluntary alcohol consumption and dietary choice. *Alcohol Alcohol.* **23**, 143–149.

[88]I. Lieblich, E. Cohen, J. R. Ganchrow, E. M. Blass, and F. Bergman (1983) Chronically elevated intake of saccharin solution induces morphine tolerance in genetically selected rats. *Science* **221**, 871–873.

[89]T. T. Gorski and M. Miller (1986) Staying sober a guide for relapse prevention. Independence, Herald House/Independence Press, MI.

[90]Alcoholics Anonymous World Services, Inc. (1975) *Living Sober: Some Methods AA Members Have Used for Not Drinking*. New York.

Alcohol Effects in Postmenopausal Women

Judith S. Gavaler
and Elaine R. Rosenblum

Introduction

The subject of alcohol effects in postmenopausal women encompasses three areas of conceptualization: The issue of *alcohol* includes both levels of consumption of alcoholic beverages as well as the alcohol and congener substances contained in alcoholic beverages. The term *effects* requires specification; the material to be discussed in this chapter will be related to endocrine effects as manifested in changes in hormone levels and their interrelationships. The term *postmenopausal* requires definition, as the endocrine changes to be discussed are menopause-specific and are not applicable to women during their reproductive years.

Alcoholic Beverage Consumption

The survey literature related to alcoholic beverage consumption patterns among postmenopausal women suggests that moderate alcohol use among postmenopausal women is common, whereas "heavy use" is somewhat rare.[1-7] The difficulty is in defining consumption cutpoints to separate moderate intake, heavy use, and alcohol abuse. As may be seen in Table 1, the cutpoints used to define heavy drinking are variable, but nonetheless

From: *Drug and Alcohol Abuse Reviews, Vol. 5: Addictive Behaviors in Women*
Ed.: R. R. Watson ©1994 Humana Press Inc., Totowa, NJ

Table 1
Alcoholic Beverage Consumption in Postmenopausal Women

Authors	Alcohol users, % of total	Age group	Definition of heavy drinking	Heavy drinkers	
				% of total	% of users
Cahalan and Cisin[1]	50	50–59	nearly every day with ≥5 drinks on most occasions	1.5	3
	44	≥60		0.9	2
O'Connell et al.[2]	75	50–59	≥4 drinks/d	2.1	2.8
	58	60–69		1.0	1.7
	59	≥70		0	0
Wechsler[3]	73	55–64	nearly every day with ≥5 drinks on most occasions	9.1	12.5
	63	≥65		3.0	4.8
NIAAA[4]	56	≥55	≥2 drinks/d	4.5	8
Gomberg[5]	50	51–60	≥2 drinks/d	4.0	8
	39	61–90		1.2	3
	39	≥71		0	0
Celentano and McQueen[6]	59	45–54	≥2 drinks/d	9.9	10.0
	59	55–64		5.2	8.9
	46	≥65		4.7	10.2
Hilton and Clark[7]	62	50–59	>1.5 drinks/d and >5 drinks/occasion at least once in a while	4.3	7
	49	≥60		1.0	2

useful. The definition of moderate drinking has now become less complex; recent guidelines recommend that moderate drinking be specified as no more than one drink a day for most women, and defines a standard drink containing 0.5 oz or 15 g of ethanol as 12 oz of beer, 5 oz of wine, or 1.5 oz of 80 proof distilled spirits.[8] A definition of alcohol abuse is inexact at best, and is usually estimated in terms of amount over time in individuals who have physical manifestations of alcohol-induced disease. Examples of alcohol abuse specifications in postmenopausal women with alcohol-induced cirrhosis include consumption from as high as >70 grams of ethanol/d for >10 yr[9] to intake of 50 g of ethanol/d for >2 yr.[10]

Consumption of alcoholic beverages is usually considered to be synonymous with intake of ethanol *per se*. Recent studies suggest, however, that the consumed congeners of alcoholic beverages may also be important, and thus should be taken into account when evaluating the effects of alcoholic beverage consumption. Specifically, recent studies have reported that both bourbon and beer contain biologically active estrogenic substances called phytoestrogens.[11–14] The endocrine effects of the consumption of both ethanol and the phytoestrogen congeners will be discussed in this chapter.

Endocrine Effects
of Alcoholic Beverage Consumption

The estrogen status of postmenopausal women and the factors that influence their estrogen levels is a subject of great interest in the scientific community because the risk of heart disease, osteoporosis, and cancers of the breast and uterus have been shown to be related to postmenopausal estrogenization. The effects of alcoholic beverage consumption on postmenopausal endocrine status can easily be assessed by first measuring steroid hormones, such as estradiol and testosterone, and the pituitary hormones, such as luteinizing hormone (LH), follicle stimulating hormone (FSH), and prolactin, and by then examining the interrelationships of the hormone with each other as well as with the variables known to be postmenopausal estrogen determinants. The literature related to alcoholic beverage consumption effects on postmenopausal endocrine status will be reviewed in this chapter.

The Postmenopausal State

The menopause is defined as the cessation of cyclic ovarian function. The menopausal state is achieved by one of two pathways. The more usual route is via a natural process during which cyclic ovarian function falters and then ceases altogether; in women experiencing a natural menopause, menopause is defined as having occurred when a full year has passed since the last menstrual period. It must further be noted that a hysterectomy without ovariectomy does not interfere with the process of natural menopause, but only eliminates menstrual bleeding making it impossible to ascertain the time of the last menstrual period as the marker of cessation of cyclic ovarian function. The other route to the menopause is via the surgical removal of the ovaries.

The hormonal status of normal postmenopausal women is characterized by estrogen deficiency and consequently elevated levels of the gonadotropins LH and FSH.[15,16] Although the postmenopausal ovary no longer produces estrogens, androgen production continues. The ovarian contribution to circulating levels of androstenedione, the precursor of estrone, is estimated to be 30%, whereas the ovarian contribution to circulating levels of testosterone, the precursor of estradiol, is estimated to be between 20 and 50%.[17-21] The availability of androgen substrate is important because the source of estrogens in postmenopausal women is from the conversion via the enzyme aromatase of androgens to estrogens. Thus the adrenal gland is also important for the estrogen status of postmenopausal women because the adrenal cortex is reported to produce up to 60% of circulating testosterone and up to 80% of androstenedione.[18,21-23]

Until fairly recently, two major variables were well established as estrogen determinants in normal postmenopausal women. Factors that influence either the activity of the androgen-converting enzyme aromatase or the availability of androgen substrate will directly influence estrogen levels.

The first major postmenopausal estrogen determinant is body fat mass. Aromatase is present in a variety of body tissue, primarily in adipose tissue; thus it is not surprising that body fat mass as estimated by body weight or the body mass index (BMI) is highly correlated with estrogen levels.[24] The second major postmenopausal estrogen determinant is the presence of the postmenopausal ovaries, which are an important source of androgens; thus it is not surprising that estrogen levels are reported to be higher in natural menopause women as compared to women who have undergone bilateral ovariectomy.[24]

There are pathological states associated with changes in estrogen levels; in patients with cirrhosis of the liver, the activity of the enzyme aromatase is reported to be increased, resulting in increased estrogen levels. In patients with adrenal insufficiency, androgen production is diminished and thus estrogen levels are decreased as a result of lower substrate availability.

Studies performed in males have suggested that alcohol may be a variable with the potential to influence estrogen levels. Specifically, aromatization is reported to be increased in alcoholic cirrhotic males.[25,26] Administration of ethanol to normal male volunteers[27] or to male experimental animals[28] has been shown to increase the conversion of androgens to estrogens and to increase the activity of the enzyme aromatase. Further, studies using isolated adrenal perfusion in male rats have shown ethanol to increase androgen production.[29] Taken together, these studies in males encouraged research designed to evaluate the possibility that alcoholic beverage consumption might be a variable capable of influencing estrogen levels and the hormonal status of postmenopausal women.[30]

The Endocrine Effects
of Alcohol Abuse in Postmenopausal Women

Although limited in numbers, there are several studies that have evaluated the endocrine status of alcoholic postmenopausal with alcohol-induced cirrhosis.[10,30–36] In all of these studies, women were receiving estrogen replacement therapy. Although not all study samples are composed exclusively of postmenopausal women or of alcoholic women with cirrhosis, the findings are markedly consistent. As may be seen in Table 2, it is clear that estradiol levels are increased and testosterone levels are decreased in alcoholic cirrhotic postmenopausal women. As mentioned in the introduction, in males, alcohol has been shown to increase the aromatization/conversion of androgens to estrogens. The estradiol to testosterone ratio can be used as an estimate of the conversion of precursor testosterone to product estradiol.[37] Thus as may also be seen in Table 2, there is evidence provided by the ratio that alcohol also increases the conversion of testosterone to estradiol in alcoholic cirrhotic postmenopausal women. As a general comment, these findings in alcoholic postmenopausal women reflect the findings in male alcoholic cirrhotics.[38]

Studies reporting the effects of alcohol abuse on the secretion of pituitary hormones in alcoholic postmenopausal women with alcohol-induced liver disease are summarized in Table 3. As was the case with the steroid hormones, the influence of alcohol abuse on levels of pituitary hormones are generally consistent. With the increase in estradiol, the decrease in both LH and FSH are expected; the absolute decrease in levels of these gonadotropins, however, is exaggerated and may reflect a direct effect of alcohol at the levels of the hypothalamus and pituitary glands.

In males, levels of prolactin are significantly increased in cirrhotic males with encephalopathy, and hyperprolactinemia in the presence of hepatic encephalopathy is associated with 100% mortality.[39–41] Dopamine is an inhibitor of prolactin secretion; thus the findings in males led to a theory of dopamine depletion and false neurotransmitter accumulation as a mechanism responsible for hepatic encephalopathy.[42] Unfortunately, when this theory was being developed and tested, women were not evaluated. Using our current dataset of 36 alcoholic cirrhotic postmenopausal women,[36]

Table 2
Steroid Estrogens in Alcoholic Postmenopausal Women

Authors	Subjects	Estradiol pg/mL	Testosterone, ng/mL	E_2:T ratio
Hugues et al.[31]	21 alcoholics[a]	39.9 ± 2.8[d]	0.40 ± 0.03[d]	
	10 controls	17.0 ± 3.0	0.60 ± 0.05	
James et al.[32]	2 cirrhotics	above normal range		
Jasonni et al.[33]	12 cirrhotics[b]	30 ± 2		
	35 controls	18 ± 1		
Carlstrom et al.[34]	21 alcoholics[c]		1.29 ± 0.13	
	63 controls		1.14 ± 0.08 (nmol/L)	
Becker et al.[10]	13 cirrhotics	63 (39–59)[d]	0.87 (0.73–1.30)	
	6 alcoholics	47 (23–59)	0.84 (0.47–1.95)	
	46 controls	42 (29–55)	0.83 (0.52–1.03)	
Gavaler and Van Thiel[35]	20 cirrhotics	39.6 ± 5.9[d]	0.44 ± 0.66[d]	127 ± 22[d]
	27 controls	27.5 ± 3.3	0.74 ± 0.08	45 ± 6
Gavaler[36]	36 cirrhotics	61.1 ± 16.9[d]	0.47 ± 0.05[d]	169 ± 43[d]
	27 controls	27.5 ± 3.3	0.47 ± 0.08	45 ± 6

[a]12 with alcoholic cirrhosis.
[b]10 of 12 with alcoholic cirrhosis.
[c]6 with alcoholic cirrhosis, 15 postmenopausal.
[d]Significantly different from controls.

Table 3
Pituitary Hormones in Alcoholic Postmenopausal Women

Authors	Subjects	Prolactin, ng/mL	LH, miu/mL	FSH, miu/mL
Hugues et al.[31]	21 alcoholics[a]	13.4 ± 2.5	15.5 ± 1.5[b]	34.5 ± 2.0[b]
	10 controls	7.2 ± 1.3	28.1 ± 3.2	76.7 ± 9.2
Becker et al.[10]	13 cirrhotics	10 (6–17)	31 (25–38)	54 (43–59)
	6 alcoholics	9 (5–12)	38 (18–49)	44 (30–68)
	46 controls	9 (24–35)	30 (24–35)	53 (44–60)
Gavaler and Van Thiel[35]	20 cirrhotics	11.8 ± 2.7[b]	7.0 ± 1.7[b]	29.3 ± 6.3[b]
	27 controls	7.2 ± 0.6	24.0 ± 2.8	63.3 ± 5.5
Gavaler[36]	36 cirrhotics	13.7 ± 2.3[b]	5.3 ± 1.4[b]	19.6 ± 4.2[b]
	27 controls	7.2 ± 0.6	24.0 ± 2.8	63.3 ± 5.5

[a]12 with alcoholic cirrhosis.
[b]Significantly different from controls.

the issue of prolactin levels among women with and without hepatic encephalopathy has been addressed. Although prolactin levels have been repeatedly found to be elevated in cirrhotic encephalopathic males, in the alcoholic postmenopausal women with alcohol-induced cirrhosis, there was no difference in prolactin levels: among the women without encephalopathy, prolactin levels were 14.3 ± 3.9 ng/mL, whereas prolactin levels were 13.1 ± 2.3 among the women with hepatic encephalopathy.[43] Gender discrepant findings such as these serve to emphasize the need to expand the research being performed in women.

With the recruitment of large study samples of alcoholic postmeno-pausal women with alcohol-induced cirrhosis, it is possible to evaluate the interrelationships of hormones with not only each other but also with measures of liver disease severity.[35,36] Figure 1 provides a striking example of the way in which the normal hormonal relationships with age are markedly disrupted. As may be seen, although all of the hormones but estradiol are significantly correlated with age, the relationship for LH, FSH, prolactin, and testosterone with age is directly opposite than that seen in the normal alcohol-abstaining women.

Further evidence of the disrupting effect of alcohol abuse on hormone relationships is summarized in Fig. 2. In contrast to the changes in the relationships of hormone levels with age in the alcoholic postmenopausal cirrhotic women, the effect on hormone interrelationships is one of obliteration; as may be seen in Fig. 2, the normal interrelationships are no longer detectable in this alcohol-abusing population. Interestingly, significant correlations become apparent with several measures of liver disease severity; such relationships have not previously been reported even in alcoholic cirrhotic males. As may be seen in Table 4, both prolactin and LH are consistently correlated with the Child's severity score,[44] as well as with albumin and total bilirubin. Such findings suggest that hormone levels, particularly LH and prolactin, may have significant prognostic value in assessing severity of liver disease in postmenopausal women with alcohol-induced cirrhosis.

Endocrine Effects
of Moderate Alcoholic Beverage Consumption
in Normal Postmenopausal Women

The issue of alcoholic beverage consumption quantitation takes on great importance when the goal is to evaluate biocorrelates of moderate use. Discrepancies in alcohol intake estimates based on method of data collection are well known to occur. The question of the degree of discordance

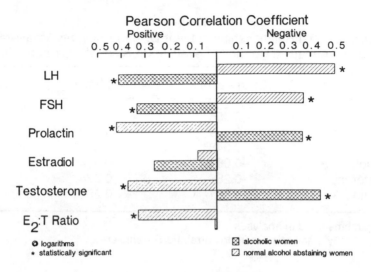

Fig. 1. Disrupted normal hormonal relationships with age in 36 alcoholic cirrhotic postmenopausal women. Pearson correlation coefficients are presented. The length of the bar represents the value of the coefficient. An asterisk denotes statistical significance.

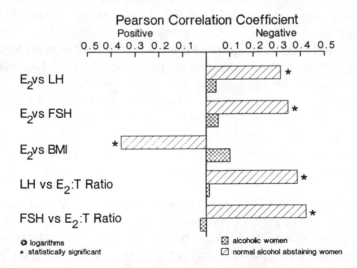

Fig. 2. Disrupted hormonal relationships in 36 alcoholic cirrhotic postmenopausal women. Pearson correlation coefficients are presented. The length of the bar represents the value of the coefficient. An asterisk denotes statistical significance.

Table 4
Correlational Relationships of Liver Disease Severity Measures
with Postmenopausal Hormone Levels in 36 Alcoholic Cirrhotic Women[a]

	Child's score	Albumin	Bilirubin
LH	-0.666^b	-0.357^b	-0.257^b
FSH	-0.539^b	-0.322^b	-0.151^b
Prolactin	0.348^b	0.347^b	0.287^b
Estradiol	-0.088	0.364^b	0.316^b
Testosterone	-0.288	0.074	-0.235
E_2:T ratio	0.101	0.281^b	0.432^b

[a]Logarithms used in analyses.
[b]Statistically significant Pearson correlation coefficient.

has been specifically addressed in a sample of normal postmenopausal women receiving no estrogen replacement therapy.[45] Alcohol consumption data in the 128 normal postmenopausal women were collected using two methods: self reported usual consumption, and 3-d food records. Fortunately, the number of women describing themselves as abstainers did not differ between the two methods ($n = 27$). Further, the amount of alcohol consumed was consistent in 65.3% of the alcohol-using women. Among the remaining 34.7%, in approximately half of the women, the self-reported usual alcohol intake overestimated the 3-d food record amount recorded; in the other half, the opposite situation occurred. Among the 92 women reporting use of wine, discrepancies in the amount estimated to be consumed were found in 22; among the 63 women indicating use of distilled spirits, discrepancies occurred in 18. For both wine and whiskey, half of the women overestimated the food-record amount in their self-report. Only 27 of the 101 normal postmenopausal women reported drinking beer; the self-report underestimated the food-record amount in 6 women, 3 of whom had not reported any use of beer.

The effect of the discrepancies on the actual estimates of alcohol consumed is shown in Table 5. As may be seen, the food-record total weekly drinks, as well as weekly drinks of both wine and whiskey, were uniformly lower than the self-reported usual consumption. Even more interesting is the difference in the strength of the correlation between estradiol and the amount of alcohol consumed using the two alcohol quantitation estimates. As may also be seen in Table 5, a stronger relationship between estradiol and the estimated amount of alcoholic beverage consumed is detected when the food-record estimate is used in the analysis. Fortunately, although the

Table 5
Discrepancies in Alcoholic Beverage Consumption
Among 101 Normal Postmenopausal Women

	Food record	Self-report	Discordant
Total drinks/wk	5.7 ± 0.6^a	4.8 ± 0.6	$35/101 = 34.7\%$
Wine drinks/wk	3.6 ± 0.5^a	3.0 ± 0.4	$22/92 = 23.9\%$
Whiskey drinks/wk	3.6 ± 0.6	2.7 ± 0.5	$18/63 = 28.6\%$

Hormone Correlations:[b] Effects of Alcohol Beverage Quantitation
in 128 Normal Postmenopausal Women

	Food record	Self-report	Intercorrelation[c]
Estradiol vs			
Total drinks/wk	$r = 0.234^a$	$r = 0.255^a$	$r = 0.826^a$
Wine drinks/wk	$r = 0.267^a$	$r = 0.288^a$	$r = 0.847^a$
Whiskey drinks/wk	$r = 0.084$	$r = 0.102$	$r = 0.775^a$

[a]Statistically significant.
[b]Pearson correlation coefficients using the logarithms of estradiol levels.
[c]Intercorrelation of the two alcohol intake measures.

self-report estimate of alcoholic beverage consumption is less strong, a significant relationship can be detected; this is important because most studies do not have the capability of using food-record data but must rely on self-reported usual consumption.

Based on the correlations of estradiol with the two alcohol consumption variables shown in Table 5, it is clear that moderate alcohol beverage consumption significantly influences postmenopausal estrogen levels. Within the guidelines that 1 drink/d is to be defined as moderate consumption,[8] the pattern of estradiol levels with levels of consumption are particularly interesting. As may be seen in Fig. 3A, estradiol concentrations increase with ascending alcohol consumption (as measured by food-record data) up to a level of 3–6 total weekly drinks, after which the estradiol concentrations plateau. This pattern suggests that there is a beneficial effect up to a limit of approx 1 drink/d, after which there is no added benefit.[30] If the postulate that alcohol *per se* increases the conversion of the androgen, testosterone, to the estrogen, estradiol, then the ratio of estradiol to testosterone should follow a pattern similar to that seen for estradiol with increasing alcoholic beverage consumption. As may be seen in Fig. 3B, the conversion/aromatization ratio does indeed demonstrate an almost superimposable pattern.

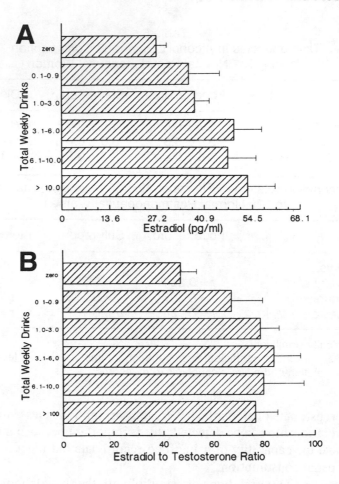

Fig. 3. **(A)** The relationship between serum estradiol levels and alcoholic beverage consumption in normal postmenopausal women. The length of the bar represents the mean level, and the bracket indicates the standard error of the mean. **(B)** The relationship between the ratio of estradiol to testosterone levels and alcoholic beverage consumption in normal postmenopausal women. The length of the bar represents the mean level, and the bracket indicates the standard error of the mean.

The next question which needs to be addressed is whether or not the findings of an association between moderate alcoholic beverage consumption and increases in estradiol levels can be reproduced in other study populations. Data are available to answer this question, and are summarized in Table 6.[46] In addition to the Pittsburgh study sample, two of three international study samples provide further evidence that moderate alcoholic beverage

Table 6
Alcoholic Beverage Consumption and Estradiol Relationships
in Normal Postmenopausal Women

	Lisbon, $n = 34$	Copenhagen, $n = 62$	Madrid, $n = 20$	Pittsburgh, $n = 128$
Alcohol users	31%	95%	75%	79%
Total drinks/wk[a]	12.4 ± 2.6	6.9 ± 0.8	5.4 ± 1.3	5.7 ± 1.3
Prevalence of consumption[a]				
2 drinks/d	18%	15%	13%	10%
3 drinks/d	18%	3%	0%	4%
4 drinks/d	0%	2%	0%	0%
Estradiol levels (pg/mL)				
abstainers	41.6 ± 2.3	35.1 ± 3.5	46.7 ± 8.6	27.5 ± 8.6
drinkers	89.0 ± 26.8[b]	68.1 ± 2.5	45.4 ± 5.5[b]	44.3 ± 5.5
Correlation of estradiol with total drinks/wk (Spearman coefficient)	$r = 0.450$[b]	$r = 0.473$[b]	$r = 0.146$	$r = 0.309$[b]

[a]Among women self-reporting alcohol use.
[b]Statistically significant.

consumption is an important determinant of postmenopausal estrogen levels in normal women. As may be seen, there is marked heterogeneity among the four groups with respect to the prevalence of alcohol use, the estimates of self-reported total weekly drinks, and the prevalence of alcohol intake at various daily consumption levels. In contrast, in three of the four study samples, estradiol concentrations are statistically higher in the normal postmenopausal women who drink than in the alcohol-abstaining women; further, even with the plateau effect noted above, the correlation of estradiol levels with total weekly drinks is statistically significant. The Madrid study sample is the "renegade" group, and cannot be ignored; the undetected or confounding variables that result in no detectable effect of alcohol consumption on estradiol levels will be interesting to examine in future studies.

The question that now needs to be addressed is whether or not there are adverse effects of moderate alcoholic beverage consumption as now defined as 1 drink/d. Effects on the liver have been evaluated in this study sample of 128 normal postmenopausal women; no alcohol-related changes were seen in two measures of liver injury and one measure of liver function.[47,48] Thus, at the levels of alcohol intake in this study group, there are no detectable adverse effects on the liver. Moderate alcohol intake has been reported to be associated with breast cancer risk; the problem is the definition of "moderate." Methodologically, when one assesses relative risk, the confidence interval (CI) around the estimate of risk must exclude a value of 1 in order to permit the risk to be termed statistically increased (or decreased). There are two studies in which risk has been evaluated at the newly defined moderate level of 1 drink/d. In neither study was the risk of breast cancer statistically increased at alcohol consumption levels in the moderate range: at 0.1–0.4 drink/d, the risk was 1.5 (95% CI: 0.9, 2.6);[49] similarly, at alcohol intake levels of 0.5–1.4 drink/d, a risk of 1.30 (95% CI: 0.98, 1.87) was reported.[50] Thus, the risk of breast cancer at alcoholic beverage consumption levels of approx 1 drink/d does not achieve statistical significance.

Perhaps the best way in which to end this section of the chapter and to put the importance of the finding of moderate alcoholic beverage consumption as an important variable that influences postmenopausal estrogen levels into context, is to briefly review the literature related to moderate alcoholic beverage consumption in postmenopausal women, which has demonstrated beneficial effects particularly related to coronary heart disease (CHD) risk. There are several studies that have reported decreased CHD risk among alcohol users;[51–54] even more interesting are the studies that have assessed CHD risk with respect to specific levels of alcoholic beverage consumption.[55,56] Specifically, the risk of death as a result of CHD has been reported to be 0.41 (95% confidence interval: 0.23, 0.71) at 0.7–1.4 drink/d,[55] whereas myocardial infarction risk has been reported to be 0.5 (95% CI: 0.3, 0.8) at alcoholic beverage consumption levels of 0.4–1.4 drink/d.[56] It is entirely possible that one of the mechanisms involved in lowering the risk in women is the increase in estrogen levels associated with such moderate alcoholic beverage consumption.

The Endocrine Effects of the Consumption of the Phytoestrogenic Congeners of Alcoholic Beverages by Normal Postmenopausal Women

As indicated in the introduction, estrogenic substances of plant origin, phytoestrogens, have been isolated and identified in the alcoholic beverages that have been investigated to date. Specifically, bourbon has been reported to contain β-sitosterol and biochanin A,[11,12] whereas beer has been reported to contain genistein and daidzen.[13] The bourbon concentrate containing the equivalent of the congeners present in one or two shots of bourbon has been shown to be capable of interacting with estrogen receptor binding sites in vitro, and, even more interesting, has been demonstrated in vivo to produce an estrogenic dose-dependent increase in uterus weight and decrease in serum LH levels in ovariectomized rats. Based on these results, we have administered a similar bourbon congener preparation to normal postmenopausal volunteers.[57,58]

Four normal postmenopausal women received the bourbon congener preparation for 4 wk; blood specimens were obtained before, weekly during the experimental period, and 1 wk after administration of the phytoestrogenic preparation has been stopped. Eight additional normal postmenopausal women were used as controls; these women provided blood specimens weekly for 4 wk. All of the women were postmenopausal, and none were or had been taking exogenous estrogen replacement therapy. The results of this experiment are summarized in Table 7. Exposure to estrogenic substances would be expected to produce a decrease in LH and FSH levels, and an increase in levels of prolactin, sex hormone binding globulin (SHBG), and high density lipoprotein (HDL). As may be seen in Table 7, there were significant differences in the two study groups with respect to the proportions of women with decreased levels of LH and FSH; the prolactin results did not achieve statistical significance. Data for the hepatic estrogen responsive proteins were not available in the controls; nevertheless, SHBG increased arithmetically, and the changes in HDL were statistically significant.

These findings of estrogenic responses to administration of bourbon phytoestrogen congeners complements studies performed in vegetarian and nonvegetarian normal postmenopausal women where an unformulated

Table 7
Changes in Pituitary Hormones and Hepatic Estrogen-Sensitive
Binding Proteins in Normal Postmenopausal Women
Administered the Phytoestrogens in Bourbon

	Subjects	Controls	p
LH decreased to <90% of baseline	3/4	0/8	0.018[a]
FSH decreased to <90% of baseline	2/4	0/8	0.021[a]
Prolactin increased to >110% of baseline	2/3	0/7	0.067[a]
SHBG increased >110% of baseline	3/4	N/A	0.10[b]
HDL increased >110% of baseline	4/4	N/A	0.05[b]

[a]Fisher's exact test.
[b]McNemar test.

hypothesis of increased phytoestrogen consumption among the vegetarian women was tested.[59,60] In these reports, compared to nonvegetarian women, vegetarian postmenopausal women had increased levels of both SHBG and HDL,[59] and increased bone mineral density.[60] Further, in a study in which normal postmenopausal were administered "estrogenic plant foods," a decrease in FSH levels and an increase in vaginal estrogenization was reported.[61] Thus it is clear that phytoestrogens, whether present in the diet or contained in consumed alcoholic beverages, are capable of exerting endocrine effects on the hormonal status of normal postmenopausal women.

Summary of Alcoholic Beverage Consumption Effects on the Endocrine Status of Postmenopausal Women

It is clear that alcohol abuse among postmenopausal women excessive enough to cause cirrhosis results in profound changes in hormonal status *per se* as well as in disruption of hormonal relationships. Interesting, for some of the hormones, there is a consistent relationship of hormone levels with various measures of liver disease severity.

Among normal postmenopausal women who drink moderately, as defined as 1 drink/d or less, there is a detectable and significant of such alcohol consumption on estradiol levels; this increase in estrogen levels can be viewed as a beneficial effect if viewed in the context of studies reporting a statistically significant reduction in heart disease risk at moderate alcoholic beverage consumption. In addition to increasing estrogen levels, which may in turn increase HDL concentrations and thus partly provide at least one mechanism for the finding of reduced CHD risk, it is also possible that the phytoestrogens present in alcoholic beverages may also play a significant role through the HDL pathway. Overall, moderate alcoholic beverage consumption among normal postmenopausal women is an area where further work is likely to be rewarding.

Acknowledgments

This work has been supported by grant AA06772 from the National Institute on Alcohol Abuse and Alcoholism. The authors thank M. J. Allan and S. Deal.

References

[1]D. Cahalan and I. H. Cisin (1968) American drinking practices: Summary of findings from a national probability sample. I. Extent of drinking by population subgroups. *Q. J. Stud. Alcohol* **29,** 130–151.

[2]B. O'Connell, R. Hudson, and G. Graves (1979) Alcohol and tobacco use, in *The Health and Social Survey of the Northwest Region of Melbourne, Melbourne, Australia.* J. Krupinsky and A. Mackenzie, eds. Health Commission of Victoria, Mental Health Division, The Institute of Mental Health Research and Post-Graduate Training, Victoria, Australia, pp. 96–111.

[3]H. Wechsler (1980) Introduction: Summary of the literature. [I. Epidemiology of male/ female drinking over the last century], in *Alcoholism and Alcohol Abuse Among Women: Research Issues.* Research Monograph No. 1, DHEW Publication No. (ADM) 80-835, National Institute on Alcohol Abuse and Alcoholism, Washington, DC, pp. 3–31.

[4]National Institute on Alcohol Abuse and Alcoholism (NIAAA) (1981) *First Statistical Compendium on Alcohol and Health.* DHHS Publication No. (ADM) 81-1115, National Institute on Alcohol Abuse and Alcoholism, Washington, DC.

[5]E. S. L. Gomberg (1982) Alcohol use and alcohol problems among the elderly, in *Special Population Issues.* Alcohol and Health Monograph No. 4, DHHS Publication No. (ADM) 82-1193, National Institute on Alcohol Abuse and Alcoholism, Washington, DC, pp. 263–290.

[6]D. D. Celentano and D. V. McQueen (1984) Alcohol consumption patterns among women in Baltimore. *J. Stud. Alcohol* **45,** 355–358.

[7]M. E. Hilton and W. B. Clark (1987) Changes in American drinking patterns and problems. *J. Stud. Alcohol* **48,** 515–522.

[8]U.S. Department of Agriculture/U.S. Department of Health and Human Services (1990) *Nutrition and Your Health: Dietary Guidelines for Americans,* 3rd ed. Home and Garden Bulletin No. 232, U.S. Department of Agriculture/U.S. Department of Health and Human Services, Washington, DC.

[9]J. N. Hugues, G. Perret, G. Adessi, T. Coste, and E. Modigliani (1978) Effects of chronic alcoholism on the pituitary-gonadal function of women during menopausal transition and in the postmenopausal period. *Biomedicine* **29,** 279–283.

[10]U. Becker, C. Gludd, S. Farholt, P. Bennett, S. Miciv, B. Svenstrup, and F. Hardt (1991) Menopausal age and sex hormones in postmenopausal women with alcoholic and non-alcoholic liver disease. *J. Hepatol.* **13,** 25–32.

[11]E. R. Rosenblum, D. H. Van Thiel, I. M. Campbell, P. K. Eagon, and J. S. Gavaler (1987) Separation and identification of phyto-estrogenic compounds from bourbon. *Alcohol Alcohol.* **1(suppl.),** 551–555.

[12]E. R. Rosenblum, D. H. Van Thiel, I. M. Campbell, and J. S. Gavaler (1991) Quantitation of β-sitosterol in bourbon. *Alcohol. Clin. Exp. Res.* **15,** 202–206.

[13]E. R. Rosenblum, D. H. Van Thiel, I. M. Campbell, and J. S. Gavaler (1993) Isolation of phytoestrogens from beer. *Alcohol. Clin. Exp. Res.* **16,** 843–845.

[14]J. S. Gavaler, E. R. Rosenblum, D. H. Van Thiel, P. K. Eagon, C. R. Pohl, I. M. Campbell, and J. Gavaler (1987) Biologically active phyto-estrogens are present in bourbon. *Alcohol. Clin. Exp. Res.* **11,** 399–406.

[15]J. S. Gavaler (1985) Effects of alcohol on endocrine function in postmenopausal women: A review. *J. Stud. Alcohol* **46,** 495–516.

[16]J. S. Gavaler (1988) Effects of moderate consumption of alcoholic beverages on endocrine function in postmenopausal women: Bases for hypotheses, in *Recent Developments in Alcoholism,* vol. 6. M. Galanter, ed. Plenum, New York, pp. 229–251.

[17]H. L. Judd, G. E. Judd, W. E. Lucas, and S. S. C. Yen (1974) Endocrine function of the postmenopausal ovary: Concentrations of androgens and estrogens in ovarian and peripheral vein blood. *J. Clin. Endocrinol. Metab.* **39,** 1020–1024.

[18]B. E. C. Nordin, R. G. Crilly, D. H. Marshall, and S. A. Barkworth (1981) Oestrogens, the menopause and the adrenopause. *J. Endocrinol.* **89,** 131–143.

[19]A. Vermeulen (1976) The hormonal activity of the postmenopausal ovary. *J. Clin. Endocrinol. Metab.* **42,** 247–253.

[20]R. J. Chang and H. L. Judd (1981) The ovary after menopause. *Clin. Obstet. Gynaecol.* **24,** 181–191.

[21]R. G. Crilly, D. H. Marshall, and B. E. C. Nordin (1980) Adrenal androgens in postmenopausal osteoporosis, in *Adrenal Androgens.* A. R. Genazzani, J. H. H. Thijssen, and P. K. Siiteri, eds. Raven, New York, pp. 241–158.

[22]J. Poortman, J. H. H. Thijssen, and F. Schwarz (1973) Adrenal androgen production and conversion to estrogens in normal postmenopausal women and in selected breast cancer patients. *J. Clin. Endocrinol. Metab.* **37,** 101–109.

[23]S. Brody, K. Carlstorm, A. Lagrelius, N. O. Lunell, and L. Rosenborg (1982) Adrenocortical steroids, bone mineral content and endometrial condition in postmenopausal women. *Maturitas* **4,** 113–122.

[24]J. S. Gavaler (1987) The determinants of estrogen levels in postmenopausal women. University Microfilms International 87-02059, Ann Arbor, MI.

[25]G. G. Gordon, J. Olivo, F. Fereidoon, and A. L. Southren (1975) Conversion of androgens to estrogens in cirrhosis of the liver. *J. Clin. Endocrinol. Metab.* **40,** 1018–1026.

[26]C. Longcope, J. H. Pratt, S. Schneider, and E. Fineberg (1984) Estrogen and androgen dynamics in liver disease. *J. Endocrinol. Invest.* **7,** 629–634.

[27]G. G. Gordon, K. Altman, A. L. Southren, E. Rubin, and C. S. Lieber (1976) Effect of alcohol (ethanol) administration on sex-hormone metabolism in normal men. *N. Engl. J. Med.* **295,** 793–797.

[28]G. G. Gordon, A. L. Southern, J. Vittek, and C. S. Lieber (1979) The effect of alcohol ingestion on hepatic aromatase activity and plasma steroid hormones in the rat. *Metabolism* **28,** 20–24.

[29]C. F. Cobb, D. H. Van Thiel, and J. S. Gavaler (1981) Isolated rat adrenal perfusion: a new method to study adrenal function. *J. Surg. Res.* **31,** 347–353.

[30]J. S. Gavaler and D. H. Van Thiel (1992) The association between moderate alcoholic beverage consumption and serum estradiol and testosterone levels in normal postmenopausal women: Relationship to the literature. *Alcohol. Clin. Exp. Res.* **16,** 87–92.

[31]J. N. Hugues, G. Coste, T. Perret, M. F. Jayle, J. Sebaoun, and E. Modigliani (1980) Hypothalamo-pituitary ovarian function in thirty women with chronic alcoholism. *Clin. Endocrinol.* **12,** 543–551.

[32]V. H. T. James, J. R. B. Green, J. B. Walker, A. Goodall, F. Short, D. L. Jones, C. T. Noel, and M. J. Reed (1982) The endocrine status of postmenopausal cirrhotic women, in *The Endocrines and the Liver.* M. Langer, L. Chiandussi, I. J. Chopra, and L. Martini, eds. Academic, New York, pp. 417–419.

[33]V. M. Jasonni, C. Bulletti, G. F. Bolelli, F. Franceschetti, M. Bonavia, P. Ciotte, and C. Flamigni (1983) Estrone sulfate, estrone and estradiol concentrations in normal and cirrhotic postmenopausal women. *Steroids* **41,** 569–573.

[34]K. Carlstrom, S. Eriksson, and G. Rannevik (1986) Sex steroids and steroid binding proteins in female alcoholic liver disease. *Acta Endocrinol.* **111,** 75–79.

[35]J. S. Gavaler and D. H. Van Thiel (1992) Hormonal status of postmenopausal women with alcohol-induced liver disease. *Hepatology* **16,** 312–319.

[36]J. S. Gavaler (1993) Effects of alcohol use and abuse on the endocrine status in expanded study samples of postmenopausal women, in *Alcohol and the Endocrine System*, S. Zakhari, ed. NIAAA Research Monograph No. 23, NIH Pub. No. 93-3533, National Institute on Alcohol Abuse and Alcoholism, Washington, DC, pp. 171–187.

[37]P. C. McDonald, P. Rombaut, and P. K. Siiteri (1967) Plasma precursors of estrogen. I. Extent of plasma conversion of 4-androstenedione to estrone in normal males and nonpregnant, normal castrated and adrenalectomized females. *J. Clin. Endocrinol. Metab.* **27,** 1103–1111.

[38]H. I. Wright, J. S. Gavaler, J. Tabasco-Minguillan, and D. H. Van Thiel (1992) Endocrine effects of alcohol abuse in males, in *Diagnosis and Treatment of Alcoholism*, 3rd ed. J. H. Mendelson and N. K. Mello, eds. McGraw-Hill, New York, pp. 341–362.

[39]C. J. McClain, J. P. Kromhout, M. K. Elson, and D. H. Van Thiel (1981) Hyperprolactinemia in portal systemic encephalopathy. *Dig. Dis. Sci.* **26,** 353–357.

[40]M. P. Sharma, S. K. Acharya, and M. G. Kamarkar (1988) Significance of prolactin levels in portosystemic encephalopathy. *J. Assoc. Physicians India* **36,** 207–209.

[41]L. De Besi, P. Zucchetta, S. Zotti, and I. Mastrogiacomo (1989) Sex hormones and sex hormone binding globulin in males with compensated and decompensated cirrhosis of the liver. *Acta Endocrinol.* **120,** 271–276.

[42]J. E. Fischer and R. J. Baldessarini (1971) False neurotransmitters and hepatic failure. *Lancet* **ii,** 75–79.

[43]J. S. Gavaler and D. H. Van Thiel (1992) Pituitary hormone patterns in 36 alcoholic cirrhotic postmenopausal women with and without encephalopathy. *Alcohol. Clin. Exp. Res.* **16,** 359.

[44]R. N. H. Pugh, I. M. Murray-Lyon, J. L. Dawson, M. C. Pietroni, and R. Williams (1973) Transection of the oesophagus for bleeding oesophageal varices. *Br. J. Surg.* **60,** 646–649.

[45]J. S. Gavaler and K. Love (1992) Detection of the relationship between moderate alcoholic beverage consumption and serum levels of estradiol in normal postmenopausal women: Effects of alcohol consumption quantitation and sample size adequacy. *J. Stud. Alcohol* **53,** 389–394.

[46]J. S. Gavaler, K. Love, D. H. Van Thiel, S. Farholt, C. Gluud, E. Monteiro, A. Galvao-Teles, T. Conton-Ortega, and V. Cuervas-Mons (1991) An international study of the relationship between alcohol consumption and postmenopausal estradiol levels, in *Advances in Biomedical Alcohol Research.* H. J. Kalant, J. M. Khanna, and Y. Israel, eds. Pergamon, New York, pp. 327–330.

[47]J. S. Gavaler (1992) Alcohol effects in postmenopausal women: Alcohol and estrogens, in *Diagnosis and Treatment of Alcoholism,* 3rd ed. J. H. Mendelson, and N. K. Mello, eds. McGraw-Hill, New York, pp. 623–638.

[48]J. S. Gavaler, R. H. Kelly, C. Wight, A. Sanghvi, J. Cauley, S. Belle, and K. Love (1988) Does moderate alcoholic beverage consumption affect liver function/injury tests in postmenopausal women? *Alcohol. Clin. Exp. Res.* **12,** 337.

[49]A. Schatzkin, D. Y. Jones, R. N. Hoover, T. P. Taylor, L. A. Brinton, R. G. Ziegler, E. B. Harvey, C. L. Carter, L. M. Lictra, M. C. Dufour, and D. B. Larson (1987) Alcohol consumption and breast cancer in the epidemiologic follow-up study of the First National Health and Nutrition Examination Survey. *N. Engl. J. Med.* **316,** 1169–1173.

[50]W. C. Willett, M. J. Stampfer, G. A. Colditz, B. A. Rosner, C. H. Hennekins, and F. E. Speizer (1987) Moderate alcohol consumption and risk of breast cancer. *N. Engl. J. Med.* **316,** 1174–1180.

[51]A. L. Klatsky, G. D. Friedman, and A. B. Siegelaub (1974) Alcohol consumption before myocardial infarction: Results from the Kaiser-Permanente epidemiologic study of myocardial infarction. *Ann. Int. Med.* **81,** 294–301.

[52]D. B. Petitti, J. Wingerd, F. Pellegrin, and S. Ramcharan (1979) Risk of vascular disease in women: Smoking, oral contraceptives, non-contraceptive estrogens and other factors. *JAMA* **242,** 1150–1154.

[53]R. K. Ross, A. Paganini-Hill, T. M. Mack, M. Arthur, and B. E. Henderson (1981) Menopausal oestrogen therapy and protection from death from ischemic heart disease. *Lancet* **i,** 858–860.

[54]K. Cullen, N.S. Stenhouse, and K. L. Wearne (1982) Alcohol and mortality in the Busselton study. *Int. J. Epidemiol.* **11,** 67–70.

[55]T. Gordon and W. B. Kannel (1983) Drinking habits and cardiovascular disease: The Framingham Study. *Am. Heart J.* **105,** 667–673.

[56]M. J. Stampfer, G. A. Colditz, W. C. Willett, F. E. Speizer, and C. H. Hennekens (1988) A prospective study of moderate alcohol consumption and the risk of coronary heart disease and stroke in women. *N. Engl. J. Med.* **319,** 267–273.

[57]J. S. Gavaler, A. Galvao-Teles, E. Monteiro, D. H. Van Thiel, and E. R. Rosenblum (1991) Clinical responses to the administration of bourbon phytoestrogens to normal postmenopausal women. *Hepatology* **14,** 193.

[58]D. H. Van Thiel, A. Galvao-Teles, E. Monteiro, E. R. Rosenblum, and J. S. Gavaler (1991) The phytoestrogens present in de-ethanolized bourbon are biologically active: a preliminary study in a postmenopausal woman. *Alcohol. Clin. Exp. Res.* **15,** 822–823.

[59]B. K. Armstrong, J. B. Brown, H. T. Clarke, D. K. Crooker, R. Hahnel, J. R. Masarei, and T. Ratajczak (1981) Diet and reproductive hormones: a study of vegetarian and nonvegetarian postmenopausal women. *J. Natl. Cancer Institute* **67,** 761–767.

[60]A. G. Marsh, T. V. Sanchez, O. Michelsen, F. L. Chaffee, and S. M. Fagal (1988) Vegetarian lifestyle and bone mineral density. *Am. J. Clin. Nutrition* **48,** 837–841.

[61]G. Wilcox, M. L. Wahlqvist, H. G. Burger, and G. Medley (1990) Oestrogenic effects of plant foods in postmenopausal women. *Br. Med. J.* **301,** 905–906.

Effects of Alcohol and Sex Hormones on Host Immune Response in Males and Females

Charles J. Grossman, Gary Roselle, Mark Nienaber, and Gary Schmitt

Introduction

The intemperate use of alcohol leads to major distortions in normal homeostasis, and results in a variety of diseases and disorders. Paramount among the effects elicited by excessive alcohol usage are abnormalities of immune system function. These are most frequently expressed as a significant depression in immune response. However, because the immune system itself is also regulated by the endocrine system, it follows that the immune dysfunctions resulting from alcohol use may also be modified by alcohol/endocrine system involvement.

Furthermore, under normal conditions, the immune response in females is more active than in males. This is commonly referred to as immunological sexual dimorphism (ISD), and results from an interplay of various factors, and especially endocrine hormones from the gonads and adrenals. These hormones are believed to play an important regulatory role during immune cell development, and also during activation of these immune effector cells.

From: *Drug and Alcohol Abuse Reviews, Vol. 5: Addictive Behaviors in Women*
Ed.: R. R. Watson ©1994 Humana Press Inc., Totowa, NJ

Thus, given the above, we might logically expect that the effects of alcohol on immune response in males and females might be expressed differently. Support for such differences will be supplied by a review of the available literature, and, in addition, hypothetical mechanisms to account for such a possible effect will also be described.

Effects of Alcohol Usage on the Immune System

Chronic use of alcohol results in significant immunological abnormalities,[1,2] including anergy to skin tests,[3,4] abnormalities in thymocyte function,[5-7] decreased numbers of circulating T-lymphocytes,[8] reduced lymphocyte antigen and mitogen responses,[1,10] a reduced IL-2 dependent proliferation of T-blast cells from both young and old mice,[10] a reduction in lymphocyte transformation and a decrease in macrophage migration inhibitory factor (MIF) production,[11-14] reduced T-cell migration,[15] and alterations in lymphocyte populations and in immune regulation.[16-18] K and NK cell response has also been reported to be reduced by ethanol[19,20] whereas Kupffer cell activity is increased.[21] The chronic alcohol syndrome is usually also associated with liver disease, and these individuals appear more susceptible to a wide spectrum of infections.[22-31] Such infectious agents include listeria,[27,31] tuberculosis,[26,30] peritonitis,[28,33,34] endocarditis,[35] pneumococcal bacteremia,[36] and viral disease.[37] Furthermore, it has been hypothesized that alcohol consumption, by reducing cell-mediated immunity, leads to malignant tumorigenesis.[38]

In animals, immune system function has also been evaluated, and abnormalities reported, after alcohol treatment for as short a duration as 3 d.[6,9,14,39-41] However, in these studies, immune response as measured by the phytohemagglutinin (PHA) mitogen-delayed cutaneous hypersensitivity assay[14,42] was related to the dosage of alcohol. It was found (Fig. 1) that treatment of rats with ethanol (5 g/kg/d) depressed the PHA skin test. However, at low levels (0.5–2.0 g/kg/d) there was a stimulation in the PHA skin test. These results suggest that low concentrations of ethanol are stimulatory on the cell-mediated immunity (CMI), whereas high concentrations are inhibitory.

An altered immune response in the chronic alcoholic has been suggested as one of the intrinsic mechanisms to explain the observed progression from alcoholic hepatitis to cirrhosis, which may proceed even after cessation of alcohol.[43,44] This is supported by the finding that increased numbers of T-helper (Th) and T-suppressor (Ts) lymphocytes, their soluble mediators, and major histocompatibility antigens, have been identified in areas

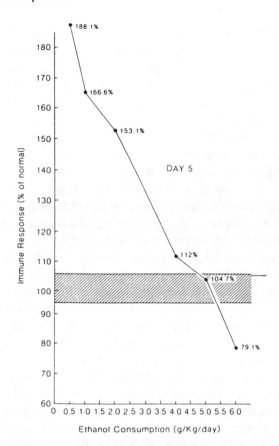

Fig. 1. Immune delayed cutaneous hypersensitivity (DCH) responses to PHA observed after 5 d of treatment with varying quantities of ethanol. Values are expressed as percent of normal (pretreatment), and hashed-in area represents the normal response (mean ±SD). Note that low doses of ethanol (0.5–2.0 g/kg) over a short period of time (5 d) resulted in significantly greater DCH responses compared to baseline ($p > 0.008$); high doses (6.0 g/kg) significantly ($p = 0.03$) depressed the DCH response. The immune responses to varying doses were linear, where $y = 190.7 - 18.4x$; $r = 0.99$; $p > 0.0001$. (Reprinted with permission from ref. 14.)

of liver necrosis and cell injury.[44,45] These findings imply that immune effector cells are involved in the injury process. Such an effect might be attributed to an autoimmune-like component because, at least on pancreatic islet cells, alcohol ingestion increased the major histocompatibility complex (MHC) expression in vivo. The suggestion is that this might then lead to the increased development of autoimmune diabetes.[46]

Certainly, the presence of hyperglobulinemia is also commonly reported in patients with alcoholic cirrhosis, and it has been suggested that this is a result of nonspecific B-cell stimulation.[47–49] On the other hand, activation of B-cells by the specific antigen dinitrophenol was shown to be reduced by low doses of alcohol.[50] Although the mechanism of this depression was not clarified, the author demonstrated that it was not owing to inhibition "of membrane depolarization induced by antigen crosslinking of the immunoglobulin receptors," and that activation of the phosphotidyl inositol pathway was not inhibited by the alcohol.[50]

The fact that in ethanol-treated rats acetaldehyde-modified proteins could elicit an immune response independent of the carrier protein supports the view that such proteins could act as neoantigens in alcoholics.[51] This effect is of additional interest given the fact that birth control pills have been shown to significantly increase the circulating levels of acetaldehyde in social-drinking females after an acute ethanol dose.[52] Certainly acetaldehyde, like ethanol, can be shown to be immunosuppressive when added to T-lymphocyte cultures at physiological concentrations for 3 d.[53] However, the immunostimulatory effects attributed to the acetaldehyde-modified proteins required in vivo treatment with ethanol for periods longer than 3 wk and up to 27 mo,[51] and this suggests that it may act to nonspecifically upregulate immune responses after long-term ethanol abuse leading to autoimmune-like disease.

The hypothesis that an autoimmune-like mechanism may either generate or further exacerbate existing alcoholic liver disease is intriguing given the observations that alcohol consumption effects lymphocyte subpopulations. In these reports, an increase in CD4 (T-helper) cells coupled with a decrease in the CD8 (T-suppressor) cells is observed in patients with alcoholic cirrhosis,[54] or in mice after ethanol feeding,[55] leading to an increased CD4/CD8 ratio.[55] We have observed a similar and significant increase in the CD4/CD8 ratio in lymphocytes prepared from rats fed an ethanol diet.[56] Furthermore, in the mouse studies, both spleen and thymic architecture are disrupted by ethanol feeding, with the thymic cortex completely destroyed, and splenic B-cells significantly reduced.[55]

Alcohol and Sex Hormones

Alcohol induces testicular atrophy in male rats[57] and ovarian failure in female rats;[58–60] increases prolactin and estradiol levels, but reduces LH levels in male rats;[61] alters pituitary–testicular interactions,[62] and the hypothalamic–pituitary–gonadal axis in humans;[63] and alters testosterone biosynthesis in male rats[64] and mice.[65]

Treatment of immature male rats with alcohol significantly effects various indices of reproductive function, including serum testosterone levels, testes weight, and number of offspring.[66] In female rats, alcohol inhibits luteinizing hormone releasing hormone (LHRH),[67] significantly increases estradiol levels after LHRH administration during the follicular phase of the menstrual cycle in women,[68] and also effects their hypothalamic–pituitary ovarian interactions.[69] Furthermore, neonatal exposure to acute ethanol significantly depresses plasma testosterone levels because it reduces testicular enzyme activity.[70] Because alcohol significantly changes gonadal steroid production,[71] it follows that alcohol depression in immune response may be mediated in part through the endocrine effects elicited by alcohol on gonadal function.

It is possible that the effects produced by alcohol on immune cell function could result from alterations in sex steroid receptors present on immune effector cells. Indeed in vivo ethanol feeding of rats has been shown to increase the mean concentration of cytosolic estrogen receptor from 35.74 to 41.75 nM ($p = 0.05$) with respect to nonethanol-fed controls, but not alter the affinity of the receptor for its ligand.[72] Furthermore, this effect was abolished by castration, which caused an increase in the receptor concentration in both the ethanol-fed (54.0 nM) and control (57.14 nM) groups.

As early as 1978, Kawanishi et al. suggested that a deficiency in T-suppressor activity might be related to alcoholic liver disease.[73] Gluud et al. expanded on this suggestion by hypothesizing that the low levels of testosterone resulting from androgenic insufficiency in males with alcoholic liver disease might lead to a reduction in suppressor cell activity.[74] This hypothesis is supported by the observation that testosterone treatment decreases the levels of immunoglobulins in patients with cirrhosis,[75] but the presence of ethanol also appears to be required to alter subpopulations.[54–56] In addition Mendenhall et al. demonstrated that anabolic steroid (oxandrolone) treatment of patients with alcoholic hepatitis was associated with a beneficial effect on long-term survival.[75]

Recently, it was reported that the structure of the androgenic steroid nucleus may determine the effect elicited on immune function. This assumption is based on the results of a study by Mendenhall et al. who treated rats with various androgens in vivo.[76] Some of these steroids (testosterone and testosterone propionate) possessed an intact steroid nucleus, whereas others (oxandrolone, stanozolol, and testolactone) possessed a steroid nucleus with various alterations. It was found that immune response, as measured by the PHA skin test, was depressed in those groups treated with steroid possessing the intact nucleus, whereas immune response was stimulated in those groups receiving the androgens with the altered nucleus. These effects may be owing, in part, to alterations in gonadal testosterone release through regulatory actions of the anabolic steroids at the hypothalamus–pituitary–gonadal axis.

Prenatal Alcohol Exposure, Sex Steroids, and Immunity

Prenatal exposure to alcohol has been well documented to cause a wide variety of developmental disorders, and alterations in levels of sex steroids may also be involved. In rats, prenatal ethanol exposure coupled with injections of the mothers with testosterone propionate resulted in significantly lower birthweights of pups.[77] This effect may be of importance given the observation that elevated levels of testosterone were present in male and female fetuses whose mothers were given ethanol for 6 d postconception.[78] This suggests that the low birth weight of the offspring might be a result of alcohol and testosterone acting synergistically.[77]

Prenatal alcohol exposure may also elicit changes in certain parameters of immune function. For example, Ewald and Huang[79] reported that chronic maternal ethanol consumption reduced the thymic weight and the number of thymic lymphocytes expressing CD4 (T-helper) and CD8 (T-suppressor) antigen in 18-d-old fetuses, as compared to pair fed controls, although the immune response of adult mice exposed to ethanol prenatally appeared normal.[80] Other investigators, however, have reported that for both animals[81] and humans,[82] prenatal exposure to ethanol may depress immune response in the adult. In the rat model, for example, such a depression of immune response owing to prenatal ethanol exposure was not detectable at 2 wk after birth, but was first detected at 6 wk after birth and was maximal up to 3 mo of age. However, by 8 mo of age the immune response had normalized.

Alcohol and Soluble Mediators

Alcohol modulation through changes in soluble mediators is not well established. In addition, little is known about differences in soluble mediator regulation of immune response in males and females. Most soluble mediators have been assessed by biological assay, so that the concentrations are a reflection of their biological functions. For example, T-cell blastogenic transformation, reflecting both T-cell activation and cellular proliferation, has been reported to be regulated by a group of lymphokines[83-85] with concomitant increases in cytotoxicity.[86-88] Macrophage migration inhibitory factor (MMIF or MIF) is observed to be decreased[40,89] after feeding ethanol to ferrets and rats, but not to guinea pigs.[7] This may represent differences in the mode and dose of ethanol treatment. Reports describing tumor necrosis factor (TNF) changes are not unanimous. Clinical features associated with acute alcoholic liver injury are nonspecific and include anorexia, muscle wasting, fever, leukocytosis, and neutrophil deposition in the liver. All of these features could, in theory, be mediated through TNF release. Anorexia is a frequent occurrence, ranging from 52–93% in patients in three studies,[90–92] and 65% in patients in a recent VA Cooperative Study on Alcoholic Hepatitis.[93]

Recently, McClain and Cohen reported on TNF activity in 16 patients with alcoholic hepatitis.[94] Basal release of TNF from peripheral monocytes was elevated in 50% of the patients and in only 12.5% of the healthy controls. In vitro stimulation of their mononuclear cells with lipopolysaccharide (LPS) resulted in more striking differences (25.3 ± 3.7 U in patients with alcoholic hepatitis vs 10.9 ± 2.4 U in healthy controls ($p < 0.005$). Similar findings in vitro of increased cytotoxicity were observed by Wickramasinghe,[95] however, Nelson and associates reported a decreased activity after LPS stimulation and after infection with *Klebsiella pneumonia*.[96,97] In addition to the obvious species and organ differences in these reports, the diverse observations may also represent differences in dose response, nutritional status, and the sex and age of the experimental subjects.

In support of McClain's findings, both Allen et al.[98] and Felver et al.[99] observed increased concentrations of both TNF alpha and IL-1. It is significant that TNF alpha but not IL-1, in the latter report, correlated significantly with survival ($p = 0.002$). Studies with IL-2 also appear conflicting. In rodents, low-dose treatment of ethanol has been reported to increase IL-2 mediated killer cell activity.[100] However, in well-nourished chronic alcoholics, Ericsson et al. saw no changes in IL-2 mediated killing.[101] On the other hand, the majority of studies employing higher ethanol intakes reported diminished IL-2 mediated NK activity.[102–107] These differences in immune response associated with differences in ethanol intake (low dose stimulation vs high dose depression) are similar to those we reported[14,42,108] utilizing delayed hypersensitivity PHA skin test response as a measure of immune reactivity. Gamma IFN in the alcoholic has been less extensively studied. Wagner et al.[109] and Chadha et al.[110] both reported that human mononuclear peripheral cells demonstrated a significant reduction in IFN gamma with impaired mitogen (Con A and PHA) stimulatory response. They concluded that this depression in IFN might contribute to the in vivo immune defect of the alcoholic.

Sex Hormones and Soluble Mediators

A large number of studies have demonstrated that sex steroids interact with lymphokines and monokines such as TNF, IL-1, IL-2, and IFN in bidirectional regulation. For example, TNF, which can enhance the immune response to T-dependent antigens,[111] and stimulate granuloma formation,[112] is decreased by hypophysectomy[113] and age, and increased in the aging rat by pituitary transplants.[114] TNF can also suppress the synthesis of cortisol and shift synthesis to increase androgen production;[115] increase follicular P production,[116,117] but not E;[116] and enhance the inhibitory effects of HCG and IL-1 on Lydig cell steroidogenesis.[118] IL-1 has also been reported to regulate and be regulated by the sex steroids estrogen and progesterone.[119-126] Certainly, IL-1 can also increase release of CRH, which upregulates the adrenal axis and downregulates the HPGT axis.[127] IL-2 can alter the ability of P to inhibit lymphocyte cluster formation,[128] and IL-2 production in culture is increased in thymocytes from androgen-resistant mice.[129] Also, elevated dehydroepiandrosterone (DHEA) can stimulate IL-2.[130] Finally, IFN gamma can inhibit FSH-stimulated P and E production in rat granulosa cells,[131] IFN treatment will decrease serum T levels in human males,[132] and block the HCG-stimulated T production in Lydig cells.[133]

Very few studies have directly attempted to learn if lymphokine/ monokine levels are different in males and females. However, it has been reported that the antibody synthesized to T-dependent antigen, lectin-induced proliferative response, and IL-2 synthesis by rat spleen cells decreased with age, and spleen cells from old females demonstrated a greater mitogen-driven response and a twofold increase in IL-2 synthesis than did spleen cells from old males.[134] A sex-related difference in LPS-induced fever development has also been demonstrated. In this model, the injection of LPS stimulates the formation of endogenous pyrogen (probably TNF). If LPS is injected into rats, it produces an attenuated febrile response in females vs males, and this difference is not present if the females are ovariectomized before LPS treatment. Furthermore, if 1-d-old females are injected with T, and 10 wk later treated with LPS, the febrile response is similar to males.[135] Finally, it has also been reported that in virus-infected mouse spleen cells in culture, IFN activity is present in spleen cells from females, but not males, and treatment with E enhances, whereas T suppresses IFN production in culture.[136]

Sex Hormones and Immune Regulation

Employing models independent of alcohol, it has been previously reported that the immune response in males is not as active as in females, both for cellular and humoral immunity.[127,137-143] Although the mechanisms that account for this immunological sexual dimorphism (ISD) are only partially understood, they appear to be mediated both during early development, and later in the adult. Early developmental mechanisms include genetic makeup leading to the early estrogens and androgens, whereas after birth a concert of hormones, including estrogens, androgens, growth hormone, and prolactin, also modulate this process.[138] In females, the more active immune response may increase longevity, but it may also elevate the frequency of autoimmune disease.[127,140] Also, sex hormones can regulate autoimmune disease. For example, in humans estrogenic oral contraceptives reduce expression of rheumatoid arthritis,[127,141,144] and in animals, estrogen replacement reduces experimental demyelinating disease.[141] Furthermore, in the autoimmune NZB Lupus Mouse model, the female develops a more severe form of autoimmune thyrotoxicosis and lupus erythematosus than the NZB male. However, if males and females are castrated early in life and given opposite hormone replacement (females + androgen, males + estrogen), then the male dies and the female is protected.[141,145–148]

Estrogens at physiological concentrations found in cycling females can act to stimulate both the cellular and humoral immune systems.[127,137–143] However, at elevated levels in pregnancy they strongly inhibit the cell-mediated system, and also partially inhibit the humoral immune system. Thus, the fetus is protected from rejection by the maternal immune system. Progestins may also be immunoinhibitory, but only in conjunction with estrogen within the immunological target tissues.[149] Furthermore, although castration results in cellular hypertrophy and hyperplasia of thymic cortex and medulla, replacement with sex steroids reverses this.[138,139,150–153] Androgens also act as immunosuppressive agents for both the cellular and humoral immune systems.[138,139,150]

Sex steroid receptors mediate these effects, and are found in most tissues of the immune system. Estrogens, androgens, and progestin receptors are located in the reticuloepithelial (RE) cells of the thymus[138,139,150–153] and spleen.[154] Estrogen and androgen receptors are also found within lymphoblasts during early maturation,[155] and expression of progestin receptors within the RE cells depends on initial priming with estrogen.[149] Thus, sex steroids modulate the process of lymphocyte development and release of thymic hormones by the immunoendocrine axes, which regulate immune response of effector-lymphocytes.[156–158]

Immunoendocrine Axes

Combined interactions between elements of the endocrine and immune systems are termed the immunoendocrine axes. Endocrine glands currently believed to be involved in regulation of immune response, include the hypothalamus–pituitary, gonads (testes, ovaries), adrenal (cortex), thymus, and

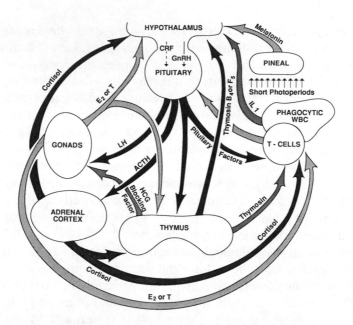

Fig. 2. Regulatory hormonal axes. Interactions of the hypothalamic–pituitary–adrenal–thymic (HPAT) axis, the hypothalamic–pituitary–gonadal–thymic (HPGT) axis, the pineal–hypothalamic–pituitary (PHP) axis, and the lymphocyte–monocyte–factor–mediated (LMFM) axis. In addition, effector immune cells (such as lymphocytes) and lymphatic organs (such as the thymus) are affected by factors (such as growth hormone and prolactin) elaborated by the pituitary. A substance from the thymus (HCG blocking factor) may also directly impact gonadal function. (Reprinted with permission from ref. *137*.)

pineal (Fig. 2), and those immunoregulatory pathways mediated by sex steroids are referred to as the hypothalamus–pituitary–gonadal (HPG) axis and also as the hypothalamus–pituitary–gonadal–thymic (HPGT) axis. Functionally, the HPG and HPGT axes act in concert, and are dependent on negative feedback by gonadal steroids (estrogens and androgens) at the level of the hypothalamus–pituitary. Such negative feedback reduces the amount of gonadotropin (FSH and LH) released, and subsequently decreases the amount of sex steroids secreted by the gonads. Reducing the amount of gonadal steroids then derepresses the thymic reticuloepithelial cells, and they increase release of thymic hormones. These thymic hormones then directly alter effector lymphocyte function, as well as feeding back to the hypothalamus to stimulate release of gonadotropin.[159–162] Sex steroids may also directly alter lymphocyte subclass development, and/or function during certain stages of their maturation within the thymic (or possibly bone marrow) micro-environment by acting on lymphocyte steroid receptors.

A Review of the Facts

Alcohol depresses many parameters of the immune response, but may also nonspecifically increase the circulating levels of immunoglobulins. Alcohol also alters lymphocyte subpopulations and increases the CD4/CD8 ratio.

1. Alcohol impacts on sex steroid hormones by altering production/release of these substances at the gonads and their action at the target cell receptors.
2. Alcohol impacts on soluble mediators generated by activated effector immune cells; increasing some and decreasing others.
3. In addition, sex steroid hormones, themselves, can impact on soluble mediators generated by activated immune cells.
4. Finally, sex steroid hormones, themselves, can function at the level of the effector lymphocyte or at the pituitary or thymus to release other hormones that will then regulate effector lymphocyte function.

Given these facts, it is not surprising that alcohol can produce a significant impact on the immune system. In addition, the effect exerted by alcohol on gonadal steroids can be envisioned to additionally affect immune system function.

Clinical Relevance

The clinical implications of the alteration of sex hormones, related to intemperate ethanol ingestion, remains unclear. However, the known effects of sex hormones on certain infectious agents and autoimmune diseases must be considered in the light of the hormonal abnormalities known to occur in alcoholics. Of particular note, in this regard, is the known feminization of alcoholic males with changes in serum testosterone concentrations and the ratio of estradiol to testosterone. Although specific clinical data are most difficult to interpret in this complex population group, certain basic information is available that may be important, as future initiatives are developed for prevention and therapy of disease in alcoholic patients.

Probably the best data relating sex hormone abnormalities to specific pathogenic organisms rests in the area of fungi. Of particular note is the stimulation of growth of *Coccidioides immitis* in the presence of clinically relevant concentrations of estradiol.[163–165] In addition, the growth of the much more common fungus, *Candida albicans*, may be promoted by estrogen as

well.[166] Conversely, conversion of *Paracoccidioides brasiliensis* from myce-
lium to yeast and conidium to yeast may be inhibited by estradiol in physiological concentrations.[167,168]

Linkage of these phenomena to human disease is not entirely clear.
However, sexual differences in clinical illness is certainly seen, particularly in female patients with *Coccidioides immitis*, both in terms of overall
clinical presentation, and more specifically, related to pregnancy.

Of additional interest is the finding of estrogen-binding receptors on
gram-negative organisms, such as *Pseudomonas aeruginosa*.[169] This patho-
gen is not uncommonly seen in patients with severe debilitating disease, as
in alcoholics with end-stage liver disease.

Of immediate interest, the issue of linkage between sex hormones
and transmission and virulence of the human immunodeficiency virus
(HIV) is gaining attention. Although there is clear documentation of differences in ease of transmission between sexes, the linkage between this
phenomenon and hormonal abnormalities is not clear. In the paper by Padian
et al., the odds of male to female transmission were significantly greater
than female to male.[170] Although this may be a purely mechanical phenomenon, Mulder et al. has reported a correlation between dehydroepiandrosterone (DHEA) and progression of disease in HIV-infected men.[171]
Specifically, DHEA level <7 nM/L was an independent predictor of disease progression. Obviously, linkage has not been made between androgenic hormone abnormalities in alcoholic males and progression of
HIV-related disease.

Alteration of a variety of clinical presentations and progression of
general autoimmune diseases has also been linked to hormone concentrations, particularly estrogen. Of particular note is the female predominance
in diseases, such as systemic lupus erythematosus (SLE), with an approx
9:1 proportion of women to men.[165] In addition, alterations are seen in
other diseases related to sex hormones, including allergic encephalomyeli-
tis in animal models,[172] hereditary angioedema,[173] and perhaps multiple
sclerosis.[174,175]

It would thus appear that although absolute linkage has not been
made among intemperate ethanol consumption, sex hormone abnormalities, and a variety of infectious and autoimmune diseases, these interrelationships may exist. The complexity of the interaction of ethanol with the
host, and the confounding difficulties of dealing with a variety of infectious
and autoimmune diseases, makes conclusive evidence difficult to accumulate. Only further careful work, particularly in animal models, will allow
final determination of the true impact of intemperate ethanol ingestion with
consequent hormonal abnormalities, and host response to these diseases.

Possible Effects of Alcohol
on Immunological Sexual Dimorphism

Because of the intimate relationship between ethanol, gonadal steroids, and immune system function, it might be expected that an alcohol-mediated immunological sexual dimorphism might be observed. Surprisingly, very few publications have attempted to address this possibility, although a limited number of investigators have directly targeted the effects of alcohol on immune response in female animals or humans. As mentioned earlier, birth control pills have been demonstrated to elevate circulating acetaldehyde levels in women,[52] and this metabolite may effect immune function. In addition, alcohol inhibits LHRH in female rats,[67] increases estradiol-mediated LHRH release in women,[68] and effects their hypothalamic-pituitary ovarian interactions.[69]

In an excellent and very recent publication by Weinberg and Jerrells,[176] the authors demonstrated that prenatal exposure to ethanol altered immune response in the male but not the female offspring. For example, "fetal ethanol-exposed males exhibited a decrease in thymocyte number as well as a decreased splenic lymphocyte proliferative response to the T-cell mitogen, Concanavalin A ..." (p. 525). This effect appeared to be a result of an inability of the lymphocytes to respond to exogenous IL-2. On the other hand, ethanol-exposed females demonstrated little or no immunological abnormalities, but did possess immunological sexual dimorphism with respect to males.

A possible sexual effect of alcohol on immune function is supported by the observed changes in the CD4/CD8 ratio reported in alcohol models.[54-56] If alcohol reduces the suppressor T-cell population, this might be viewed as a prerequisite leading to an autoimmune type disease state. This is not a new hypothesis and has been discussed in detail from the standpoint of classic autoimmune diseases like lupus and rheumatoid arthritis.[127] In this view, lesions during development lead to abnormalities in T-suppressor cell function that promote the autoimmune disease in the adult. Sex steroids, glucocorticoids, and other hormones (prolactin, GH, thymic hormones, and so on) as well as the genotype, all impact the cells during development in the microenvironment (Fig. 3). In addition, various hormones also can affect function of the lymphocyte subpopulations in the adult (Fig. 4).

Given all we currently know regarding alcohol and hormones, it is quite probable that the effects elicited by alcohol on the immune response may function via similar pathways both during development and in the adult. Such mechanisms may also be mediated by a concert of hormones

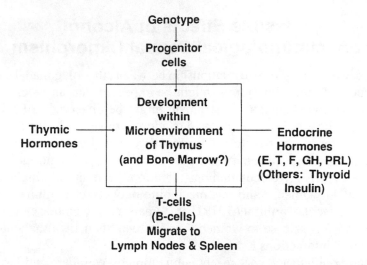

Fig. 3. Factors that influence the maturation of effector lymphocytes in the microenvironment of the thymus and bone marrow. (Reprinted with permission from: C. J. Grossman (1990) *Prog. Neuroendocrinol. Immunol.* **3,** 75–82.)

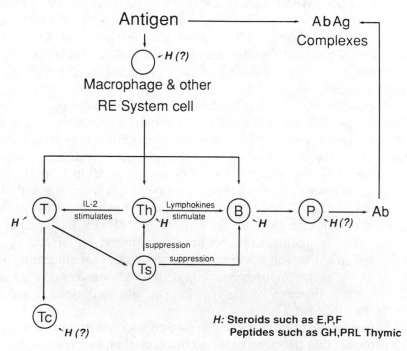

Fig. 4. Steps involved in the activation of effector lymphocytes after antigen stimulation. As can be seen, hormones are thought to impact at each stage of this process. (Reprinted with permission from ref. *127.*)

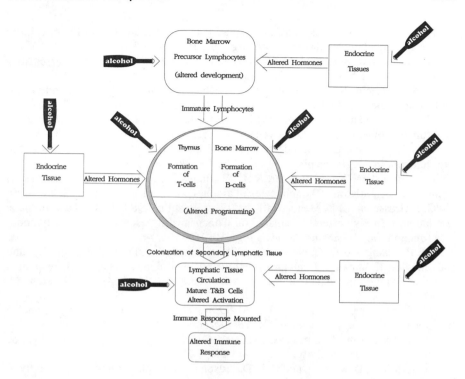

Fig. 5. Alcohol is believed to modify immune response by acting at all levels. As can be seen, the effects of alcohol can be expressed during the earliest stages of immune cell development. Furthermore, later stages, during which the programming of T and B lymphocytes takes place, may also be affected by alcohol. Normally the steps leading to a fully functional immune system are under the control of endocrine hormones from the gonads. Because alcohol can adversely modify steroid hormone production by gonadal tissue, it is possible that this may provide an additional mechanism whereby alcohol perturbs immune response.

that impact on the immune effector cells. In Fig. 5, we have outlined the various components that may be involved, and we suggest that the outcome may be expressed differently in males and females owing to the differences in hormone environment.

References

[1]T. R. Jerrells, C. A. Marietta, M. J. Eckardt, E. Majchrowicz, and F. F. Weight (1986) Effects of ethanol administration on parameters of immunocompetency in rats. *J. Leukocyte Biol.* **39,** 499–510.

[2]T. R. Jerrells (1991) Immunodeficiency associated with ethanol abuse, in *Drugs of Abuse, Immunity and Immunodeficiency.* H. Friedman, S. Specter, and T. W. Klein, eds., Plenum, NY, pp. 229–236.

[3]M. R. Berenyi, B. Straus, and D. Cruz (1974) In vitro and in vivo studies of cellular immunity in alcoholic cirrhosis. Am. J. Dig. Dis. 19, 199–205.

[4]B. Straus, M. R. Berenyi, J. M. Huang, and E. Straus (1971) Delayed hypersensitivity in alcoholic cirrhosis. Am. J. Dig. Dis. 16, 509–516.

[5]I. M. Bernstein, K. H. Webster, R. C. Williams Jr., and R. G. Strickland (1974) Reduction in circulating T lymphocytes in alcoholic liver disease. Lancet 2, 488–490.

[6]G. A. Roselle and C. L. Mendenhall (1982) Alterations of in vitro human lymphocyte function by ethanol, acetaldehyde and acetate. J. Clin. Lab. Immun. 9, 33–37.

[7]G. A. Roselle and C. L. Mendenhall (1984) Ethanol-induced alterations in lymphocyte function in the guinea pig. Alcohol. Clin. Exp. Res. 8, 62–67.

[8]I. M. Bernstein, K. H. Webster, R. C. Williams Jr., and R. G. Strickland (1974) Reduction in circulating T lymphocytes in alcoholic liver disease. Lancet 2, 488–490.

[9]C. J. Grossman, C. L. Mendenhall, and G. A. Roselle (1988) Alcohol and immune regulation, I. In vivo effects of ethanol on Concanavalin A sensitive thymic lymphocyte function. Int. J. Immunopharmacology 10, 187–195.

[10]M. P. Chang and D. C. Norman (1990) Immunocytotoxicity of alcohol in young and old mice. II. Impaired T cell proliferation and T cell-dependent antibody responses of young and old mice fed ethanol-containing liquid diet. Mech. Ageing Develop. 57, 175–186.

[11]R. K. Zetterman, T. Chen, and C. M. Leevy (1974) Role of altered lymphocyte function in alcoholic liver disease. Gastroenterology 67, 837.

[12]R. K. Zetterman, A. Luisada-Opper, and C. M. Leevy (1973) Alcoholic hyaline and cellular immune reactivity. Gastroenterology 65, 578.

[13]A. A. Mihas, D. M. Bull, and C. S. Davidson (1974) Cellular immune reactivity to liver tissue in alcoholic hepatitis. Gastroenterology 67, 816.

[14]N. E. Dehne, C. L. Mendenhall, G. A. Roselle, and C. J. Grossman (1989) Cell mediated immune responses associated with short term alcohol intake; time course and dose dependency. Alcohol. Clin. Exp. Res. 13, 201–205.

[15]R. M. Kaelllin, A. Semerjian, D. M. Center, and J. Bernardo (1984) Influence of ethanol on human T-lymphocyte migration. J. Lab. Clin. Med. 104, 752–760.

[16]R. K. Zetterman and C. M. Leevy (1975) Immunologic reactivity and alcoholic liver disease. Bull. NY Acad. Med. 51, 533–544.

[17]W. I. Smith Jr., D. H. Van-Thiel, T. Whiteside, B. Janoson, J. Magovern, T. Puet, and B. S. Rabin (1980) Altered immunity in male patients with alcoholic liver disease: evidence for defective immune regulation. Alcohol. Clin. Exp. Res. 4, 199–206.

[18]G. A. Roselle, C. L. Mendenhall, C. J. Grossman, and R. E. Weesner (1988) Lymphocyte subset alterations in patients with alcoholic hepatitis. J. Clin. Lab. Immunol. 26, 169–173.

[19]R. Schnabel, M. Bokor, G. Malatinsky, and T. Gram (1990) Killer-cell activity in alcohol-originated diseases of the liver, and the effect of alcohol on the K-cell function under in vitro conditions. Acta Med. Hung. 47, 189–199.

[20]S. E. Blank, D. A. Duncan, and G. G. Meadows (1991) Suppression of natural killer cell activity by ethanol consumption and food restriction. Alcohol. Clin. Exp. Res. 15, 16–22.

[21]H. Eguchi, P. A. McCuskey, and R. S. McCuskey (1991) Kupffer cell activity and hepatic microvascular events after acute ethanol ingestion in mice. Hepatology 13, 751–757.

[22]F. Paronetto (1981) Immunologic factors in alcoholic liver disease. *Semin. Liver Dis.* **1**, 232–243.

[23]R. N. MacSween and R. S. Anthony (1982) Immune mechanisms in alcoholic liver disease. *J. Clin. Lab. Immunol.* **9**, 1–5.

[24]R. R. MacGregor (1986) Alcohol and immune defense. *JAMA* **256**, 1474–1479.

[25]J. P. Nolan (1965) Alcohol as a factor in the illness of university service patients. *Am. J. Med. Sci.* **40**, 135–142.

[26]R. J. Rhodes, G. H. Hames, and M. D. Campbell (1969) The problem of alcoholism among hospitalized tuberculous patients. Report of a national questionnaire survey. *Am. Rev. Resp. Dis.* **99**, 440–442.

[27]L. A. Busch (1971) Human listeriosis in the United States, 1967–1969. *J. Infect. Dis.* **123**, 328–332.

[28]H. O. Conn and J. M. Fessel (1971) Spontaneous bacterial peritonitis in cirrhosis: variations on a theme. *Med. Baltimore* **50**, 161–197.

[29]A. Lavetter, J. M. Leedom, A. W. Mathies Jr., D. Ivler, and P. F. Wehrle (1971) Meningitis due to Listeria monocytogenes. A review of 25 cases. *N. Engl. J. Med.* **285**, 598–603.

[30]A. O. Feingold (1976) Association of tuberculosis with alcoholism. *South. Med. J.* **69**, 1336,1337.

[31](1985) Surveillance and assessment of alcohol-related mortality—United States, 1980. *Morbidity Mortality Weekly Rep.* **34**, 161–163.

[32]C. E. Cherubin, J. S. Marr, M. F. Sierra, and S. Becker (1981) Listeria and gram-negative bacillary meningitis in New York City, 1972–1979. Frequent causes of meningitis in adults. *Am. J. Med.* **71**, 199–209.

[33]J. P. Correia and H. O. Conn (1975) Spontaneous bacterial peritonitis in cirrhosis: endemic or epidemic? *Med. Clin. North Am.* **59**, 963–981.

[34]M. Epstein, F. M. Calia, and G. J. Gabuzda (1968) Pneumococcal peritonitis in patients with postnecrotic cirrhosis. *N. Engl. J. Med.* **278**, 69–73.

[35]T. T. Yoshikawa and A. D. Schwabe (1968) Bacterial endocarditis and cirrhosis of the liver. *Am. J. Dig. Dis.* **13**, 664–668.

[36]C. C. Davis, M. A. Mellencamp, and L. C. Preheim (1991) A model of pneumococcal pneumonia in chronically intoxicated rats. *J. Infect. Dis.* **163**, 799–805.

[37]J. Cotte, F. Forestier, A. M. Quero, P. Bourrinet, and A. German (1982) The effect of alcohol ingestion on the susceptibility of mice to viral infections. *Alcohol. Clin. Exp. Res.* **6**, 239–246.

[38]G. A. Roselle, C. L. Mendenhall, and C. J. Grossman (1991) Ethanol and overall immunoregulation, in *Drugs of Abuse and Immune Function*. R. R. Watson, ed. CRC, Boca Raton, FL, pp. 186–197.

[39]J. I. Tennenbaum, R. D. Ruppert, R. L. Pierre, and N. J. Greenberger (1969) The effect of chronic alcohol administration on the immune responsiveness of rats. *J. Allergy* **44**, 272–281.

[40]G. A. Roselle, C. L. Mendenhall, A. Muhelman, and A. Chedid (1986) The ferrets: a new model of oral ethanol injury involving the liver, bone marrow and peripheral blood lymphocytes. *Alcohol. Clin. Exp. Res.* **10**, 279–284.

[41]R. M. Kaelin, A. Semerjian, D. M. Center, and J. Bernardo (1984) Influence of ethanol on human T-lymphocyte migration. *J. Lab. Clin. Med.* **104**, 752–760.

[42]C. L. Mendenhall, C. J. Grossman, G. A. Roselle, S. J. Ghosn, T. Y. Coyt, S. Thompson, and N. E. Dehne (1989) Phytohemagglutinin skin test response to evaluate in vivo cellular immune function in rats. *Proc. Soc. Exp. Biol. Med.* **190,** 117.

[43]C. M. Leevy, R. K. Zetterman, and T. Chen (1975) The lymphocyte and liver diseases of the alcoholic, in *Alcoholic Liver Pathology,* J. M. Khanna, Y. Israel, and H. Kalant, eds. Alcoholism and Drug Addiction Research Foundation of Ontario, Toronto, Canada, pp. 157–170.

[44]L. Si, T. L. Whiteside, R. R. Schade, and D. Van-Thiel (1983) Lymphocyte subsets studied with monoclonal antibodies in liver tissues of patients with alcoholic liver disease. *Alcohol. Clin. Exp. Res.* **7,** 431–435.

[45]G. Holdstock, W. B. Ershler, and E. L. Krawitt (1982) Demonstration of non-specific B-cell stimulation in patients with cirrhosis. *Gut* **23,** 724–728.

[46]B. Ruhland, L. Walker, A. O. Wollitser, and C. M. Peterson (1991) Ethanol influences class I and class II MHC antigen expression on human fetal islet-like cell clusters. *Alcohol. Clin. Exp. Res.* **15,** 745–747.

[47]G. Pomier-Layrargues, P.-M. Huet, G. Richer, D. Marleau, and A. Viallet (1980) Hyperglobulinemia in alcoholic cirrhosis. Relationship with portal hypertension and intrahepatic portal-systemic shunting as assessed by Kupffer cell uptake. *Dig. Dis. Sci.* **25,** 489–493.

[48]S. R. Berger, R. A. Helms, and D. M. Bull (1979) Cirrhotic hyperglobulinemia: increased rates of immunoglobulin synthesis by circulating lymphoid cells. *Dig. Dis. Sci.* **24,** 741–745.

[49]I. D. Wilson, G. Onstad, and R. C. Williams Jr. (1969) Serum immunoglobulin concentrations in patients with alcoholic liver disease. *Gastroenterology* **57,** 59–67.

[50]M. Aldo-Benson (1989) Mechanisms of alcohol-induced suppression of B-cell response. *Alcohol. Clin. Exp. Res.* **13,** 469–475.

[51]S. Worrall, J. De Jersey, B. C. Shanley, and P. A. Wilce (1989) Ethanol induces the production of antibodies to acetaldehyde-modified epitopes in rats. *Alcohol Alcohol.* **24,** 217–223.

[52]C. M. Jeavons and A. R. Zeuber (1984) Effects of elevated female sex steroids on ethanol and acetaldehyde metabolism in humans. *Alcohol. Clin. Exp. Res.* **8,** 352–358.

[53]G. A. Roselle and C. L. Mendenhall (1982) Alteration of in vitro human lymphocyte function by ethanol, acetaldehyde and acetate. *J. Clin. Lab. Immunol.* **9,** 33–37.

[54]C. Muller, H. Wolf, J. Gottlicher, and M. M. Eibl (1991) Helper-inducer and suppressor-inducer lymphocyte subsets in alcoholic cirrhosis. *Scand. J. Gastroenterol.* **26,** 295–301.

[55]A. J. Saad and T. R. Jerrells (1991) Flow cytometric and immunohistochemical evaluation of ethanol-induced changes in splenic and thymic lymphoid cell populations. *Alcohol. Clin. Exp. Res.* **15,** 796–803.

[56]C. J. Grossman, personal communication.

[57]D. H. Van-Thiel, J. S. Gavaler, C. F. Cobb, R. J. Sherins, and R. Lester (1979) Alcohol-induced testicular atrophy in the adult male rat. *Endocrinology* **105,** 888–895.

[58]D. H. Van-Thiel, J. S. Gavaler, and R. Lester (1978) Ethanol: a gonadal toxin in the female. *Drug Alcohol Depend.* **2,** 373–380.

[59]D. H. Van-Thiel, J. S. Gavaler, and R. Lester (1978) Alcohol-induced ovarian failure in the rat. *J. Clin. Invest.* **61,** 624–632.

[60]V. Rettori, C. W. Skelley, S. M. McCann, and W. L. Dees (1987) Detrimental effects of short-term ethanol exposure on reproductive function in the female rat. *Biol. Reprod.* **37,** 1089–1096.

[61]A. I. Esquifino, A. Mateos, C. Martin, J. M. Canovas, and J. Fermoso (1989) Time-dependent effect of alcohol on the hypothalamic-hypophyseal-testicular function in the rat. *Alcohol. Clin. Exp. Res.* **13,** 219–223.

[62]I. Salonen and I. Huhtaniemi (1990) Effects of chronic ethanol diet on pituitary-testicular function of the rat. *Biol. Reprod.* **42,** 55–62.

[63]T. W. Boyden and R. W. Pamenter (1983) Effects of ethanol on the male hypothalamic-pituitary-gonadal axis. *Endocr. Rev.* **4,** 389–395.

[64]J. Ellingboe and C. C. Varanelli (1979) Ethanol inhibits testosterone biosynthesis by direct action on Leydig cells. *Res. Commun. Chem. Pathol. Pharmacol.* **24,** 87–102.

[65]F. M. Badr, A. Bartke, S. Dalterio, and W. Bulger (1977) Suppression of testosterone production by ethyl alcohol. Possible mode of action. *Steroids* **30,** 647–655.

[66]T. J. Cicero, M. L. Adams, L. O'Connor, B. Nock, E. R. Meyer, and D. Wozniak (1990) Influence of chronic alcohol administration on reproductive indices of puberty and sexual maturation in male rats and the development of their progeny. *J. Pharm. Exp. Therapeut.* **255,** 707–715.

[67]J. K. Hiney and W. L. Dees (1991) Ethanol inhibits luteinizing hormone-releasing hormone release from the median eminence of prepubertal female rats in vitro: investigation of its actions on norepinephrine and prostaglandin-E2. *Endocrinology* **128,** 1404–1408.

[68]J. H. Mendelson, N. K. Mello, S. K. Teoh, and J. Ellingboe (1989) Alcohol effects on luteinizing hormone releasing hormone-stimulated anterior pituitary and gonadal hormones in women. *J. Pharm. Exp. Therapeut.* **250,** 902–909.

[69]J. N. Hugues, T. Coste, G. Perret, M. F. Jayle, J. Sebaoun, and E. Modigliani (1980) Hypothalamo-pituitary ovarian function in thirty-one women with chronic alcoholism. *Clin. Endocrinol.* **12,** 543–551.

[70]W. R. Kelce, V. K. Ganjam, and P. K. Rudeen (1990) Inhibition of testicular steroidogenesis in the neonatal rat following acute ethanol exposure. *Alcohol* **7,** 75–80.

[71]G. G. Gordon and A. L. Southren (1977) Metabolic effects of alcohol on the endocrine system, in *Metabolic Aspects of Alcohol.* C. S. Lieber, ed. University Park Press, Baltimore, MD, pp. 249–293.

[72]G.A. Roselle, C. L. Mendenhall, and C. J. Grossman (1993) Ethanol, sex steroids and lymphokine activity in a rat model of dietary ethanol consumption. Submitted to *Alcohol. Clin. Exp. Res.*

[73]H. Kawanishi, H. Tavassolie, E. Schervish, and R. P. MacDermott (1978) Deficiency of suppressor lymphocyte activity in chronic active alcoholic liver disease. *Gastroenterology* **74,** 1128 (abstract).

[74]C. Gluud, U. Tage-Jensen, M. Bahnsen, O. Dietrichson, and A. Svejgaard (1981) Autoantibodies, histocompatibility antigens and testosterone in males with alcoholic liver cirrhosis. *Clin. Exp. Immunol.* **44,** 31–37.

[75]C. L. Mendenhall, S. Anderson, P. Garcia-Pont, S. Goldberg, T. Kiernan, L. B. Seeff, M. Sorrell, C. Tamburro, R. Weesner, R. Zetterman, A. Chedid, T. Chen, and L. Rabin (1984) Short-term and long-term survival in patients with alcoholic hepatitis treated with oxandrolone and prednisolone. *N. Engl. J. Med.* **311,** 1464–1470.

[76]C. L. Mendenhall, C. J. Grossman, G. A. Roselle, Z. Hertelendy, S. J. Ghosn, K. Lamping, and K. Martin (1990) Anabolic steroid effects on immune function: Differences between analogues. *J. Ster. Biochem. Mol. Biol.* **37,** 71–76.

[77]R. F. McGivern (1989) Low birthweight in rats induced by prenatal exposure to testosterone combined with alcohol, pair-feeding or stress. *Teratology* **40,** 335–338.

[78]I. L. Dahlgren, C. J. P. Eriksson, B. Gustafsson, C. Harthon, E. Hard, and K. Larsson (1989) Effect of chronic and acute ethanol treatment during pregnancy and early postnatal ages on testosterone levels and sexual behavior. *Pharmacol. Biochem. Behav.* **33,** 867–873.

[79]S. J. Ewald and C. Huang (1990) Lymphocyte populations and immune response in mice prenatally exposed to ethanol, in *Alcohol, Immunomodulation, and AIDS.* D. Seminara, R. R. Watson, and A. Pawlowski, eds. Liss, New York, pp. 191–200.

[80]S. J. Ewald, C. Huang, and L. Bray (1991) Effects of prenatal alcohol exposure on lymphocyte populations in mice, in *Drugs of Abuse, Immunity and Immunodeficiency.* H. Friedman, S. Specter, and T. W. Klein, eds., Plenum, New York, pp. 237–244.

[81]D. C. Norman, M.-P. Chang, S. C. Castle, J. E. Van Zuylen, and A. N. Taylor (1989) Diminished proliferative response of Con A-blast cells to interleukin 2 in rats exposed to ethanol in utero. *Alcohol. Clin. Exp. Res.* **13,** 69–72.

[82]S. Johnson, R. Knight, D. J. Marmer, and R. Steele (1981) Immune deficiency in fetal alcohol syndrome. *Ped. Res.* **15,** 908–911.

[83]J. Lundy, J. H. Raaf, S. Deakins, H. J. Wanebo, D. A. Jacobs, T. Lee, D. Jacobowitz, C. Spear, and H. F. Oettgen (1975) The acute and chronic effects of alcohol on the human immune system. *Surg. Gynecol. Obstet.* **141,** 212–218.

[84]T. Chen and C. M. Leevy (1976) Lymphocyte proliferation inhibitory factor (PIF) in alcoholic liver disease. *Clin. Exp. Immunol.* **26,** 42–45.

[85]J. A. Prieto and M. G. Mutchnick (1980) Suppressor T-cell activity (SCA) in acute and chronic alcoholic liver disease. *Gastroenterology* **79,** 1046.

[86]A. M. Cochrane, A. Moussouros, B. Portmann, I. G. McFarlane, A. D. Thomson, A. L. Eddleston, and R. Williams (1977) Lymphocyte cytotoxicity for isolated hepatocytes in alcoholic liver disease. *Gastroenterology* **72,** 918–923

[87]A. Facchini, G. F. Stefanini, M. Bernardi, F. Miglio, G. Gasbarrini, and G. Labo (1978) Lymphocytotoxicity test against rabbit hepatocytes in chronic liver diseases. *Gut* **19,** 189–193.

[88]M. G. Mutchnick, A. Missirian, and A. G. Johnson (1980) Lymphocyte cytotoxicity in human liver disease using rat hepatocyte monolayer cultures. *Clin. Immunol. Immunopathol.* **16,** 423–437.

[89]G. A. Roselle, C. L. Mendenhall, and C. J. Grossman (1993) Ethanol and sex steroids II. The effects of migration inhibitory factor activity. Submitted *Alcohol. Clin. Exp. Res.*

[90]D. H. Gregory and D. F. Levi (1972) The clinical-pathologic spectrum of alcoholic hepatitis. *Am. J. Dig. Dis.* **17,** 479–488.

[91]A. A. Mihas, W. G. Doos, and J. G. Spenney (1978) Alcoholic hepatitis—a clinical and pathological study of 142 cases. *J. Chronic Dis.* **31,** 461–472.

[92]J. Green, S. Mistilis, and L. Schiff (1963) Acute alcoholic hepatitis: a clinical study of fifty cases. *Arch. Int. Med.* **112,** 67–78.

[93]C. L. Mendenhall, S. Anderson, P. Garcia-Pont, S. Goldberg, T. Kiernan, L. Seeff, M. Sorrell, C. Tamburro, R. Weesner, R. Zetterman, A. Chedid, T. Chen, and L. Rabin (1984) Short-term and long-term survival in patients treated with oxandrolone and prednisolone. *N. Engl. J. Med.* **311,** 1464–1470.

[94]C. J. McClain and D. A. Cohen (1989) Increased tumor necrosis factor production by monocytes in alcoholic hepatitis. *Hepatology* **9,** 349–351.

[95]S. N. Wickramasinghe (1985) Rates of metabolism of ethanol to acetate by human neutrophil precursors and macrophages. *Alcohol Alcohol.* **20,** 299–303.

[96]S. Nelson, G. Bagby, and W. R. Summer (1989) Alcohol suppresses lipopolysaccharide-induced tumor necrosis factor activity in serum and lung. *Life Sci.* **44,** 673–676.

[97]S. Nelson, G. Bagby, and W. Summer (1989) Alcohol suppresses tumor necrosis factor and lung host defenses. *Alcohol. Clin. Exp. Res.* **13,** 330.

[98]J. I. Allen and A. Khoruts (1989) Increased plasma tumor necrosis factor and interleukin-1 in patients with alcoholic liver disease. *Hepatology* **10,** 649.

[99]M. E. Felver, E. Mezey, M. McGuire, M. C. Mitchell, H. F. Herlong, G. A. Veech, and R. L. Veech (1990) Plasma tumor necrosis factor alpha predicts decreased long-term survival in severe alcoholic hepatitis. *Alcohol. Clin. Exp. Res.* **14,** 255–259.

[100]Q. B. Saxena, R. K. Saxena, and W. H. Adler (1981) Regulation of natural killer activity in vivo: part IV—high natural killer activity in alcohol drinking mice. *Indian J. Exp. Biol.* **19,** 1001–1006.

[101]C. D. Ericsson, S. Kohl, L. K. Pickering, J. Davis, G. S. Glass, and L. A. Faillace (1980) Mechanisms of host defense in well nourished patients with chronic alcoholism. *Alcohol. Clin. Exp. Res.* **4,** 261–265.

[102]S. Saxena, K. T. Nouri-Aria, M. G. Anderson, A. L. Eddleston, and R. Williams (1986) Interleukin 2 activity in chronic liver disease and the effect of in vitro alpha-interferon. *Clin. Exp. Immunol.* **63,** 541–548.

[103]M. Suthanthiran, S. D. Solomon, P. S. Williams, A. L. Rubin, A. Novogrodsky, and K. H. Stenzel (1984) Hydroxyl radical scavengers inhibit human natural killer cell activity. *Nature* **307,** 276–278.

[104]N. H. Stacey (1984) Inhibition of antibody-dependent cell-mediated cytotoxicity by ethanol. *Immunopharmacology* **8,** 155–161.

[105]S. S. Ristow, J. R. Starkey, and G. M. Hass (1982) Inhibition of natural killer cell activity in vitro by alcohols. *Biochem. Biophys. Res. Commun.* **105,** 1315–1321.

[106]A. S. Walia, K. M. Pruitt, J. D. Rodgers, and E. W. Lamon (1987) In vitro effect of ethanol on cell-mediated cytotoxicity by murine spleen cells. *Immunopharmacology* **13,** 11–24.

[107]R. M. Abdallah, J. R. Starkey, and G. G. Meadows (1988) Toxicity of chronic high alcohol intake on mouse natural killer cell activity. *Res. Commun. Chem. Pathol. Pharmacol.* **59,** 245–258.

[108]C. L. Mendenhall, C. J. Grossman, G. A. Roselle, S. Ghosn, P. S. Gartside, S. D. Rouster, P. B. R. K. Chalasani, G. Schmitt, K. Martin, and K. Lamping (1990) Host response to Mycobacterium (BCG) infection in the alcoholic. *Gastroenterology* **99,** 1723–1726.

[109]F. Wagner, R. Fink, R. Hart, C. Lersch, H. Dancygier, and M. Classen (1992) *J. Stud. Alcohol* **53,** 277–280.

[110]K. C. Chadha, R. B. Whitney, M. K. Cummings, M. Norman, M. Windle, and I. Stadler (1990) Evaluation of interferon system among chronic alcoholics. *Prog. Clin. Biol. Res.* **325,** 123–133.

[111]P. Ghiara, D. Boraschi, L. Nencioni, P. Ghezzi, and A. Tagliabue (1987) Enhancement of in vivo immune response by tumor necrosis factor. *J. Immunol.* **139,** 3676–3679.

[112]V. Kindler, A. P. Sappino, G. E. Grau, P. F. Piguet, and P. Vassalli (1989) The inducing role of tumor necrosis factor in the development of bactericidal granulomas during BCG infection. *Cell* **56,** 731–740.

[113]C. K. Edwards, R. M. Lorence, D. M. Dunham, S. Arkins, L. M Yunger, J. A. Greager, R. J. Walter, R. Dantzer, and K. W. Kelley (1991) Hypophysectomy inhibits the synthesis of tumor necrosis factor alpha by rat macrophages: partial restoration by exogenous growth hormone or interferon gamma. *Endocrinology* **128,** 986–989.

[114]D. R. Davila, C. K. Edwards III, S. Arkins, J. Simon, and K. W. Kelley (1990) Interferon-gamma-induced priming for secretion of superoxide anion and tumor necrosis factor-alpha declines in macrophages from aged rats. *FASEB J.* **4**, 2906–2911.

[115]M. Jaattela, V. Ilvesmaki, R. Voutilainen, U. H. Stenman, and E. Saksela (1991) Tumor necrosis factor as a potent inhibitor of adrenocorticotropin-induced cortisol production and steroidogenic P450 enzyme gene expression in cultured human fetal adrenal cells. *Endocrinology* **128**, 623–629.

[116]K. F. Roby and P. F. Terranova (1988) Tumor necrosis factor alpha alters follicular steroidogenesis in vitro. *Endocrinology* **123**, 2952–2954.

[117]K. F. Roby and P. F. Terranova (1990) Effects of tumor necrosis factor-alpha in vitro on steroidogenesis of healthy and atretic follicles of the rat: theca as a target. *Endocrinology* **126**, 2711–2718.

[118]J. H. Calkins, H. Guo, M. M. Sigel, and T. Lin (1990) Differential effects of recombinant interleukin-1 alpha and beta on Leydig cell function. *Biochem. Biophys. Res. Commun.* **166**, 1313–1318.

[119]J. H. Calkins, M. M. Sigel, H. R. Nankin, and T. Lin (1988) Interleukin-1 inhibits Leydig cell steroidogenesis in primary culture. *Endocrinology* **123**, 1605–1610.

[120]B. C. Fauser, A. B. Galway, and A. J. Hsueh (1989) Inhibitory actions of interleukin-1 beta on steroidogenesis in primary cultures of neonatal rat testicular cells. *Acta Endocrinol. Copenh.* **120**, 401–408.

[121]S.-K. Hu, Y. L. Mitcho, and N. C. Rath (1988) Effect of estradiol on interleukin 1 synthesis by macrophages. *Int. J. Immunopharmacol.* **10**, 247–252.

[122]M. L. Polan, A. Daniele, and A. Kuo (1988) Gonadal steroids modulate human monocyte interleukin-1 (IL-1) activity. *Fertil. Steril.* **49**, 964–968.

[123]M. L. Polan, A. Kuo, J. Loukides, and K. Bottomly (1990) Cultured human luteal peripheral monocytes secrete increased levels of interleukin-1. *J. Clin. Endrcrinol. Metab.* **70**, 480–484.

[124]M. L. Polan, J. Loukides, P. Nelson, S. Carding, M. Diamond, A. Walsh, and K. Bottomly (1989) Progesterone and estradiol modulate interleukin-1 beta messenger ribonucleic acid levels in cultured human peripheral monocytes. *J. Clin. Endrcrinol. Metab.* **69**, 1200–1206.

[125]J. G. Cannon and C. A. Dinarello (1985) Increased plasma interleukin-1 activity in women after ovulation. *Science* **227**, 1247–1249.

[126]P. S. Kalra, A. Sahu, and S. P. Kalra (1990) Interleukin-1 inhibits the ovarian steroid-induced luteinizing hormone surge and release of hypothalamic luteinizing hormone-releasing hormone in rats. *Endocrinology* **126**, 2145–2152.

[127]C. J. Grossman, G. A. Roselle, and C. L. Mendenhall (1991) Sex steroid regulation of autoimmunity. *J. Ster. Biochem. Mol. Biol.* **40**, 649–659.

[128]P. Van-Vlasselaer, J. Goebels, and M. Vandeputte (1986) Inhibition of lymphocyte aggregation by progesterone. *J. Reprod. Immunol.* **9**, 111–121.

[129]N. J. Olsen and W. J. Kovacs (1989) Increased thymic size and thymocyte interleukin 2 production in androgen-resistant mice. *Scand. J. Immunol.* **29**, 733–738.

[130]R. A. Daynes, D. J. Dudley, and B. A. Araneo (1990) Regulation of murine lymphokine production in vivo. II. Dehydroepiandrosterone is a natural enhancer of interleukin 2 synthesis by helper T cells. *Eur. J. Immunol.* **20**, 793–802.

[131]W. C. Gorospe, T. Tuchel, and B. G. Kasson (1988) Gamma-interferon inhibits rat granulosa cell differentiation in culture. *Biochem. Biophys. Res. Commun.* **157**, 891–897.

[132]M. Orava, K. Cantell, and R. Vihko (1986) Treatment with preparations of human leukocyte interferon decreases serum testosterone concentrations in men. *Int. J. Cancer* **38**, 295,296.

[133]M. Orava, R. Voutilainen, and R. Vihko (1989) Interferon-gamma inhibits steroidogenesis and accumulation of mRNA of the steroidogenic enzymes P450scc and P450c17 in cultured porcine Leydig cells. *Mol. Endocrinol.* **3**, 887–894.

[134]D. R. Davila and K. W. Kelley (1988) Sex differences in lectin-induced interleukin-2 synthesis in aging rats. *Mech. Ageing Dev.* **44**, 231–240.

[135]N. Murakami and T. Ono (1987) Sex-related differences in fever development of rats. *Am. J. Physiol.* **252**, R284–R289.

[136]R. Ishikawa and N. J. Bigley (1990) Sex hormone modulation of interferon (IFN) alpha/beta and gamma production by mouse spleen cell subsets following picornavirus infection. *Viral Immunol.* **3**, 225–236.

[137]C. J. Grossman (1989) Possible underlying mechanisms of sexual dimorphism in the immune response, fact and hypothesis. *J. Ster. Biochem.* **34**, 241–251.

[138]C. J. Grossman (1984) Regulation of the immune system by sex steroids. *Endocrinol. Rev.* **5**, 435–455.

[139]C. J. Grossman (1985) Interactions between the gonadal steroids and the immune system. *Science* **227**, 257–261.

[140]C. J. Grossman (1988) The importance of hormones in the regulation of the immune system. *Immunol. Allergy Pract.* **10**, 21–29.

[141]C. J. Grossman and G. A. Roselle (1986) The control of immune response by endocrine factors and the clinical significance of such regulation. *Prog. Clin. Biochem. Med.* **4**, 9–56.

[142]C. J. Grossman (1989) Stress and the immune response: interactions of peptides, gonadal steroids and the immune system, in *Frontiers of Stress Research*. H. Weiner, D. Hellhammer, R. Murison, and I. Florin, eds. Hans Huber, Stuttgard, Germany, pp. 181–190.

[143]C. J. Grossman (1990) Immunoendocrinology, in *Basic and Clinical Endocrinology*. F. S. Greenspan and P. H. Forsham, eds. Lang, New York, pp. 40–52.

[144]C. J. Grossman (1991) The effect of oral contraceptives on immune function in HIV positive women. A talk presented at National Institute of Child Health and Human Development. *NIH.* (Personal communication).

[145]J. R. Roubinian, R. Papoian, and N. Talal (1977) Androgenic hormones modulate autoantibody responses and improve survival in murine lupus. *J. Clin. Invest.* **59**, 1066–1070.

[146]J. R. Roubinian, N. Talal, J. S. Greenspan, J. R. Goodman, and P. K. Siiteri (1978) Effect of castration and sex hormone treatment on survival, anti-nucleic acid antibodies, and glomerulonephritis in NZB/NZW F1 mice. *J. Exp. Med.* **147**, 1568–1583.

[147]J. R. Roubinian, N. Talal, J. S. Greenspan, J. R. Goodman, and P. K. Siiteri (1979) Delayed androgen treatment prolongs survival in murine lupus. *J. Clin. Invest.* **63**, 902–911.

[148]J. Roubinian, N. Talal, P. K. Siiteri, and J. A. Sadakian (1979) Sex hormone modulation of autoimmunity in NZB/NZW mice. *Arthritis Rheum.* **22**, 1162–1169.

[149]H. Fujii-Hanamoto, C. J. Grossman, G. A. Roselle, C. L. Mendenhall, and K. Seiki (1990) Nuclear progestin receptors in rat thymic tissue. *Thymus* **15**, 31–45.

[150]C. J. Grossman, L. J. Sholiton, and P. Nathan (1979) Rat thymic estrogen receptor-I. preparation, location and physiochemical properties. *J. Ster. Biochem.* **11**, 1233–1240.

[151]C. J. Grossman, L. J. Sholiton, G. C. Blaha, and P. Nathan (1979) Rat thymic estrogen receptor- II. physiological properties. *J. Ster. Biochem.* **11,** 1241–1246.

[152]C. J. Grossman, P. Nathan, B. B. Taylor, and L. J. Sholiton (1979) Rat thymic dihydrotestosterone receptor: preparation, location and physiochemical properties. *Steroids* **34,** 539–553.

[153]C. J. Grossman, L. J. Sholiton, and J. A. Helmsworth (1983) Characteristics of the cytoplasmic and nuclear dihydrotestosterone receptors of human thymic tissue. *Steroids* **42,** 11–22.

[154]C. J. Grossman and Y. Haruki (1991) Personal communication.

[155]A. Gulino, I. Screpanti, M. R. Torrisi, and L. Frati (1985) Estrogen receptors and estrogen sensitivity of fetal thymocytes are restricted to blast lymphoid cells. *Endocrinology* **117,** 47–54.

[156]C. J. Grossman, L. J. Sholiton, and G. A. Roselle (1982) Estradiol regulation of thymic lymphocyte function in the rat: mediation by serum thymic factors. *J. Ster. Biochem.* **16,** 683–690.

[157]C. J. Grossman and G. A. Roselle (1983) The interrelationship of the HPG-thymic axis and immune system regulation. *J. Ster. Biochem.* **19,** 461–467.

[158]C. J. Grossman, L. J. Sholiton, and G. A. Roselle (1983) Dihydrotestosterone regulation of thymocyte function in the rat—mediation by serum factors. *J. Ster. Biochem.* **19,** 1459–1467.

[159]M. Dardenne, W. Savino, D. Duval, D. Kaiserlian, J. Hassid, and J. F. Bach (1986) Thymic hormone-containing cells. VII. Adrenals and gonads control the in vivo secretion of thymulin and its plasmatic inhibitor. *J. Immunol.* **136,** 1303–1308.

[160]R. W. Rebar, I. C. Morandini, M. F. Silva de Sa, G. F. Erickson, and J. E. Petze (1981) The importance of the thymus gland for normal reproductive function in mice, in *Dynamics of Ovarian Function*. N. V. Schwarts and M. Hunzicker-Dunn, eds. Raven, New York, pp. 285–290.

[161]R. W. Rebar, A. Miyake, G. F. Erickson, T. L. K. Low, and A. L. Goldstein (1983) The influence of the thymus gland on reproductive function: a hypothalamic site of action, in *Factors Regulating Ovarian Function*. G. S. Greenwald and P. R. Terranova, eds. Raven, New York, pp. 465–469.

[162]R. W. Rebar, A. Miyake, T. L. Low, and A. L. Goldstein (1981) Thymosin stimulates secretion of luteinizing hormone-releasing factor. *Science* **214,** 669–671.

[163]D. J. Drutz, M. Huppert, S. H. Sun, and W. L. McGuire (1981) Human sex hormones stimulate the growth and maturation of *Coccidioides immitis*. *Infect. Immun.* **32,** 897–907.

[164]B. Styrt and B. Sugarman (1991) Estrogens and infection. *Rev. Infect. Dis.* **13,** 1139–1150.

[165]C. J. Grossman and G. A. Roselle (1986) The control of immune response by endocrine factors and the clinical significance of such regulation. *Prog. Clin. Biochem. Med.* **4,** 9–56.

[166]P. C. Braun (1989) Influence of corticosterone and estradiol on the metabolic activities of *Candida albicans* (abstract F104), in *Abstracts of the 1989 Annual Meeting of the American Society for Microbiology*. J. A. Morello and J. E. Domer, eds. American Society for Microbiology, Washington, DC, p. 475.

[167]D. S. Loose, E. P. Stover, A. Restrepo, D. A. Stevens, and D. Feldman (1983) Estradiol binds to a receptor-like cytosol binding protein and initiates a biological response in *Paracoccidioides brasiliensis*. *Proc. Natl. Acad. Sci. USA* **80,** 7659–7663.

[168]M. E. Salazar, A. Restrepo, and D. A. Stevens (1988) Inhibition by estrogens of conidium-to-yeast conversion in the fungus *Paracoccidioides brasiliensis. Infect. Immun.* **56,** 771–773.

[169]S. S. Rowland, N. Bashirlahi, and W. A. Falkler Jr. (1989) Studies of an estrogen-binding protein in *Pseudomonas aeruginosa* (abstract D149), in *Abstracts of the 1989 Annual Meeting of the American Society for Microbiology.* J. A. Morello and J. E. Domer, eds. American Society for Microbiology, Washington DC, p. 107.

[170]N. S. Padian, S. C. Shiboski, and N. P. Jewell (1991) Female-to-male transmission of human immunodeficiency virus. *JAMA* **266,** 1164–1167.

[171]J. W. Mulder, P. H. J. Frissen, P. Krijnen, E. Endert, F. de Wolf, J. Goudsmit, J. G. Masterson, and J. M. Lange (1992) Dehydroepiandrosterone as predictor for progression to AIDS in asymptomatic human immunodeficiency virus-infected men. *J. Infect. Dis.* **165,** 413–418.

[172]B. G. Arnason and D. P. Richman (1969) Effect of oral contraceptives on experimental demyelinating disease. *Arch. Neurol.* **21,** 103.

[173]M. Frank (1979) Effect of sex hormones on the complement related clinical disorder of hereditary angioedema. *Arth. Rheum.* **22,** 1295.

[174]H. G. Miller and K. Schepira (1959) Etiological aspects of multiple sclerosis. *Br. Med. J.* **17,** 37.

[175]J. Miller (1961) The influence of pregnancy or disseminated sclerosis. *Proc. Roy. Soc. Med.* **54,** 4.

[176]J. Weinberg and T. R. Jerrells (1991) Suppression of immune responsiveness: sex differences in prenatal ethanol effects. *Alcohol. Clin. Exp. Res.* **15,** 525–531.

Women, Recovery Groups, and "Love Addiction"

Janice Haaken

The concept of relationships as *addictive* has achieved broad currency in the popular clinical literature over the past decade. Books on love addiction and codependence now fill self-help sections of bookstores, and therapeutic gurus promote workshops offering relief from these compulsive forms of desire. In addition, an array of recovery groups for love addicts and codependents have formed, providing a widening audience for this burgeoning literature.

Of the many recovery groups that have developed out of the alcoholism and chemical dependency fields, Adult Children of Alcoholics (ACOA) has been particularly active in promoting groups for codependents. An extension of the concept of relationship addiction, codependence is conceived as a disease or personality disorder associated with a family history of alcoholism.[1-3] ACOA, a 12-step program that developed out of the Alcoholics Anonymous (AA) and Al-Anon traditions, describes codependence as the pathology of attachments based on caretaking and excessive responsibility for others, the emotional legacy of adult children of dysfunctional families. This focus on what is most commonly constructed as a feminine malady accounts for the growing appeal of ACOA groups among women, who constitute approx 80% of the membership.* The growth of these groups since ACOA's inception in the late 1970s has been phenomenal; thousands of

---

Note: A similar version of this chapter was published in *Free Associations (London)* **25**, 1992.

*This estimate is based on interviews with local and national ACOA organizers, and is consistent with my own observations at the meetings I attended in the Portland, Oregon area.

From: *Drug and Alcohol Abuse Reviews, Vol. 5: Addictive Behaviors in Women*
Ed.: R. R. Watson ©1994 Humana Press Inc., Totowa, NJ

groups now exist around the United States, particularly in the West where publishers claim that demand for ACOA literature is also particularly strong. These recovery groups, whether ACOA or the more recent group, Codependents Anonymous, are all based on the 12-step philosophy of AA (*see* Table 1).

Both concepts—love addiction and codependence—are based on an extension of the disease model of addiction advanced by Alcoholics Anonymous to conflictual interpersonal dependencies. Although some use the terms interchangeably, codependence refers to a more general pattern of behavior, i.e., a personality disorder based on a preoccupation with the needs of others. Whereas the love addict becomes over-involved in dyadic relationships, the codependent may manifest her/his disease through a tendency to take responsibility for the feelings and well-being of others in myriad interpersonal contexts. The codependence literature provides more clinical elaboration of the malady of relationship addiction, introducing a broad constellation of pathological behaviors and etiological explanations associated with an identity based on caretaking and overinvolvement in relationships.

The analysis presented here is grounded in two sets of theoretical and practical concerns. As a psychoanalytic clinician, I have been interested in the therapeutic potential and limits of the constructs associated with the recovery movement.[4,5] ACOA groups are of particular interest because they go beyond the narrow behavioral objectives of AA groups, i.e., to provide group support both in maintaining sobriety and in instilling greater responsibility in the alcoholic. As a social psychological phenomenon, ACOA groups are significant because they apply the AA philosophy and the disease model of addiction to interpersonal problems, extending these ideas far beyond the primary addictions, i.e., drug and alcohol.

My therapeutic interest in recovery groups, and in ACOA groups as a specific case example, is not based on conceiving of them as watered-down therapy, for although these groups have become the treatment of choice for many, they are not a substitute for the detailed self-exploration and interpretive process of psychotherapy. The extent to which they provide the equivalent of psychotherapy, however, should not be the main criterion for judging their therapeutic and social value. In critiquing them, I focus on both what is of value in ACOA groups, as well as their limitations. But given the evangelical tone of the claims of these new 12-step adherents, and the steady stream of testimonials that appear increasingly on bookshelves and in the media, my primary interest has been in critically addressing their more problematic aspects.

My other interest in this contemporary phenomenon is grounded in feminist politics and a current debate within feminism over "postfeminist"

Table 1
The 12 Steps of Alcoholics Anonymous

1. We admitted we were powerless over alcohol (in some ACOA groups, "relationships" is substituted for alcohol).
2. We came to believe that a Power greater than ourselves could restore us to sanity.
3. We made a decision to turn our will and our lives over the care of God as we understood Him.
4. We made a searching and fearless moral inventory of ourselves.
5. We admitted to God, to ourselves, and to another human being, the exact nature of our wrongs.
6. We were entirely ready to have God remove all these defects of character.
7. We humbly asked Him to remove our shortcomings.
8. We made a list of all persons we had harmed, and became willing to make amends to them all.
9. We made direct amends to such people wherever possible, except when to do so would injure them or others.
10. We continued to take personal inventory and when we were wrong promptly admitted it.
11. We sought through prayer and meditation to improve our conscious contact with God as we understood Him, praying only for knowledge of His will for us and the power to carry it out.
12. Having had a spiritual awakening as a result of these steps, we tried to carry this message to alcoholics, and to practice these principles in all our affairs.

thought (for discussion, *see* Stacy[6]). Postfeminism refers to those ideals and understandings that informed the women's movement, i.e., equality between men and women and the importance of women's self-determination, which have been depoliticized with the decline of an activist women's movement. Like much of the popular literature on intimacy and relationships, ACOA groups attract primarily women and draw implicitly on a feminist critique of gender roles. They stress the importance of egalitarian relationships with men and provide support for women's emancipatory struggles against personal domination, offering a challenge to traditional institutions, particularly the family.

At the same time, feminist critics have argued that much of the contemporary recovery literature, promoted through groups such as ACOA, offers narrow psychological explanations of feminine pathology, consistent with the conservatism of the 1980s. Betty Tallen,[7] for instance, pointed out that codependence has become big business, a new rubric for promoting treatment of "women's ailments" and for exploiting the insecurities and oppressive conditions that dominate women's lives. Harriet Goldhor Lerner[8] argued that although the literature legitimizes women's pursuit of greater autonomy, it identifies dependency conflicts as stemming from women's "disease," thereby depoliticizing the difficulties that pervade women's lives.

Although Tallen and Goldhor Lerner viewed the opportunism of these new moral entrepreneurs as a major problem, neither explored the basis of women's identification with the recovery literature. Nor do such feminist critics explore the extent to which self-diagnosis, as one of the bases of 12-step group participation, represents a different phenomenon from the labeling of women imposed by the medical establishment.

The following discussion begins by examining the concept of addiction in the work of Robin Norwood, a psychotherapist and author who has influenced how women's difficulties are articulated in ACOA groups. My critique draws on psychodynamic and feminist perspectives in suggesting how the ideas and explanations offered by Norwood resonate with the experiences of many contemporary women. The analysis that follows from this critique situates ACOA groups within the historical context of the Al-Anon tradition, the precursor to ACOA. ACOA's formation as a 12-step program separate from AA and Al-Anon is discussed within the context of changing gender roles and emerging discourses on the family. Finally, a case example of ACOA group meetings is presented, based on participant-observation of meetings I attended in the Portland, Oregon area. This approach provided a means of gaining access to how members of recovery groups, such as ACOA, appropriate the literature on addiction in understanding interpersonal problems, and how they apply this literature within the context of the groups. In addition to attending eight ACOA and four Al-Anon meetings, I discussed both programs with participants and group leaders as opportunities arose outside of the scheduled meetings. Al-Anon meetings were included because joint participation in Al-Anon or AA groups is recommended in ACOA literature as an initiation into the 12-step philosophy and the disease concept of alcoholism.

Relationship Addiction and Women

Robin Norwood's popularly acclaimed books, *Women Who Love Too Much*[9] and *Letters from Women Who Love Too Much*,[10] are used as guiding texts in many ACOA groups. In ACOA meetings specifically organized for "people who love too much" or in women-only groups, members some-

times take turns reading passages. Norwood's books have also been important in popularizing the notion of relationship addiction. Her stance on relationship addiction, implicitly challenging feminist assumptions about abuse,
is summarized as follows:

> Women who are being abused physically can best be understood and
> treated when they are recognized as being relationship addicted. They
> are afflicted with a progressive and ultimately fatal disease that must
> be taken as seriously by them and those who treat them as any other
> life-threatening form of addiction. The only women I've personally
> known to recover from this particularly dramatic and deadly variety of
> relationship addiction have done so through being involved with one
> Twelve-step program or another, usually Alcoholics Anonymous or
> Al-Anon. (p. 327)[10]

Norwood's accounts of addictive love are not limited to physically
abused women, although the theme of a feminine identity based on caretaking
and stoical tolerance for abuse runs through her stories of women's lives.
The unequal division of emotional labor, where women carry the primary
responsibility for the "emotional work" of relationships, is also a central
theme and a basis for the broad appeal of Norwood's books among women.
In my own clinical experience, Norwood's message that women should "stop
taking care of other people" and "start taking care of themselves"—a repe-
titive incantation in contemporary self-help literature generally—speaks to
the emotional deprivation and disappointment so many women experience
in relationships with men.

Although many feminists would reject Norwood's claim that women
are often drawn to destructive and self-destructive men, she clearly described
a problem that has been difficult for feminists to address. The women
Norwood described recall their sense of excitement or challenge in being
with unpredictable, irresponsible men. She also noted the grandiose component of this feminine, self-sacrificing position in relationships. Norwood
minimized the social context of abuse, e.g., the myriad ways in which men
are encouraged to act out against women, and the emotional costs of women's
economic dependency on men. However, she correctly suggested that there
can be an emotionally rewarding component of destructive relationships
for women. Norwood did not resurrect "female masochism" to explain
women's psychological identification with abusive and self-destructive men.
Instead, she recognized the impulses for mastery and control behind the
tendency to recreate the traumatic relationships of childhood. Women do
not simply invite abuse from men in order to recreate the past. However, in
seeking a new resolution to situations that are associated with childhood
memories of destructive vulnerability and lack of control, women do become

vulnerable to situations that recall the past. Women who "love too much" become self-sacrificing and overly nurturing as a means of controlling a chaotic and disturbing inner and outer world. Norwood also stressed the futility of these efforts for women. Although there is pleasure in becoming "the strong woman in charge of a man's welfare," and in finding "someone who needed me enough not to go away," women are ultimately absorbed by these relationships in a way that leaves them empty. Moreover, focusing on men—and the need to repair them—can serve as a defense against being conscious of one's own personal interests and difficulties in the world.

Ultimately, Norwood medicalized women's overdependency on emotionally or physically abusive men, seeing it as a disease process, not analogous to addiction, but an actual addiction. She elaborated on the parallel, stressing the common urgency and progressive nature of all addictions:

> The first step in treating a woman with this problem is to help her realize that, like any addict, she is suffering from a *disease process* [Norwood's emphasis] that is identifiable, is progressive without treatment, and that responds well to specific treatment ... To wait for (the addicted woman) to figure out on her own that she is a woman who loves too much, whose disease is becoming progressively severe and may very well ultimately cost her life, is as inappropriate as listening to all the typical symptoms of any other disease and then expecting the patient to guess her condition and her treatment. (p. 205)[9]

Norwood has contributed to the current popularity of addiction theory in explaining a broad range of miseries over which people feel little control. The comparison between a physical dependency and emotional dependency on another person is compelling because it suggests an underlying causal unity behind seemingly disparate forms of human behavior. Although there is a sense of urgency in Norwood's equation of emotional problems and pernicious disease (and this is clearly intended to mobilize anxiety and to challenge existing defenses), she also offered a reassuring message of hope and salvation. Norwood told women that they are very sick, but that they can be made well.

There are problematic implications, both etiologically and therapeutically, to this notion of an underlying congruence among addictive processes. There are ongoing debates about what constitutes addiction to drugs and alcohol, and whether or not addiction should be conceived as a disease process, i.e., of having an identifiable etiology and a predictable course or progression through successive stages.[11-13] There is considerable evidence that alcoholism, for example, is not inevitably a progressive condition. Many alcoholics stabilize their intake of alcohol or return to moderate drinking after a period of abstinence.[14,15]

Although a review of the debates on addiction falls outside the scope of this chapter, the psychiatric literature does suggest that there are no clearly identifiable dynamics nor consistent etiological factors underlying drug or alcohol dependency.[16-18] But regardless of how we conceive of the regressive component of chemical or alcohol addiction, there are myriad problems in extending these formulations to the interactive pressures and dependencies of relationships. If addiction implies a regressive retreat from the object relational world, where the drug becomes the substitute object, the women that Norwood described do not achieve whatever euphoria that might be expected in a logical extension of addiction theory. Whatever the pathology that underlies these conflicted attachments, it exists in a world of real human connection requiring some capacity for ego functioning and normal dependency alongside of the pathology.

On the other hand, there is a certain phenomenological congruity to compulsive forms of desire, whether the object is alcohol, drugs, or people.[19,20] To describe something or someone as addictive is to express the power of infantile longings and the emergence of an archaic split between exciting and persecutory objects. Falling in love has been described as a drug, and alcohol has been described as a faithful lover. In both experiences the euphoria of union contains the memory of an idealized, gratifying, comforting object, and the heightened narcissism derived from it. It also awakens the experience of infantile ambivalence, and the sense of terror and loss when the exciting object is withdrawn.

For women in abusive relationships, the abusive partner can come to represent the split-off bad part of herself, which she can only experience through her tie with an external, phallic representation of badness. Abused wives also often recognize, both consciously and unconsciously, the desperate dependencies behind their husbands' abusive behavior, and they do experience themselves as powerful objects of desire, particularly during the husband's repentant moments—as he attempts to recover her love and approval.

Literature on alcoholism includes this experience of vacillation between the god-like and the demonic properties of alcohol—its simultaneously exaltive, life-enhancing and poisonous life-destroying powers.[21] Norwood's literature on tortured relationships similarly captures this ambivalent split-off world dominated by angels and devils. But these dependency relationships are forged out of domination, where the power of the "slave" is derived from understanding the vulnerability and infantile dependency of the "master." Most of the women Norwood described are not passively abused; they tolerate periods of abuse but generally view their partners as weak and needy. Unconsciously, the woman may experience the man's rage and abuse as justifiable in that she, as well as the man, may fear the power of the pre-Oedipal, maternal object within herself, and her own capacity to engulf.[22,23]

Norwood told women that the devil is really within themselves, a message that does represent a potentially important insight. But she also told women that there are no meaningful distinctions between victim and perpetrator, between the drug addict who lives for his next fix and the relationship addict who lives in order to fix. It is a message based on archaic truths, and archaic truths alone. On an archaic level, there is a sense in which all tortured dependencies—whether their external objects are people or substances—evoke disturbing and primitive object- and self-representations. But archaic truths must always be understood alongside their ego-developmental and object-relational elaborations. Norwood missed the complexity of the developmental processes underlying "excessive caretaking" for women, focusing exclusively on pathology. As feminist theorists have argued, the maternal object represents an ideal based on caretaking and empathic concern for others, as well as regression and merger.[23,24]

Addiction, in Norwood's model, represents a reified, reductionistic rendering of psychodynamic psychology, packaged for mass marketing. To accept this world of social and psychological equivalents, where victim and perpetrator, addict and caretaker, are no different pathologically is to accept an undifferentiated world. There are no meaningful distinctions here between pleasures associated with some relational capacity, which, nonetheless, contain primitive or regressed components, and those severely regressed, autistic states associated with advanced drug or alcohol addiction. In Norwood's theorizing, these distinctions are conceived of as mere stages along the same disease continuum, with each stage advancing in an equivalent way.

The disease model offered by Norwood simultaneously expressed the drama of intrapsychic life and empties out its richness and symbolic complexity. It is a world where the secular metaphors of medicine, of the "bad" appearing as an invasive disease agent, are combined with archaic fantasies of religious redemption. Both these worlds are reduced to concretized, hypostatized meanings.

The therapeutic approach Norwood described is confrontive and directive rather than interpretive. This approach views the symptomatology as the direct manifestation of a disease that must be directly controlled, rather than as a symbolically mediated means of expressing conflict. In the drug and alcohol field, there has been some basis for this behavioral approach, i.e., focusing on abstinence as a necessary condition to further treatment, in that alcoholics often do poorly in insight-oriented treatment.[25] But the problems in treating addicts are related to these patients' difficulties in withstanding the deprivation and frustration of treatment without resorting to regressive withdrawal through substance abuse. The narcissistic and sociopathic character disorders associated with some forms of alcoholism and drug addiction also mitigate against forming a strong working alliance and attachment to a therapist. Most of the women who fall within Norwood's typology differ in crucial ways from many substance abusers in that they are able to form attachments, albeit conflictual and destructive.

Historical Continuities and Discontinuities

Al-Anon, an organization formed in the United States in 1951 by the wife of one of the founders of AA, was the prototype of the many recovery groups of the 1980s.[26] ACOA is patterned after the Al-Anon model and its focus on the problems of significant others in the lives of addicted individuals. The emergence of Al-Anon in the early 1950s, and the particular character of its literature, expressed some of the contradictions of women's lives during the postwar period, particularly of women whose lives did not conform to normative ideals of domesticity. The gender ideology of the 1950s polarized and heightened conceptions of femininity and masculinity, as men returned from the war to resume their jobs, and women workers were displaced. This social contract called for women to provide emotional and physical support in exchange for economic dependency on men. But this romantic ideal of family life and harmonious gender reciprocity belied the continuing discontent of many women and their resistance to the restoration of domesticated femininity, temporarily suspended by the war effort. The 1950s' cult of domesticity only thinly veiled the problems inherent in creating a haven of family togetherness in a world dominated by cold war repression, on the one hand, and commodified visions of personal happiness on the other.[27]

The early Al-Anon literature expresses the conflict many women married to alcoholics experienced between holding the family together and not conforming to the normative ideal of femininity and companionable marriage. Although many middle class women struggled with the problem that "had no name," as Betty Friedan called it in *The Feminine Mystique*,[28] the more palpable problems of Al-Anon members required naming. These were the problems of women who were married to men who had "hit bottom"—who had failed to deliver on the American postwar promise of upward mobility achieved through conventional notions of masculine success.

For Al-Anon members, there was a disquieting recognition that they were the functional heads of their households, and that thus they were running the risk of becoming "masculinized." A central theme in the early literature was that of the "proud wife" who is "trying to run things," and the woman who derives "ego" gratification from the position of control she comes to assume through her alcoholic husband's disabilities.[29]

For the Al-Anon member, learning about the disease of alcoholism involved a reconstruction of her husband's problems, and her own relationship to those problems. Al-Anon encouraged, through the disease concept of alcoholism, a dissociation of the husband's destructive behavior from his essential nature as a "good husband." Understanding alcoholism as a disease permitted these women to split off the abuse and neglect that they experienced, and to view these as manifestations of the disease for which the husband was not responsible. One of the 12 steps for Al-Anon members in the 1950s required that "I admit that I was wrong in my understanding of an alcoholic, being thankful that it is an illness instead of pure cussedness" (p. 25).[29] Wives were encouraged to adopt a stoical detachment, to root out pride and selfishness in their own character, and not to "permit natural fear and worry to show through their shining shields of hope" (p. 138).[29]

Al-Anon was the progenitor of some of the unifying ideas behind contemporary recovery groups for women, specifically in recognizing the role of the wife as an "enabler" of the husband's alcoholism. The essential insight behind the enabler construct, or what is referred to in ACOA as codependence, emerged out of treatment of alcoholics. Family members, typically the wives of alcoholics, inadvertently supported the very behavior they were ostensibly trying to control. By intervening and protecting the alcoholic, e.g., cleaning up messes, lying to the alcoholic's boss, and paying unpaid bills, the wife was compensating for her spouse's irresponsibility and loss of control. However, these very attempts at restoring control had the effect of preventing the alcoholic from experiencing the uncomfortable consequences of his behavior. As the wife increasingly took over areas of the alcoholic's life and functioning, the alcoholic's tendency to deny the destructiveness of his behavior intensified.

Al-Anon meetings did provide space for women to give voice to impulses deemed subversive by standards of the time, while providing interpretations for those impulses consistent with the AA philosophy. For instance, the recognition by early Al-Anon members that they could find subversive pleasure in feeling superior to the men they married also entailed confessing the errors of their ways and working to restore the conventional order of family life, with the husband as the rightful head of the family.

ACOA: The Ambivalent Daughter of AA and Al-Anon

The early AA and Al-Anon literature emerged out of the experiences of alcoholic men and their wives and their attempts to find recovery through their own efforts and the support of fellow sufferers. ACOA, not formally affiliated with AA or Al-Anon, emerged in the early 1980s as its rebellious progeny. The founders of ACOA had grown up in the Al-Anon family groups, including Alateen and Alatot and, although not breaking from the 12-step program, they were the first alcohol-related 12-step group to become formally independent of AA.[30] ACOA does not have an organizationally approved literature as does Al-Anon, and groups draw extensively on the love addiction and codependence literature in meetings. ACOA groups have adopted a less structured and less regimented approach to meetings, combining the 12-steps and an evolving "laundry list" of ACOA traits and characteristics, as well as the ACOA "bill of rights" and "affirmations." The meetings stress more open expression of feelings than typically characterizes Al-Anon groups, including expression of hostility toward parents.[26] Al-Anon offers groups for adult children as well, but these groups are much less variable in format and content than are ACOA groups.[31]

ACOA groups represent a continuation of the human potential movement, as well as a departure from this tradition. Unlike the personal growth marathons that flourished in the 1970s, opening up new entrepreneurial opportunities for slick consultants and highly paid therapeutic gurus, ACOA groups are democratically run by participants, and group services are free. Whereas the personal growth marathons sold quick-fix, feel-good, instant mental health, ACOA groups stress the ongoing process of understanding and dealing with emotional pain. Personal growth marathons, grounded in the practices and ideas of humanistic psychology, denied the determinative influence of the past, and offered a solipsistic vision of self-creation and self-determination. The message of ACOA groups, on the other hand, is one of accepting limits, conflict, and the formative power and constraints of the past.

Although drawing on much of the language of the human potential movement, e.g., the need for "personal affirmation," "getting in touch with my feelings," "taking risks," ACOA groups open up a much more disturbing domain of American family life than did the personal growth marathons of the previous decade. ACOA participants share a sense of felt urgency and anguish, and a deep disappointment and disillusionment with family life. The use of kinship terms in describing relationships within the groups, e.g., "brothers and sisters in recovery," represents a desire for a more stable therapeutic community than is offered in other therapeutic groups or marathons, and a search for alternative forms of community.

There is some confusion over who actually founded the early "adult child" groups, or ACA groups, which were the precursors to the official organization that took the acronym of ACOA. Claudia Black and Stephanie Brown first coined the term "adult children of alcoholics" when publicly describing in 1979 their clinical work with alcoholic families.[30] During this same period, two women therapists in New York City initiated support groups for ACAs.[26] Tony Allen, who first developed the "laundry list" used so extensively in ACOA meetings, has recently claimed the mantle of cofounder, explaining that he initially had rejected the leadership role "thrust upon him" by the fledgling groups formed in New York City in the late 1970s.[32]

Although most of the ACA literature credits both men and women as influencing the development of adult child organizations and literature, women are clearly leading authorities in the movement. The emotionally injured children of alcoholics (COAs) described by Margaret Cork in *The Forgotten Children*[33] became the not-to-be forgotten daughters who launched the ACA movement of the early 1980s. Sharon Wegscheider,[1] Claudia Black,[34] Cathleen Brooks,[35] and Janet Woititz[2] brought public attention to the problems of adult children, eclipsing the COA organizations that promoted child advocacy and chartered new organizations during the same period.[30]

As a social phenomenon, ACA was shaped by the social movements of the 1960s and 1970s that challenged normative gender roles and the ideal of family-togetherness-at-any-cost. ACA literature articulates the feeling of emotional abandonment and lack of control that women often experience in relationships, themes that also resonate with the emerging literature associated with the men's movement. The ACA literature speaks to the emotional legacy of daughters who identify with their mothers' sense of wearisome responsibility for others. Even though it describes the dysfunctional family as sharing a common disease for which neither parent is individually responsible, ACA literature, like much of the literature on family pathology, implicates women more fully than men in family pathology.[36] Woititz, for example, described the children as being more sympathetic to the alcoholic father than to the nonalcoholic mother.[2] Whereas the father is described as often "everything you wanted a father to be" when he is sober, the mother is viewed as more fundamentally unhappy. "Even with all of his problems, you may have preferred your father. Because she was grouchy and irritable, acting as if she had the weight of the world upon her shoulders" (p. 9).[2] When the mother is alcoholic, Woititz continued, the father may have helped out with domestic chores "but you felt peculiar about it, because you knew it wasn't his job, and he was doing it to make up for the fact that your mother was drunk. In the end, you probably took over the things that mothers usually do" (p. 10).[2] Although she acknowledged the COA's tendency to blame the mother, the tendency of Woititz to validate all of the child's feelings—a tendency common to ACA literature generally—does not permit a distinction between the position of the mother in the unconscious (as the ambivalent object of infantile dependency) and her historical reality.[37]

Addiction Theory and Ideology

Clearly, much of the appeal of ACOA groups is in their capacity to reduce the tremendous sense of isolation and hopelessness felt by many in American society. In much of the adult child literature, the term addiction is a metaphor for both human excess (particularly an excessive desire for control) and the experience of powerlessness and profound social isolation. As both metaphor and reality, the concept of addiction has come to occupy a larger and larger terrain in American popular psychology.

Schaef distinguished between substance addictions, e.g., dependency on alcohol, drugs, nicotine, or food, and process addictions, e.g., consuming interest in working, gambling, sex, shopping, religion, marriage, or emotional states, such as worry or excitement.[38] In many cities in the United States, there are 12-step programs for each of these compulsive ailments, and many adherents circulate among the various problem-specific groups. The prototypical addiction refers to reliance on alcohol or drugs to achieve a sense of emotional control, as well as the paradoxical loss of control, which is both a consequence and symptom of the addictive process. But in ACOA literature, the addictive process has come to refer to any and all human excesses—"any process over which we are powerless" and "anything we are not *willing* to give up."[39]

As a feminist and adherent of the AA philosophy, Schaef linked addiction and women's oppression.[38] She described, in apocalyptic terms, the deterioration of American society, and attributes its moral, economic, and social decay to the "addictive system." Schaef went on to argue that the addictive system is really the "White male system," a system that has all of the characteristics of an alcoholic, e.g., dependent, controlling, self-centered, greedy, and exploitive of others.

Schaef's analysis represents an attempt to identify societal origins of addictions, and points to the pervasive moral emptiness of consumer society and organizational life in the United States. Her analysis also suggests there are myriad ways women "take in" and support destructive tendencies in men. However, Schaef's arguments reduce all of the problems of contemporary society to psychological sickness and to a vaguely understood tendency toward "addictive thinking." Her outspoken moral outrage and sense of urgency have inspired many feminist adherents of the AA philosophy.

By combining the AA message with broadly defined social and psychological anxieties, proponents of recovery groups, such as ACOA, have expanded the popular appeal of the AA philosophy to young adults and middle aged people alike. The membership of AA, as well as that of the more recent recovery groups, also has shifted over the past few decades from a lower class to a middle class constituency, and has attracted higher functioning individuals who have not yet "hit bottom."[40]

The pietistic emphasis on clean living as a positive value and as a concept of moral reform also appeals to middle class adherents, because it resonates with the political climate of the United States in the 1980s. The drug culture and sexual experimentation that flourished in the counter-culture and youth movements of the 1960s and 1970s did naively celebrate impulsivity but failed to recognize the potentially self-destructive components and limitations of hedonistic visions of freedom. Current public anxieties over AIDS, which is often associated with the dangers of sexual experimentation, and drug and alcohol abuse, which is linked with increases in crime and a general breakdown in the social order, are based on real social problems. But in the absence of social movements offering real analyses or meaningful alternatives to the current social and economic crises of American society, groups that claim that our social ills are a result of excesses and moral laxity strike a receptive chord.

The appeal of the AA message is also related to scaled-down expectations. For example, the serenity prayer, offered at most 12-step meetings, including ACOA, beseeches members to "accept the things I cannot change" and "the courage to change the things I can." Messages of personal empowerment and "giving ourselves permission to be successful" combine with "turning our will over to God" and "living one day at a time." Just as America has fallen from a position of control and domination in the world, and has had to give up the heady vision of continued prosperity, the addict is understood as suffering from an excessive desire for control and an exuberant confidence that belies the underlying self-destructiveness and the inevitability of a crash—of hitting bottom.

But like so much of contemporary American thought, the ideology of recovery groups is mixed and contradictory. On the one hand, there is an implicit critique of American society, and an emphasis on the social basis of human suffering. Recovery groups based on the 12-step model emphasize many good commitments, such as rotation of leadership tasks, the equal value of participants' contributions, and nonhierarchical group processes.

The groups attempt to restore a sense of the potential for goodness in people and a commonality of purpose through which members can transcend the limits of individual experience.

On the other hand, recovery groups establish unity against the "exciting, bad" objects of desire, i.e., alcohol, and other people, by idealizing self-control and by shunning "excesses." In AA, being a "dry drunk" means exhibiting the expansiveness and excessive, unrealistic optimism members come to associate with the alcoholic state. In the ACOA groups I attended, the terms dry drunk, addict, and "co" (codependent) were applied to myriad behaviors that participants felt to be in some way excessive.

Since ACOA groups are based on an assumed equivalence of addictive processes, any and all forms of excess come to signal the underlying disease process generally, serving as reminder of the common affliction and the futility of a final cure. To be "in recovery" or to be "working the program" means more than mere abstinence. It represents the idealized, self-purifying activity of the group and the addicted individual's dependency on the 12-step program to maintain internal cohesion and stability.

This puritanical group ideal is both psychologically and politically conservative. On both levels, it pathologizes the rebellious component of various excesses and idealizes self-purification and splitting off of disruptive aspects of both the self and the society. It discourages differentiated understanding of the various reasons for compulsive disorders and the specific meaning of the various objects of compulsive human desire. The groups establish a community of the afflicted—but one based on undifferentiated understanding of both individual and social pathology.

The disease concept of alcoholism, a central tenet of addiction theory, serves a defensive function for ACOA participants, and, like a neurotic symptom, allows the expression and acting out of repressed experience while simultaneously distorting and rerepressing the original conflict. The disease of alcoholism, which is a unifying theme in the backgrounds of ACOA participants, represents all that was sick and bad in the group's collective past. The disease metaphor carries the connotation of an impersonal, invasive, destructive experience, as well as a sense of hopelessness and doom. But it also reifies these experiences, and serves as a defense against real understanding. It is the addiction that is understood to be the singular cause of one's past and current misery. At one ACOA meeting I attended, for example, a woman responded to another woman's story of sexual abuse by her father by offering that "of course he abused you—he was an alcoholic."

It is important to recognize, however, the truth behind the metaphorical understanding of alcohol addiction as a spiritual sickness, while, at the time, stressing the defensive function of the metaphor. What inheres in various descriptions of the addictive or dysfunctional family is the anguish and uncertainty of growing up in a world where the adults were confused, repressive, and out of control. For ACOA participants, the parents' drinking comes to be understood as a spiritual problem because it is associated with moral apathy, social isolation, and hopelessness about the world and the future. As a result, many children of alcoholics have difficulty relying on stable, comforting internal objects.

The notion of alcoholism as a disease permits group members to locate and isolate the bad as essentially external from the self, as a pathogenic agent that was taken in but can be ritually expelled. The concept of addiction similarly serves as a kind of conceptual container into which everything that is troublesome within oneself and the world, past and present, is placed.

The Groups

Although ACOA groups vary in their specific thematic focus and level of enthusiasm, there is a surprising degree of uniformity and orderliness to the meetings. The leader plays a nominal role in guiding the process of the group. The first third of the meeting is structured by reading the AA 12 steps and 12 traditions, followed by ACOA's "laundry list" describing the nature of the group's collective pathology, and a list of personal rights and affirmations. These readings set the tone for the remainder of the meeting, which consists of voluntary sharing of experiences, beginning with the leader, and concluding with the serenity prayer and a rousing cheer for the group, i.e., "Come back, it works!"

ACOA groups go much further than AA and Al-Anon in claiming to offer a therapeutic and reparative experience for group members—a place where members are encouraged to talk about painful experiences in the past and present, and to experience the restorative acceptance and support of the group. Confession before the group is emphasized as an initial step toward recovery from the injurious effects of growing up in a dysfunctional family. Members are free, however, to speak or to remain silent during meetings. Criticism or concern expressed by new members about the program—which is quite common—is superficially permitted but not really "taken in" by the group. The normative understanding is that such reservations about the program are part of the "denial" associated with both the disease and the early phase of recovery, and will pass.

The clinical literature on adult children of alcoholics is consistent with the themes voiced at ACOA meetings. The literature describes the experience of "not really being seen" as children, of a pseudo-mutuality and estrangement that underlied the pretense of family togetherness.[41,42] Real human contact often took the forms of overt violence, severe punishment, or personal humiliation. The families of many ACOA members were unable to deal with real conflict in a purposeful way. The alternative, then, to violent confrontation was a phobic avoidance of all conflict. Descriptions of family history offered at meetings suggest that primitive defenses, such as repression, denial, and splitting, became the dominant modes of managing feelings and conflicts.

Although seeming to offer a reparative experience for many of these injurious relationships, many key principles and processes of ACOA groups are a reenactment of the very pathology that the groups purportedly overcome. Group members take turns briefly sharing their private experiences and feelings but the prohibition on "crosstalk," i.e., participants' responding to the one who is sharing, prevents any meaningful interaction within the group. Although the crosstalk rule does permit the group to maintain stability and emotional safety, it also disallows meaningful interaction. An indiscriminant openness is cultivated, in which members are encouraged to express very private experiences within a group where other people often come and go as strangers. This undermines any potential for learning, through experiences with others, what makes situations or other people emotionally safe or trustworthy.

Pseudo-mutuality is cultivated within ACOA groups whereby group members are assumed to share a common personality disorder, i.e., relationship addiction or codependence, and the description of this disorder offered at group meetings is intended to explain the life difficulties of group members. Aspects of this description of fears and excesses that presumably characterize the group apply to many, if not most people. However, the specificity of what these fears and excesses mean to people, and those experiences that give rise to them, are negated by the shopping list of symptoms that circulates in the group.

Groups based on common afflictions can provide a means of mitigating the narcissist injuries associated with personal adversity.[11] The group experience anoints the sufferer with special healing powers and a mission in life through "carrying the message to others," step 12 in the recovery program. There is a valuable component of this idealizing capacity of the groups, particularly in aiding participants in adopting defenses that permit greater relational connectedness, and diminish impulsivity and acting out.

In AA and Al-Anon, the groups are unified through the members' tormented relationship with alcohol. In ACOA, the group is unified by sharing a common personality disorder—a more problematic basis for group identity. Although the psychodynamic implications of alcohol dependency and its relation to the specific problems of individual members is obscured in

AA, the groups' pragmatic, behavioral approach to sobriety limit its potential invasiveness. Group identity is based on a common affliction, which still permits other areas of self-definition and self-understanding. Depressed participants do sometimes feel shamed by other members who accuse them of self-pity (in AA parlance, the "poor me's" or "sitting on the pity pot"). But AA's focus on difficulties with alcohol cultivates an awareness, among members, of the group's limitations and specificity.

The idea that groups share a common personality disorder, the premise of ACOA, encourages merger with the group while denying the specificity of members' experiences. The groups provide a means of "naming the problem"—of labeling the various problems and anxieties of members. But in attempting to explain so much, the groups ultimately explain very little.

The structure and ideology of ACOA groups provide a means of emotionally containing the disturbing, "bad" impulses of group members, but the appeal is to regressive modes of control and reasoning, much like the appeal in a great deal of religious thought. Recognizing one's disease, like accepting original sin, is understood to mean relinquishing human pride and negating human agency in the world. Finding redemption means yielding to an imagined perfect parent who can protect us from the torment of our own desires and limitations, the damaged humanity of other people, and our own disappointing efforts to change them.

ACOA groups encourage members to express their anger and disappointment, but to then move, ritualistically, to a stance of forgiveness and acquiescence. Drawing on the AA 12 traditions, ACOA groups stress that essential to recovery from a "relationship addiction" is recognizing that "I need to concentrate not so much on what needs to change in the world as on what needs to be changed in me and my attitudes:" This vision of health and inner peace involves renouncing struggle and conflict. "When confronted by a foe, praise him, bless him, let him go."[43] This message clearly fails to provide a meaningful way of distinguishing between rational and irrational aggression and confrontation, and fails to offer a healthy way of thinking about human reparative efforts in the world.

Conclusions

Relationship addiction and codependence are presented in the popular clinical literature as conditions with varying symptoms, but ones based on an underlying disease shared by all sufferers. According to the literature, it originates in an equivalently understood repressive, addictive family system, it progresses in an equivalent way toward ultimate self-destruction, and it requires the same redemptive solution. The person who attempts to hold the family together is the same as the alcoholic who abandons it; the person who depends on drugs for a sense of well-being is the same as the one who depends on people for these same feelings. Although the literature does reject the repressive moral categories of the past, it provides a morally and psychologically impoverished substitute world devoid of the tensions inherent in differentiated consciousness.

Recovery groups, such as ACOA, that draw extensively on the concept of addiction, do offer comfort and hope to individuals who share a common experience of feeling overwhelmed and out of control. The groups provide a place and language for talking about emotional pain and the feeling of loss of control in a society that provides so little space for this. Recovery groups reduce the sense of isolation and aloneness so common in American society, and convey hope and a commonality of purpose through which members can transcend the limits of individual experience.[44]

On the other hand, the contemporary literature on relationship addiction, and the recovery groups that draw on this literature, pathologize caretaker dilemmas and vastly oversimplify problems of human dependency and interdependency. The message that codependents must disinvest in unrewarding relationships is particularly compelling for women today who continue to carry the traditional burdens of caretaking responsibilities and whose entry into the paid workforce has, to some degree, intensified these burdens. Although women have gained some measure of autonomy and freedom from enforced dependencies on men and family life, conditions of daily life have not permitted a real emancipation from the old division of domestic and emotional labor. The old social contract between the sexes has unraveled, and, as of yet, new forms of reciprocity and healthy interdependence between men and women have not been sufficiently realized. The codependence literature vastly oversimplifies these problems of dependency and interdependency, on both the social and individual levels.

The construct of relationship addiction embraces much of humanity in a common psychopathological net. Although this concept articulates concerns that are common to many in this society, and points to the need for sociological and cultural explanations for psychopathology, it assimilates a great deal in attempting to offer one simple construct to explain the multifarious existential, social, and psychopathological bases of human emotional suffering.

We do need theories and ideas that speak to core human dilemmas and to the commonalities in human emotional suffering. But as clinical work has become increasingly guided by narrowly defined specialties on the one hand, and ad hoc eclecticism, such as addiction models, on the other, the potential for broad-based theorizing has diminished. Clinicians who are not anchored in broad-based, theoretically developed traditions are tremendously vulnerable to clinical trends and popular literature that "pull it all together" conceptually. The addiction label becomes a broad conceptual container into which myriad life difficulties and internal and external pressures are placed. The message is compelling because it seems to provide, for both the therapists who draw on the literature and the individuals who identify with the disease, deliverance from the difficult task of separating out what is internal and what is external, what is healthy and emotionally useful, and what is pathological and emotionally destructive in worrisome, conflictual, interpersonal relationships.

References

[1]S. Wegscheider (1981) *Another Chance.* Science and Behavior Books, Palo Alto, CA.

[2]J. G. Woititz (1983) *Adult Children of Alcoholics.* Health Communications, Deerfield Beach, FL.

[3]T. Cermak (1986) *Diagnosing and Treating Co-Dependence.* Johnson Institute, Minneapolis, MN.

[4]J. Haaken (1990) A critical analysis of the codependence construct. *Psychiatry* **53,** 396-406.

[5]J. Haaken (1993) From Al-Anon to ACOA: Co-dependence and the reconstruction of caregiving. *Signs: Journal of Woman, Culture and Society* **18,** 321–345.

[6]J. Stacy (1987) Sexism by a subtler name? *Socialist Rev.* **96,** 7–28.

[7]B. S. Tallen (1990) Co-dependency: A feminist critique. *Sojourner: The Women's Forum.* April, p. 20.

[8]H. Goldhor Lerner (1990) Problems for profit? *Women's Review of Books.* April, pp. 15,16.

[9]R. Norwood (1986) *Women Who Love Too Much.* Simon and Schuster, New York.

[10]R. Norwood (1988) *Letters from Women Who Love Too Much.* Simon and Schuster, New York.

[11]P. Antze (1987) Symbolic action in Alcoholics Anonymous, in *Constructive Drinking; Perspectives on Drink from Anthropology.* M. Douglas, ed. Cambridge University Press, New York.

[12]C. MacAndrew (1968) On the notion that certain persons who are given to drunkenness suffer from a disease called alcoholism, in *New Concepts In Mental Illness.* S. Plot and R. Edgerton, eds. Doubleday, New York.

[13]R. Reinert (1968) The concept of alcoholism as a disease. *Bull. Menninger Clin.* **32,** 21–25.

[14]D. L. Davies (1962) Normal drinking in recovered alcohol addicts. *Q. J. Stud. Alcohol* **22,** 94–104.

[15]R. Smart (1978) Spontaneous recovery in alcoholics: A review and analysis of the available research. *Q. J. Stud. Alcohol* **38,** 123–164.

[16]R. E. Meyer (1986) *Psychopathology and Addictive Disorders.* Guilford, New York.

[17]S. M. Mirin (1984) *Substance Abuse and Psychopathology.* American Psychiatric Press, Washington, DC.

[18]B. J. Rounsaville, Z. S. Dolinsky, T. F. Babor, and R. E. Meyer (1987) Psychopathology as a predictor of treatment outcome in alcoholics. *Arch. Gen. Psychiatry* **44,** 505–513.

[19]S. Peele and A. Brodsky (1975) *Love and Addiction.* Taplinger, New York.

[20]J. Simon (1982) Love: Addiction or road to self-realization, a second look. *Am. J. Psychoanal.* **42,** 252–262.

[21]R. Wilmot (1985) Euphoria. *J. Drug Issues* **15,** 155–191.

[22]J. Benjamin (1988) *The Bonds of Love: Psychoanalysis, Feminism, and the Problem of Domination.* Pantheon, New York.

[23]N. Chodorow (1978) *The Reproduction of Mothering: Psychoanalysis and the Sociology of Gender.* University of California Press, Berkeley, CA.

[24]C. Gilligan (1982) *In a Different Voice: Psychological Theory and Women's Development.* Harvard University Press, Cambridge, MA.

[25]R. Weiss and S. Mirin (1989) The dual diagnosis alcoholic: evaluation and treatment. *Psychiatr. Ann.* **19,** 261–265.

[26]E. Marlin (1987) *Hope: New Choices and Recovery Strategies for Adult Children of Alcoholics.* Harper and Row, New York.

[27]E. May (1988) *Homeward Bound.* Basic Books, New York.

[28]B. Friedan (1963) *The Feminine Mystique.* W. W. Norton, New York.

[29]Al-Anon (1986) *First Steps: Al-Anon, 35 Years of Beginnings.* Al-Anon Family Group Headquarters, New York.

[30]S. B. Jacobson (1991) The recovery movement: from children of alcoholics to co-dependency. Paper presented at the National Consensus Symposium on Children of Alcoholics and Co-Dependence, October. Warrenton, VA.

[31]S. Brown (1992) Personal communication.

[32]D. Wolter (1990) The founding of ACoA. *Phoenix: Recovery, Renewal, Growth.* November, pp. 14–21.

[33]A. M. Cork (1969) *The Forgotten Children.* Paperjacks, Unionville, ON, Canada.

[34]C. Black (1981) *It Will Never Happen to Me.* M.A.C., Denver, CO.

[35]C. Brooks (1982;1989) *The Secret Everyone Knows.* Hazeldon Foundation, Center City, MN.

[36]B. Thorne (1982) Feminist rethinking of the family: an overview, in *Rethinking the Family: Some Feminist Questions.* B. Thorne and M. Yalom, eds. Longman, New York, pp. 1–24.

[37]N. Chodorow and S. Contratto (1982) The fantasy of the perfect mother, in *Rethinking the Family: Some Feminist Questions.* B. Thorne and M. Yalom, eds. Longman, New York, pp. 54–71.

[38]A. W. Schaef (1987) *When Society Becomes an Addict.* Harper and Row, San Francisco.

[39]Portland ACOA Intergroup (1988) *ACOA Knews???* vol. 5, Portland, OR.

[40]E. Kurtz (1979) *Not-God: A History of Alcoholics Anonymous.* Hazeldon Foundation, Center City, MN.

[41]R. Ackerman (1978) *Children of Alcoholics: A Guide for Educators, Therapists and Parents.* Learning Publications, Holmes Beach, FL.

[42]B. L. Wood (1987) *Children of Alcoholism: The Struggle for Intimacy and Self in Adult Life.* New York University Press, New York.

[43]Alcoholics Anonymous (1976) *Alcoholics Anonymous,* 3rd ed., Alcoholics Anonymous World Services, New York.

[44]C. Cutter and H. Cutter (1987) Experience and change in Al-Anon family groups: Adult Children of Alcoholics. *J. Stud. Alcohol* **48,** 29–32.

Sexuality Issues
of Chemically Dependent
Women

Janet M. Teets

Introduction

The meaning of sexuality encompasses a broad range of experiences and feelings. This chapter expands on Reiss' (1986) idea that two characteristics are key to sexuality: physical pleasure and self-disclosure.[1] Sexuality, then, is that drive of each individual to seek intimacy, a reciprocal self-disclosure with another human being, while also seeking sensual bodily pleasure. Sometimes the expression of intimacy takes precedence over sensual pleasure; at other times sensual pleasure is primarily expressed. Other factors must be considered as integral parts of sexuality, such as how one plays one's gender role, body image, sexual orientation, and biological functioning. All these factors, in turn, are mediated and affected by one's culture, in the broad sense, society, and in the more narrow sense, one's community, subgroups, and family. The complex interrelationship between those factors profoundly influences how one expresses one's own sexuality.

For women, sexuality is the fabric on which the self-concept is interwoven and developed. A chemically dependent woman's sexuality is often deeply affected by many experiences: the stigma of being a drunken/using woman in a society that still condemns her more than a man, dysfunctional family relationships, and destructive childhood sexual encounters that set

From: *Drug and Alcohol Abuse Reviews, Vol. 5: Addictive Behaviors in Women*
Ed.: R. R. Watson ©1994 Humana Press Inc., Totowa, NJ

the tone for later dysfunctional intimacy. In addition, the drug/alcohol-seeking lifestyle makes her vulnerable to other destructive experiences that are often played out in a sexual way.

This chapter will address sexuality issues of chemically dependent women. The term chemical dependency is used to mean dependency on alcohol and/or drugs. Current literature will be presented about those issues affecting sexuality of the chemically dependent woman: sexual abuse, rape, violence from one's intimate partner, sexual behavior while using, sexual orientation, gender role enactment, and sexual health problems. Recommendations for treatment will also be addressed. In addition, the author's perspective on sexuality issues formed from facilitating group discussions on sexuality with recovering chemically dependent women will also be presented.

Childhood Sexual Abuse

A number of researchers have found that chemically dependent women were victims of childhood sexual abuse. This abuse came from both within the family and outside the family.

The incidence of incest experienced by chemically dependent women in one treatment facility was reported to be 53% as revealed through extensive sexuality questionnaires.[2] Benward and Densen-Gerber found that of 118 women who were interviewed using a standardized format by female treatment staff 44% were victims of incest.[3] A comparison of 35 alcoholic women and a paired group of nonalcoholic controls in another study indicated that the alcoholics were significantly more likely to have experienced incestual abuse than the controls.[4] Incest was experienced by 34% of the alcoholics compared to 16% of the controls.

In a large study of adolescent girls who had been treated for substance abuse ($N = 597$), 35.2% responded yes during follow-up interviews to the question of whether someone in their family had sexually abused them.[5] In addition, 58 girls in the sample had previously told counselors of sexual abuse experiences, but denied sexual abuse in the follow-up interviews, and thus were not included in the study results. This discrepancy in revealing traumatic sexual encounters in the family may point to the importance of trust when asking such a sensitive question, particularly of young subjects. Another study asked 117 women who were attending Alcoholics Anonymous to respond on self-administered questionnaires to questions regarding childhood incest.[6] Of that group, 29 (24.7%) had had a childhood incest experience.

Other studies do not differentiate between intrafamilial and extrafamilial sexual abuse. In a study comparing family backgrounds of drug-addicted women ($N = 28$) with nonaddicted women ($N = 22$), 67% of drug-addicted women stated they had been sexually assaulted in comparison to 15% of nonaddicted women.[7] The data was collected through the use of verbally administered questionnaires. These sexual assaults included incest and rapes, much of it occurring before the women reached adulthood. Another study reported that during unstructured group discussions on sexuality, recovering chemically dependent women frequently spoke of incest and other childhood sexual abuse they had experienced.[8]

A study by Sullivan on alcoholic nurses found that 18% of the 139 recovering nurses reported having been sexually molested, but it is not clear whether the molestation occurred in childhood or adulthood or who the molesters were.[9] The study by Sterne et al. identified a neighbor as being the second most frequent perpetrator of sexual abuse, next to father, but it is unclear, again, if the molestations all occurred in childhood, or if some occurred in adulthood.[2]

Two studies were conducted that found an association between heavy drinking or using and childhood sexual and/or physical abuse. The first study investigated the association between a history of physical and sexual abuse and alcoholic drinking behavior among psychiatric out-patient women.[10] A sample of 118 women coming to the clinic for the first time completed self-rating questionnaires that included the Michigan Alcoholism Screening Test (MAST) and questions about physical and sexual abuse. From this sample, 14% of the women were categorized as heavy drinkers as defined by MAST results. The women with a history of physical and sexual abuse had significantly higher scores on the MAST than those with no history of abuse. Even when the first abuse occurred before the age of 18 and there was no recent abuse, the high MAST scores continued, suggesting, the authors felt, that early physical or sexual abuse may be associated with current levels of alcohol use. The second study investigated the relationship between sexual abuse and substance abuse in an adolescent psychiatric clinic group and found similar results.[11] Forty-eight adolescents, male and female, being treated in an in-patient psychiatric unit and who had been sexually abused were matched with other in-patient adolescents who were not sexually abused. Self-report questionnaires on alcohol and drug use were completed by the adolescents; data from the questionnaires were combined with information from parents, school personnel, and a drug counselor interview on substance use. The results showed that significantly more of the sexually abused adolescents made regular use of cocaine and stimulants, drank or used drugs more often, and were drunk or high more often than the control group. Again, there seems to be an association between substance use and being sexually abused.

The incidence of sexual abuse experienced by chemically dependent females, then, has ranged from 67–24.7% of the samples studied. The method of data collection has varied, from self-report questionnaires to interviews with a counselor, which may account for some differences in percentages. The relationship of sexual abuse to a woman's chemical dependency is still unclear, as the studies have not delineated well when chemical dependency began in relation to the sexual abuse. Complicating the picture, too, is the fact that women who have experienced sexual abuse as children are more likely to be revictimized sexually later on in life,[12] and the drug-using lifestyle makes the woman more vulnerable to sexual assault.

Rape

Chemically dependent women not only are likely to have experienced sexual molestation while growing up, but also are more likely to be victims of rape or attempted rape as adults. Teets' analysis of sexuality topics discussed by recovering chemically dependent women revealed that rape was a common experience for these women.[8] Ethnographic interviews of 10 Black women who used crack also revealed that 3 of the 10 had been raped by men who smoke crack.[13] An interview study currently being conducted by the author, which asks if after the age of 14 the woman had ever been forced to have any kind of sexual intercourse, and if they had ever been the victim of a rape or attempted rape, has resulted in the finding that of 54 women interviewed, 33 (61%) had been raped, and 18 (33%) were on the receiving end of an attempted rape but were able to call for help or fight off the offender. Only five of the 54 women had not been the victim of rape or attempted rape. At least 17 (51.5%) of the rape victims said they had been raped more than once, some numerous times. In addition, 12 of the sample responded that they had experienced unwanted sexual advances because of being drunk, high, or asleep. Although this does not fit a legal definition of rape, it certainly indicates sexual exploitation. The average age of this sample is 30.8 yr, and the average number of years the subjects have been using alcohol/drugs is 13.5 yr. Clearly, rape for this group of long-time chemically dependent women was a common experience.

Winick and Levine explained an annual marathon therapy conducted with drug-dependent women in a therapeutic community who are also survivors of rape.[14] They stated that the percentage of women who are self-reported victims of rape in their facility over the years has ranged from 18–44%. The fact that the percentage of women who reported being raped is less than found in the author's study may be owing to differences in seeking the information. Chemically dependent women need to be asked about rape after they are comfortable and trusting of treatment.

Sexual Behavior
While Using/Drinking

Sexual behavior while using or drinking is an area that has been addressed by some researchers. A classic study by Beckman discovered that alcoholic women reported they wanted intercourse most when drinking, enjoyed it most when drinking, and were more likely to engage in intercourse when drinking than the nonalcoholic controls.[15] Almost three-fourths of chemically dependent women said they always or frequently used alcohol or other drugs in conjunction with sexual activity in another study.[2] Covington and Kohen pointed out from their study of 35 recovering alcoholic women that the alcoholic women used alcohol more frequently with sexual experiences than the control group.[4] In fact, these subjects believed that alcohol contributed to good sexual experiences. Teets found, in her sexuality group discussions, that women commonly said they had never had sex while sober.[8] Thus, as chemically dependent women face recovery, they have fears and concerns about having sex while sober, especially in light of the fact that they may believe that using is necessary for sexual responsiveness.

Some chemically dependent women are apt to change sexual partners frequently. An interview study that asked about the sexual behavior of intravenous drug users ($N = 142$) found that 21.8% of the female intravenous drug users revealed they had had sex with three or more partners in the past 12 mo.[16] Another study that interviewed 91 Black and Latino women in methadone clinics found that only 9% had had sex with more than one partner over the last 3 mo.[17] This study did find that those who reported shooting up intravenous drugs more frequently had more sexual partners, and those women who used cocaine had more sexual partners than women using other drugs. Washton and Stone-Washton believed that cocaine is strongly connected to compulsive sexuality because many users experience strong sexual stimulation from cocaine.[18] However, it has also been found to be more common among drug-dependent men than women.[18] The effect of cocaine use on women's sexual responsiveness has not been researched. The Sterne et al. study also found that almost half of their sample said they had had two or more sexual partners per year for the last 5 yr.[2]

Another sexual behavior sometimes employed by drug-dependent women is that of trading sex for drugs or money. The Feucht et al. study found that 25% of the drug-dependent White women and 28% of the drug-dependent Black women said they had exchanged sex for drugs or money.[16] Trading sex for crack was a common occurrence according to the 10 women interviewed in the Carlson and Siegal ethnographic study.[13] Of the 10 women, 7 admitted to performing sexual favors in exchange for crack.

The number of chemically dependent women who engaged in prostitution seems to vary from study to study. In the Carlson and Siegal study, 3 of the 10 women had had a history of prostitution before accepting crack in place of money.[13] Only 8% of the sample of chemically dependent women studied by Sterne et al. said they had a history of prostitution.[2] However, a recent study of adolescent delinquents points to an opposite finding regarding prostitution.[19] On-the-street interviews were conducted with 600 "seriously delinquent" (defined as having committed a minimum of 10 major crimes or 100 lesser crimes during the year before interview) adolescents in Miami, Florida. All of the adolescents were current drug users, and 91% of the sample were using some form of cocaine at least three times a week. Of the 100 females interviewed, 87 reported a median of 200 acts of prostitution. Their results also suggest that those female delinquents who started using drugs early in life and used drugs heavily were very likely to become engaged in prostitution. An ethnographic study of prostitutes designed to learn about beliefs and behaviors that place them at risk for HIV transmission recruited most of their subjects from methadone maintenance programs.[20] All of the sample, 15 women, had been or were current intravenous drug users. Although no conclusion can be made about drug abusing women also being prostitutes or about prostitutes using drugs from this study, it points out that many prostitutes do indeed use drugs.

It may be that the number of years of chemical dependency influences the numbers of sexual partners a woman will have or whether she turns to prostitution or using sex for drugs. Certainly as a woman becomes more heavily addicted, financial resources often dwindle, and paying for one's addiction becomes more difficult. Sex is one commodity women can sell. As a woman endeavors to recover from her addiction, her past sexual behaviors may engender much shame and guilt and she worries whether she can avoid these old patterns of behavior as she faces sobriety.

Battering From One's Intimate Partner

Being the recipient of beatings from one's significant other probably occurs more frequently among chemically dependent women than among the general population of women. Miller et al. conducted interviews with alcoholic women ($N = 45$) and women from a random household population ($N = 40$) to learn whether spouses of alcoholic women are more violent than spouses of women in the general population, whether there are certain types of violence alcoholic women are more likely to receive, and the contribution of spousal violence to the development of alcohol problems in women.[21] They found that the alcoholic women were more likely to report higher levels of conflict with spouses, more negative verbal interaction, and more moderate and severe violence than the nonalcoholic group. A fourth of the alcoholic women had been recipients of the more severe violent use of hitting, kicking, or punching with a fist compared to 5% of the control group. Miller et al. were uncertain, however, as to the relationship between the violence and the woman's alcoholism. They suggested that it may be a complex relationship: that an alcoholic woman, by being negatively labeled, is perceived as being a more socially acceptable target of spousal violence, and that perhaps victimization leads to the development of alcoholism for women.

A study that specifically addressed the relationship between cocaine use and violence among men and women was done by Goldstein et al.[22] In their ethnographic studies, 133 female and 152 male drug users and distributors were interviewed once a week for at least 8 wk to identify the nature, scope, and drug-relatedness to all violence perpetrated or experienced during the 8 wk. They concluded that the majority of violent events for the females occurred in the context of nondrug-related disputes involving spouses and lovers. In contrast to male drug users who were more likely to be perpetrators of violence with an increase in cocaine use, women using large amounts of cocaine or using it on a regular basis were more likely to be victims of violence.

Gender Role Enactment

There has been some earlier research on the sex (gender) role enactment of the alcoholic woman. Wilsnack found that some alcoholic women see a traditional feminine role as gratifying on a conscious level, but on an unconscious level behave in a more traditionally masculine way, such as being independent or assertive.[23] Because of this discrepancy, Wilsnack felt alcoholic women were experiencing stress because they were not fulfilling society's female role expectations. According to Sandmaier, who interviewed over 50 recovering female alcoholics, they generally fell into one of two patterns: women who strongly identified with the traditional feminine role through life, and those that rejected the role.[24] For both groups Sandmaier says there was conflict for the woman regarding her sex-role fulfillment. There was no comparison to a control group, however, in the Sandmaier study.

In a later study, Conte et al. examined the personality and coping differences between alcoholic women being treated in an inpatient setting (N = 17) and nonalcoholic women seen on an outpatient basis for medical screening ($N = 23$) in comparison with similar groups of alcoholic and nonalcoholic men.[25] The subjects were administered a battery of instruments designed to measure coping styles and personality variables. The alcoholic women were found to rate themselves as more submissive, more passive, and more depressed, and were considerably more conflicted about themselves than the nonalcoholic women and the alcoholic men. The researchers suggested that the reason may be that drinking for women still carries some stigma, in that intoxication for a woman is socially unacceptable, whereas for a man it may be considered "macho." Gomberg reported that alcoholic women have trouble seeing themselves as autonomous, but instead see themselves only in relation to others.[26] There has been little recent research on sex-role enactment among chemically dependent women.

Sexual Orientation

Although the question of sexual orientation of chemically dependent women has not been examined as a separate issue in detail, questions about sexual preference have been asked in some of the previously mentioned studies. In the Beckman study 20% of the alcoholic women ($N = 120$) reported they had had a sexual experience with someone of the same sex compared to 4% of the nonalcoholic normals ($N = 119$) and 13% of the nonalcoholic women in treatment for psychological problems ($N = 118$).[15] When answering the question of how they consider themselves, however, 6% of the alcoholic women said they were homosexual and 3% said they were bisexual; this compared to 2–3% of both the normal and in-treatment nonalcoholic women who considered themselves homosexual and the 2–3% that considered themselves bisexual.

In the Covington and Kohen study, 37% of their sample of 35 recovering women responded that they were bisexual and 5% said they were lesbian.[4] The study reported by Sterne et al. found that 29% of their female chemically dependent sample said their sexual preference was lesbian, 3% said bisexual, 61% said heterosexual, and 7% said they were uncertain.[2] The study of sexual problems in chemically dependent nurses by Sullivan found that of the 122 female chemically dependent nurses 7% responded that they were homosexual, compared to 2% of the control group of 385 nondependent nurses.[27] In studying sexual behavior of intravenous drug users, 4.3% of the White and 10.8% of the Black women reported some homosexual activity in the past 12 mo.[16]

Differences in how the question of sexual orientation is asked probably affects the responses received. It appears that among chemically dependent women there is a higher percentage of lesbian and bisexual women than among nonchemically dependent women, but it may also be true that through drinking and using drugs, women may engage in a wider variety of sexual behavior. Among the gay/lesbian and bisexual population, the rates of alcoholism have been estimated to be three times that of the general population.[28]

Women's Sexual Health Issues

Chemically dependent women seem to experience a variety of health problems that affect their sexuality. One of the areas, physiological functioning of the reproductive organs, was investigated in the Beckman study.[15] The alcoholic women were significantly more likely to report problems in getting pregnant than the nonalcoholic normals and the nonalcoholic women being treated for psychological problems. Both alcoholics and those being treated for psychological problems reported more menstrual or "other female problems" than the control group; the other female problems were not delineated in the study. The alcoholic women were also more likely to report drinking more than usual during their premenstruum than the other two groups, although the researcher suggested this finding should be viewed with caution.

Wilsnack reported on research conducted in the 1970s that suggested alcoholic women experienced sexual dysfunction, although she concluded that most of these studies showed a variety of methodological concerns.[29] Wilsnack concluded that sexual dysfunction may be an antecedent to alcoholism as well as a consequence of excessive drinking. The Covington and Kohen study learned that the alcoholic women reported more sexual dysfunction than the controls, which included lack of sexual interest and sexual arousal, decreased lubrication, and fewer orgasms.[4] Furthermore, 79% of the alcoholic women reported they experienced sexual dysfunction before their alcoholism, 85% reported it was experienced during their alcoholism, and 74% said they were experiencing sexual dysfunctions during sobriety. A study by Sullivan also reported that recovering chemically dependent nurses admitted to more sexual dysfunction than the control group.[27]

Is there a relationship between sexual dysfunctions and childhood sexual abuse among chemically dependent women? A study that investigated physical and psychosocial symptoms of adult incest survivors points to an association between sexual dysfunctions and incest.[30] Data on past sexual history and current symptoms were collected from the clinical charts of women who had come to crisis centers. From this data, 132 women were identified as having been sexually abused by a family member but not reporting or being treated for it. Thirty-seven percent of the survivors of incest reported sexual dysfunction compared to 1.2% of a control group. One difficulty with this study, however, is that many of the incest survivors also received other kinds of abuse as children, and 73.5% were raped as adults, which confounds the association between incest and sexual dysfunction.

Chemically dependent women experience a variety of health problems that may be related to their using lifestyle. Mondanero wrote that addicted women may experience infertility secondary to anovulation that is a result of drug use or pelvic inflammatory disease.[31] She also said that chemically dependent women may experience unplanned pregnancies or be unaware of becoming pregnant because of irregular periods or not paying attention to changes in their bodies because of their drug use. Female drug abusers may experience urinary tract infections, sexually transmitted diseases, and other medical conditions related to their drug use. They need services, Mondanaro said, for family planning and gynecological problems, and yet drug-dependent women often feel discrimination from health care providers who do not enjoy caring for them.

AIDS prevention has been cited as another important area of health concern for chemically dependent women because of their risk behaviors such as intravenous drug use, sharing of needles and multiple sex partners.[16,19,32] Other factors known to exist in drug abusers such as poor nutrition, use of drugs known to suppress the immune system, repeated infections, and stress also contribute to an increased risk for AIDS transmission for the chemically dependent woman.[32]

Seeking abortions for unwanted pregnancies may also be more common among chemically dependent women. The Sterne et al. study reported that 44% of their female chemically dependent sample had had an abortion, and >80% reported gynecological concerns such as yeast infections, irregular menstrual periods, crabs, or gonnorrhea.[2] The Sullivan study also found that the recovering chemically dependent nurses reported significantly more abortions and miscarriages than the control group of nurses.[27]

Thus the need for health care services for chemically dependent women is considerably more than just their need for treatment of addiction. Besides gynecological and medical services, they often need education in how to best care for themselves. They may also have unresolved feelings about past abortions and physical damage they have done to their bodies.

Treatment Recommendations

There is little research that investigates the importance of including the issue of sexuality in treatment programs for women with chemical dependency. Several authors have stated that sexuality issues must be addressed based on experiences in their own treatment programs. Schaefer and Evans outlined a rather detailed approach to the area of sexuality for chemically dependent women.[33] They stressed that sexuality should be addressed in women-only groups, using a structured format of lectures and information, along with group exercises and individual assignments. Among the topics to be addressed are socialization of the female role, reclaiming sexual power, genitalia (parts and function), childhood and adolescent sexuality, boundary clarification, sexual abuse, effects of chemical dependency on female sexuality, sexual identity issues, and integrating spirituality and sexuality.

Others who underscore the need to address many areas of sexuality are Mondanaro et al.[34] The topic areas specifically mentioned include: sexual dysfunctions, sexual abuse, dysfunctional family systems, effects of drugs on sexuality, sexuality information and education, and defining healthy sexuality and intimacy. Equally important, they said, however, is that counselors need to learn to be comfortable with their own sexuality, increase their knowledge about sexual functioning and sociocultural factors affecting women's sexuality, be at ease in using sexual terminology, and have an openness to a variety of sexual expression.

In agreement are Mandel and North regarding treatment needs in the area of sexuality.[35] They added that chemically dependent women also need to do values clarification work regarding female sexuality and sex roles, and grief work around issues of guilt, shame, and loss associated with alcoholism and female identity. They also suggested that consciousness-raising women only groups, based on a feminist model, can be effective in helping women maintain sobriety.

Bollerud stated that some chemically dependent women are experiencing posttraumatic stress disorder related to their past physical and sexual abuse.[36] In her view, the treatment approach should address:

1. A cognitive understanding of the nature of violence and its impact on women, with a discussion of posttraumatic stress included;
2. Individual treatment that allows discussion of the abuse in detail;
3. Group experiences that will allow women to share their shame, isolation, and powerlessness in an effort to increase their sense of empowerment; and
4. Aftercare that includes the expected AA involvement as well as outpatient psychotherapeutic self-help groups for women.

Some counselors in the field of chemical dependency treatment believe, in fact, that not aggressively treating childhood trauma issues leads to relapse for the chemically dependent woman. Young wrote that "one of the greatest unacknowledged contributors to recidivism in alcoholism and other addictions may be the failure to identify and treat underlying childhood sexual abuse issues" (p. 249).[37] In the initial abstinent phase Young postulated that the woman who experienced sexual abuse is at risk for relapse in four ways:

memories that were unknown to the woman begin to surface, feelings associated with the abuse begin to emerge as do other feelings as well, the
demands of living are now faced without the aid of addictive behaviors,
and other addictive behaviors may emerge. Young suggested that in addition to treating the disease of addiction, a treatment process that focuses on
the sexual abuse must also be initiated. However, she noted that this is a
sensitive area because if the woman is rushed into exploration of the sexual
abuse, that in itself can lead to relapse. After childhood sexual abuse issues
are identified, Young felt recovery must proceed along two pathways: supporting the individual in her abstinence, and working through the sexual
trauma in abuse-focused groups and in individual work with a counselor.

Root agreed with Young that there is a substantial role of sexual victimization in "treatment failures" for those substance-abusing women who
were victimized.[38] She believed that addiction to drugs, alcohol, or food may
play a role in relieving the symptoms of posttraumatic responses to victimization, and for that reason raised the issue of whether it is realistic to insist
that the addiction must be treated first. If addictive behaviors are seen as a
coping response to the trauma, then it follows that the woman needs to concurrently develop alternate coping responses as she strives to become abstinent.
During treatment when the woman begins to deal with sexual victimization, she often feels worse because she is no longer using chemicals to numb
the feelings associated with the victimization. Root suggested that the therapist warn the individual that a flood of feelings may result during treatment, and provide hope for getting better, since the sense of betrayal at
feeling worse during treatment of the victimization will mimic those feelings of betrayal inherent in the childhood trauma. According to Root:

> This is not to suggest that women should cope with past trauma by
> turning to alcohol, drugs, or food. Rather, it is to question prevailing
> approaches to addiction, rooted in a narrow specialization, that almost
> invariably make abstinence from substance abuse the priority in treat-
> ment. These methods of coping have adaptive qualities for some women
> who do not have a repertoire of positive skills for coping with the nega-
> tive affect, images, and cognitions accompanying unresolved sexual
> trauma. (p. 546)[38]

Preventing relapse among public-sector chemically dependent women
was addressed by Weiner et al.[39] Although sexuality was not singled out as
an important area, within their recommendations are sexuality issues mentioned previously: dependency on others, particularly men, and family issues, such as physical, emotional, and/or sexual abuse. These authors also
emphasized the need for this socioeconomic group of women to develop
better coping skills, particularly in the area of vocational or work training.

All of these issues have a major impact on the woman's self-esteem. They pointed out that the common treatment issues of public-sector women are complex and interrelated. It might be argued that all the issues of treatment are interrelated for all women, no matter the socioeconomic class, and what differs are the interventions needed to increase coping with whatever individual problems the woman experiences.

Sexuality Groups

For the past 5 years, I have conducted weekly group meetings on sexuality with recovering chemically dependent women living in a halfway house as a volunteer staff member. These have been unstructured group discussions with no preset agenda. My role has been one of facilitator, as I have found that the women attending the group will bring forth issues of concern to them. For the first 2 years I kept content notes on each meeting in order to better understand their sexuality issues.[8] The content notes were then condensed into topics, and the number of times the topics were discussed was tabulated. The top seven topics discussed were: incest and other childhood sexual abuse, rape, having sex while sober, values regarding sexual intimacy in one's recovering life, battering, women's sexual health concerns, and coping strategies. The areas that emerged correspond mostly with those addressed in this chapter from other researchers and clinicians. One exception is that of the area of sexual dysfunctions. This may be because although some women stated they hated sex or had no interest in it, this dislike was discussed in relation to their perceived reasons for it, such as sexual abuse or the effect of drugs on their sexual desires, and sexual dysfunction was not presented as a major concern. Lesbianism was discussed occasionally, especially if some of the women present were lesbian and wanted to use the group setting to increase other women's understanding of being lesbian, or to bring it out in the open in a safe way. Gender role enactment was discussed within the context of other topics such as battering or what expectations are of women in our society, and what was learned from parents regarding those expectations.

Over the 5 years of facilitating the sexuality group discussions, I have continued to lead the group in an unstructured manner. As a volunteer staff member who only sees the women once a week and consults with the staff briefly during that time, this approach has worked well. The women take a fair amount of responsibility for the group, and know they will be asked what is important to talk about today regarding sexuality. I have become sensitive to the important issues of abuse and am not reluctant to pick up on a clue that alludes to abuse in order to give the woman an opportunity to ventilate and to receive support from her peers. Sometimes a group member will have a topic already picked out for the group meeting when we start; occasionally they have chosen a topic to discuss the week before, which allows us all time to reflect on that topic before discussion. More structured meetings with set agendas may work as well, but it is important that the method not be one primarily of didactic teaching, as sexuality is an area of such profound affect. Certainly, teaching the facts regarding an area, clearing up of misconceptions, and giving information should be included as the need arises; however, using the mode of lecture would probably inhibit women from discussing the sensitive areas of incest, rape, and their shame and guilt regarding past sexual experiences. The facilitator of sexuality groups must be comfortable with sexuality, knowledgeable of women's reproductive and sexual health issues, and able to hear explicit sexual and abuse talk without shock or judgment. That person must also be skilled at facilitating the group's support to individual members' pain as it is expressed.

Summary

Several issues regarding sexuality for chemically dependent women have been identified from the research and from clinicians. Our knowledge is still new in this area, particularly in regard to evaluation of treatment that includes sexuality in the treatment process. More work needs to be done in investigating the extent of sexuality concerns for chemically dependent women, and what factors influence those concerns. For example, do some substances used affect women's sexual behavior more than others? Does the length of chemical dependency affect sexuality concerns? Will an aggressive approach to treating sexual abuse decrease relapse among drug-dependent women? Nonetheless, even before our knowledge is extended, it is imperative that treatment programs address sexuality issues for their chemically dependent women. Men probably need to discuss and resolve sexuality issues as well. However, it is apparent that sexuality plays a significant role in a woman's addiction, perhaps as contributor, perhaps as consequence, or perhaps as both. Too often because of discomfort with the topic, or a fear of treading on too private areas, that important essence of a person is ignored. Treating all of a woman means acknowledging and confronting the role sexuality has played in her addiction. Recovery may depend on it.

References

[1] I. Reiss (1986) *Journal into Sexuality: An Exploratory Voyage.* Prentice-Hall, Englewood Cliffs, NJ.

[2] M. Sterne, S. Schaefer, and S. Evans (1983) Women's sexuality and alcoholism, in *Alcoholism: Analysis of a World-Wide Problem.* P. Golding, ed. MTP, Lancaster, England, pp. 421–425.

[3]J. Benward and J. Densen-Gerber (1977) Incest as a causative factor in antisocial behavior: an exploratory study. *Contemp. Drug Problems* **4**, 323–340.

[4]S. Covington and J. Kohen (1984) Women, alcohol, and sexuality. *Adv. Alcohol Subst. Abuse* **4**, 41–56.

[5]G. Edwall, N. Hoffmann, and P. Harrison (1989) Psychological correlates of sexual abuse in adolescent girls in chemical dependency treatment. *Adolescence* **24**, 277–288.

[6]J. Kovack (1986) Incest as a treatment issue for alcoholic women. *Alcohol. Treatment Q.* **3**, 1–15.

[7]T. Hagan (1988) A retrospective search for the etiology of drug abuse: a background comparison of a drug-addicted population of women and a control group of non-addicted women, in *Problems of Drug Dependence 1987, Proceedings of the 49th Annual Scientific Meetings*. L. Harris, ed. National Institute on Drug Abuse, Bethesda, MD, pp. 254–261.

[8]J. Teets (1990) What women talk about: sexuality issues of chemically dependent women. *J. Psychosocial Nursing Ment. Health Serv.* **28**, 4–7.

[9]E. Sullivan (1987) A descriptive study of nurses recovering from chemical dependency. *Arch. Psychiatr. Nursing* **1**, 194–200.

[10]C. Swett Jr., C. Cohen, J. Surrey, A. Compaine, and R. Chavez (1991) High rates of alcohol use and history of physical and sexual abuse among women outpatients. *Am. J. Drug Alcohol Abuse* **17**, 49–60.

[11]M. Singer and M. Petchers (1989) The relationship between sexual abuse and substance abuse among psychiatrically hospitalized adolescents. *Child Abuse Neglect* **13**, 319–325.

[12]D. Russell (1986) *The Secret Trauma: Incest in the Lives of Girls and Women.* Basic, New York.

[13]R. Carlson and H. Siegal (1991) The crack life: an ethnographic overview of crack use and sexual behavior among African-Americans in a midwest metropolitan city. *J. Psychoactive Drugs* **23**, 11–20.

[14]C. Winick and A. Levine (1992) Treating rape survivors in a therapeutic community. *J. Psychoactive Drugs* **24**, 49–55.

[15]L. Beckman (1979) Reported effects of alcohol on the sexual feelings and behavior of women alcoholics and nonalcoholics. *J. Stud. Alcohol* **40**, 272–282.

[16]T. Feucht, R. Stephens, and S. Roman (1990) The sexual behavior of intravenous drug users: assessing the risk of sexual transmission of HIV[1]. *J. Drug Issues* **20**, 195–213.

[17]R. Schilling, N. El-Bassel, L. Gilbert, and S. Schinke (1991) Correlates of drug use, sexual behavior, and attitudes toward safer sex among African-American and Hispanic women in methadone maintenance. *J. Drug Issues* **21**, 685–698.

[18]A. Washton and N. Stone-Washton (1990) Abstinence and relapse in outpatient cocaine addicts. *J. Psychoactive Drugs* **22**, 135–147.

[19]J. Inciardi, A. Pottieger, M. Forney, D. Chitwood, and D. McBride (1991) Prostitution, IV drug use, and sex-for-crack exchanges among serious delinquents: risk for HIV infection. *Criminology* **29**, 221–235.

[20]M. Shedlin (1990) An ethnographic approach to understanding HIV high-risk behaviors: prostitution and drug abuse. *NIDA* **93**, 134–149.

[21]B. Miller, W. Downs, and D. Gondoli (1989) Spousal violence among alcoholic women as compared to a random household sample of women. *J. Stud. Alcohol* **50**, 533–540.

²²P. Goldstein, P. Bellucci, B. Spunt, and T. Miller (1991) Volume of cocaine use and violence: a comparison between men and women. *J. Drug Issues* **21**, 345–367.

²³S. Wilsnack (1973) Sex role identity in female alcoholics. *J. Abnorm. Psychol.* **82**, 253–261.

²⁴M. Sandmaier (1980) *The Invisible Alcoholics: Women and Alcohol Abuse in America.* McGraw-Hill, New York.

²⁵H. Conte, R. Plutchik, S. Picard, M. Galanter, and J. Jacoby (1991) Sex differences in personality traits and coping styles of hospitalized alcoholics. *J. Stud. Alcohol* **52**, 26–32.

²⁶E. Gomberg (1982/83) How women recover: experience and research observations. *Alcohol Health Res. World* **7**, 28–40.

²⁷E. Sullivan (1988) Associations between chemical dependency and sexual problems in nurses. *J. Interpersonal Violence* **3**, 326–330.

²⁸S. Schaefer, S. Evans, and E. Coleman (1988) Sexual orientation concerns among chemically dependent individuals, in *Chemical Dependency and Intimacy Dysfunction.* E. Coleman, ed. Haworth, New York, pp. 121–140.

²⁹S. Wilsnack (1984) Drinking, sexuality, and sexual dysfunction in women, in *Alcohol Problems in Women: Antecedents, Consequences and Intervention.* S. Wilsnack and L. Beckman, eds. Guilford, New York, pp. 189–227.

³⁰B. Brown and C. Garrison (1990) Patterns of symptomatology of adult women incest survivors. *West. J. Nursing Res.* **12**, 587–600.

³¹J. Mondanaro (1981) Reproductive health concerns for the treatment of drug dependent women, in *Treatment Services for Drug Dependent women*, vol. I. B. Reed, G. Beschner, and J. Mondanaro, eds. National Institute on Drug Abuse, Bethesda, MD, pp. 258–281.

³²J. Mondanaro (1987) Strategies for AIDS prevention: motivating health behavior in drug dependent women. *J. Psychoactive Drugs* **19**, 143–149.

³³S. Schaefer and S. Evans (1988) Women, sexuality and the process of recovery, in *Chemical Dependency and Intimacy Dysfunction.* E. Coleman, ed. Haworth, New York, pp. 91–120.

³⁴J. Mondanaro, M. Wedenoja, J. Densen-Gerber, J. Elahi, M. Mason, and A. Redmond (1982) Sexuality and fear of intimacy as barriers to recovery for drug dependent women, in *Treatment Services for Drug Dependent Women*, vol. II. B. Reed, G. Beschner and J. Mondanaro eds. National Institute on Drug Abuse, Bethesda, MD, pp. 303–357.

³⁵L. Mandel and S. North (1982) Sex roles, sexuality and the recovering woman alcoholic: program issues. *J. Psychoactive Drugs* **14**, 163–166.

³⁶K. Bollerud (1990) A model for the treatment of trauma-related syndromes among chemically dependent inpatient women. *J. Subst. Abuse Treatment* **7**, 83–87.

³⁷E. Young (1990) The role of incest issues in relapse. *J. Psychoactive Drugs* **22**, 249–258.

³⁸M. Root (1989) Treatment failures: the role of sexual victimization in women's addictive behavior. *Am. J. Orthopsychiatry* **59**, 542–549.

³⁹H. Weiner, M. Wallen, and G. Zankowski (1990) Culture and social class as intervening variables in relapse prevention with chemically dependent women. *J. Psychoactive Drugs* **22**, 239–248.

Women
and Substance Abuse

A General Review

Barbara W. Lex

Introduction

This chapter is a selective review of information about substance abuse effects in women. Because data summarized here are drawn from cross-sectional studies, treated prevalence studies, and laboratory experiments, it is necessary to recognize certain caveats. In all likelihood, complex biological factors influence individual vulnerability, and environmental aspects also shape behavior but may shift over time.[1] Assumptions about factors that influence drinking and drug use behavior as well as definitions of problem drinking, alcohol abuse, alcoholism, drug use, and drug abuse vary across time and studies. Further, specifications of cutoff points for hazardous quantities or frequencies of alcohol intake (e.g., "heavy drinking") also vary considerably and rarely are adjusted for gender. Men and women may require different questions in interviews, but often questions pertinent to women are simply added to those used for men. More regrettably, in some cases data may be obtained from men and women, but results are then combined.

To date, information about alcohol effects is more readily available than information about effects of other substances. It should be recognized,

From: *Drug and Alcohol Abuse Reviews, Vol. 5: Addictive Behaviors in Women*
Ed.: R. R. Watson ©1994 Humana Press Inc., Totowa, NJ

however, that women in clinical populations are likely to be using alcohol concurrently with other substances. Accordingly, sole discussion of alcohol abuse or dependence is unlikely to reflect clinical reality. In addition, few investigators have obtained information about women's reproductive function, although all abused substances have an impact on the female reproductive system at some juncture in the hypothalamic–pituitary–gonadal axis.

Severity of Problems

Alcohol problems in women received little systematic attention until the last two decades. Neglect of women's alcohol problems occurred largely because of beliefs that sociocultural factors protected women from alcohol abuse, or that alcohol dependence was similar in men and women, or that alcoholic women were more deviant, psychologically disturbed, and difficult to study and treat.[2–6] It is now apparent that age, drinking patterns, and symptoms of alcohol dependence differ between women and men.[3,4,7–10] There are numerous reviews of the characteristics of female alcoholics and comparisons of gender differences between male and female alcoholics.[4,5,11–18] Onset of drinking problems in women occurs 4–8 yr later than in men,[13,19–21] but alcohol-dependent women also drink less frequently and consume less alcohol,[10,19,21] report having fewer binges and less continuous drinking,[10,11,21] recall fewer blackouts, morning drinking, and delirium tremens episodes,[21,22] and report that before coming to treatment they had shorter drinking histories.[12,13,23]

Thus, alcohol problems may appear to be less severe for women. However, recent reports implicate alcohol abuse in the development of serious gynecological and obstetric dysfunctions,[24–26] as well as with more rapid development of cardiovascular, gastrointestinal, and liver diseases.[4,27–29] Alcohol can also seriously affect the developing fetus.[30] Further, women who have alcohol problems are at risk for polysubstance use, including use of such dependency-producing substances as psychotropic prescription medications, marijuana, and cocaine.[3,4,31]

Course of Illness in Women and Men

The course of alcohol dependence differs in men and women. Women with alcohol problems report heavy drinking at a later age, drinking smaller quantities, engaging in solitary drinking, having a higher frequency of tranquilizer use, experiencing more psychiatric treatment, and being less likely to have encounters with the criminal justice system.[32] In addition to a family history of alcohol problems, women are more likely to have spouses with alcohol problems.

A popular term for the apparently accelerated course of symptom severity in alcoholic women is "telescoping." Thus, in a sample of 30 men and 16 women studied by Orford and Keddie, the median number of years since problem onset was 11 for men vs 3.6 for women.[33] Alcohol consumed on a typical heavy drinking day was 220 g for men vs 120 g for women, both highly significant differences. Further, the dominant pattern of drinking for women in the 6 mo prior to obtaining treatment was regular drinking vs sporadic drinking, whereas half the men reported regular drinking, and the other half, binge drinking. Similarly, 8 men and 8 women had significant differences in years of heavy drinking (2.6 ± 2.7 for women vs 9.1 ± 5.3 for men), and in their consumption during a recent typical week (171.3 ± 82.9 alcohol "units" for men vs 90.3 ± 49.1 for women).[34] A study of 54 men vs 67 women found similar results.[35] Comparable patterns of abbreviated time-course and less consumption were also observed for female opiate addicts.[36]

Parrella and Filstead developed an early-onset severity index, whereby development of alcohol dependence is represented as a sequence of progressively serious behaviors and consequences.[37] Events that occur earlier are less severe or disruptive, and each event is a benchmark indicating development of a more serious stage in alcohol dependence. Subjects were 1940 alcoholics, 72% males (1392) and 28% females (548), admitted to an inpatient facility between November 1981 and December 1983. Women were significantly older for all age of onset variables, including age regular drunkenness began, age patient realized alcohol gave relief of withdrawal symptoms, age that a significant other first identified the alcohol problem, age patient first tried to stop drinking, and age patient realized that alcohol use was a problem. Roughly one-half (48%) of men and one-third (31%) of women reported regular drunkenness before age 25, and one-fourth of the men (24%) had tried to stop drinking at or before age 25, vs less than one-fifth of the women (18%). Among subjects with early onset, a greater percentage of women attained severe levels of alcohol problems. Thus development of alcohol dependence followed a sequence. It was also important that the authors indicated different cutoff points for early onset for men and for women.[37] One prior conclusion from this study is that occurrence of these milestones by age 25 is associated with more rapid progression to severe alcohol problems for women.

Alcohol and Other Drug Effects on Reproductive Function in Women

It has long been known that alcoholism is associated with severe disruption of reproductive function in men. Impotence, low testosterone levels, testicular atrophy, gynecomastia, and diminished sexual interest are consistently reported. Until very recently, however, there has been relatively little research on alcohol effects on reproductive function in women.

Interpretation of data is complicated because most reports are from studies of alcoholic women admitted to hospitals for liver disease, pancreatitis, or other medical disorders. These conditions could cause menstrual cycle disturbances independently of alcohol. The adverse effects of chronic alcohol abuse on reproductive function of the hypothalamic–pituitary–gonadal axis may be a result of direct toxic effects of alcohol on the hypothalamus, pituitary or ovaries, or a combination of these pathophysiological processes. Studies of acute alcohol effects on pituitary gonadotrophin secretion have been carried out under basal conditions during the follicular or luteal phase of the menstrual cycle.[38] Acute alcohol intake did not produce any significant changes in plasma levels of pituitary gonadotrophins in women.

Hugues and colleagues studied hypothalamo–pituitary function in 31 alcoholic women aged 29–66 yr with chronic pancreatitis or liver cirrhosis.[39] The majority (67%) also were amenorrheic: four women had severe oligomenorrhea, six had mild oligomenorrhea or cycles of normal length. *In toto*, five distinct patterns of hypothalamo–pituitary ovarian activity were discerned. Normal menopause was seen in eight of the amenorrheic patients. Women in this group had low estrogen levels, high basal gonadotrophin secretion, and a distinct luteinizing hormone releasing hormone (LHRH)-induced gonadotrophin response. Five women comprised a second group with hypothalamic amenorrhea associated with low estrogen output, low gonadotrophin levels, and adequate response to LHRH. In the third group were eight perimenopausal women aged 43–51 yr, characterized by adequate estradiol levels with a preferential follicular stimulating hormone (FSH) increase. Some subjects could still respond to ovarian stimulation, whereas for others estrogen status remained normal. Six women had inadequate luteal phase, and five women had anovulation related to a defect in cyclic control of gonadotrophin secretion.

Other studies have approached the question of reproductive compromise by screening obstetric–gynecological treatment populations for alcohol-related problems. Russell and Bigler screened 499 women seen in an obstetric–gynecological outpatient clinic at a general hospital in Buffalo.[40] Patients responded to a self-administered questionnaire encompassing 31 variables: 8 sociodemographic characteristics, 1 regarding tobacco smoking, 12 alcohol use queries, and 10 alcohol-related problems. Criteria for alcohol-related problems were reports of heavy alcohol consumption (QFV), whereby heavy drinking was defined as consumption of three or more drinks/d (regardless of quantity) two to three times/mo and five or more drinks on more than one-half of all drinking occasions. Reports of heavy drinking ranged from 10–14%.

A combination of factors was required to identify all heavy drinkers in the sample. Individuals who were identified as problem drinkers by counselors rather than through screening procedures were more likely to be younger (mean 26.0 ± 12.0 yr) women who consumed a mean of 2.5 ± 1.8 oz of alcohol/episode. The young women who had avoided adverse social consequences of heavy alcohol intake had no work or steady social involvements to interfere with drinking, and they associated with people who did not criticize high intake. Behaviors most frequently endorsed were having a blackout (55%), feeling a need to cut down on drinking (48%), reporting that parents had drinking problems (42%), seeking help for emotional problems (33%), experiencing family problems associated with one's own drinking (28%), having friends or relatives express concern about their drinking (25%), having siblings with a drinking problem (23%), receiving a physician's advice to cease drinking (21%), and having a husband with a drinking problem (18%). The rate of heavy drinking was higher in gynecological patients (19%) than in obstetric patients (11%), and heavy drinkers constituted 18% of the combined samples. Heavy alcohol consumption in patients under age 40 was also associated with gastrointestinal pain and obesity, experiencing one or more physical complaints, or one or more psychological problems.

Halliday and colleagues replicated this work by analyzing data from two private practices in the Boston metropolitan area, a general practice providing gynecological care and a clinic for premenstrual syndrome patients.[28] In the general gynecological practice 185 women between the ages of 18 and 44 were screened for patterns of alcohol consumption. Approximately 21% had symptoms of amenorrhea, dysmenorrhea, irregular bleeding, infertility, and pelvic pain, and 16% had excessive alcohol intake or were alcohol dependent. Of the remaining 147 women, 33% reported concerns about alcohol use. The second sample included 96 women seeking medical care for premenstrual syndrome. Over half (51%) reported concerns related to alcohol. The rate of alcohol abuse and alcohol dependence in the general gynecology treatment group was 12%, and 21% in the premenstrual syndrome group.

Women who sought care for premenstrual syndrome typically were older, had more education, and experienced more unemployment. The two groups were similar in terms of race (98% White), marital status, parity, participation in stable relationships, and sexual preference. Results of a logistic regression analysis that controlled for age, education, and employment status found a highly significant association between premenstrual syndrome and alcohol abuse. However, the study did not examine any cause-and-effect relationships between obstetric/gynecological problems and alcohol abuse.

These clinical findings confirm results from a cross-sectional study of women's alcohol use[29] in which 917 women were queried about the prevalence of dysmenorrhea, heavy menstrual flow, and premenstrual discomfort. Severity of menstrual distress symptoms linearly increased with amount of alcohol consumption. Further, women who drank at least 1.5 oz/d of absolute alcohol had higher rates of gynecological surgery other than hysterectomy. Miscarriage, stillbirths, and premature births occurred to women who had greater alcohol intake, as well as with women who were classified "temporary abstainers." There are several possible interpretations of this latter finding:[41] women with gynecological dysfunction may find alcohol effects unpleasant and consequently abstain, increased health consciousness might be responsible for both sensitivity to potential medical problems and a greater likelihood of abstaining from alcohol, or women who have had gynecological problems may have consulted physicians who instructed them to limit alcohol use. Clinical confirmation of increased rates of menstrual problems, hysterectomies, abortions, and miscarriages in alcoholic vs control women was reported from Denmark,[42] but alcoholic women also had significantly greater numbers of pregnancies. This latter finding was also reported by Smith and Asch.[43]

It is generally reported that one out of every six couples experiences an infertility problem, and women seeking help for obstetric and gynecological problems appear to have a higher than expected rate of substance abuse problems. Results from a 1988 cross-sectional survey found that 9% of women of childbearing age (15–44 yr) had used marijuana or cocaine during the month before the study.[44] Busch and colleagues conducted a mail questionnaire study of two groups of women diagnosed with infertility problems or pelvic pain.[45] Items in the questionnaire included type and amount of alcohol and drug consumption and patterns of use, the Michigan Alcoholism Screening Test (MAST),[46] and a comparable inventory for drug dependence that included 21 questions. Subjects also identified the date of onset of use of various substances as well as dates of onsets of the pelvic pain or infertility problems.

A total of 23 women (31%) in the study had either a potential or probable alcohol and/or drug use problem. On the basis of alcohol use and MAST scores, 16 (or 70%) were identified as having an alcohol problem. In the total sample, 11 other women (15%) had potential or probable drug dependence problems, and an additional 5% had combined alcohol and drug dependency problems. More than one psychoactive drug was used by the 11 women with drug dependence problems, including marijuana, cocaine, narcotic analgesics, tranquilizers and hypnotics, or stimulants. Marijuana was the most frequently consumed substance, and four patients reported smoking marijuana one or more times/d. Most of the women who reported using mood-altering drugs used several types of drugs. Analgesic drug use was reported by more pelvic pain subjects than infertility subjects, and many reported use of analgesics during menses. A higher rate of infertility was associated with a larger percentage reporting alcohol problems (23.2%). More importantly, 13 out of 74 (18%) reported that use of alcohol and/or mood-altering substances increased after onset of pelvic pain or infertility.[45]

Alcohol disrupts the hypothalamic–pituitary–gonadal axis in both men and in women.[47] Pathophysiologic effects of chronic alcohol intake on reproductive function may be the result of direct toxic effects of alcohol on the hypothalamus, pituitary, or ovaries, or of interaction effects related to estrogen and progesterone. Some major alcohol-related disorders of the female reproductive system include amenorrhea, anovulation, luteal phase dysfunction, ovarian atrophy, spontaneous abortion, and early menopause. Postmortem studies of alcoholic women have found evidence of ovarian atrophy. Derangements of female reproductive function also are reported for cocaine, marijuana, and opiate users. Cocaine, marijuana, and opiates have been associated with amenorrhea, anovulation, and spontaneous abortion, whereas cocaine and opiates are linked to hyperprolactinemia, and marijuana and opiates, with luteal phase dysfunction.[47]

Endocrine profiles were obtained for 18 women aged 17–58 yr receiving court-ordered treatment for alcohol or polysubstance dependence under civil commitment in a Massachusetts hospital.[38] According to DSM-III-R criteria, 12 women were diagnosed as alcohol dependent or abusers, and their alcohol consumption ranged from 42–324 g/d, and 6 women were diagnosed as polysubstance dependent. Besides alcohol (84–830 g/d), cocaine was the most frequently abused drug followed by tranquilizers, sedatives, marijuana, amphetamines, and opiates. All women received a thorough physical examination and laboratory studies including blood hemogram and chemistry.[38] All were detoxified and showed no abstinence signs when samples were obtained for LH, FSH, prolactin, estradiol, progesterone, and cortisol analysis.

No single profile of derangements was observed. Independent of amount and duration of alcohol use, 50% of the alcoholic women had hyperprolactinemia, and one patient had secondary amenorrhea with a normal prolactin level and low levels of LH and estradiol. Two polysubstance-dependent women had hyperprolactinemia, and one had secondary amenorrhea with normal prolactin but low LH, FSH, and estradiol. Although specific mechanisms of alcohol and drug effects on reproductive dysfunction have yet to be determined, hyperprolactinemia may cause amenorrhea and disruptions of the menstrual cycle. In another report of this sample, polysubstance-dependent women recalled beginning sexual activity at an earlier age (mean = 15.7 ± 2.6 yr) than alcohol-dependent women (mean = 18.6 ± 3.3 yr).[48] Although 50% of alcohol-dependent women had had no live births, one polysubstance-dependent woman reported 12 conceptions, resulting in 6 live births, 1 stillbirth, and 5 spontaneous abortions. Thus, the effects of substance use on reproductive capacity are far from clear and, in all likelihood are influenced by other environmental factors, such as nutrition or trauma.

Mortality

A prospective follow-up study examined predictors of mortality in alcoholic women.[49] Feighner criteria were used to ascertain alcoholism in 103 women who had been admitted to psychiatric hospitals (one public and one private) during 1967 and 1968. Mean age at admission was 44 yr (range: 18–67 yr), mean number of years drinking prior to admission was 9 (range: 1–38 yr), and three-fourths of the women had had previous inpatient admissions for alcohol problems. The sample included 44% who were married, 49% separated, divorced, or widowed, and 7% who had never married. In 1979 and 1980, all but three (lost) subjects were restudied. A total of 21 women were deceased.

In comparison with the overall female population in the city of St. Louis, excess mortality in alcoholic women yielded a ratio of 4.5:1. Approximately 75% of the original population was White. A higher mortality rate was observed for Black women (42%) vs White women (28%). Alcoholic women also were significantly younger at time of death (mean age 51.0 yr) than women in the city of St. Louis (mean age 66.5 yr). The largest numbers of deaths were attributed to pancreatitis, liver cirrhosis, and other liver disorders (29%), and deaths from these causes occurred at a mean age of 44.9 yr (range: 32–59 yr). Violence and accidents accounted for 26% of deaths, at a mean age of 49.5 yr (range: 28–70 yr). Deaths in these categories were more than double the overall rate for White women (ratio 20:8) as for Black women (ratio 8:4). Only two deaths were identified as suicides by violent means, but two additional women who overdosed on combinations of alcohol and prescription medications may also have been suicidal. Another three deaths were accidental, attributed to fires related to smoking and drinking. The one homicide was a case in which a 54-yr-old woman was stabbed by a male drinking companion.

Four variables—age at admission for treatment, onset of alcoholism before age 30, a primary diagnosis of antisocial personality, and frequent binge drinking—classified 75% of the sample. Liver cirrhosis, delirium tremens, convulsions, and severity of alcoholism, as measured by the number of symptoms and by daily drinking, unemployment, and poor marital history added little to the overall variance. More global variables of duration and intensity of alcohol abuse were better predictors of mortality than highly specific alcohol-related symptoms. Only abstinence was associated with reduced mortality. Women who identified themselves as "social" drinkers had a higher proportion of deaths, and their death rate was comparable to those of sporadic/variable drinkers (20% vs 17%). The greatest number of deaths (54%) occurred among women who continued to drink steadily and in high volume.

Physical Sequelae
of Alcohol and Drug Abuse and Dependence

Gender differences in ethanol metabolism and hepatotoxicity have been summarized by Van Thiel and Gavaler.[24] These include interactions of sex hormones with alcohol intake rates, alcohol absorption, alcohol metabolism, and alcohol-induced liver disease. Alcohol is water soluble, does not require digestion, and enters the body by diffusion from the stomach and intestine. After absorption, alcohol is distributed in total body water and oxidized almost completely within the liver. Only small amounts are excreted unmetabolized in breath, urine, and perspiration. Since no specific feedback regulation of ethanol metabolism is known, it is believed that metabolism continues until all alcohol is exhausted.

Alcohol delays gastric emptying into the small intestine, but once emptied it is rapidly absorbed. Men and women have different rates of gastric emptying and transport within the intestines, and pregnancy and menstrual cycle phase can effect these factors in women. During pregnancy and the luteal menstrual cycle phase, higher progesterone levels are associated with delayed gastric emptying and intestinal transit; no comparable changes have been identified in men.[26]

Men and women also differ in the volume of distribution (V_d) of alcohol and other drugs. Volume of distribution is determined by the dose divided by the attained plasma concentration. Since they have a larger concentration of lipid tissue, women have smaller volumes of distribution for water-soluble alcohol and larger volumes of distribution for lipid-soluble drugs such as D^9-THC, the major psychoactive compound in marijuana. Plasma concentration is related directly to dose. Metabolism of alcohol, as well as other drugs, occurs in the liver. Alcohol dehydrogenase (ADH) accounts for 80–85% of the metabolism of alcohol. The remainder of metabolism is effected by the microsomal mixed-function oxidase or microsomal ethanol-oxidizing system (MEOS). The ADH system metabolizes alcohol at concentrations approx 1.0 mM, whereas the MEOS system metabolizes at 10 mM or higher alcohol concentrations. MEOS activity is greater in livers of chronic alcoholics as well as in individuals who use cross-tolerant drugs such as benzodiazepines or barbiturates, but availability of ADH is not influenced by alcohol intake or other pharmacological effects.

A recent review of sex differences in alcohol metabolism argued for important differences in total body water that affect the volume of alcohol distribution.[26] These observations partially explain the apparently greater degrees of liver damage that occur in women, whereby alcohol concentrations for women are greater than those obtained for men at the same dose peak. The sex hormones estradiol and testosterone also affect alcohol metabolism. Overall, females have increased ability to reduce ethanol, whereas males have increased oxidation. For a wide variety of drugs, including caffeine, estrogen administration and the use of oral contraceptives diminishes drug metabolism in the liver.

Van Thiel and Gavaler cited over 10 reports of gender-related differences in the incidence of alcohol-induced liver disease.[26] Women experience double the rate of cirrhosis with comparable age at onset of cirrhosis. Several investigators have concluded that the cutoff point for hazardous consumption in women lies well within the range of moderate consumption in men.[50] Moreover, the extent of alcohol-related liver damage sustained by women appears to continue despite abstinence.[26]

A recent study reported that higher blood alcohol levels (BALs) in women could be attributed to gender differences in "first-pass" or initial metabolism and oxidation by gastric tissue.[51] Endoscopic gastric biopsies indicated less gastric alcohol dehydrogenase activity in female social drinkers, and almost none in female alcoholics. Although this study did not address specific underlying mechanisms, it reinforces the notion that different consumption cutoffs may apply to women and men. This work must be questioned,[52] and at this time a difference in gastric oxidation cannot account for "telescoping" associated with use of other substances, such as opiates.

Psychosocial Sequelae
of Alcohol and Drug Abuse and Dependence

The 1985 National Household Survey on Drug Abuse, sponsored by the National Institute on Drug Abuse and the National Institute on Alcohol Abuse and Alcoholism oversampled Blacks, Hispanics, and persons under age 35, with a 83.5% response rate, yielding 8038 interviews.[53] Robbins examined gender differences in psychosocial problems associated with alcohol and other drug use.[54] Data were drawn from the 1985 National Household Survey on Drug Abuse,[53] and the study analyzed 17 psychosocial sequelae of substance use. It was concluded that intrapsychic problems are stronger predictors of alcohol abuse in women, and that problems in social functioning are stronger predictors in men. Gender differences could be explained by men's greater consumption and frequency of intoxication.

Some have hypothesized that the differential psychosocial consequences of substance use in women derive in part from biological factors, including alcohol metabolism.[54] Further, since women make higher use of psychoactive prescription drugs, some of which are cross-tolerant with alcohol, vulnerability to alcohol-drug interactions is likely to stem from liver clearance rates. Differences in the social enactment of gender-related social behaviors are also thought to have negative consequences for women, since substance use is popularly believed to be more stigmatizing for women. Some have alleged that the potential compromise of women's sexual chastity or nurturing childcare responsibilities underlies the greater stigma that accords to females who use substances. These observations have been noted historically as well as cross-culturally.

It also has been argued that men and women have different styles of deviant behavior.[54] Deviance expressed by men is said to be directed toward others and antisocial in content. In contrast, deviance expressed by women is thought to be channeled into internalized distress and manifested in emotional upset. It is reasoned that women make stronger efforts to hide substance use, to use substances at the behest or in the company of a male partner, to curtail alcohol and drug use except when caretaking expectations are in abeyance, and to strive to behave in "feminine" social roles despite alcohol or drug effects.[54] It can be argued that for these reasons women who use alcohol and other drugs report greater depression, anxiety, and guilt, whereas more men report alcohol- and drug-related employment problems, belligerence, and legal problems. These generalizations are also reflected in the greater frequency of referrals for treatment that follow alcohol-related legal, financial, or job problems in men.

Another hypothesis asserts that consumption patterns are converging for women and men. This hypothesis remains controversial and is related to an ideological debate. Epidemiological data on alcohol and other drug use consumption patterns in recent years yield little support for the idea that consumption behavior by all women and men is similar; however, there is evidence that younger age groups exhibit less gender difference in consumption patterns. Robbins contended that the increased prevalence of drinking by women stems from fewer abstainers rather than more numerous heavy drinkers.[54] Convergence in consequences of substance abuse may exhibit greater similarity for men and for women in certain sectors of society. Popular opinion has not accepted greater alcohol and drug consumption by women. For example, the criminal justice system alters the severity and swiftness with which arrests, jeopardy of employment, and referral for child abuse become more common.

Factor analysis groups the 17 drug- or alcohol-related problems into three factors. Intrapsychic problems related to substance use included: being depressed or losing interest in activities; feeling alone and isolated; feeling anxious; feeling irritable; feeling suspicious and mistrustful; and having increased difficulty in contending with personal problems. Difficulties in social functioning and carrying out role expectations, the second factor, included: having trouble at school or on the job; having trouble with the police; having serious financial problems; failure to consume four or more regular meals; and needing to obtain emergency medical help. The third factor reflected consequences of substance use episodes, including: disputes with family or friends; driving unsafely; inability to remember behavior (blackouts); and clouded thinking. Effects of alcohol, marijuana, and cocaine use were also associated with these problems.

Gender affected frequency distributions for the 17 problems. The most frequently named effects were: confused thinking (10% of men and 6% of women), driving unsafely (11% of men and 4% of women), disputes with family or friends (8% of men and 5% of women), blackouts (8% of men and 4% of women), depression or loss of interest in activities (7% of men and 5% of women), and feeling anxious and irritable (7% of men and 4% of women). The least frequent consequence was having to obtain emergency medical help (1% of men and <1% of women). Men reported more drug related psychological problems and problems in social functioning, with Whites reporting more problems than Blacks or Hispanics.

The most psychological problems were reported by younger age groups (18–25 yr), whereas persons over age 35 reported the least psychological problems. Although more psychological problems were reported by young White females ages 12–17 yr, the highest score for social problems was reported by young adult White males ages 18–25 yr. Young White girls (age 12–17 yr), however, had more problems with social functioning than any category of males. Overall, the data generally supported the "styles of pathology" hypothesis. Of the 17 problems, 12 showed gender differences. Women reported themselves more diffusely affected by intrapsychic factors, such as depression, feeling suspicious or distrustful, and feeling irritable. On the other hand, men had more serious external problems with trouble at school or on the job, impaired driving, money problems, criminal justice encounters, and the need for emergency medical help. Also, more men reported feeling unable to contend with their personal problems. Unanticipated findings included greater vulnerability in women to belligerence associated with alcohol, marijuana, and cocaine use. Missing four or more regular meals, purportedly related to uncontrolled or binge consumption, was more frequent among women and associated with cocaine use, possibly suggesting that for some women cocaine consumption may be used to limit food intake.

Further analysis indicated that alcohol, marijuana, and cocaine use explained nearly 80% of the gender differences in social problems. Men used more alcohol and other substances, which explained their higher frequency of problems in social functioning. In this sample, alcohol intoxication accounted for more gender difference than use of illicit drugs.[54]

However, it should be noted that the nature of the sample surveyed, a cross-sectional sample of persons residing in households, may underrepresent the effects of marijuana and cocaine on individuals not living in conventional domestic settings. Studies of incarcerated or hospitalized populations of both men and women might have yielded different results. Thus, the sociological interpretation may be correct, insofar as conclusions were drawn from observations of a less deviant or severely impaired population. Robbins[54] also wondered whether women's greater vulnerability to disputes with their family and friends reflected a gender difference in expected behavior or reflected greater stigma and social disapproval directed toward women who abuse substances. Another factor could be that women who abuse alcohol and other drugs are more likely to have families that include other substance abusers, thus generating greater family conflict and dysfunction. Women are also more likely to use substances in the company of substance abusing spouses or mates.[54] This observation is apt and also may contribute to domestic discord.

Contributing Factors

Family History of Alcoholism

Alcoholism in women is more strongly correlated with a family history of alcohol problems than is alcoholism in men.[55–57] Haver studied effects of parental alcohol consumption patterns and attitudes toward alcohol use on treatment outcome.[58] Of 44 women, 50% reported alcoholic fathers, 14% reported alcoholic mothers, and three women had alcoholism in both parents. The approximate ratio of female to male alcoholics in mother's family was 1:2, and in father's family, 1:3.5. Positive family history of alcoholism was correlated with younger age at drinking onset, but was statistically significant only for alcoholism in father and first degree relatives. Parental ambivalence about alcohol use was not associated with outcome, but total number of alcoholic first degree relatives and number of alcoholic relatives in mother's family was associated with poor outcome. However, there was no assessment of possible influences from maternal alcohol intake during gestation. Anecdotally, several of the women reported having a high tolerance for alcohol when they had begun to use alcohol.

It has been argued that familial and genetic factors in inheritance of alcoholism cluster into at least two clinically identifiable alcohol dependence syndromes. A large-scale adoption study in Sweden used information from hospital, clinic, and registry records to identify two types of alcoholism in men.[59] One subtype (Type I) was identified as "milieu-limited," as expression of alcoholism occurred later and was related to interplay with environmental factors, whereas the second type, designated as "male-limited" (Type II), was generally associated with early onset of alcohol-related problems and was accompanied by impulsivity, risk taking, and criminality. From these studies it was also alleged that genetic factors in women with family histories of alcoholism are differentially expressed. Alcoholism in women with milieu-limited alcoholic fathers was shaped by environmental conditions, such as exposure to alcohol or social status of the adoptive father superimposed on a biological substrate. In contrast, the female counterpart of male-limited alcoholism was said to be expressed primarily as somatization.[59] Somatic concerns typically included complaints of abdominal, back, or neck pains, but did not necessarily accompany alcohol problems. Further, in the Swedish adoption studies the highest prevalence of alcoholic relatives in the backgrounds of alcohol-dependent women was found among women with alcoholic mothers.[7] It should be noted, however, that the typologies that emerged were drawn from records of work absences, illness treatments, and alcohol problems and did not include information collected directly from either male or female probands.

Evidence for changes in contributions of familial, nonfamilial, and genetic risk factors in transmission of alcoholism has been drawn from cross-sectional surveys and studies of the families of alcoholic probands. Epidemiologic Catchment Area (ECA) data for two sites showed increased prevalence of alcoholism and decreased age of onset in males and females.[8,60] In response to these findings, data from an ongoing family study of alcoholic probands and their first degree relatives in St. Louis were analyzed to identify the impact of secular trends on alcoholism prevalence, age of onset, and transmissibility.[61]

Using Feighner criteria,[62] Reich and Cloninger studied 60 female and 240 male alcoholics, their parents, siblings, and offspring ($N = 831$).[61] Alcoholism rates for sons and daughters of probands were higher than rates for their fathers and mothers, and male and female probands had similar numbers of first degree alcoholic relatives. Lifetime prevalence of alcoholism was calculated at about 12.3% for males and 4% for females (for persons born before 1940), and at about 22% for males and 10% for females born since 1955.[61] Thus, age of onset and lifetime prevalence for women had more than doubled and could be approaching that of men, with higher increases in the children of alcoholics. Comparison of age of onset for Type I (over 25 yr) vs Type II alcoholism suggested that there was an overall increase in prevalence of Type II alcoholism.[61] Other analysts[63] also support the contention that alcohol dependence in women has gradually increased during the last three decades. Although not addressed in the Swedish studies, a combination of familial, genetic, and environmental factors are also significant for intercurrent polysubstance use.[3] In the United States intercurrent alcohol dependence with other drug abuse or dependence is an established clinical reality for both women and men.

Assortative Mating

Numerous investigators have reported differential patterns of mate selection in alcoholic women and men. One of the earliest studies reported that the differential sex ratio of alcoholic men to women contributed to assortative mating, with one out of ten women likely to marry an alcoholic man, in contrast to 1 out of 50 men marrying an alcoholic woman.[64] Bromet and Moos calculated rates for alcoholic men ($N = 210$) and women ($N = 82$) and found that 51% of currently married women and 18% of currently married men had alcoholic spouses.[32] It was suggested that exposure to a heavy drinking mate might serve as an environmental vector for transmission of heavy drinking from one mate to another.

In a recent study of 64 women with alcohol problems admitted to three treatment units in Oslo, Norway, 51% (33 women) attributed the etiology of their drinking problems to conjugal partners. However, the effects of a heavy drinking partner were bimodal. Thirty-two percent of the sample attributed their escalated alcohol consumption as a strategy to *maintain* a relationship with an alcoholic partner, whereas another 18% attributed onset of alcohol problems to escalated drinking that resulted from *abandonment* by an alcoholic partner. In the first instance, women were attached to alcoholic partners and escalated drinking over time in order to join the partner to cement a deteriorating relationship. Case material from the second group indicated that loss of a partner prompted a catastrophic and self-destructive reaction in which women engaged in heavy alcohol consumption as a part of a pattern of withdrawing from friends, work, and social contacts in general.[65]

Whitehead and Layne examined patterns of alcohol consumption in Canadian men and women between ages 15 and 29 yr.[50] Self-report consumption information was obtained and adjusted for body weight. Heavy drinking for men was defined as six drinks, whereas the cutoff for heavy drinking for women averaged 4.5 drinks. In this group, 60% of women had never been married, 35% were married, and 4% had been divorced or separated. In contrast, for the same age groups 70% of males reported that they had never married, 26% had been married, and 2% had been divorced or separated. Overall, married individuals between ages 15 and 29 had the lowest rates of heavy drinking. However, 16% of unmarried males and females were heavy drinkers, with the highest rates of heavy drinking in divorced or separated men or women (28%). Thus, marital status was clearly associated with heavy alcohol consumption by men and women. This study found employment outside the home a protective factor for married women, and student status protected both males and females from heavy drinking. For older males, those who were both married and unemployed had the highest rates of heavy drinking (20%), similar to males who were single and unemployed (18%). Thus, in this Canadian sample, rates of heavy consumption were similar for males and females irrespective of age, sex, occupation, and marital status. This study did not examine assortative mating *per se*, but indicates a secular trend toward convergence in heavy drinking patterns between males and females when the criterion for heavy drinking is adjusted according to gender.

A recent review reasoned that assortative mating rates between male and female alcoholics are similar when adjusted for the differential in alcoholism rates between them.[66] Contradictory viewpoints can be reconciled on the basis of methodology, especially for criteria for inclusion in the "alcoholic" category. Definitions range from loosely defined "problem drinking" or "alcoholism" to more specific RDC criteria.[67] The literature on opiate addiction is similarly inconsistent. Given differences in age, ethnic group, and historical factors, various investigators have asserted that male heroin addicts, for example, have no mates, have brittle relationships with mates, have relationships with mates that resemble relationships with mothers, and, in general, have sabotaging relationships with mates.[68]

Stressful Life Events

Excessive alcohol consumption may function as both a cause and result of stressful life experiences, marital problems, employment problems, physical illness, or depression. Consumption rates may fluctuate through time and, thus, are inadequate to predict alcohol intake. Further, the effects of excessive drinking may be age-specific, circumscribed by events, delayed, or accumulate over time. Certain life stages, such as young adulthood, are generally associated with increased alcohol intake and women may react to unusual events or stressful experiences by increasing alcohol intake.

Wilsnack and coworkers[29,41] obtained retrospective data from a strati-fied sample of 917 women studied in a cross-sectional survey in 1981. The sample included 500 moderate to heavy drinking women (consuming four or more drinks/wk), 378 lighter drinking or abstinent women, and 39 self-reported former problem drinkers. All were over age 21 and none resided in institutional settings. Demographic characteristics of the women surveyed corresponded to those of the general female population of the United States in 1980, including occupational categories, racial distributions, and educa-tional levels. Respondents answered questions about alcohol consumption, drinking context, problems associated with drinking, symptoms of alcohol dependence, attitudes and beliefs about drinking, family history, self-con-cept and role performance, stressful life experiences, social support, anxi-ety and depressive symptoms, reproductive problems, sexual experience, use of drugs in addition to alcohol, and participation in antisocial behav-iors. Respondents also provided data on lifetime changes in drinking, includ-ing age at onset of alcohol use, frequency of alcohol use, and quantity of consumption. They were asked at what ages their drinking patterns changed and how quantity and frequency changed. The questionnaire provided an opportunity to describe six different drinking history stages, but only 2% of the sample reported as many as five stages.

Median age of respondents was 42. Only 28% reported lifetime abstinence from alcohol. The median age for initiating drinking was 18 yr and 87% of nonabstainers had begun drinking by age 21. Of women who had drunk more than minimally in the preceding year, a majority (57%) had experi-enced at least one problem consequence of drinking. Problems and symp-toms were typically recognized early in adult life. One out of five women who consumed alcohol had at some time worried about the possibility of a drinking problem. Chronic heavy drinking and general concerns about per-sonal drinking habits were less frequent, and tended to develop later than specific problems or symptoms.

Comparisons were made among age cohorts. Particular emphasis was placed on identifying women who had begun drinking prior to age 25 and later engaged in heavy drinking, as well as on identifying women who had experienced adverse consequences prior to age 25. Early onset of heavy drinking and adverse consequences were more common for younger women and may reflect an actual acceleration of drinking experience and alcohol abuse among young women. Despite the fact there had been little change in young women's drinking during the past decade, symptoms of alcohol depen-dence are more commonly and frequently reported by all women drinkers. Contemporary women drink more openly, thus, their drinking may be less protected. However, young women may be more acquainted with detrimental effects of alcohol on health and behavior.

Evidence indicated that women had not simply forgotten their past drinking behavior and recalled changes in their drinking patterns over time. Only one-fourth of current drinkers said that they had been drinking at the same level since they began to use alcohol, a comparable number reported increased consumption over time, and 10% reported reductions with no increases. Almost half of the current drinkers (42%) reported prior fluctuations in drinking, indicating that these assessments had face validity.

Health-related events were recalled readily and 98% of the women answered pertinent questions, with 93% able to recall age of first occurrence. Median ages for first experiences of four different reproductive problems typically occurred during their mid-20s. Miscarriage or stillbirth was reported by 28% of women who had ever been pregnant. Premature delivery also occurred in mid-20s as did birth of a baby with birth defects and infertility lasting for at least 1 yr duration. On average, regular use of marijuana occurred at age 18, depressive episodes occurred at an average of age 27, and regular tranquilizer use occurred about age 37.

Since it is commonly believed that stress from reproductive problems is related to drinking levels, these variables were compared. Reproductive problems were not very strongly related to consumption in excess of a 24-drinks/wk threshold. The majority of women who reported drinking in association with stressful life-events stated that drinking increased after the event. This relationship held across different age cohorts. Increased drinking usually occurred one decade or more later than a reproductive problem.

Gomberg and Schilit examined the question of whether alcoholic women drink heavily because they are relatively isolated, or whether isolation is a consequence of drinking.[69] A study of 301 women alcoholics in treatment examined social consequences of alcoholism and the impact of heavy drinking in women's social networks. Women with alcohol problems were criticized and rejected by family and friends. Consequences included serious family quarrels, decreased communication with parents or other relatives, anger from family or friends, diminished frequency of contact with friends, perceived criticism from friends, avoidance of nondrinking friends, association with other heavy drinkers, suspicion and distrust of people, solitary activities, increased loneliness, and solitary drinking.

Age differences in social network behaviors were related to consequences of drinking. Alcoholic women in their 20s more frequently reported that they cut themselves off from friends who did not drink heavily, maintained contact with heavy drinking companions, and felt suspicious and distrustful. Younger women also reported more rejection by family and friends. Accordingly, it appears unlikely that alcoholic women are passive victims of aggression and rejection.

However, perceptions may be distorted, as alcohol abuse is often denied for many years. It is also possible that any link between stressful life-events and increased alcohol consumption may reflect the activities of a subgroup of alcoholics who behave impulsively and aggressively and are thus likely to promote both excessive drinking and adverse consequences.[70] It has been suggested that women may be more likely to attribute heavy drinking to causes that elicit sympathy as opposed to censure, especially because of the stigmatized attitudes directed toward heavy drinking females.[70,71] Allan and Cooke interviewed a general population sample of 230 women about their alcohol consumption and recent life-events.[70] There was no evidence that women in general responded to life-events with heavy and uncontrolled drinking. The middle-aged cohort, considered to be at high risk, was comprised of moderate alcohol users who consumed about three drinks/wk, in contrast to men of similar age who consumed about 36 drinks/wk. It was also argued that attribution of drinking to life problems may discourage alcohol treatment and promote use of prescription drugs to ameliorate dysphoria or other emotional distress.

Remy and colleagues studied the impact of life-events on 86 male and 35 female alcoholics ages 20–60 yr.[72] It was hypothesized that gender would affect the type of events considered to be important. Subjects were patients in internal medicine, gastroenterology, and psychiatric units, and a control group of 60 moderate alcohol users matched by age and sex was drawn from an occupational health center. Each subject indicated which of 48 events on a check-list had occurred during their lifetimes. The extent of adaptation prompted by each event was rated on a scale that ranged between 1 and 6. Scale items endorsed more than five times and by at least four subjects identified 29 items for men and 20 for women. These items were then intercorrelated.

For male alcoholics, 20 out of a possible 144 pairs of events were significantly associated, in contrast to only four associations for control men. Among alcoholic women, 17 out of 125 possible pairs of events were significantly correlated, but no events were significantly correlated for control women. Data for alcoholic men indicated strong intercorrelations among conjunctions of three events: marriage, sexual difficulties, and arguments with spouse. Alcoholic men additionally cited work-related events. For alcoholic women, two main sequences of events emerged. The first focused on changes in working conditions, social activities, marital relations, and lifestyle, whereas the second focused on family troubles, including changes in family stability, sexual difficulties, stillbirth or abortion, death of a close relative, and ending a job.

Patterns were evaluated according to the extent of impact. Three clusters of events were observed for alcoholic men. The first included events
with social connotations, such as those resulting from unemployment, change
in physical appearance, change in family get-togethers, and change in social
activities. The second cluster identified events with family connotations,
such as change in working conditions or hours, increase in arguments with
spouse, birth of a child, or minor illness. A third cluster included events
with more personal meaning, ending a job as a result of occurrence of an
accident or hospitalization, a change in religious activities, and sexual difficulties. Relationships were more complicated for alcoholic women, with
eight clusters of events identified. Changes in residence were intercorrelated
with sexual difficulties and divorce, marriage, birth of a child, and minor
illness; changes in family get-togethers were intercorrelated with unwanted
pregnancy and ending work; sexual difficulties were associated with death
of a close relative and moving; the birth of a child was linked to marriage
and minor financial problems; minor illness was linked with marriage and
departure of a child from home; changes in working conditions were associated with serious illness or accident and to injury or hospitalization; and
injury or hospitalization was associated with change in working conditions
and change in physical appearance.

It was concluded from these findings that women have a more frag-
mented view of life-events. Cause-and-effect or temporal relationships identified as significant included changes in place of residence, sexual difficulty,
divorce, marriage, financial problems, birth of a child, serious illness or
accident, injury or hospitalization, and change of working conditions. Thus,
it appears that women used private life-events as indicators for assessing
the impact of other events. On the other hand, men accorded greater importance to work events and judged the impact of other events in terms of
effects on their occupational life. Interestingly, employed women did not
rate events in the same manner as employed men.

Alcoholics viewed life-events more interdependently. Alcoholic men
may have responded to events that marked their inability to fulfill their
occupational roles and function as "breadwinners," whereas women were
more likely to focus on events that compromised their role as "homemakers." There were indications that alcoholic women may tend to inflate the
importance of their role as mother and housewife and men their roles as
"breadwinners."

For women, although the two concepts are usually not carefully distinguished, psychological conflicts in either female gender identity (individual perception of one's sex status) or in performance of the female sex
role (specific expectations of behavior associated with one's sex status)[73]

have been alleged to somehow precipitate alcohol problems.[74,75] However, the ways in which these behaviors might be linked to alcohol abuse have not been completely explained.[76] Nor is there any obvious link between known male-female differences in biological capacity, such as strength, information processing, or reproductive capacity, and development of alcohol problems.[73] Instead, it has often been intuitively assumed that mutually exclusive expectations and behavioral norms are inherent in incompletely described different male and female sex roles and that for some women these ill-defined polar differences somehow promote or perpetuate excessive use of alcohol.

Kroft and Leichner[77] administered standardized questionnaires that measured sex-role conflicts, sex-role beliefs, sex-role satisfaction, and depression to 46 institutionalized alcoholic women, 29 female alcoholics in remission, 61 social drinkers, and 24 abstainers. Social drinkers and alcoholics in remission were significantly more "untraditional" than abstainers, but alcoholics were only slightly more "traditional" than social drinkers. Thus, alcoholism was associated with relatively traditional sex-role beliefs.

It was suggested that alcoholic women seemed to value traditional feminine roles, but their inability to perform as expected could be one source of chronic tension and anxiety promoting excess alcohol consumption. However, to some extent all groups studied experienced sex-role conflict. Interestingly, all women expressed a desire to act in more "masculine" ways than they perceived themselves, whereas there was little difference between their real and ideal "feminine" self-image. Sex-role satisfaction scores indicated little difference among the groups, although abstinent alcoholic women reported more dissatisfaction with their roles as "wife/girlfriend." In consonance with a number of other studies, alcoholic women were found to be more depressed than nonalcoholic women, indicating that depressive symptoms may be integrally involved in the interpersonal conflicts of alcoholic women. Women might have used alcohol to palliate stress associated with dissatisfaction, or alcohol effects might have masked interpersonal conflicts. Thus, interpersonal conflicts might have a stronger association with the etiology of excessive drinking than intrapsychic conflicts.

Gender Differences in Drug Dependence

A series of reports examined sex differences in addict careers of 546 male and female clients in methadone maintenance programs in southern California.[78–81] At admission women were approx 26 yr of age vs 29 yr for men. Both women and men averaged about 10.5 yr of education. Roughly 90% of men and women had been arrested, with their first arrest at approx

16.5 and 18.5 yr, respectively. About 80% of men and women were married and about 85% had lived with a partner in consensual union, with an average number of 2.5 children. Significantly, about 15% of women, but no men, reported initiation into drug use by a spouse or common-law partner. Instead, men were more likely to initiate use within a group context. More women reported that they were initiated into drug use by a daily user. However, no men reported living with an addicted woman prior to their initiation to opiates.

Approximately 60% of men used marijuana, and 40% drank daily. White males were more likely to deal drugs than White females, but Hispanic women were more likely to be involved in drug dealing than Hispanic men. Overall, more men than women reported having been a gang member and having school problems. Male addicts were also arrested at younger ages, were more frequently incarcerated for more than 30 d, and were more likely to be on probation.

Over 25% of the sample began daily heroin use within the first 3 wk of initial use and about 25% became dependent within one month of their first use. Overall, women took less time to develop dependence, and many became dependent within 1 mo. The mean number of total months from initiation into opiate use to opiate dependence was 14 mo for women and 21 mo for men.

The pattern of differential time to dependence is consistent with findings from other studies. During the interval between initiation of use to dependence, women were likely to sharply curtail nonopiate drug use and slightly decrease alcohol use. It was conjectured that women replace use of other drugs with heroin, whereas men continue to experiment with many drugs simultaneously. Women and men seemed to follow similar opiate use patterns, but for women addiction careers seemed "compressed" into a shorter cycle.[78]

Women reported shorter durations of consistent daily use (23 mo vs 32 mo). About one-third of men and women had ever abstained. Men were abstinent for longer intervals (approx 8 mo) than women (approx 3.5 mo), but men were more frequently incarcerated. Female opiate users entered treatment after significantly less time, averaging about 5 yr from first drug use to admission to a methadone maintenance program, vs about 8 yr for men.

Influence of an opiate-using partner was a strong factor perpetuating opiate use for women. Women were most likely to attribute their use to social reasons, especially use by a partner (approx 36%), but about 10% of men and women reported social use by friends as a major social reason for using opiates. For about 50% of men and 30% of women, other sustaining factors were related to liking the "high" and developing tolerance. Men also cited ready availability or cheap price of heroin, although women were more likely to be supplied with heroin.

Opiate Addicts

Kosten and colleagues studied 522 treated opiate addicts, including 126 (24%) women.[36] Both men and women first used opiates at approximately age 18 and typical duration of opiate use (9 yr) was similar. Using RDC criteria,[67] intercurrent psychiatric diagnoses differed by gender, with women having more dysphoric and anxiety disorders (64 vs 49%), and more men having antisocial personality disorders (30 vs 17%). The majority of men and women were in the age group 26–35 yr (55 and 63%) followed by the 18–25 yr age range (25 and 28%). Most had completed high school, and roughly 20% had education beyond high school. Men were more likely to have full-time employment, but were also more likely to be unmarried.

Approximately 16% of men and about 20% of women reported their father having had a history of alcoholism and family history of paternal depression was approximately double (10%) for women. Family history of psychological disorders in mothers was about 7% for males and females and a history of depression in mothers was around 10% for both men and women. Women were less likely (about 3%) than men (7%) to report alcoholism in a sibling. The rate of drug addiction in siblings, however, was about 25% for both men and women. Women were twice as likely to have received their first psychiatric treatment by age 15 (10%). In contrast to about 30% of men, roughly 15% of women had experienced school failure, although rates for school behavior problems were about 50% for men and women. With regard to other problems, males had approximately double the arrest rate (11%) of women (6%) and women were slightly more likely (40%) than men (32%) to have experienced severe family disruption. On the Addiction Severity Index,[82] the rating for legal problems was similar for men and for women (3.3). Ratings for family and social problems (3.4) and substance abuse problems were also comparable (5.4). However, women had a severity rating of 4.0 for intercurrent psychological problems, whereas men averaged 3.3. Women also had higher scores for medical problems (2.5 vs 1.5), but employment problems were comparable, averaging 3.3.

This study also investigated whether parental alcoholism was associated with addict alcoholism.[36] In 522 treated addicts with an overall rate of alcoholism of 35%, 17.6% of fathers and 5.8% of mothers were alcoholic. The maternal alcoholism rate was higher (9.7%) in alcoholic addicts than among nonalcoholic addicts (3.8%). Some generalized vulnerability for substance abuse may be transmitted from alcoholic parents to their off-spring.[36] Interestingly, parental alcoholism was more strongly associated with proband's alcoholism in the case of antisocial personality in female addicts and with affective disorder in alcoholic male addicts.

Cocaine Users

There is comparatively little information concerning differences between male and female cocaine users. One recent study[83] compared sociodemographic characteristics, reasons for cocaine use, drug effects, depressive symptoms, and psychiatric diagnoses in 95 men (74%) and 34 women (26%) hospitalized for cocaine abuse. Women were significantly younger than men at time of first drug use (mean age 15.6 vs 18.5 yr) and age of first substance abuse treatment (mean 24.6 vs 29.1 yr) and had used cocaine for a significantly shorter period of time (mean 3.7 vs 5.4 yr). Men and women were similar in their mean total years of drug use (10.2 vs 9.0 yr), years of heavy drug use (5.2 vs 4.3), number of different drugs used during the previous 30 d (3.5 vs 4.4), and amount of cocaine used during the past 6 mo (106.3 vs 107.5), but differed in the amount of money that they had spent on cocaine during the past 6 mo ($9375 vs $3050). More men were married (40 vs 21%), but more women lived with a drug dependent partner (36 vs 21%). More men were employed (78 vs 50%) and had professional, executive, or sales jobs (61 vs 20%).

Women were more likely to have an axis I DSM-III-R diagnosis in addition to substance abuse, especially depression, whereas only men had antisocial personality disorder. Of patients with depression, women reported more depression than men on the Hamilton Depression Rating Scale (HDRS) at admission, at 2 wk after admission, and at 4 wk after admission. For patients who had no diagnosis of major depression at admission, HDRS scores were similar for men and women at admission, but women had per-sistent elevated scores at 2 and at 4 wk post-admission.

Women gave four reasons for cocaine use: depression, feeling unso-ciable, family and job pressures, and health problems. Overall, men cited more intoxication effects from cocaine and were more likely to report that cocaine decreased libido (67 vs 38%). For men and women cocaine had similar effects on aggression, appetite, anxiety, and mood. However, women reported significantly less guilt as a cocaine effect (47 vs 23%). Most men and women (57%) reported they used cocaine to increase sociability.

Involvement with a drug-dependent partner may have contributed to the more rapid development of addiction in some women,[83] as cohabiting with a cocaine-using partner was more frequently reported by women. This observation also was made for female opioid addicts,[84] and alcoholics.[85]

Marijuana Smokers

Two laboratory studies investigated marijuana self-administration in young men[86] and women.[87] Subjects were classified as either "moderate" or "heavy" users based on drug-use history interviews and self-report questionnaire data. Moderate smokers had used marijuana more than five times/ mo but less than daily during the previous year, whereas heavy smokers had used marijuana five or more times/wk during the previous year.

Subjects were studied on a research unit for 35 d in groups of three or four that included both moderate and heavy smokers. Study protocols included three phases: A 7-d drug-free baseline phase; a 21-d drug acquisition period during which marijuana cigarets could be purchased on a free-choice basis; and a 7-d postdrug phase. During all study phases subjects could work for points at a simple operant task that earned 50 cents per one-half hour of effort. During the 21-d acquisition period, points earned could either be exchanged directly for marijuana (50 cents/cigaret) or accumulated until the conclusion of the study, added to points earned during the baseline periods, and exchanged for money.

Male heavy smokers consumed about four cigarets/d at the beginning of the 21-d marijuana smoking intervals and their consumption increased to about 6.5 cigarets/d by the end, whereas male moderate smokers consumed about two cigarets/d at the beginning and increased to about three cigarets/d.[86] In sharp contrast, daily marijuana consumption for female heavy smokers averaged 3.5 cigarets/d and 1.4 cigarets/d for female moderate smokers (87). No significant linear increases in marijuana smoking were apparent for women. Although heavy smoking women used significantly more marijuana than moderate smoking women, their smoking patterns showed more fluctuation. Over 21 d marijuana consumption showed a negligible decrease for heavy smokers and a negligible increase for moderate smokers. Marijuana use by female heavy smokers fluctuated daily because no subject smoked on all 21 d. Female moderate marijuana smokers also did not smoke every day, but their average daily use hovered around the overall mean.

Thus, there may be distinct patterns of marijuana use for men and women. Women's marijuana smoking patterns may reflect social influences, such as the temporal pattern of weekday vs weekend smoking.[88] However, fluctuations also could be related to the greater amount of lipid tissue in females, which can store and gradually release D^9-THC. To complicate interpretations further, data for women also indicated that moderate smokers increased their smoking on days when they reported heightened unpleasant moods such as anger.[87]

Another study series used daily diaries to obtain prospective reports of alcohol and marijuana consumption by female marijuana smokers, and alcohol and marijuana consumption by female social drinkers.[89,90] A study of 30 female marijuana smokers (mean age 26.4 yr) obtained daily questionnaires for three consecutive menstrual cycles (roughly 90 d/subject, ≥98% completion rate). Subjects recorded the quantities and times of alcohol and marijuana consumption, episodes of sexual activity, and occurrence of unusual life-events.[89] Temporal variables significantly affected both marijuana and alcohol consumption. On weekdays marijuana use occurred earlier in the day, but significantly greater marijuana use and more concordant alcohol and marijuana use occurred on weekends. Older women (ages 26 to 30 yr) exhibited more concordant alcohol and marijuana use than younger women (ages 21 to 25 yr). Significant differences in alcohol use also distinguished heavy from light marijuana smokers, but neither sexual activity nor unusual events were associated with concordant alcohol and marijuana consumption in all subjects.[89]

Female marijuana smokers were divided into two groups. On days of marijuana use, heavy smokers consumed between 1.8 and 7.6 marijuana cigarets, whereas light smokers consumed between 0.4 and 1.5 marijuana cigarets. Heavy smokers reported greater daily alcohol use, more days of concordant alcohol and marijuana use, greater frequency of morning marijuana smoking, and greater frequency of smoking in the morning, afternoon, and evening. Heavy marijuana smokers smoked marijuana more frequently on days when unusual events occurred, but showed no weekday vs weekend effect. More heavy marijuana smokers also had a history of tobacco cigaret smoking (89).

Heavy marijuana smokers tended to be slightly younger than light smokers and were significantly younger when they had begun to smoke marijuana. Light marijuana smokers were four times more likely to attribute a search for insight and understanding as a reason for their marijuana use. No significant differences were found between the two groups for age at first alcohol use, age at first sexual intercourse, years of regular alcohol or marijuana use, years of education, or reported lifetime use of hallucinogens, tranquilizers, or cocaine. The patterns of consumption and sexual activity were similar for heavy and light marijuana smokers.[89]

A study of female social drinkers used a similar prospective method as well as daily diary records of consumption patterns and mood states (roughly 90 d/subject, ≥98% completion rate). Heavy drinkers (mean ≥ 1.80 drinks/d) were significantly more likely to smoke marijuana than moderate drinkers (mean ≤ 1.75 drinks/d). Heavy drinkers also smoked significantly more marijuana. In this sample of social drinkers neither age nor frequency of sexual activity were related to patterns of alcohol or marijuana consumption.[90]

Investigation of mood states for 30 female marijuana smokers[91] also found differences between heavy and light users. Potential predictors of eight mood scores were examined for young women who smoked marijuana and drank alcohol in the community. Again, prospective data were obtained from diary questionnaires submitted daily during three consecutive menstrual cycles.

Heavy users smoked a mean of 2.1 marijuana cigarets/d across the three menstrual cycles, whereas light users smoked a mean of 0.6 marijuana cigarets/d. Marijuana and alcohol were consumed on the same day by heavy users on 41% of study days, and by light users on 29% of study days. Unusual or stressful events occurred on 22% of all study days for 29 subjects. Sexual activity was recorded on 28% of all study days by 24 subjects. No difference in sexual activity frequency for heavy vs light users was found.

A multiple regression analysis examined interaction effects of six predictor variables (heavy use, consumption of both marijuana and alcohol, occurrence of unusual events, sexual activity, menses, and weekdays vs weekends). Heavy marijuana smokers had lower scores on friendliness, elation, and vigor and higher scores on tension, anger, fatigue, and confusion. Thus, being a heavy marijuana smoker influenced all mood scores except depression. Days of both smoking marijuana and consuming alcohol were associated with changes in increased scores for friendliness and vigor and decreased scores for tension and fatigue. Days of sexual activity did not affect negative moods, but did increase friendliness, elation, and vigor. In contrast, on days of unusual events, increased tension, depression, anger, and confusion, but not fatigue, were unrelated to positive moods. Only elation was significantly lower on weekdays than weekends and only menstruation influenced moods by increasing fatigue.[91]

Decreased elation scores reported by heavy marijuana smoking women may indicate that, for women who smoke marijuana heavily, marijuana smoking becomes associated with decreased euphoria.[91] Similar findings for young men were reported by Mirin and coworkers.[92] However, absence of changes in depression scores for female heavy marijuana users was an unanticipated finding that differed from increased depression reported by male heavy marijuana users.[92] Our measure of stress, "unusual events," was significantly associated with increased negative moods but unrelated to positive moods. Increased tension, depression, anger, and confusion were reported on days of stress.[91] A study by Bruns and Geist has found that stress, inherent in labeled events "good" and "bad" may differentially affect adolescent females and males, as females generally assigned significantly higher scores to the acute effects of stressors.[93]

Longitudinal Studies of Marijuana Users

Kandel and coworkers conducted longitudinal studies of substance use among individuals who were first identified in high school during 1971 and 1972.[94,95] In 1980 and 1981, 83% of the original 1651 adolescents were reinterviewed at ages 24 to 25. The majority of respondents had used marijuana, 78% and 69% of young men and women, respectively. Further, 37% of males and 24% of females reported using cocaine. Psychedelics had been used by 32% of males and 19% of females, stimulants had been used by 30% of males and 19% of females, and 20% of males and 15% of females had used minor tranquilizers (such as benzodiazepines) without prescription. Thus, 90% of individuals in this cohort who had used marijuana at least 1000 times in their lives had also used other illicit drugs. In addition, 79% who had used marijuana more than 100 times (but less than 1000 times) reported use of illicit drugs, 51% of those who had used marijuana less than 100 times but more than 10 times used illicit drugs, 16% of those who had used marijuana between one and nine times also used other illicit drugs, and only 6% of adolescents who had never used marijuana reported use of illicit drugs. This relationship was strongly log-linear, yielding a correlation of .995 between increasing marijuana use and use of other illicit drugs. Consequently, it was difficult to disentangle marijuana effects from effects of other substance use, including cigarets and alcohol.

Job instability was associated with marijuana and other illicit drug use by both males and females. The amount of marijuana consumption at the initial survey predicted an increased number of unemployed intervals at follow-up. Illicit drug use also affected performance of adult family roles, predicting lower rates of marriage for women and yielding positive correlations with divorce or separation among both women and men and with abortions among women. Women's use of illicit drugs, other than marijuana, by ages 15 or 16 predicted subsequent use of prescribed psychoactive medications. It was concluded that use of illicit drugs other than marijuana during adolescence may palliate feelings of depression.[96]

Marijuana users were found to be heavily involved in social relationships where marijuana use was common. Men's marijuana consumption within the last 12 mo was associated with divorce, separation, or never being married. Male marijuana users were also more than likely to report having automobile accidents. Of women who had used marijuana four or more times/wk during the past year, 96% reported that most or all of their friends used marijuana.[94] Among women living with a spouse or partner, one could observe the "husband effect"; that is, a male spouse or partner's use had a strong main effect on women's marijuana use. This effect was greater than peer's use and the use of other illicit drugs.

Kandel concluded that interpersonal factors are more significant for women's marijuana use.[94] Kandel proposed that men are likely to be involved in several different types of social networks and in friendships where prevailing behaviors and values are different from those favored by their spouses or partners. In contradistinction, women may be engaged in more circumscribed and less variable social activities. Marijuana use requires a permissive social context in both adolescence and young adulthood. For women involved with a partner, not only the partner but friends provide important influences on continued marijuana smoking.

Women and Treatment

Overall Comparisons

Over the last two decades patterns of substance use have shifted.[3] Alcohol-dependent men still outnumber alcohol-dependent women,[60] but more prescription medications are used by women.[97] There are numerous studies of treatment of women with alcohol problems, although their quality and utility is uneven.[98] Several studies have examined women's social histories, personality, and motivation characteristics, but fewer studies have focused on biological variables. Further, prevalence rates may have been underestimated for women. It has been suggested that women are less likely to use conventional alcoholism treatment facilities and more likely to seek help from private physicians. Some also argue that women's drinking may remain more covert than that of men, that women are actively dissuaded by partners—often themselves heavy drinkers—from seeking treatment, and that available treatment facilities fail to adequately accommodate problems presented by female alcoholics.

One study of 60 alcoholic and 60 nonalcoholic women compared six psychosocial characteristics, including number of alcoholic first-degree relatives, number of health-related problems, depression scores, self-esteem scores, traditional social role perception, and perceived adequacy in meeting expectations of significant others.[99] Alcoholic women were recruited from Alcoholics Anonymous and inpatient and outpatient facilities. The riterion for selection was utilization of some alcoholism treatment modality. Mean length of sobriety was 35 d and no one was abstinent more than 90 d. Mean age was 35.7 yr and mean number of years married was 11.1. In contrast to 80% of women in the control group, only 23% of the alcoholic women were married and 92% of control women, vs 67% of the alcoholic women, had been married at least once. Significantly more nonalcoholic women (78% vs 25%) were employed and had more formal education (mean 15.8 vs 13.1 yr).[99]

Alcoholic women had more relatives (gender unspecified) with drinking problems (6.5 vs 1.5) and a greater number of health problems (8.2 vs 2.7). In addition, alcoholic women had higher depression scores (8.1 vs 4.1) and lower self-esteem scores (mean 25.3 vs 32.7) and rated themselves as less conforming with typical expectations for feminine behavior (score 54.3 vs 57.0). Alcoholic women also perceived greater differences between expectations of their significant others vs the extent to which their behavior matched expectations (3.2 vs 4.1).

A discriminant function analysis accurately classified 92% of alcoholic and nonalcoholic women.[99] Self-esteem and depression variables had limited ability to distinguish alcoholic women. However, having numerous health problems and alcoholic first degree relatives contributed strongly to the equation. Although subjects were not not screened for DSM-III axis I diagnoses, findings are reminiscent of the characteristics of daughters of alcoholic fathers described by Cloninger, Bohman, and colleagues.[7,8,100]

Gender Bias in Treatment and Outcome Studies

It has been suggested that since more men than women are alcoholic or heavy drinkers, women are excluded from studies since their numbers are small and inclusion might generate unstable statistics, or that follow-up studies of women may be complicated because their names may change following divorce or marriage. Vannicelli and Nash evaluated 259 studies published between 1972 and 1980 to assess whether sex bias contributed to underrepresentation of women.[101] Data were pooled for over 64,000 men and women. In comparisons that separately analyzed males and females at most 2459 or 7.8% were female. Close to 80% of the 259 studies had male first authors and 13.4% of all individuals studied by women were female, in contrast to only 4.3% studied by men. Female investigators were also more likely to conduct follow-up studies.

Vannicelli also identified three barriers to efficacious alcoholism treatment for women.[102] First, were expectancies that women do not profit from treatment because they are more depressed, experience mood swings, and are self-centered. Second, traditionally stereotyped sex role expectancies limited beliefs in female alcoholics' potential for change. Lastly, lack of information about prognosis for alcoholic women has led to the assumption that their treatment is ineffective.

Providers infantilize female alcoholics, thus undercutting their strength and growth. Further, lack of research precludes development of a scientific basis for designing treatment for women. Data are insufficient to evaluate individual therapy vs group therapy, the value of family therapy, the need for women to be treated separately or in mixed groups, or the impact of a female vs male therapist.[102]

Patterns of Compliance

It is believed that female alcoholics are difficult to engage in treatment, highly ambivalent about treatment, and have poor motivation. Duckert noted that women with alcohol problems are less likely to seek alcoholism treatment, but are more likely to seek specific help for marital problems, family problems, physical illness, or emotional problems that they do not attribute to alcohol abuse.[103] Attrition rates during the first month of treatment ranged from 28–80%. Moreover, women who dropped out had a poor prognosis.

In Great Britain, local Councils on Alcohol have adopted an approach that departs from the typical medical model and are believed to be more successful in attracting problem-drinking women. Counselors are volunteers, services do not include either detoxification or direct access to psychiatric or medical care, and self-referrals constitute the major proportion of those who seek help. Female counselors are available to female clients, which may reduce stigma, appointment scheduling is flexible, and individual counseling is emphasized. Accordingly, results from these services contrast with services which require a referral from a general practitioner, the courts, or employers.

Allan and Phil studied 112 men and women with drinking problems enrolled by a community-based volunteer agency over a 6-mo period.[104] About one-half (52%) were married, about 25% were separated or divorced, and the remainder (21%) were single. Ages ranged from 18–65 yrs with a mean of 40 yr and 61% of the clients were employed. Of the sample, 27% came to the clinic only once. After 4 wk, 37 more dropped out and by 6 mo another 29% had dropped out. After 6 mo only 7% were still in treatment. Further, 72% did not respond to any follow-up contacts. Formal discharge occurred for 21% of the sample, thus leaving the remaining 7% in need of additional services. Only men (11% of original referrals) attended the clinic for 6 mo or more. Women were more likely to participate in only one interview (35 vs 21%). Men had a mean of 4.7 sessions during 6 wk, whereas women had an average of 3.3 sessions over 4.5 wk.

Referral source was important, but gender of counselors did not affect retention (78% of women were assigned to female counselors). About one-half (49%) were self-referrals, with the remainder referred by general practitioners, hospitals, and shelters. Persons referred from agencies remained in treatment longer, with 14% of agency-referred clients in treatment after 6 mo vs only 1.8% of self-referrals. Age, marital status, or employment status did not affect retention. Referrals from shelters, employers, or courts had an average of 6.1 appointments over 9.1 wk, whereas self-referrals attended 3.4 sessions over 3.7 wk. In contrast to 80% of self-referred clients, only half of the clients referred from coercive sources spontaneously left treatment.

Only two women were referred by coercive sources (employers). Since the vast majority of women were self-referrals, or were referred by noncoercive sources, their high attrition rate may be associated with low motivation as opposed to greater pathology. Since the majority of clients may be seen only once, the initial interview should be a thorough evaluation with results incorporated into an individualized treatment plan.

Thom[105] examined barriers to help-seeking in 25 men and 25 women who were new admissions referred to an alcohol clinic. Women and men were similar in age (43.1 vs 42.4 yr). They did not differ significantly in number living with a spouse or mate, divorced, widowed, separated, or married; in number living with children under age 16, living in rented or owner occupied homes, living with relatives; in number employed; and in number having education beyond the statutory age for leaving school.

Most women felt that their heavy alcohol consumption was a legitimate response to personal problems and did not perceive that heavy intake might further complicate their problems. They shared a belief that drinking for the sake of drinking was the major reason that people should have alcohol treatment, thus denying that their clinic referral was appropriate. A major obstacle for men was concern that they had a problem which could not be resolved without assistance. Men typically believed that they should be able to control their drinking and found it difficult to ask for help. Some men acknowledged concern that their coworkers would think that they were lacking in masculinity if it became generally known they were attending an alcohol treatment clinic. Thus, women objected to being labeled as in need of alcohol treatment, whereas men were concerned that they would be labeled in need of psychiatric care.

Few (four women and no men) reported practical problems that made it difficult to attend the clinic. Childcare was not a salient issue, but clients felt awkward about obtaining time off from work. An equal number of men and women ($N = 5$) were afraid of the hospital. These fears included shame and embarrassment about discussing personal problems, fear and lack of knowledge about treatment requirements, fear of being told never to drink again, and fear of the physician as an authority figure.

This study also examined reasons for referral.[106] Half of men and women had first sought treatment within the previous year. Similar numbers of men ($N = 16$) and women ($N = 14$) were referred to the alcohol clinic by general practitioners. However, almost double the number of women ($N = 9$ vs $N = 5$) were referred to the alcohol clinic from an emergency clinic, suggesting that women may delay treatment until health problems become urgent.

Only three men and six women failed to report a significant life-event in the year prior to the interview. No men, but eight women reported experiencing physical violence. Ten men vs two women reported job loss, and ten men vs six women reported serious health problems. An equal number of men and women ($N = 5$) had problems with the law, and those experiencing death of a significant other were similar (five men and four women). Smaller numbers reported loss of a child (three men and three women), marital dissolution (three men and two women), and suicide attempts (one man and four women). Two men vs five women reported becoming homeless. Serious health problems, marital breakup, loss of child, and violence by respondents influenced help-seeking, whereas patients did not necessarily perceive job loss, deaths, legal problems, loss of adult significant others, experiencing violence, becoming homeless, having an accident, or attempting suicide, as precipitants to alcohol treatment.

For men, marital disruption or threat of separation was a more frequent precipitant ($N = 9$) than for women ($N = 2$). Intriguingly, two men and three women reported that an encouraging event prompted them to feel worthy and to have hope for the future, thus reinforcing the need for alcohol treatment. The influence of significant others also provided encouragement to seek help. More men ($N = 13$) than women ($N = 4$) attributed this influence to a spouse, whereas more women ($N = 6$) than men ($N = 3$) reported positive influence from their children. Four men and five women reported that friends encouraged treatment and eight men vs five women reported that a general practitioner encouraged treatment. Only women reported that other relatives or coworkers encouraged treatment.

Health problems were cited by 15 men and 14 women, but only women ($N = 3$) reported drug use as a health problem. Fourteen women vs eight men reported depression and five women vs one man reported generalized anxiety or panic attacks. For men, major reasons for entry into treatment included worries about health, possible marital breakup, fear of losing children, or fear of job loss. Women were less likely to be in stable living arrangements and most frequently reported pressure from others and worries about their health as prompts to enter treatment. However, whereas men saw encouragement from others as a positive factor, women were more likely to see clinic attendance as a way of escaping unpleasant pressure from others, but did not expect any concomitant changes in their lives.

Engagement in Treatment

Robinson conducted a qualitative study of factors involved in successful interventions for alcohol-dependent women.[107] Eighteen recovering alcoholic women were identified through various community programs, but no systematic sampling was undertaken. Five women had been inpatients in psychiatric units and four of them had not received help with their alcohol problem during their hospitalizations. Five women also reported treatment with therapists who were either unapprised of the existence of an alcohol dependence problem or unable to provide appropriate intervention. In addition, six women had physicians who gave no assistance. Further, women who sought treatment from physicians and other psychiatrists reported receiving psychoactive medications that in some instances supplanted alcohol dependence.

Of the 18 women, 17 found Alcoholics Anonymous a source of social support. Other social supports, however, appeared to be highly individual, ranging from encouragement from close friends ($N = 4$), boyfriend, spouse, or parents, to individual problems such as threat of prosecution, threat of jail, or job loss. Perceived barriers to treatment were also highly individual, including desire for anonymity, lack of information, alcohol-dependent spouse ($N = 2$), drug-dependent child, threat of divorce, monetary support from parents, fear of prosecution, refusal of spouse to pay medical expenses, and unpredictable work schedule. Women reported that family members and friends most frequently talked, nagged, or otherwise showed concern ($N = 10$), showed anger or disgust ($N = 4$), or denied the problem ($N = 3$), but humiliation and embarrassment rarely prompted women to seek treatment. Employers typically made no response or imposed sanctions ($N = 5$).

Beckman and coworkers[35,108] investigated effects of sociodemographic, personal, and contextual characteristics of women and men in treatment settings. Women's typically lower levels of disposable income and paucity of other economic resources were potentially major obstacles to obtaining treatment.

Women were more likely than men to acknowledge problems with family, friends, and finances. Roughly one-half (48%) of women reported having had one or more types of treatment-related problems, in contrast to one-fifth (20%) of men. Men and women had similar concerns about health and expectations of medical care and were similar in their scores for locus of control scales. Both men and women received limited encouragement from sources other than family and friends. Over 20% of women reported opposition from family and friends during the month prior to treatment, but only one man reported opposition, from a drinking companion. Finally, women were three times more likely than men to report that they needed childcare, but the rates were actually very small (6 vs 2%). There also was a tendency for women to report that they felt a need for educational counseling.

A step-wise discriminant function analysis examined 12 independent variables, including health perceptions, health locus of control, drinking-related problems, negative effects of obtaining treatment, and negative effects of not obtaining treatment. Other variables included satisfaction with treatment, perceived success of treatment, and beliefs about family or genetic contributions to alcoholism. Findings generally supported the contention that women experience more difficulties in entering treatment, but that family therapy and environmental intervention strategies counterbalanced these obstacles. Women also may have had more difficulties than men in establishing trust in their alcohol counselor or therapist. A third important factor for women was primary affective disorder. Accurate differential diagnosis is especially important because management and treatment of depression and of alcohol dependence require different strategies. A recent review by Turnbull[98] examined the possible confounding that results from lack of differentiation between primary and secondary alcoholism. Turnbull reported that up to one-third of all women with alcohol problems may have a primary diagnosis of depression. It is generally believed that alcohol treatment can proceed accordingly after a distinction has been made between manifestations of intercurrent disorders.

A current study[109] examined prevalence rates of intercurrent disorders in male ($N = 260$) and female ($N = 241$) patients with alcohol and drug problems. Diagnoses were made using the NIMH Diagnostic Interview Schedule (DIS). Individuals with polysubstance dependence had higher rates of intercurrent psychiatric disorders. Women and men did not differ in overall rates for cognitive impairment, schizophrenia, and affective disorders. Women had higher rates of anxiety, bulimia, and psychosexual disorders, an unexpected finding. In all likelihood these findings reflect use of the DIS, since disorders such as bulimia have only been recognized within the past decade.

Treatment Outcome

There appears to be little evidence indicating poorer prognosis for women in comparison with men.[102] Vannicelli and Nash[101] recalculated outcome data for 23 of the 259 studies that had differentiated between male and female alcoholics. According to these investigations there is no scientific evidence that women respond poorly to treatment, as 78% (18 studies) showed no differences in outcome, 4 studies showed better outcome for women, and no studies showed better outcome for men.

Concerns about social conditions peculiar to women as mothers have promoted development of all-female treatment programs, several of which provide childcare or are targeted toward pregnant women. Duckert reviewed treatment outcomes for programs specifically targeted to women.[103] Results indicated that improvement rates ranged from 20% to close to 60%.

Herr and Pettinati[110] presented outcome data for 48 homemakers and 24 employed women who had received inpatient alcoholism treatment in a psychiatric hospital in a 28-d program. Average age at admission was 43 yr. At admission, 24 women (one-third) had been working outside of the home, while the remainder ($N = 48$) were homemakers. More homemakers were married (85 vs 33%), while more working women were divorced or separated (42 vs 8%). Homemakers reported longer drinking histories (mean 9.2 vs 5.8 yr). Adjustment was categorized as good, poor, or inconsistent.

Outcome was assessed at the end of 4 yr. Although approximately one-half of the homemakers and employed women maintained a good adjustment over the 4-yr interval, 24% of homemakers vs 14% of employed women showed a poor adjustment. At follow-up, 60% of homemakers still functioned as homemakers and 59% of employed women were still in the labor force. In comparison with 7 of 13 women who maintained the same occupation, 9 of the 10 women who changed occupation were improved at follow-up. A smaller number of women (three homemakers and three women in the labor force) did not change marital status at the time they changed occupations, suggesting that improvement in adjustment might be more related to change in occupation but independent from change in marital status. However, change in occupation cannot be considered as a single variable, since it might prompt reallocation of leisure time, or may be a consequence, rather than a reason, for improvement.

A series of reports by Haver[55,58,111] presented data from a follow-up study of 44 Norwegian women treated for alcohol problems between 1970 and 1980. Follow-up interviews occurred approx 6.5 yr after first admission when the mean age of the women was 32.2 yr. Exactly one-half of the women reported that violence had occurred between their parents or between a parent and themselves. In the majority of cases, fathers abused mothers, followed by fathers abusing patients, mothers abusing patients, and mothers abusing fathers. Twenty-four women reported that one or both parents were alcoholic. Alcoholism was more frequently associated with intrafamilial violence. At treatment, 80% of the women had had at least one male partner, 57% had lived with an alcohol abuser, and 18% had experienced domestic violence. Four women had a history of residing with one or more partners who were alcoholic, violent, or both.

The experience of physical abuse by her father or of witnessing abuse of her mother by her father was significantly correlated with the number of violent partners that a patient had during the follow-up interval. Thus, the more these female patients had violent experiences during childhood, the greater the likelihood of violent relationships in their adult lives. In contrast, during the follow-up interval, women who had no family history of childhood violence were more likely to break off relationships with a violent partner. A multiple regression analysis indicated that childhood violence experiences explained 11% of variance in outcome. Having a violent partner after treatment increased the explained variance to 25%. Significant associations were also observed among childhood violence experiences, violence of a cohabiting partner, and antisocial and/or borderline personality disorders. Personality disorders added an additional 9% to the explained outcome in variance. Childhood violence may promote symptoms reminiscent of posttraumatic stress disorder, and these aftereffects may contribute to a woman's inability to cope with life problems. Thus, the combination of adult and childhood violence contributed significantly to poor outcome.

The same 44 women were evaluated for alcohol consumption during the year prior to follow-up interview.[58] All of the women had consumed alcohol, but by the time of follow-up, their alcohol consumption differed. Twelve women consumed about the average amount of alcohol (2 L/yr) reported for women in the Norwegian population, seven women drank <7 L/yr, and the remainder (39% or 17 women) were heavy drinkers whose consumption ranged from 8–180 L in a year's span. Almost all of the women who consumed more than 20 cL of pure alcohol (roughly two-thirds of a bottle of spirits) on any single drinking day met one or more criteria for pathological alcohol use. In contrast, no women who reported consuming <14 cL met any criteria for pathological alcohol abuse. Four women shifted from moderate to heavy drinking and four women shifted from heavy drinking to moderate drinking. Among the abstainers, all relapsed one or more times following treatment.

At follow-up, long-term abstainers included six women who changed their identities to nondrinkers by informing their drinking partners that they chose to abstain, by avoiding situations in which other people drank, by attending self-help groups, or through religious participation. Interestingly, even long-term abstainers relapsed into heavy drinking when prompted by a life crisis. Although these factors could be consequences and not predictors, typical life crises were divorce or removal of children from the household. Thirty-seven percent (16) of the women were short-term abstainers who attempted to remain sober but could not maintain sobriety over the entire follow-up interval. These 16 women appeared to be able to respond to responsibilities such as holding a job or caring for children by reducing their drinking frequency. A shift to social drinking was reported by 39% (17) women, although a check of registry records indicated that only eight had provided accurate information. Abstinence for these women occurred months or years after treatment. Life situations changed for the better, with some separating from heavy drinkers and living either with sons or daughters, a new partner, or by themselves. Average consumption of alcohol by social drinkers ranged from one or two glasses to four to six glasses per occasion. Of the four women who maintained heavy drinking following treatment two retained jobs while two had unstable employment.

Goldstein and coworkers[112] summarized outcome evaluations for substance abuse treatment, which included studies of programs designed primarily for alcohol dependence treatment and studies of programs designed primarily for other drug abuse treatment. Information was drawn from a data bank of program evaluations. The major criterion for inclusion was reported findings for a minimum of 10 patients. A total of 2231 studies were included, with 18.2% ($N = 182$) focused on alcoholism treatment and 10.5% ($N = 234$) focused on drug abuse. All studies included information about both intervention and outcome variables.

Goldstein and colleagues noted that few studies focused on program quality such as therapist training, appropriateness of technique, or the importance of the program in a community. In comparison with results from alcohol abuse treatment programs and treatment programs for other psychological disorders, roughly 50% of the 234 studies of drug abuse treatment had weak designs, including absence of control subject comparisons. Alcohol treatment studies used both random and matched control groups (roughly 40% of studies). Analyses beyond descriptive statistics were most frequently used for alcoholism studies (45%), next frequently used in other mental health treatment studies (41.5%), but least frequently used in drug abuse treatment research (26.5%). One-third of all studies in the databank did not specify gender and 20.9% of alcoholism treatment outcome studies failed to note gender. In almost half (49.5%) of the alcohol studies all patients were male, whereas only 20.5% of drug abuse treatment programs reported data from only men, and outcome studies of general mental health treatment programs had the lowest rate for all male populations (14%). With regard to ethnicity, drug abuse treatment programs were more likely to report the proportion of Black patients in their populations (15.9% as opposed to 2.2% of alcohol studies and 2.7% of general mental health studies).

In a test–retest design, examining follow-up 6 mo after admission, McLellan and colleagues[113] reported on efficacy of treatment using the

Addiction Severity Index (ASI).[82] Information was obtained from three treatment sites:

1. A Veterans Administration outpatient clinic sample (N = 57 males),
2. 15 male and 22 male alcohol-dependent patients and 15 female and 8 male drug-dependent patients at a private clinic, and
3. 11 male and 10 male alcohol-dependent patients and 24 female and 19 male drug-dependent patients from a rehabilitation facility.

Follow-up interviews at 6 mo postadmission used the ASI. However, only 84% (N = 151) of the patients could be contacted for follow-up interviews. The best predictor of a patient's overall status at follow-up was the ASI psychiatric severity rating at treatment admission. It should be noted, however, that these findings were generalized to both male and female patients in both the alcohol and drug abuse treatment samples.

Beck and colleagues[114] assessed hopelessness using the Beck Hopelessness Scale, which was administered to 20 alcoholic and 20 heroin addicted women engaged in outpatient treatment at a large community mental health center. The classification estimates yielded by analysis for test samples correctly assigned 18 out of 20 women to their type of substance abuse.

The Beck Hopelessness Scale is a 20-item self-report instrument that evaluates negative future expectancies. Total scores can range from 0–20, with yes or no answers for each question. The mean hopelessness score for alcohol-dependent women was 7.3, and 8.3 for heroin-dependent women. The means indicated moderate levels of hopelessness for both groups. However, answers provided by alcohol-dependent women indicated that they perceived a better chance for succeeding in the future. Five items distinguished between alcohol-dependent women and heroin-addicted women, including expected quality of life 10 yr hence, accomplishments, future success, inability to attain goals, and anticipation of future pleasant events. Alcohol-dependent women were more hopeful about the content of the next decade and expected greater success in the future in general.[114] Although the authors interpreted these results as an argument for cognitive therapy focused toward rectifying dysfunctional thoughts, it is also possible that heroin-dependent women may have experienced more adverse consequences of substance abuse and, accordingly, made a realistic assessment of their possible futures.

Brunswick and Messeri studied response to treatment in 43 male and 26 female young adult Black heroin users.[115] As measured by abstinence, treatment had a significantly greater effect on women. However, women had entered treatment later than men, and had higher rates of fertility, school dropout, and resort to "hustling" to support their addiction. One possible interpretation of women's more favorable treatment outcome may stem from helpful social supports provided by therapeutic relationships.

Underhill identified numerous factors relevant to treatment programs for women.[116] According to Underhill, the greater societal stigma attached to women with alcohol problems manifests itself in lower self-esteem, a factor that persists as women recover. For this reason, highly confrontative techniques were considered counterproductive. She also emphasized that information about the concept of learned helplessness, assertiveness and recognition of negative affect, such as anger, should be a portion of education for women involved in alcohol treatment programs. Other relevant issues include prevalence of sexual abuse, including incest, physical abuse, and sexual assault. It has been estimated that the prevalence of these events in the histories of women seeking treatment for substance abuse dependence may range from 40–74%. Some have argued that women's unique experiences are best treated in the context of same sex groups, whereas others contend that the shared experience of substance abuse can be effectively handled in groups including both men and women. Others have also suggested that men are more expressive of emotional problems in mixed groups and accordingly receive nurturing support from women, the net result being that men improve whereas women do not. This topic requires additional consideration.

Conclusions

A number of factors can be repeatedly identified among problems related to substance abuse in men and women. These include sociocultural factors, biological factors, and pharmacologic effects of substances. All of these factors can and do interact to exacerbate substance abuse problems.

1. Predisposing cultural factors. There is evidence for and against cause-and-effect relationships between life crises and substance use. Accordingly, those who counsel women experiencing stress should be aware of potential risk for substance abuse. Preventative strategies would include increasing awareness of human tendencies to alleviate psychic pain through use of alcohol or drugs, and providing alternative means for problem solving. It is also important to examine the social influence of male partners, to consider the environmental distortions that accompany a family history of alcoholism or other substance abuse, and to assess the impact of life stressors. Socioeconomic factors and social class status also cannot be discounted.
2. Predisposing biological risk factors. There is evidence that biological factors, which include effects of family history of alcoholism and other substance abuse, comorbidity with other psychological disorders, such as

depression, anxiety, and eating disorders, as well as reproductive dysfunctions, have a role in promotion and perpetuation of women's substance abuse. Further, the dysphoria that accompanies heavy consumption also has a significant impact on psychosocial factors. The disruption of reproductive function associated with excessive intake is an additional burden. Socioeconomic status, as reflected in nutritional status, also can exert an influence on biological factors as well as pharmacological effects.

3. Predisposing pharmacological factors. While pharmacological effects of substances may appear more clear-cut than sociocultural or biological factors, all intersect. Reproductive dysfunction may be pre-existing, as in some cases of infertility, but also may be exacerbated by substance abuse.[47] Family history of alcoholism may affect perception of sensitivity to alcohol and other substances,[10,90] and also may alter mood states associated with consumption.[117] In one key study, Birnbaum and coworkers found that even social drinkers who became abstinent during a 90-d study reported improved moods after cessation of drinking.[118] Comorbidity with other psychological disorders is also important.[1,83,98,109,119]

With all of these interacting factors, it is important to choose appropriate junctures for intervention. One salient issue pertains to family history of alcoholism. It has been asserted that close to 28 million individuals in the United States,[120,121] slightly more than half of whom may be female,[56] constitute a large population at risk for alcohol and substance abuse. Since this legacy can include domestic violence, and is believed by some to foster associations with men who also have substance abuse problems, the sheer magnitude of this population invites educational initiatives.

Further, Cloninger and coworkers have argued that the prevalence of family history of alcoholism is increasing in response to a secular trend that has been facilitated by greater overall alcohol consumption in American society.[8] Reich and coworkers suggested there is increasing prevalence of Type II alcoholism in young women.[61] There may be a relationship between inheritance of Type II alcoholism and reproductive dysfunction since daughters of Type II alcoholic men have increased abdominal pain.[8,59,122] Our own work with women civilly committed to receive treatment[38,48] found a substantial number of women with both family history of alcoholism, polysubstance dependence, hormonal disruption and reproductive dysfunction, lower socioeconomic status, and encounters with the criminal justice system. Some of them had been victims of violence, including rape and incest, and all had experienced heavy consumption and accompanying dysphoria. However, the optimal time to intervene was much earlier in their lifetime.

Strategies for prevention of child abuse related to substance-abuse include strengthening the system of prenatal care delivery that is targeted to high-risk communities. In addition, there may be positive benefits to alcohol and drug prevention programs targeted to 11th and 12th graders. However, since young women who drop out of school may be at higher risk, special attention through outreach should be addressed to their needs. Moreover, reproductive dysfunctions accompany use of alcohol, marijuana, cocaine, and opiates.[38,47,48] Other efforts require increased access to prenatal care, especially for minority women, as well as ongoing healthcare, social services, daycare, and employment, and financial assistance services.

Necessary Research

The following suggested topics are by no means exhaustive, but point in directions that can further illuminate gender differences in substance abuse:

1. It is imperative to establish a useful database for substance abuse research and intervention programs. Differentiation of subjects by gender in cross-sectional, point prevalence, treated prevalence, longitudinal, and outcome studies is a basic need.
2. Effects of substances on the neuroendocrine system in both women and men must be studied in order to address a poorly explored topic that is likely to prove integral in treatment as awareness of dysfunctions increases.
3. More individuals are presenting for treatment with dual diagnoses, either polysubstance use and/or another axis I disorder, or an axis II disorder, especially antisocial personality disorder. Substance use by patients with other DSM–III–R categories of psychological disorders will continue to require greater attention, and use of alcohol or other substances to palliate psychological distress will continue to require study. Such patients require thorough comprehensive evaluation and treatment. Basic epidemiological and laboratory research can examine efficacy of various treatment modalities via analysis of outcome data.
4. Both familial/genetic and environmental variables are important factors in substance use by women and men. However, "nature–nurture" discussions engender fruitless debate since substance abuse is multidetermined and a major strategy for analysis should examine a broad spectrum of factors of which there is limited understanding.
5. It is unlikely that the substances used, substance consumption patterns, research strategies, or treatment approaches will attain equilibrium. Changing patterns of substance use will present a continuing challenge to clinicians that can be met in part by ongoing epidemiological and laboratory research.
6. Substance use affects all life areas and costs to individuals and society for rehabilitation are almost incalculable. Contributions to knowledge about primary prevention should be a goal for both basic and applied scientists and treatment specialists. Cooperation among all whose work touches on substance abuse is a prerequisite, since clinicians and applied scientists both interpret and guide treatment and research needs.

Acknowledgments

This work was supported in part by grants AA 06252 and AA 06792 from the National Institute on Alcohol Abuse and Alcoholism and DA 02905, DA 04059, DA 00101, DA 00064, and DA 04870 from the National Institute on Drug Abuse. Carol Buchanan prepared the manuscript, Lynne Wighton assisted with the references, and Jennifer Stevens provided editorial assistance.

References

[1]N. K. Mello (1983) Etiological theories of alcoholism, in *Advances in Substance Abuse*, vol 3. N. K. Mello, ed. JAI, Greenwich, CT, pp. 271–312.

[2]K. M. Fillmore (1984) "When angels fall;" Women's drinking as cultural preoccupation and as reality, in *Alcohol Problems in Women: Antecedents, Consequences, and Intervention*. S. C. Wilsnack and L. J. Beckman, eds. Guilford, New York, pp. 7–36.

[3]R. L. Clayton, H. L. Voss, C. Robbins, and W. F. Skinner (1986) Gender differences in drug use: An epidemiological perspective, in *Women and Drugs: A New Era for Research*. B. A. Ray and M. C. Braude, eds. US Government Printing Office, Washington, DC, pp. 80–99.

[4]B. W. Lex (1985) Alcohol problems in special populations, in *The Diagnosis and Treatment of Alcoholism*, 2nd ed. J. H. Mendelson and N. K. Mello, eds. McGraw-Hill, New York, pp. 89–187.

[5]N. K. Mello (1980) Some behavioral and biological aspects of alcohol problems in women, in *Alcohol and Drug Problems in Women*. O. J. Kalant, ed. Plenum, New York, pp. 263–312.

[6]J. Mondanaro (1989) *Chemically Dependent Women: Assessment and Treatment*. D. C. Heath, Lexington, MA.

[7]M. Bohman, S. Sigvardsson, and C. R. Cloninger (1981) Maternal inheritance of alcohol abuse cross-fostering analysis of adopted women. *Arch. Gen. Psychiatry* **38,** 965–969.

[8]C. R. Cloninger, S. Sigvardsson, T. Reich, and M. Bohman (1986) Inheritance risk to develop alcoholism, in *Genetic and Biological Markers in Drug Abuse and Alcoholism*. M. C. Braude and H. M. Chao, eds. US Government Printing Office, Washington, DC, pp. 86–96.

[9]M. N. Hesselbrock, V. M. Hesselbrock, and T. F. Babor (1984) Antisocial behavior, psychopathology and problem drinking in the natural history of alcoholism, in *Longitudinal Research in Alcoholism*. D. W. Goodwin, K. T. V. Dusen, and S. A. Mednick, eds. Kluwer-Nijhoff, Boston, pp. 197–214.

[10]M. A. Schuckit (1984) Subjective responses to alcohol in sons of alcoholics and control subjects. *Arch. Gen. Psychiatry* **42,** 879–884.

[11]K. W. Wanberg and J. L. Horn (1970) Alcoholism symptom pattern of men and women. *Q. J. Stud. Alcohol* **31,** 40–61.

[12]J. Curlee (1970) A comparison of male and female patients at an alcoholism treatment center. *J. Psychol.* **74,** 239–247.

[13]L. J. Beckman (1976) Alcoholism problems and women: An overview, in *Alcoholism Problems in Women and Children*. M. Greenblatt, and M. A. Schuckit, eds. Grune & Stratton, New York, pp. 65–96.

[14]M. A. Schuckit and E. R. Morrissey (1976) Alcoholism in women: Some clinical and social perspectives with an emphasis on possible subtypes, in *Alcoholism Problems in Women and Children.* M. Greenblatt and M. A. Schuckit, eds. Grune & Stratton, New York, pp. 5–35.

[15]S. Waller and B. Lorch (1978) Social and psychological characteristics of alcoholics: A male-female comparison. *Int. J. Addict.* **13,** 201–212.

[16]S. Blume (1980) Clinical research: Casefinding, diagnosis, treatment and rehabilitation, in *Alcohol and Women.* US Government Printing Office, Washington, DC, pp. 121–149.

[17]E. S. Gomberg (1980) Risk factors related to alcohol problems among women, in *Alcohol and Women.* US Government Printing Office, Washington, DC, pp. 83–120.

[18]H. B. Braiker (1982) The diagnosis and treatment of alcoholism in women, in *Special Population Issues.* US Government Printing Office, Washington, DC, pp. 111–139.

[19]J. L. Horn and K. W. Wanberg (1969) Symptoms patterns related to excessive use of alcohol. *Q. J. Stud. Alcohol* **30,** 35-38.

[20]N. H. Rathod and I. G. Thompson (1971) Women alcoholics: Clinical study. *Q. J. Stud. Alcohol* **32,** 45–52.

[21]J. Rimmer, F. N. Pitts, T. Reich, and G. Winokur (1971) Alcoholism II: Sex, socioeconomic status, and race in two hospitalized samples. *Q. J. Stud. Alcohol* **32,** 942–952.

[22]J. S. Tamerin, A. Tolor, and B. Harrington (1976) Sex differences in alcoholics: A comparison of male and female alcoholics, self and spouse perceptions. *Am. J. Drug Alcohol Abuse* **3,** 457–472.

[23]L. Dahlgren (1978) Female alcoholics III. Development and pattern of problem drinking. *Act. Pscychiat. Scand.* **57,** 325–335.

[24]J. S. Gavaler (1988) Effects of moderate consumption of alcoholic beverages on endocrine function in post-menoposal women: Bases for hypotheses, in *Recent Developments in Alcoholism*, vol. 6. M. Galanter, ed. Plenum, New York, pp. 229–251.

[25]N. K. Mello (1988) Effects of alcohol abuse on reproductive function in women, in *Recent Developments in Alcoholism,* vol. 6. M. Galanter, ed. Plenum, New York, pp. 253–276.

[26]D. H. Van Theil and J. S. Gavaler (1988) Ethanol metabolism and hepatotoxicity: Does sex make a difference? in *Recent Developments in Alcoholism*, vol. 6. M. Galanter, ed. Plenum, New York, pp. 291–304.

[27]S. B. Blume (1986) Women and alcohol: A review. *JAMA* **256,** 1467–1470.

[28]A. Halliday, B. Booker, P. Cleary, M. Aronson, and T. Delbanco (1986) Alcohol abuse in women seeking gynecologic care. *Obstet. Gynec.* **68,** 322–326.

[29]S. C. Wilsnack, R. W. Wilsnack, and A. D. Klassen (1984) Drinking and drinking problems among women in a U.S. national survey. *Alcohol. Health Res. World* **9,** 3–13.

[30]S. E. Fisher and P. I. Karl (1988) Maternal ethanol use and selective fetal malnutrition, in *Recent Developments in Alcoholism*, vol. 6. M. Galanter, ed. Plenum, New York, pp. 277–289.

[31]M. J. Kreek (1987) Multiple drug abuse patterns and medical consequences, in *Psychopharmacology: The Third Generation of Progress.* H. Y. Meltzer, ed. Raven, New York, pp. 1597–1604.

[32]E. Bromet and R. Moos (1976) Sex and marital status in relation to the characteristics of alcoholics. *J. Stud. Alcohol* **37,** 1302–1312.

[33]J. Orford and A. Keddie (1985) Gender differences in the functions and effects of moderate and excessive drinking. *Br. J. Clin. Psychol.* **24,** 265–279.

[34]S. Crawford and D. Ryder (1986) A study of sex differences in cognitive impairment in alcoholics using traditional and computer-based tests. *Drug Alcohol Depend.* **18,** 369–375.

[35]L. J. Beckman and H. Amaro (1986) Personal and social difficulties faced by women and men entering alcoholism treatment. *J. Stud. Alcohol* **47,** 135–145.

[36]T. R. Kosten, B. J. Rounsaville, and H. D. Kleber (1985) Parental alcoholism in opioid addicts. *J. Nerv. Mental Dis.* **173,** 461–469.

[37]D. P. Parrella and W. J. Filstead (1988) Definition of onset in the development of onset-based alcoholism typologies. *J. Stud. Alcohol* **49,** 85–92.

[38]S. K. Teoh, B. W. Lex, J. Cochin, J. H. Mendelson, and N. K. Mello (1989) Anterior pituitary gonadal and adrenal hormones in women with alcohol and polydrug abuse, 60th Anniversary Fifty-First Annual Scientific Meeting Abstracts, The Committee on Problems of Drug Dependence, Inc., Keystone, CO.

[39]J. N. Hugues, T. Coste, G. Pettet, M. F. Jayle, J. Sebaoun, and E. Modigliani (1980) Hypothalamo-pituitary ovarian function in thirty-one women with chronic alcoholism. *Clin. Endocrinol.* **12,** 543–551.

[40]M. Russell and L. Bigler (1979) Screening for alcohol-related problems in an outpatient obstretric-gynecologic clinic. *Am. J. Obstet. Gynec.* **134,** 4–12.

[41]R. W. Wilsnack, A. D. Klassen, and S. C. Wilsnack (1986) Retrospective analysis of lifetime changes in women's drinking behavior. *Adv. Alcohol Subst. Abuse* **5,** 9–28.

[42]U. Becker, H. Tønnesen, N. Kaas-Claesson, and C. Gluud (1989) Menstrual disturbances and fertility in chronic alcoholic women. *Drug Alcohol Depend.* **24,** 75–82.

[43]C. G. Smith and R. H. Asch (1987) Drug abuse and reproduction. *Fertility Sterility* **48,** 355–373.

[44]National Institute on Drug Abuse (1989) National household survey on drug abuse: 1988 cross-sectional data, in *HHS News,* August, 1989. U.S. Department of Health and Human Services, Washington, DC, pp. 1–4.

[45]D. Busch, A. B. McBride, and L. M. Benaventura (1986) Chemical dependency in women: The link to ob/gyn problems. *J. Psychosoc. Nurs.* **24,** 26–30.

[46]M. L. Selzer (1971) The Michigan Alcoholism Screening Test: The quest for a new diagnostic instrument. *Am. J. Psychiatry* **127,** 1653–1658.

[47]N. K. Mello, J. H. Mendelson, and S. K. Teoh (1989) Neuroendorine consequences of alcohol abuse in women. *Ann. NY Acad. Sci.* **562,** 211–240.

[48]B. W. Lex, S. K. Teoh, I. Lagomasino, N. K. Mello, and J. H. Mendelson (1990) Characteristics of women receiving mandated treatment for alcohol or polysubstance dependence in Massachusetts. *Drug Alcohol Depend.* **25,** 13–20.

[49]E. M. Smith, C. R. Cloninger, and S. Bradford (1983) Predictors of mortality in alcoholic women: A prospective follow-up study. *Alcohol. Clin. Exp. Res.* **7,** 237–243.

[50]P. C. Whitehead and N. Layne (1987) Young female Canadian drinkers: Employment, marital status and heavy drinking. *Br. J. Addict.* **82,** 169–174.

[51]M. Frezza, C. di Padova, G. Pozzato, M. Terpin, E. Baraona, and C. S. Lieber (1990) The role of decreased gastric alcohol dehydrogenase activity and first-pass metabolism. *N. Engl. J. Med.* **322,** 95–99.

[52]J. B. Whitfield, G. A. Starmer, and N. G. Martin (1990) Alcohol metabolism in men and women. *Alcohol Clin. Exp. Res.* **14,** 785–786.

[53]National Institute on Drug Abuse (1985) National Household Survey on Drug Abuse: Main Findings 1985. US Government Printing Office, Washington, DC.

[54]C. Robbins (1989) Sex differences in psychosocial consequences of alcohol and drug abuse. *J. Health Soc. Behav.* **30,** 117–130.

[55]B. Haver (1987) Female alcoholic V: The relationship between family history of alcoholism and outcome 3-10 years after treatment. *Act. Psychiat. Scand.* **76,** 21–27.

[56]L. Midanik (1983) Familial alcoholism and problem drinking in a national drinking practices survey. *Addict. Behav.* **8,** 133–141.

[57]T. McKenna and R. Pickens (1981) Alcoholic children of alcoholics. *J. Stud. Alcohol* **42,** 1021–1029.

[58]B. Haver (1987) Female alcoholics IV: The relationship between family violence and outcome 3-10 years after treatment. *Act. Psychiat. Scand.* **75,** 449–455.

[59]C. R. Cloninger, M. Bohman, S. Sigvardsson, and A. L. von Knorring (1985) Psychopathology in adopted-out children of alcoholics: The Stockholm adoption study, in *Recent Developments in Alcoholism*, vol. 6. M. Galanter, ed. Plenum, New York, pp. 37–51.

[60]L. N. Robins, J. E. Helzer, M. M. Weissman, H. Orvaschel, E. Gruenberg, J. D. Burker Jr., and D. A. Regier (1984) Lifetime prevalence of specific psychiatric disorders in three sites. *Arch. Gen. Psychiatry* **41,** 949–958.

[61]T. Reich, C. R. Cloninger, P. Van Eerdewegh, J. P. Rice, and J. Mullaney (1988) Secular trends in the familial transmission of alcoholism. *Alcohol. Clin. Exp. Res.* **12,** 458–464.

[62]J. Feighner, E. Robins, and S. B. Guze (1972) Diagnostic criteria for use in psychiatric research. *Arch. Gen. Psychiatry* **26,** 57–63.

[63]M. M. Kilbey and J. P. Sobeck (1988) Epidemiology of alcoholism, in *Women and Health Psychology*. C. B. Travis, ed. Erlbaum, Hillsdale, NJ, pp. 91–107.

[64]E. S. Lisansky (1957) Alcoholism in women: Social and psychological concomitants. *Q. J. Stud. Alcohol* **18,** 588–623.

[65]S. Vaglum and P. Vaglum (1987) Partner relations and the development of alcoholism in female psychiatric patients. *Act. Psychiat. Scand.* **76,** 499–506.

[66]T. Jacob and D. A. Bremer (1986) Assortative mating among men and women alcoholics. *J. Stud. Alcohol* **47,** 219–222.

[67]R. L. Spitzer, J. Endicott, and E. Robins (1978) *Research Diagnostic Criteria (RDC) for a Selected Group of Functional Disorders*. New York State Psychiatric Institute, New York.

[68]B. W. Lex (1990) Male heroin addicts and their female mates: Impact on disorder and recovery. *J. Subst. Abuse* **2,** 147–175.

[69]E. S. L. Gomberg and R. Schilit (1985) Social isolation and passivity of women alcoholics. *Alcohol Alcohol.* **20,** 313–314.

[70]C. A. Allan and D. Cooke (1986) Women, life events and drinking problems. *Br. J. Psychiatry* **148,** 462.

[71]E. R. Morrisey and M. A. Schuckit (1978) Stressful life events and alcohol problems among women seen at a detoxication center. *J. Stud. Alcohol* **39,** 1559–1576.

[72]M. Remy, S. Soukup-Stepan, and A. Tatossian (1987) A new use of life event questionnaires: Study of the life events world of a population of male and female alcoholics. *Soc. Psychiatry* **22,** 49–57.

[73]J. Leland (1982) Sex roles, family organization, and alcohol abuse, in *Alcohol and the Family*. J. Orford and J. Harwin, eds. Croom Helm, London, pp. 88–113.

[74]L. J. Beckman (1975) Women alcoholics: A review of social psychological studies. *J. Stud. Alcohol* **36,** 799–823.

[75]J. Scida and M. Vannicelli (1979) Sex-role conflict and women's drinking. *J. Stud. Alcohol* **40,** 28–44.

[76]G. Knupfer (1982) Problems associated with drunkenness in women: Some research issues, in *Special Population Issues*. US Government Printing Office, Washington, DC, pp. 3–39.

[77]C. Kroft and P. Leichner (1987) Sex-role conflicts in alcoholic women. *Int. J. Addict.* **22,** 685–693.

[78]Y. I. Hser, M. D. Anglin, and W. McGlothlin (1987) Sex differences in addict careers. 1. Initiation of use. *Am. J. Drug Alcohol Abuse* **13,** 33–57.

[79]M. D. Anglin, Y. I. Hser, and W. H. McGlothlin (1987) Sex differences in addict careers. 2. Becoming addicted. *Am. J. Drug Alcohol Abuse* **13,** 59–71.

[80]Y. I. Hser, M. D. Anglin, and M. W. Booth (1987) Sex differences in addict careers. 3. Addiction. *Am. J. Drug Alcohol Abuse* **13,** 231–251.

[81]M. D. Anglin, Y. I. Hser, and M. W. Booth (1987) Sex differences in addict careers. 4. Treatment. *Am J Drug Alcohol Abuse* **13,** 253–280.

[82]A. T. McLellan, L. Luborsky, G. E. Woody, and C. P. O'Brien (1980) An improved diagnostic evaluation instrument for substance abuse patients. The addiction severity index. *J. Nerv. Mental Dis.* **168,** 26–33.

[83]M. L. Griffin, R. D. Weiss, S. M. Mirin, and U. Lange (1989) A comparison of male and female cocaine abusers. *Arch. Gen. Psychiatry* **46,** 122–126.

[84]T. R. Kosten, B. J. Rounsaville, and H. D. Kleber (1986) Ethnic and gender differences among opiate addicts. *Int. J. Addict.* **20,** 1143–1162.

[85]M. N. Hesselbrock, R. E. Meyer, and J. J. Keener (1985) Psychopathology in hospitalized alcoholics. *Arch. Gen. Psychiatry* **42,** 1050–1055.

[86]T. F. Babor, J. H. Mendelson, I. Greenberg, and J. C. Kuehnle (1975) Marihuana consumption and tolerance to physiological and subjective effects. *Arch. Gen. Psychiatry* **32,** 1548–1552.

[87]T. F. Babor, B. W. Lex, J. H. Mendelson, and N. K. Mello (1984) Marijuana, effect and tolerance: A study of subchronic self-administration in women, in *Problems of Drug Dependence 1983*. L. S. Harris, ed. US Government Printing Office, Washington, DC, pp. 199–204.

[88]B. W. Lex, S. L. Palmieri, N. K. Mello, and J. H. Mendelson (1987) Alcohol use, marijuana smoking, and sexual activity in women. *Alcohol* **5,** 21–25.

[89]B. W. Lex, M. L. Griffin, N. K. Mello, and J. H. Mendelson (1986) Concordant alcohol and marihuana use in women. *Alcohol* **3,** 193–200.

[90]B. W. Lex, S. E. Lukas, N. E. Greenwald, and J. H. Mendelson (1988) Alcohol-induced changes in body sway in women at risk for alcoholism: A pilot study. *J. Stud. Alcohol.* **49,** 346–356.

[91]B. W. Lex, M. L. Griffin, N. K. Mello, and J. H. Mendelson (1989) Alcohol, marijuana, and mood states in young women. *Int. J. Addict.* **24,** 405–424.

[92]S. Mirin, L. Shapiro, R. Meyer, R. Pillard, and S. Fisher (1971) Casual versus heavy use of marijuana: A redefinition of the marijuana problem. *Am. J. Psychiatry* **127,** 1134–1140.

[93]C. Bruns and C. Geist (1984) Stressful life events and drug use among adolescents. *J. Human Stress* **10,** 135–139.

[94]D. B. Kandel (1984) Marijuana users in young adulthood. *Arch. Gen. Psychiatry* **41,** 200–209.

95D. B. Kandel, M. Davies, D. Karus, and K. Yamaguchi (1986) The consequences in your adulthood of adolescent drug involvement. *Arch. Gen. Psychiatry* **43,** 746–754.

96S. Paton, R. Kessler, and D. Kandell (1977) Depressive mood and illicit drug use: A longitudinal analysis. *J. Genet. Psychol.* **131,** 267–289.

97E. M. Corrigan (1985) Gender differences in alcohol and other drug use. *Addict. Behav.* **10,** 313–317.

98J. E. Turnbull (1988) Primary and secondary alcoholic women. *Soc. Casework J. Contemp. Soc. Work* **69,** 290–297.

99L. Y. Silvia, G. T. Sorell, and N. A. Busch-Rossnagel (1988) Biopsychosocial discriminators of alcoholic and nonalcoholic women. *J. Subst. Abuse* **1,** 55–65.

100M. Bohman, C. R. Cloninger, A.-L. von Knorring, and S. Sigvardsson (1984) An adoption study of somatoform disorder. III. Cross-fostering analysis and genetic relationship to alcoholism and criminality. *Arch. Gen. Psychiatry* **41,** 872–878.

101M. Vannicelli and L. Nash (1984) Effect of sex bias on women's studies on alcoholism. *Alcohol Clin. Exp. Res.* **8,** 334–336.

102M. Vannicelli (1984) Barriers to treatment of alcoholic women. *Subst. Alcohol Actions/Misuses* **5,** 29–37.

103F. Duckert (1987) Recruitment into treatment and effects of treatment for female problem drinkers. *Addict. Behav.* **12,** 137–150.

104C. Allan and M. Phil (1987) Seeking help for drinking problems from a community-based voluntary agency: Patterns of compliance amongst men and women. *Br. J. Addict.* **82,** 1143–1147.

105B. Thom (1986) Sex differences in help-seeking for alcohol problems: 1. The barriers to help-seeking. *Br. J. Addict.* **81,** 777–786.

106B. Thom (1987) Sex differences in help-seeking for alcohol problems: 2. Entry into treatment. *Br. J. Addict.* **82,** 989–997.

107S. D. Robinson (1984) Women and alcohol abuse—factors involved in successful interventions. *Int. J. Addict.* **19,** 601–611.

108L. J. Beckman and K. M. Kocel (1982) The treatment-delivery system and alcohol abuse in women: social policy implications. *J. Soc. Issues* **38,** 139–151.

109H. E. Ross, F. B. Glaser, and S. Stiansy (1988) Sex differences in the prevalence of psychiatric disorders in patients with alcohol and drug problems. *Br. J. Addict.* **83,** 1179–1192.

110B. M. Herr and H. M. Pettinati (1984) Long term outcome in working and homemaking alcoholic women. *Alcohol Clin. Exp. Res.* **8,** 576–579.

111B. Haver (1987) Female alcoholics: III. Patterns of consumption 3–10 years after treatment. *Acta Psychiatr. Scand.* **75,** 397–404.

112M. S. Goldstein, M. Surber, and D. M. Wilner (1984) Outcome evaluations in substance abuse: A comparison of alcoholism, drug abuse and other mental health interventions. *Int. J. Addict.* **19,** 479–502.

113A. T. McLellan, L. Luborsky, and C. P. O'Brien (1986) Alcohol and drug abuse treatment in three different populations: Is there improvement and is it predictable? *Am. J. Drug Alcohol Abuse* **12,** 101–120.

114A. T. Beck, R. A. Steer, and B. F. Shaw (1984) Hopelessness in alcohol- and heroin-dependent women. *J. Clin. Psychol.* **40,** 602–606.

115A. F. Brunswick and P. A. Messeri (1986) Pathways to heroin abstinence: A longitudinal study of urban Black youth. *Adv. Alcohol Subst. Abuse* **5,** 103–122.

[116]B. L. Underhill (1986) Issues relevant to aftercare programs for women. *Alcohol Health Res. World* **11,** 46–48.

[117]B. W. Lex (1990) Anthropological insights on substance abuse. Paper presented at annual meeting of the American Anthropological Association, Washington, DC.

[118]L. M. Birnbaum, T. H. Taylor, and E. S. Parker (1983) Alcohol and sober mood state in female social drinkers. *Alcohol. Clin. Exp. Res.* **7,** 362–368.

[119]N. K. Mello (1983) A behavioral analysis of the reinforcing properties of alcohol and other drugs in man, in *The Pathogenesis of Alcoholism, Biological Factors*, vol. 7. B. Kissin and H. Begleiter, eds. Plenum, New York, pp. 133–198.

[120]M. Woodside (1988) Research on children of alcoholics: Past and future. *Br. J. Addict.* **83,** 785–792.

[121]M. Russell, C. Henderson, and S. B. Blume (1985) *Children of Alcoholics: A Review of the Literature.* Children of Alcoholics Foundation, New York.

[122]C. R. Cloninger, B. Bohman, and S. Sigvardsson (1981) Inheritance of alcohol abuse cross-fostering analysis of adopted men. *Arch. Gen Psychiatry* **38,** 861–868.

Service Needs of Injection Drug Users

Gender and Racial Differences

Diane A. Mathis,* Helen A. Navaline, David S. Metzger, and Jerome J. Platt

Introduction

A number of recent investigations have focused on the treatment needs of injection drug users (IDUs); especially with regard to gender and ethnic/racial differences. The results of those studies indicate that female IDUs represent a large portion of the addicted population, and have particular treatment needs that differ from their male counterparts. In addition, those treatment needs often vary among ethnic and racial groups. In order to elucidate the service needs of IDUs, data is presented from a recent study that compares the gender and racial differences in characteristics and service utilization of subjects in methadone treatment. The results of that study parallel other research, and indicate that gender and racial differences are important factors to consider in the development of effective treatment programs.

Female Opiate Use

Historical Perspective

Opiate addiction among women is not a new phenomenon. Significant numbers of women were addicted to powdered morphine sulfate and other opiates during the late 1800s. In fact, during this period, the number of

*Deceased.

From: *Drug and Alcohol Abuse Reviews, Vol. 5: Addictive Behaviors in Women*
Ed.: R. R. Watson ©1994 Humana Press Inc., Totowa, NJ

women addicted to opiates was nearly twice the number of addicted men.[1-3] Generally, this opiate use by females occurred under the advice of a physician for the treatment of physical or psychological disorders, or as self-medication with the patent medicines and "tonics" that were then widely available.[4] Following the passage of the Harrison Act in 1914, which outlawed the previously widespread use of nonprescription opiates, the opiate addict's social role was changed; it was now criminalized. This change was followed by a substantial shift in the gender of the opiate addict population. After 1914, the number of women using opiates decreased, and the overwhelming majority of new addicts were men.

Current Estimates of Frequency

However, since the 1960s, reports indicate that opiate use has increased at a higher rate among women than among men.[5] The actual number of female opiate users in the population is unknown, and estimated from the frequency of female IDUs in drug treatment. Until about 1970, the proportion of female opiate users in treatment was approx 20%; by the mid 1980s, this number had increased to 30%.[6] However, as discussed later in this chapter, the percentage of women in treatment for opiate addiction may be an underestimate of the proportion of women iv drug users in the general population.[7]

Methadone Treatment Services

Goals

Methadone treatment has become a primary modality for the treatment of chronic opiate dependence. Its purpose now extends beyond merely reducing opiate and other drug use, into areas of social and vocational rehabilitation,[8] as well as psychological stabilization.[9] Thus, methadone programs must deal with various levels of problem severity within a wide range of physical, psychological, and social problems.

Shortcomings

Although a number of services and adjunctive therapies have been attempted as potential aids in treating a range of needs for the IDU, investigations directed at the efficacy of these services and therapies,[10-15] have shown that two important problems confront the field: (1) available services are often not utilized by patients; and (2) services that are delivered may not meet the client's needs.[16,17] Thus, an increasing amount of investigative attention has been directed at developing methods for matching program treatments with the addict's needs.[18] Particular interest has been focused on identifying the needs of gender and racial subgroups within the overall patient population.[19-21]

The Need for Gender and Racial Typologies

HIV Infection and Transmission

One reason for a focus on subgroups within the IDU treatment population has been the outcome of studies directed at identifying those at risk for HIV infection and transmission. With the advent of the AIDS epidemic and the implementation of the National AIDS Demonstration Research (NADR) programs throughout the United States, female IDUs have been increasingly identified as a population that requires significant attention. In 1987, the Centers for Disease Control reported that among all females who have AIDS, 50% contracted it through iv drug use. In addition, HIV seropositivity for female IDUs is significantly higher among Black addicts than among other racial or ethnic groups,[22,23] and their death rate in 1988 was nine times the rate of White women.[24]

As IDUs, women are not only at high risk for contracting AIDS; but, they are also at high risk for spreading it through sexual activity or childbirth. HIV seropositivity transmitted through heterosexual contact is reported with increasing frequency.[25-28] In addition, infants born to HIV-infected mothers have an estimated 65% risk of being HIV-infected.[29] Black children represent more than half of all pediatric AIDS cases, and the vast majority of these Black children contracted AIDS from their infected mothers.[22,30]

Methadone Program Design and Utilization

An outcome of investigations that specifically focused on female IDUs was the growing realization that females were not utilizing treatment services, and that methadone programs may not be providing the specific services that meet the needs of female addicts. As suggested earlier, determinations of the proportion of female IDUs in the general population that are based on the percentage of females in treatment may underestimate the actual frequency of female iv drug use; i.e., females are apparently underrepresented in the treatment population.[7] The reason for this underrepresentation may reflect a general inadequacy of methadone treatment programs to serve the needs of female IDUs.[31,32]

For example, female addicts frequently have more psychological symptoms of distress than male addicts.[33-35] Yet, Ball and Ross[16] reported that psychiatric services were not commonly received among their overall sample of IDUs in methadone treatment. In addition, females entering drug treatment often leave the program before any beneficial effects can be obtained,[36,37] and several studies describe female addicts as more difficult to treat than males.[38] But, the tendency for females to reject treatment, and the problems encountered in treating them, may be due to inappropriate or inadequate services that do not meet the specific needs of the female addict.[39]

Investigating Treatment Needs

Overall Findings

Considering the outcome of prior studies that have focused on the female IDU, several patterns emerge. Females tend to begin opiate use at a later age, but enter treatment earlier in their drug career than males do.[40,41,43] The psychosocial characteristics of drug-abusing females differ from those of drug-abusing males.[42–45] Females also tend to have higher rates of separation and divorce,[46] but are more likely to have childcare responsibilities.[46] At the same time, they have fewer economic and social supports, and are more likely to be unemployed and receive welfare.[40]

The Present Study

Despite the recent focus on gender and racial differences among IDUs, a thorough understanding of these differences is still needed. The study described below was conducted in order to investigate the characteristics and treatment needs of IDUs in methadone treatment. Its purposes were to differentiate between the overall typology and service utilization of male and female subjects, plus examine the differences between Black and White subjects. The results of this study, taken together with previous findings, provides an extensive characterization of the differences in treatment needs among these subgroups.

Method

Subjects

For the overall sample, subjects were 479 patients from five methadone maintenance clinics located in Philadelphia and southern New Jersey. These participants were 67.8% male and 32.2% female. The sample included 198 Blacks (73.2% male and 26.8% female), 241 Whites (64.7% males and 35.3% females), as well as 37 Hispanics (59.5% male and 40.5% female) and 3 subjects from the "Other" racial category (66.7% male and 33.3% female). This overall sample was used to analyze gender differences in the characteristics of participants in methadone treatment. For the analysis of racial differences, the sample was limited to 439 (198 Blacks, and 241 Whites).

Procedure

Recruitment of Participants

Recruitment in each of these programs was accomplished by research staff using similar procedures. Initially, administrative staff were contacted and fully briefed on the study objectives and methods. Then, counselors and other staff members were contacted to ensure that they had a clear understanding of the study. The next step involved informing patients of the study through a series of procedures, including posting notices and distributing project descriptions. Research staff were scheduled to stand near the methadone window during dispensing hours for 1 wk prior to recruiting interested subjects. This procedure gave staff the opportunity to see all patients and discuss the details of study participation with them. After recruitment, subjects were scheduled for their first data-collection session.

Questionnaire Data Collection

Each data-collection session included a group of 6–10 subjects who completed an extensive self-report questionnaire that measured basic demographics, education, sources of financial support, legal involvements, familial characteristics, substance abuse and treatment, and psychological symptomology. Psychological symptoms were also measured using the SCL-90 and Beck Depression Inventory. Data collection sessions were conducted under the supervision of research technical staff, who explained the study, secured informed consent, reviewed and monitored the rules for questionnaire completion, assisted those with language limitations, and maintained an orderly data-collection atmosphere. All subjects were paid $10.00 for the time they devoted to the study. Data collection sessions usually lasted for 1 h. Data concerning AIDS-risk behavior were collected during 6-mo follow-up sessions, and were obtained from 409 subjects.

Personal Interviews

In addition to the questionnaires, data were also collected using personal interviews with a randomly selected group of 165 participants. Selection for the personal interviews took place following the completion of all questionnaires in each clinic. Once selected, subjects were interviewed at 6 mo after initial participation in the study. Each interview included the Addiction Severity Index (ASI), and a series of questions regarding treatment services.

Data Analysis

Categorical data were analyzed by chi-square (χ^2) test of significance. Interval data were analyzed by two-tailed, Student's *t*-test for unrelated samples. When a difference between frequencies (χ^2) or means (*t*-test) exceeded the critical value of $p < .05$, it was considered to be significant. For monthly income, differences between the median incomes were tested.

Results

Women comprised about one-third (32.2%) of this sample. There were no overall or gender differences in racial composition or educational level of the sample. Subjects had completed an average of 11 yr education, with the majority (59%) having a high school diploma or GED.

Demographics

Age

The average age of the overall sample was approx 37 yr; however, females were younger than males. The average age of both Black females (36.9) and males (40.6), and White females (32.3) and males (35.7) were significantly different ($p < .01$).

Employment

Less than 30% of the subjects were currently employed. Significantly fewer White women had worked in the past year than White men ($p < .05$; *see* Table 1). For those subjects who were employed, the majority were satisfied with their job. However, significantly more White females than White males reported job satisfaction ($p < .05$); the same trend was observed among Blacks, but the gender difference was not significant. White females were significantly less likely than White males to report looking for work ($p < .01$), or wanting employment, ($p < .01$).

Sources of Financial Support

Overall, public assistance was the most frequently reported source of income for all subjects. However, White females relied on it significantly more frequently than White males ($p < .01$). Employment as a source of income was reported second most frequently, and by significantly more White males than White females ($p < .05$). Money from other sources (i.e., not from employment, welfare, social security, unemployment, or family and friends) was reported significantly more frequently by White females than White males ($p < .05$).

Criminal Involvement

For all measures of criminal involvement, males scored higher than females (Table 2). Significant differences between White males and females were found for the ASI Legal Composite Score ($p < .05$; Table 3). A large majority of the subjects reported prior arrests. Significant differences were obtained between males and females for the number of times arrested ($p < .01$). However, gender differences in having ever been arrested were only found among Whites ($p < .01$).

In addition, most subjects reported prior imprisonment. Significantly more males than females reported having ever been incarcerated ($p < .01$), and males were incarcerated for a longer period of time than females ($p < .01$). These differences were constant for both Blacks and Whites.

Table 1

Education, Employment, and Income Sources for Methadone Patients
by Race and Gender

	Black				White			
	Female		Male		Female		Male	
	%/M	(N)[a]	%/M	(N)	%/M	(N)	%/M	(N)
Highest grade								
completed (M)	11.1	(52)	11.2	(144)	11.5	(85)	11.7	(156)
Diploma (%)	39.6	(53)	55.2	(145)	71.8	(85)	73.7	(156)
Currently employed (%)	17.3	(52)	20.7	(145)	36.9	(84)	48.1	(154)
If working:								
Hours working/wk (M)	41.4	(8)	34.8	(29)	33.4	(30)	37.6	(68)*
Years at present								
job (M)	2.0	(7)	4.1	(19)*	3.5	(21)	5.0	(49)
Happy with job (%)	100	(9)	76.7	(30)	90.0	(30)	75.3	(73)
Employed past yr (%)	55.8	(52)	61.7	(141)	63.9	(83)	77.1	(153)*
Desire to work		(50)		(135)		(80)		(145)**
Not at all (%)	6.0		6.7		8.8		5.5	
Somewhat (%)	20.0		17.8		35.0		18.6	
Very much (%)	74.0		75.6		56.3		75.9	
Looking for work (%)	69.8	(43)	75.4	(114)	48.3	(58)	76.1	(92)**
Income[b]	322.0	(48)	196.0	(140)**	434.0	(76)	600.0	(137)
Sources of income		(50)		(143)		(80)		(152)
Job (%)	14.0		24.5		36.3		53.9*	
Welfare (%)	82.0		69.2		56.3		40.1*	
SSI (%)	6.0		8.4		7.5		7.9	
Unemployment (%)	0		2.1		1.3		3.3	
Family/friends (%)	2.0		1.4		7.5		5.3	
Others (%)	6.0		9.1		21.3		7.9**	
Receive food								
stamps (%)	75.0	(36)	65.6	(90)	50.6	(77)	39.2	(143)

[a]Overall sample size is 439. Smaller sample sizes for individual variables are a result of missing data.

[b]Income represents median ($) received per month. The median was chosen for this analysis because of a skewed distribution.

Symbols for level of significance in this and subsequent tables are: $*p < .05$; $**p < .01$.

Arrest rates for drug-related charges did not differ between males and females for the overall sample; however, Black males had been arrested on these charges significantly more often than Black females ($p < .01$). In contrast, court-ordered drug treatment was reported by more White males than White females ($p < .05$), but not for Black subjects. Gender and racial differences in arrest rates for alcohol-related problems were also obtained;

Table 2
Criminal Behaviors of Methadone Patients
by Race and Gender

| | Black | | | | White | | | |
| | Female | | Male | | Female | | Male | |
	%/M	(N)[a]	%/M	(N)	%/M	(N)	%/M	(N)
Ever arrested (%)	80.8	(52)	90.3	(145)	72.9	(85)	89.1	(156)**
Number lifetime arrests (M)	4.4	(48)	9.7	(133)**	4.0	(76)	6.9	(143)*
Arrests during past year (M)	.2	(49)	.5	(142)**	.6	(80)	.5	(148)
Ever incarcerated (%)	57.7	(52)	82.8	(145)**	39.3	(84)	64.7	(156)**
Months incarcerated (M)	14.6	(30)	33.3	(115)**	9.1	(28)	22.7	(85)**
Arrests on drug charges (M)	.8	(48)	3.5	(138)**	2.8	(79)	3.3	(148)
Arrested for drunk driving (%)	3.8	(52)	4.2	(144)	14.1	(85)	25.0	(156)*
Other alcohol related arrests(%)	3.8	(52)	11.8	(144)	7.1	(85)	21.8	(156)**
Court ordered to treatment (%)								
Currently	23.1	(52)	32.6	(144)	23.5	(85)	39.1	(156)*
Ever	1.9	(52)	3.4	(145)	5.9	(85)	6.4	(156)

[a]*See* footnote to Table 1.

Table 3
Average ASI Scores of Methadone Patients by Race and Gender

| | Black | | White | |
| | Female | Male | Female | Male |
	(N= 21)[a]	(N= 64)	(N= 30)	(N= 42)
Medical[b]	.41	.37	.38	.39
Employment	.88	.78	.67	.66
Legal	.08	.15	.08	.16*
Alcohol use	.10	.14	.03	.10**
Drug use	.24	.28	.30	.36*
Family/Social	.21	.19	.25	.30
Psychiatric	.28	.18*	.26	.30

[a]*See* footnote to Table 1.
[b]Composite scores are derived from Addiction Severity Index during a 6-mo follow-up interview.

only White males had been arrested significantly more often than their female counterparts ($p < .01$).

Family Status and Background

Current Status

Marital Status. The majority of the sample was unmarried. As shown in Table 4, though no overall significant differences were obtained between males and females for marital status, more White males tended to be single; more White females tended to be separated or divorced ($p < .05$).

Living Arrangement. Less than one-quarter of this sample lived alone; most lived with their minor children and/or spouse/sexual partner, followed by parents or other relatives. However, the racial differences in living arrangement of males and females differed significantly ($p < .01$). Black males tended to live alone; Black females tended to live with a sex partner.

Overall, females had more children living with them than males had ($p < .01$). This gender difference was true for both Blacks and Whites. White females also supported more children than White males did ($p < .01$). The number of children supported by males and females did not differ for Blacks.

Familial Relationships. For a majority of subjects, parents were still living. Significantly more Black females than Black males reported that their mothers were still alive ($p < .05$; Table 5). More females also reported that their fathers were living ($p < .01$); however, more females than males also did not know if their father was living.

With regard to the quality of relationship with their parents, more males reported that their relationship with their mother was excellent or good; more White females than White males reported that it was fair or that they had had no contact with her ($p < .01$). In addition, more White males reported that the relationship with their father was good; more White females reported no contact with him ($p < .05$).

Childhood Experiences

Living Arrangements. With regard to childhood experiences in living arrangements, generally no differences between male and female IDUs (regardless of race) were obtained, with one exception. Both Black and White females reported more frequently than males that they had lived in a foster home ($p < .01$).

Relatives with Alcohol Problems. For the overall sample, problems with alcohol among respondent's relatives were more prevalent than drug problems. Most of these relatives were members of the respondent's nuclear family, and fathers with alcohol problems were cited most often. More White

Table 4
Sociodemographic Characteristics of Methadone Patients by Race and Gender

| | Black | | | | White | | | |
| | Female | | Male | | Female | | Male | |
	%/M	(N)[a]	%/M	(N)	%/M	(N)	%/M	(N)
Household composition		(49)		(143)**		(77)		(151)
Alone (%)	16.3		33.6		13.0		15.9	
w/ Spouse (%)	16.3		17.5		28.6		23.8	
w/ Sex partner (%)	20.4		12.6		23.4		13.2	
w/ Parents (%)	10.2		16.8		19.5		35.1	
w/ Friends (%)	14.3		9.8		7.8		7.9	
w/ Relatives (%)	14.3		9.8		5.2		2.6	
w/ Adult children (%)	8.2		0		2.6		1.3	
Marital status		(52)		(145)		(85)		(156)*
Single (%)	40.4		37.2		22.4		39.1	
Married (%)	19.2		20.7		27.1		27.6	
Separated/divorced (%)	32.7		39.3		43.5		30.8	
Widowed (%)	7.7		2.8		7.1		2.6	
Number/children (M)	2.4	(51)	2.5	(139)	1.6	(84)	1.2	(144)**
Number/children								
you support (M)	1.7	(50)	1.2	(133)	1.4	(82)	.9	(144)**
Children living w/you (%)	71.7	(53)	36.8	(144)**	73.8	(84)	31.6	(152)**

[a]See footnote to Table 1.

females than White males ($p < .01$) reported having relatives, especially mothers or sisters ($p < .01$), with alcohol problems; Black females, more frequently than Black males, reported that they had a brother with an alcohol problem ($p < .05$).

Relatives with Drug Problems. The majority of participants reported that they had at least one family member with a drug problem; a substantial proportion reported having more than one. Most of the reported relatives with a drug problem were members of the respondent's nuclear family, with brothers and sisters cited most often. Regardless of race, more females than males reported having a sister with a drug problem ($p < .01$).

Initiation and Frequency of Substance Abuse

Drugs

Significant gender and racial differences were obtained regarding reasons for initiation of drug use ($p < .05$; Table 6). White males reported more often than White females that they started in order to "feel part of the crowd"

Table 5
Familial Relationship and Background
of Methadone Patients by Race and Gender

	Black				White			
	Female		Male		Female		Male	
	%/M	(N)[a]	%/M	(N)	%/M	(N)	%/M	(N)
Quality of marital relationship		(20)		(48)		(34)		(66)
Excellent	15.0		18.8		17.6		15.2	
Good	35.0		41.7		44.1		33.3	
Fair	20.0		27.1		14.7		33.3	
Poor	30.0		12.5		23.5		18.2	
Mother living		(53)		(145)*		(85)		(155)
Yes	77.4		63.4		80.0		83.2	
No	20.8		36.6		18.8		16.8	
Don't know	1.9		0		1.2		0	
Maternal relationship		(42)		(101)		(70)		(131)**
Excellent	42.9		43.6		25.7		35.9	
Good	26.2		42.6		34.3		43.5	
Fair	21.4		10.9		21.4		12.2	
Poor	2.4		0		8.6		7.6	
No contact	7.1		3.0		10.0		.8	
Father living		(53)		(145)		(85)		(155)
Yes	47.2		41.4		64.7		60.6	
No	43.4		54.5		30.6		38.1	
Don't know	9.4		4.1		4.7		1.3	
Paternal relationship		(34)		(76)		(61)		(103)*
Excellent	17.6		22.4		14.8		22.3	
Good	29.4		32.9		26.2		35.0	
Fair	14.7		23.7		21.3		22.3	
Poor	14.7		2.6		9.8		10.7	
No contact	23.5		18.4		27.9		9.7	
Relatives w/drug problem	69.8	(53)	49.0	(145)**	61.9	(84)	48.4	(155)*
Mother	10.0		8.4		19.5		6.5**	
Father	26.0		23.8		39.0		26.1*	
Sister	20.0		11.2		14.6		4.6**	
Brother	30.0		14.0*		22.0		13.7	
Aunt/uncle	26.0		14.7		30.5		22.9	
Son/daughter	4.0		.7		0		0	
As a child, lived:								
Other relatives	43.4	(53)	40.3	(144)	30.6	(85)	25.0	(156)
In foster home	19.1	(47)	4.1	(123)**	7.1	(84)	.7	(146)*
In group home	2.1	(47)	.8	(123)	1.2	(84)	1.4	(146)
In treatment center	2.1	(47)	3.3	(123)	3.6	(84)	5.5	(146)
In detention center	2.1	(47)	10.6	(123)	13.1	(84)	7.5	(146)
Adopted	6.3	(48)	2.3	(128)	3.6	(83)	4.6	(151)

[a]*See* footnote to Table 1.

Table 6
Drug Use History of Methadone Patients by Race and Gender

	Black				White			
	Female		Male		Female		Male	
	%/M	(N)[a]	%/M	(N)	%/M	(N)	%/M	(N)
Age at first use								
Alcohol (M)	16.6	(48)	15.1	(134)*	14.7	(76)	13.4	(148)**
Marijuana (M)	17.9	(44)	17.1	(132)	15.8	(77)	15.0	(151)
Heroin (M)	20.4	(53)	19.8	(143)	20.5	(83)	18.3	(155)**
Average lifetime use								
Heroin (M)	143.4	(21)	170.9	(65)	89.3	(30)	130	(43)*
Cocaine (M)	25.2	(21)	43.1	(64)	14.4	(30)	29.5	(43)
Amphetamines (M)	5.7	(21)	13.4	(65)	29.5	(30)	36.0	(43)
Sedatives (M)	23.2	(21)	15.9	(65)	60.3	(29)	93.3	(43)*
Barbiturates (M)	2.9	(21)	0	(65)	22.5	(30)	38.0	(43)
Other opiates (M)	17.7	(21)	18.7	(65)	56.1	(29)	91.0	(43)*
Methadone (M)	83.5	(21)	75.6	(65)	52.7	(30)	109.4	(43)**
Alcohol (M)	55.7	(20)	90.2	(64)	87.0	(30)	134.5	(43)*
Alcohol								
to intoxication (M)	15.8	(20)	60.2	(63)**	40.1	(30)	70.9	(43)
Why began using drugs		(22)		(71)		(42)		(86)*
To feel part								
of the crowd (%)	45.5		42.3		35.7		53.5	
To relax (%)	31.8		16.9		40.5		16.3	
For the fun of it (%)	22.7		25.4		16.7		25.6	
Boredom (%)	0		15.5		7.1		4.7	

[a]*See* footnote to Table 1.

or "for the fun of it." Blacks did not differ in reporting these motives. In comparison to males, females (especially White females) more often reported that they initiated drug use in order to relax.

Regardless of race, males had used heroin ($p < .01$), methadone ($p < .05$), and cocaine ($p < .05$) more often throughout their lifetime than females. Within racial groupings, White males had started using heroin at an earlier age than females ($p < .01$). Black males and females did not differ in their age of first heroin use. For frequency of drug use during the immediately preceding month (Table 7), the only differences found were for cannabis and cocaine. Males of both races had used cannabis more frequently than females ($p < .05$), and White males had used cocaine more frequently than their female counterparts ($p < .05$).

Table 7
Frequency of Drug Use During Past Month
Among Methadone Patients by Race and Gender

	Black				White			
	Female		Male		Female		Male	
	%/M	(N)[a]	%/M	(N)	%/M	(N)	%/M	(N)
Heroin		(51)		(142)		(82)		(151)
Daily	11.8		11.3		2.4		9.9	
Few times/wk	13.7		11.3		8.5		7.3	
Few times	37.3		29.6		23.2		18.5	
Not at all	37.3		47.9		65.9		64.2	
Cocaine		(51)		(142)		(82)		(152)*
Daily	19.6		10.6		2.4		.7	
Few times/wk	19.6		21.1		2.4		12.5	
Few times	29.4		30.3		19.5		23.7	
Not at all	31.4		38.0		75.6		63.2	
Amphetamine		(50)		(143)		(84)		(153)
Daily	0		.7		0		.7	
Few times/wk	2.0		0		0		0	
A few times	0		6.3		2.4		1.3	
Not at all	98.0		93.0		97.6		98.0	
Valium		(51)		(143)		(85)		(155)
Daily	2.0		4.9		10.6		16.8	
Few times/wk	5.9		9.1		9.4		6.5	
Few times	25.5		22.4		24.7		23.9	
Not at all	66.7		63.6		55.3		52.9	
Marijuana		(51)		(143)		(83)		(154)
Daily	9.8		7.0		4.8		4.5	
Few times/wk	5.9		8.4		6.0		7.8	
Few times	27.5		31.5		20.5		29.9	
Not at all	56.9		53.1		68.7		57.8	
Alcohol		(51)		(143)		(83)		(155)**
Daily	7.8		8.4		0		9.0	
Few times/wk	9.8		18.9		6.0		10.3	
Few times	29.4		32.9		22.9		26.5	
Not at all	52.9		39.9		71.1		54.2	

[a]*See* footnote to Table 1.

Alcohol

ASI alcohol use scores were higher for White males than White females ($p < .01$), but did not differ among Blacks. Regardless of race, males reported that they started alcohol use at an earlier age than females reported ($p < .01$). Black males also reported that they had been more frequently intoxicated with alcohol over their lifetime than Black females reported ($p < .01$). For alcohol use during the preceding month, White females reported that they had drank more often than White males reported drinking ($p < .01$).

Drug Treatment

Overall, the age when subjects first felt that they had a drug problem did not differ for males and females, except among White subjects ($p < .01$). As shown in Table 8, White females first felt that they had a drug problem at a later age than White males. In addition, Black females had tried to stop using drugs without entering treatment significantly less often than Black males ($p < .01$).

Previous Utilization

For both races, there were no gender differences for when subjects first started treatment nor for what type of treatment program they initially entered. However, White females had entered detoxification, residential, and inpatient treatment less often than White males did ($p < .01$).

Current Utilization

Regardless of race, females had spent significantly less time at the clinic during each visit ($p < .05$). In addition, White females had been in their current methadone treatment program for significantly less time than White males ($p < .05$; Table 9). For Blacks, there were no gender differences in length of time in current treatment.

Psychopathology

For the whole sample, subjects showed elevated symptoms of psychopathology compared to the general population. For example, all scores on the SCL-90 (except phobic anxiety) were at least 1 SD above the norm. The analysis of gender differences in psychiatric symptomology (*see* Table 10), showed that Black females reported significantly more symptoms on the SCL-90 than did Black males ($p < .01$); and no differences between White females and males were obtained. However, with regard to depression, females, regardless of race, scored significantly higher on the SCL-90 Depression Scale ($p < .01$ for Blacks; $p < .05$ for Whites), and on the Beck Total Depression Scale ($p < .05$).

AIDS-Risk Behavior

Needle Use

There were no gender or racial differences in the frequency of injecting drugs in the past 6 mo (*see* Table 11). However, White females had shared needles significantly less often, and had used new needles signifi-

Table 8
Treatment-Related Characteristics of Methadone Patients
by Race and Gender

	Black		White	
	Female	Male	Female	Male
	%/M (N)[a]	%/M (N)	%/M (N)	%/M (N)
Age recognized				
drug problem (M)	23.3 (53)	23.2 (143)	22.2 (85)	20.9 (156)*
Age first entered				
treatment (M)	27.5 (53)	29.2 (143)	24.3 (84)	23.4 (152)
First treatment utilized	(53)	(143)	(85)	(155)
Methadone (%)	73.6	74.8	65.9	64.5
Residential (%)	9.4	4.9	7.1	10.3
Outpatient (%)	1.9	4.2	11.8	9.0
Inpatient (%)	13.2	12.6	14.1	17.4
Frequency of treatment (M)				
Stopping on own	5.2 (50)	10.6 (127)**	7.8 (69)	12.8 (124)
Methadone	2.6 (52)	2.9 (145)	2.7 (85)	3.1 (155)
Residential	.7 (49)	.9 (136)	.9 (80)	1.4 (142)**
Outpatient	.9 (52)	.9 (138)	.7 (81)	.9 (147)
AA	.8 (48)	.5 (129)	3.2 (77)	2.6 (139)
NA	.9 (47)	.6 (135)	4.2 (79)	1.8 (144)
Detox	1.7 (50)	1.9 (139)	1.9 (82)	3.0 (150)**
Inpatient	1.1 (48)	1.2 (139)	1.1 (82)	2.2 (152)**
Treatment that helped				
you most:	(51)	(143)	(82)	(154)
Methadone (%)	88.2	81.1	81.7	81.8
Residential (%)	3.9	7.7	3.7	6.5
Outpatient (%)	2.0	3.5	3.7	1.3
Inpatient (%)	3.9	7.7	7.3	5.8
NA (%)	0	2.8	2.4	3.9
Stopping on own (%)	7.8	3.5	8.5	4.5

[a]*See* footnote to Table 1.

cantly more often than White males ($p < .05$). Though the same trend was found for Black females, this difference was not significant. In addition, females, regardless of race, were more likely than males to report that it was not difficult to obtain new needles ($p < .01$).

Condom Use

No significant gender or racial differences in condom use were reported. However, White females were least likely to report that they always used condoms.

Table 9
Clinic Service Utilization of Methadone Patients
by Race and Gender

	Black		White	
	Female	Male	Female	Male
	%/M (N)[a]	%/M (N)	%/M (N)	%/M (N)
Months at clinic (M)	28.8 (52)	31.9 (140)	24.6 (84)	33.1 (148)**
Average methadone dose (M)	46.4 (44)	46.2 (110)	50.7 (81)	53.7 (143)
Current dose:	(50)	(145)	(83)	(150)
About right	56.0	57.9	62.7	54.0
Not enough	44.0	35.9	28.9	40.0
Too much	0	6.2	8.4	6.0
Have take home privileges	26.9 (52)	39.2 (143)	28.2 (85)	27.6 (152)
Satisfied with clinic services	70.2 (47)	66.0 (144)	75.6 (82)	82.0 (150)
Most helpful clinic service:	(51)	(144)	(82)	(149)
Doctor	3.9	7.6	3.7	6.0
Medication	51.0	51.4	73.2	73.2
Individual counseling	60.8	56.3	51.2	43.0
Job counseling	0	.7	1.2	1.3
Group counseling	9.8	4.9	4.9	3.4
How long you expect to attend program:	(50)	(141)	(80)	(147)
Forever	6.0	10.6	5.0	14.3
Several years	26.0	26.2	17.5	20.4
About a year	44.0	47.5	52.5	49.7
Few months or less	24.0	15.6	25.0	15.6

[a]*See* footnote to Table 1.

HIV Testing

Significantly more White females than White males reported being tested for HIV seropositivity ($p < .05$). The general trend was similar among Blacks, though not significant. As shown in Table 11, the significant gender difference in reporting HIV testing among Whites was apparently due to fewer White males being tested.

Discussion

Consistent with past research, the present data clearly demonstrate that female addicts in methadone treatment have specific treatment needs. As discussed below, females have not only different patterns of addiction, psy-

Table 10
Psychiatric Symptomology Among Methadone Patients
by Race and Gender

	Black				White			
	Female		Male		Female		Male	
	%/M	(N)[a]	%/M	(N)	%/M	(N)	%/M	(N)
Beck Depression Inventory Score	15.19	(53)	13.94	(145)	16.91	(85)	15.3	(156)
SCL-90 Scale Scores:								
GSI[b]		(51)	.60	(139)**	.97	(81)	.87	(153)
Somatization	1.02	(51)	.68	(137)**	1.07	(82)	.90	(154)
Obsessive/compulsive	1.00	(49)	.68	(139)*	.98	(83)	.97	(154)
Interpersonal sensitivity	.98	(51)	.54	(139)**	.93	(83)	.80	(152)
Depression	1.14	(52)	.72	(138)**	1.41	(81)	1.20	(153)
Anxiety	.83	(51)	.53	(139)**	.93	(81)	.89	(155)
Hostility	.83	(52)	.57	(139)*	.92	(81)	.76	(155)
Phobic anxiety	.46	(52)	.25	(139)*	.35	(81)	.40	(152)
Paranoid ideation	1.07	(53)	.71	(141)*	.94	(81)	.92	(156)
Psychoticism	.79	(50)	.44	(141)*	.56	(81)	.50	(156)

[a]*See* footnote to Table 1.
[b]General Symptom Inventory.

chopathology, and dysfunctional family backgrounds, but also greater needs for childcare, and fewer financial resources. Despite these pressing treatment needs, the females in this study used fewer residential and inpatient programs than had males, had spent less time than males at their methadone clinic, and had spent less time in their current methadone treatment program.

The reason for this lack of treatment utilization is unclear. Some authors suggest that it may be due to the female IDUs socioeconomic class. Generally, female IDUs have fewer financial resources and consequently are less likely to seek help from professional or social service agencies.[47] However, as discussed below, lack of utilization may result not only from methadone treatment services that do not meet the needs of female IDUs,[31,32] but also from increased childcare responsibilities that preclude participation in treatment programs, and the difficulty of accessing a population that is rarely even forced into treatment legally. The following discussion will examine some of the important parameters that distinguish female addicts from their male counterparts, and that demand treatment intervention.

Table 11
HIV-Risk Behaviors of Methadone Patients by Race and Gender

	Black				White			
	Female		Male		Female		Male	
	%/M	(N)[a]	%/M	(N)	%/M	(N)	%/M	(N)
Injected drugs	60.6	(33)	67.2	(119)	50.9	(55)	62.6	(99)
Shared needles	25.0	(20)	23.8	(80)	35.7	(28)	40.3	(62)
Times shared needles (M)	3.2	(34)	.7	(119)	.5	(57)	1.6	(98)*
Used new needles		(19)		(80)		(27)		(62)*
All the time	73.7		56.3		59.3		22.6	
Most of the time	21.1		32.5		29.6		48.4	
Half of the time	0		6.3		7.4		16.1	
Less than half of the time	5.3		3.8		3.7		6.5	
Never	0		1.3		0		6.5	
Difficult to get new needles	5.0	(20)	13.8	(80)	21.4	(28)	25.8	(62)
Condom use		(34)		(112)		(51)		(98)
Always	20.6		19.6		9.8		16.3	
Most of the time	8.8		11.6		13.7		6.1	
Half of the time	0		7.1		3.9		4.1	
Less than half of the time	5.9		11.6		5.9		14.3	
Never	64.7		50.0		66.7		59.2	
Tested for HIV	64.7	(34)	53.0	(117)	58.9	(56)	41.8	(98)*

[a]Data are derived from a 6-mo follow-up sample of 376 subjects. Smaller sample sizes for individual variables are a result of missing data.

Criminal Activity

Gender Differences

Criminal activity is common among heroin addicts. For addicts in methadone treatment, the frequency of prior arrests has been reported to range from 83%,[48] to 87%.[49] However, as illustrated in the present and other data,[46] criminal involvement is more frequent for males than for females. Compared to females, males had higher ASI Legal Composite Scores, more arrests, had been jailed more frequently, and had spent more time in jail.

Implications for Treatment Involvement

Many of the criminal involvements for heroin addicts are drug-related. For example, among a sample of heroin addicts, 85% of those who had been arrested had been charged with a drug offense.[50] Among a British sample of 208 addicts, 52% had been convicted of at least one drug offense. Furthermore, 95% of that sample admitted to illegal possession of drugs, and

50% admitted to selling drugs during the prior 3 mo.[51] One consequence of drug-related arrests can be court-ordered drug treatment. In the present study, mandatory participation in drug treatment occurred significantly more often for males. Thus, the gender difference seen in criminal activity may actually reduce the likelihood of court-ordered treatment for females.

Certainly, criminal activity cannot be encouraged as an avenue for seeking drug treatment. Nevertheless, arrest, imprisonment, and court-order treatment are all factors that can contribute to treatment intervention in the addict population. Because females are not arrested as frequently as males, legal interventions are less likely to occur. Thus, the lower level of criminal activity found among females may be an additional barrier that restricts the female addict from being detected and treated. In addition, because the husband or sexual partner of a female addict generally tends to also be drug-dependent,[52,53] the high arrest and imprisonment rate among male addicts also contributes to reduced financial support and unstable social support systems for the female addict.

Pattern of Drug Addiction

Current Drug Use

In the present study, the frequency of current drug use among male and female IDUs did not differ, with some exceptions. Black subjects tended to use heroin and cocaine more often than White subjects,[46] and Black females used cocaine the most often. In addition females used cannabis significantly less often than males, regardless of race.[40,46]

Onset of Problematic Drug Use

Though the frequency of drug use did not differ at the time these subjects were in treatment, female addicts differed from males in the pattern of their addict careers. In the present sample, females had initiated drug use at a later age, and used drugs for a shorter period of time. These findings support a number of reports suggesting that drug abuse may become more problematic for females at a faster rate than it does for males.[40,41,43] In addition, though the female subjects in the present study had used drugs for a shorter period of time than the male subjects, they initially entered treatment for drug addiction at approximately the same age, and were participating in their current methadone program at a younger age than their male counterparts.[40]

The present results also suggest that, once drug use is initiated, the White female may be more susceptible to a rapid onset of addiction and problematic drug abuse than either gender of Blacks, or White males. Though females from both racial groups did not differ in age of initial drug use, the average time between drug-use initiation and problem recognition was the shortest for White females (1.7 yr).

Initiation of Drug Use

The results of this study suggest that gender differences in reported reasons for starting to use drugs may be due to underlying racial differences. Most studies report that males more than females initiate drug use in order to satisfy curiosity or gain peer acceptance.[40,53] In the present study, these differences were only found for White subjects. No gender differences in curiosity (i.e., "for the fun of it"), or peer acceptance were found among Blacks. Other reports suggest that females begin using drugs in order to relieve psychological distress.[53] Support for this suggestion is implied by the current finding that females of both races reported more frequently than males that they began using drugs in order to relax.

Though the present study did not investigate the influence of the IDUs sexual partner on initiation of drug abuse, the literature consistently shows that female IDUs are more likely than males to have a sexual partner who is an iv drug user,[28,46] and that partner is frequently part of their initiation into drug use. For example, in a series of studies that examined gender and ethnic differences among 567 White and Hispanic addicts in methadone treatment, female IDUs reported more frequently than males that initiation of iv drug use was strongly influenced by their IDU sexual partners.[20,40]

AIDS-Risk Behavior

Condom Use

Because female IDUs are more likely than their male counterpart to have a sexual partner who is also an iv drug user, they are at high risk for HIV infection. In a study of 457 IDUs that examined gender and ethnic differences in AIDS-risk sexual behavior, a large majority of subjects did not use condoms, and females were no more likely than males to use condoms.[28] In that study, White males were the least likely group to report condom use. However, males participating in the present study were not less likely than females to use condoms; in fact, the least likely group to report condom use was White females.

Needle Use

Few studies have been conducted that focus on gender differences in iv drug use practices that place the subject at high risk for HIV infection. However, in the present study, we examined gender differences in many of these AIDS-risk behaviors. As shown in Table 11, few differences between males and females, regardless of race, were found. However, White females shared needles significantly less often and used new needles significantly more often than White males. Among Blacks, these differences were not significant, but the same trend was found. When these subjects were asked if it was difficult to obtain new needles, significantly more males reported this difficulty.

HIV Testing

The results of the present study also indicated that White females were more likely than White males to have been tested for HIV infection. This racial difference was due to the low percentage of White males that had been tested. Among Blacks, the same general trend was observed, though the gender differences were not significant.

Thus, the present results indicate that interventions designed to reduce AIDS high-risk behaviors need to be increased. These interventions must be focused on both males and females, and designed to alter the specific sexual and drug-use behaviors that can transmit HIV infection.

Psychological Symptoms

Using the SCL-90 and Beck Depression Inventory, this sample of IDUs reported elevated symptoms of psychological distress, and female subjects reported substantially more psychological distress than their male counterparts. These findings are in agreement with other studies.[54] For example, Kosten et al.[46] suggested that female IDUs in treatment have higher current and lifetime rates of anxiety disorders than male IDUs. In that study, females also exhibited higher rates of depression, and scored significantly higher than males on the ASI Psychiatric Composite score. The results of the present study also support previous findings that Black males report the lowest levels of psychological symptomology.[40]

It could be argued that these results are biased by the self-report nature of the assessment, and may be affected by a respondent's willingness to reveal symptomology. Thus, the elevated scores of females could reflect a greater tendency to disclose symptoms;[55] lower scores by males, and Black males in particular, could reflect denial or increased motivation to hide symptoms. However, the present findings are in close agreement with other reports that utilized the MMPI, which can identify subjects who are not answering honestly. Those reports have also demonstrated significant degrees of psychopathology among narcotic addicts.[56,57,59] The proportion of pathological MMPI profiles among heroin users has been reported to range from 88[58] to 94%.[56,57] For females, one report obtained pathological profiles for 79% of street addicts and 82% of prison addicts.[59] In addition, an early report[35] examined gender differences in MMPI profiles among 120 institutionalized addicts. Women scored significantly higher on scales for depression and suspiciousness. Furthermore, in comparison to White addicts, Black addicts have also shown significantly less psychopathology on MMPI profiles.[60,61]

Thus, the present findings, taken together with previous data, indicate that psychopathology and psychological distress is common among IDUs, especially among females. This increased pathology and distress is an important consideration for designing treatment interventions. In addition, a more thorough understanding of gender differences among addicts is needed. For example, though the pattern of more rapid addiction and treatment entry may reflect gender-specific physiological responses to drug action and metabolism,[43] this pattern may also be a result of differences in underlying psychopathology, or background and familial characteristics.

Family and Interpersonal Relationships
Dysfunctional Backgrounds

A number of authors have examined the childhood experiences and family environment of drug addicts, and have found a correlation between dysfunctional backgrounds and the development of drug addiction.[62] For example, more addicts than nonaddicts have reported an unhappy childhood, physical punishment, and parental separation.[63] In addition, more dysfunctional and abusive backgrounds have been reported for female addicts than for male addicts.[46,64,65] Though the present study did not directly address these particular childhood experiences, the results did indicate that in comparison to males, significantly more females reported that they had lived in a foster home during childhood. This finding agrees with other reports that female addicts have more disrupted and dysfunctional family backgrounds than male addicts do.[46,66]

A number of studies also suggest that heroin addicts did not establish positive relationships with their parents.[62] The paternal relationship has received particular attention. Compared to users of other drugs, heroin addicts have been shown to have especially poor relationships with their fathers,[67,68] who are reported as emotionally distant or hostile parents.[2] Quality of paternal relationship has not been fully examined for female addicts. However, among the present sample of IDUs in methadone treatment, more females than males reported that they did not know if their father was still living, or that they had no contact with him. More females also reported that they had no contact with their mother. This latter finding lends support to previous reports that female IDUs are more likely to have poor maternal relationships.[20]

Familial Drug/Alcohol Problems

A number of findings, together with the results of this study, suggest that parental dysfunction may be a major contributing factor to female addiction, and correlated psychopathology. In one study, 85% of a heroin-addicted sample reported considerably less opportunity for establishing normal relationships during childhood due to familial pathology, such as alcoholism, and physical or psychiatric illness.[69] Indeed, drug and alcohol addiction are often reported as part of the addict's family background, regardless of gender.[62]

In the present study, the majority of participants reported that they had at least one family member with a drug problem; a substantial proportion reported having more than one. Similar to findings by Rosenbaum[52,53] females reported having relatives with a drug problem significantly more often than males did, especially a drug-addicted sibling. These IDUs also reported that problems with alcohol among relatives were more prevalent than drug problems. Most of the relatives were members of the respondent's nuclear family, and fathers with alcohol problems were cited most often. More females than males reported relatives with alcohol problems; but they more frequently reported that their mother was alcoholic. This latter finding may contribute to the greater frequency of females reporting no contact with their mother, as well as the greater tendency to be placed in foster care.

Thus, the psychopathology, childhood, and family background of the female addicts described in this and other studies, strongly suggest that special attention and effort must be directed toward the psychological functioning of female addicts in treatment. The need for general psychological services is apparent from the reports of psychological distress among female addicts. The importance of a specific focus on the effects of parental drug and alcohol addiction, as well as parental rejection and loss, is also apparent from the female addict's disproportionate experience with these events.

One reason that a direct focus on treating the long-term effects of an abusive/dysfunctional family is important for the female addict is that it may improve the stability of her current social support systems. Dysfunctional childhood relationships usually lead to dysfunctional adult relationships. In turn, unstable marital and family relationships put the female addict at increased risk for loss of financial and emotional support.

Marital Status

Most addicts do not have stable marital relationships. For example, among a British sample of heroin addicts seeking drug treatment, only 20% were married and living with their spouses, and a full 34% reported no ongoing sexual relationship.[51] In a study of heroin addicts in New Orleans, only 29% were married to or living with a sexual partner.[71] In the present study, less than 20% of the sample were currently married, and over a third of the sample had never married.

However, less than one-quarter of this sample lived alone; most lived with their minor children/sexual-partner, parents, or other relatives. More males tended to live alone, and more females (especially Blacks) tended to live with a sex partner or children.[40] Though these results parallel another report that White females are the least likely to be single,[46] that report also suggested that female IDUs were more likely to be separated or divorced; whereas, White males tended to be single. For this sample of subjects, White females (but not Black females) were most likely to be separated or divorced. The likelihood of being single did not differ between White males, or either gender of Blacks.

Even when addicts are married, the quality of marital relationship is often poor, and has a high incidence of separation and divorce. One report indicated that, compared to a general drug-using population, heroin-users have the highest percentage of divorces and poor marriages.[68] Another report found that 70% of married addicts were separated, and virtually all the subjects felt tension and sexual frustration in their marriage.[69] In the present study, of the subjects who were married, almost half of them described their marital relationship as only fair or poor.

The reason for the high incidence of marital instability and discord among addicts may be a result of several factors. Certainly negative childhood experiences unstable family backgrounds, psychopathology, and the effects of drug addiction itself are contributing factors. Nevertheless, services that address the problem of unstable living arrangements and sexual relationships are obviously necessary. The need for such services are required not only for the addict, but also for their children.

Parenting

Within the overall society, responsibility for childrearing is generally assumed by females; within addict populations, this responsibility does not differ. For example, in the present study significantly more females had children living with them than males did. With regard to responsibility for dependent children, the results of other studies are similar to the present ones: Female IDUs of both races are most likely to be responsible; White male IDUs are the least likely.[46] This responsibility may have profound affects on the female IDU. First, responsibility for the care of dependent children may restrict her entry and retention in treatment programs.

In addition, given that these women are IDUs, lack past and present social support systems, and report significant psychological distress, their parenting abilities must certainly be compromised. Left untreated, the problems of the female IDU will quite likely create a dysfunctional environment for their children. That dysfunctional family environment, which includes a drug-addicted parent, puts the child at high risk for not only psychological distress, but also initiating and continuing their own drug use.[71,72] Thus, treatment services for female IDUs that provide effective parental guidance are needed for two purposes: (1) train the IDU in their parental responsibilities; and (2) protect the child from the effects of inadequate parenting.

However, in order to provide adequate treatment for the female IDU with children, services that provide her only with parental guidance are not sufficient; they must also provide her with adequate childcare that allows her to not only enter and remain in treatment, but also work outside the home. In the present study, females financially supported significantly more children than males did. However, as described below, their employment rate was significantly lower.

Employment

Unemployment among heroin addicts has always been higher than the nonaddict population. In the 1970s, approx 50%[51] to 75%[73] of addicts in treatment were reported to be unemployed. In the present study, less than 30% of all subjects were employed. But, female IDUs had worked significantly less than males. This finding is in agreement with Goldsmith et al.,[70] who reported that female addicts had poorer employment records than male addicts.[46] Not surprisingly, the present findings also showed that females received significantly less monthly income than their male counterparts, and significantly more income from public assistance.[40]

Because females have more demands on them for childcare responsibility than males do, their high rate of unemployment is not surprising. Provision of adequate childcare services that would provide female IDUs with the time needed to seek, gain, and keep employment could help alleviate their substantial unemployment problem.

However, the provision of childcare services alone may not be adequate to increase employment among female IDUs. These subjects were also less likely than males to be looking for work, and reported more frequently that they did not want employment. Unwillingness to seek and not desiring employment may only reflect the practical considerations of childcare responsibilities, and these attitudes may change once childcare services are made available. However, these attitudes may also reflect underlying psychopathology and vocational maladjustment. Vocational instability is common among IDUs,[74,75] and treatment programs that are specifically designed to address the problems of the IDU in the job environment are necessary adjuncts to addiction therapy.[8] For the female, vocational programs should also be designed to address the gender-specific problems that they confront in the work environment.

Treatment Considerations

In order to increase the effectiveness of substance abuse treatment for women, the actual typology of female methadone clients needs to be considered carefully. Thus, the characteristics of women who become involved in services, the patterns of that service utilization, and the full range of services and treatments most commonly offered to them must be identified. In addition, in order to serve not only the female addict, but also the male addict, the gender differences in these characteristics must be understood. Finally, because many recent reports have suggested that cultural and racial differences may interact with gender differences,[20,76] the specific needs of women in terms of race or cultural background must be considered.

In this chapter we have examined gender differences by race. There is growing recognition among treatment providers that effective interventions must be responsive to a broad range of social, economic, and in particular, psychological problems typically associated with opiate dependence. These ancillary problems do not disappear with the cessation of drug use. Consequently, patients must learn to resolve and cope with difficulties that may predate their addiction and will certainly be present during their recovery. If not addressed, these problems will complicate treatment and increase the likelihood of relapse. Therefore, treatment needs of methadone patients extend well beyond the need to eliminate drug use. This holistic approach demands that treatment services be designed with sensitivity to patients' race and gender as these factors often influence social roles and expectations.

Conclusion

Female IDUs need to utilize more services in drug treatment programs than they currently do, and more services that address their needs must be made available to them. Because females have more severe patterns of addiction, psychopathology, and dysfunctional family backgrounds, psychological treatment programs must be developed that are specifically designed to address these problems. Though female IDUs may represent only 30% of the drug treatment population, they are much more likely to have childcare responsibilities. Left untreated, her addiction and associated problems will necessarily impact on those children. In addition, because of her responsibilities for childcare, she has less opportunity to participate in treatment programs, and has fewer financial resources. If a major effort is made to provide sufficient childcare and vocational services for the female IDU, this pattern of poverty, maladjustment, and drug addiction may be altered.

Acknowledgments

This work was supported by grant No. 92-530-ADA-00 from the New Jersey State Department of Health, and grant Nos. RO1-DA03456 and RO1-DA05186 from the National Institute on Drug Abuse. We also wish to express our gratitude to S. Chestnut for her assistance in preparing this manuscript.

References

[1]E. M. Brecher (1972) *Licit and Illicit Drugs.* Little, Brown, Boston.

[2]I. Chein, D. L. Gerard, R. S. Lee, and E. Rosenfeld (1964) *The Road to h: Narcotics, Delinquency and Social Policy.* Basic, New York.

[3]C. Terry and M. Pellens (1970) The extent of chronic opiate abuse in the United States prior to 1921, in *The Epidemiology of Opiate Addiction in the United States.* J. Ball and C. D. Chambers, eds. Thomas, Springfield, IL, pp. 36–67.

[4]Institute of Medicine. (1990) *Treating Drug Problems, vol. 1: A Study of the Evolution, Effectiveness, and Financing of Public and Private Drug Treatment Systems.* National Academy, Washington, DC.

[5]M. R. Burt, T. J. Glynn, and B. J. Sowder (1979) *An Investigation of the Characteristics of Drug Abusing Women.* DHEW Pub. No. (ADM)80-917. NIDA, Rockville, MD.

[6]H. M. Ginzburg, S. H. Weiss, M. G. Macdonald, and R. L. Hubbard (1985) HTLV III exposure among drug users. *Cancer Res.* **45,** 4605s–4608s.

[7]B. G. Reed (1985) Drug misuse and dependency in women: The meaning and implications of being considered a special population or minority group. *Int. J. Addict.* **20,** 13–62.

[8]D. S. Metzger and J. J. Platt (1990) Solving vocational problems for addicts in treatment, in *The Effectiveness of Drug Abuse Treatment: Dutch and American Perspectives.* J. J. Platt, C. D. Kaplan, and P. J. McKim, eds. Krieger, Malabar, FL, pp. 101–112.

[9]B. S. Brown (1990) The American addiction scene, in *The Effectiveness of Drug Abuse Treatment: Dutch and American Perspectives.* J. J. Platt, C. D. Kaplan, and P. J. McKim, eds. Krieger, Malabar, FL, pp. 3–14.

[10]J. H. Jaffe (1979) The swinging pendulum: The treatment of drug users in America, in *Handbook on Drug Abuse.* R. L. Dupont, A. Goldstein, and J. O'Donnell, eds. NIDA, Rockville, MD, pp. 3–16.

[11]J. H. Jaffe (1985) Drug dependence: Opioids, nonnarcotics, nicotine (tobacco), and caffeine, in *Comprehensive Textbook of Psychiatry, V,* vol. 1. H. I. Kaplan and B. J. Sadock, eds. Williams and Wilkins, Baltimore, pp. 642–686.

[12]J. C. Marsh, M. E. Colten, and M. B. Tucker (1982) Women, drugs and alcohol: New perspectives. *J. Soc. Issues* **38,** 1–7.

[13]A. T. McLellan, A. I. Alterman, J. Cacciola, D. Metzger, and C. P. O'Brien (1992) A new measure of substance abuse treatment: Initial studies of the treatment services review. *J. Nerv. Ment. Disord.* **180,** 101–110.

[14]A. T. McLellan, C. P. O'Brien, R. Kron, A. I. Alterman, and K. A. Druley (1980) Matching substance abuse patients to appropriate treatments: A conceptual and methodological approach. *Drug Alcohol Dep.* **5,** 189–195.

[15]A. T. McLellan, C. P. O'Brien, D. Metzger, A. I. Alterman, J. Cornish, and H. Urschel (1992) Is substance abuse treatment effective—compared to what? in *Addictive States.* C. P. O'Brien and J. Jaffe, eds. Raven, New York, pp. 231–252.

[16]J. C. Ball and A. Ross (1991) *The Effectiveness of Methadone Maintenance Treatment.* Springer Verlag, New York.

[17]G. W. Joe, D. D. Simpson, and R. L. Hubbard (1991) Unmet service needs in methadone maintenance. *Int. J. Addict.* **26,** 1–22.

[18]J. C. Ball and E. Corty (1990) Policy issues pertaining to the treatment of heroin addicts in the United States—with particular reference to methadone maintenance therapy, in *The Effectiveness of Drug Abuse Treatment: Dutch and American Perspectives.* J. J. Platt, C. D. Kaplan, and P. J. McKim, eds. Krieger, Malabar, FL, pp. 61–70.

[19]J. B. Cohen, L. B. Hauer, and C. B. Wofsy (1989) Women and IV drugs: Parenteral and heterosexual transmission of Human Immunodeficiency Virus. *J. Drug Issues* **19,** 39–56.

[20]Y.-I. Hser, M. D. Anglin, and W. McGlothlin (1987) Sex differences in addict careers 1: Initiation of use. *Am. J. Drug Alcohol Abuse* **13,** 33–57.

[21]S. C. Wilsnack and R. W. Wilsnack (1990) Women and substance abuse: Research directions for the 1990s. *Psychology Addict. Behav.* **4(suppl.),** 46–49.

[22]D. K. Lewis and J. K. Watters (1989) Human Immunodeficiency Virus seroprevalence in female intravenous drug users: The puzzle of black women's risk. *Soc. Sci. Med.* **29,** 1071–1076.

[23]E. E. Schoenbaum, P. A. Selwyn, R. S. Klein, M. F. Rogers, K. Freeman, and G. H. Friedland (1986) Prevalence of and risk factors associated with HTLV- III/LAV antibodies among intravenous drug abusers in methadone program in New York City. Abstract presented at second International Conference on AIDS, Paris.

[24]S. Y. Chu, J. W. Buehler, and R. L. Berkelman (1990) Impact of the human immunodeficiency virus epidemic on mortality in women of reproductive age. *JAMA* **264,** 225–229.

[25]C. A. Campbell (1990) Women and AIDs. *Soc. Sci. Med.* **30,** 407–415.

[26]K. K. Holmes, J. M. Karon, and J. Kreiss (1990) The increasing frequency of heterosexually acquired AIDs in the United States, 1983–88. *Am. J. Public. Health* **80,** 858–862.

[27]D. K. Lewis and J. K. Watters (1988) HIV seroprevalance and needle sharing among heterosexual intravenous drug users: Ethnic gender comparisons. *Am. J. Public Health* **78,** 1499.

[28]D. K. Lewis and J. K. Watters (1991) Sexual risk behavior among heterosexual intravenous drug users: Ethnic and gender variations. *AIDS* **5,** 77–83.

[29]Centers for Disease Control. (1985) Recommendations for assisting in the prevention of perinatal transmission of Human T-Lymphotrophic Virus-Type III/Lymphadenopathy Associated Virus and Acquired Immunodeficiency Syndrome. *Morbidity Mortality Weekly Rep.* **34,** 721–726, 731–732.

[30]M. E. Guinan and A. Hardy (1987) Epidemiology of AIDS in women in the United States. *JAMA* **257,** 2039–2042.

[31]G. Beschner and P. Thompson (1981) *Women and Drug Abuse Treatment: Needs and Services.* DHHS Pub. No. (ADM)81-1057. NIDA, Rockville, MD.

[32]N. Naierman, B. Savage, B. Haskins, J. Lear, H. Chase, K. Marvelle, and R. Lamothe (1979) An assessment of sex discrimination in the delivery of health development services. Final Report, Office of Civil Rights (ABT Associates), Contract HEN-100-78-0137, Washington, DC.

[33]G. DeLeon and N. Jainchill (1980) Female drug abusers: Social and psychological status 2 years after treatment in a therapeutic community. Paper presented at the National Alcohol and Drug Conference, Washington, DC.

[34]N. Jainchill and G. DeLeon (1979) Are female drug abusers more deviant? Paper presented at the meeting of the Eastern Psychological Association, Philadelphia.

[35]R. Olson (1964) MMPI sex differences in narcotic addicts. *J. Gen. Psychiatry* **71,** 157–266.

[36]R. Moise and B. G. Reed (1982) Issues in treatment of heroin addicted women. *Int. J. Addict.* **17,** 109–139.

[37]R. Moise, B. G. Reed, and C. Conell (1981) Women in drug abuse treatment programs: Factors that influence retention at very early and later stages in two treatment modalities: A summary. *Int. J. Addict.* **16,** 1295–1300.

[38]L. J. Beckman (1978) The psychosocial characteristics of alcoholic women. *Drug Abuse Alcohol Rev.* **1,** 1–12.

[39]T. Doshan and C. Bursch (1982) Women and substance abuse: Critical issues in treatment design. *J. Drug Educ.* **12,** 229–239.

[40]M. D. Anglin, Y. Hser, and M. W. Booth (1987) Sex differences in addict careers 4: Treatment. *Am. J. Drug Alcohol Abuse* **13,** 253–280.

[41]E. H. Ellinwood, W. G. Smith, and G. E. Vaillant (1966) Narcotic addictions in males and females: A comparison. *Int. J. Addict.* **1,** 33–45.

[42]J. E. Prather and L. S. Fidell (1978) Drug use and abuse among women: An overview. *Int. J. Addict.* **13,** 863–885.

[43]C. Robbins (1989) Sex differences in psychosocial consequences of alcohol and drug abuse. *J. Health Soc. Behav.* **30,** 117–130.

[44]F. Suffet and R. Brotman (1976) Female drug use: Some observations. *Int. J. Addict.* **11,** 19–33.

[45]P. B. Sutker (1981) Drug dependent women: An overview of the literature, in *Treatment Services for Dependent Women*, vol. 1. DHHS Pub. No. (ADM)81-1177. NIDA, Rockville, MD, pp. 25–51.

[46]T. R. Kosten, B. J. Rounsaville, and H. D. Kleber (1985) Ethnic and gender differences among opiate addicts. *Int. J. Addict.* **20,** 1143–1162.

[47]J. C. Marsh and N. A. Miller (1985) Female clients in substance abuse treatment. *Int. J. Addict.* **20,** 995–1019.

[48]G. Nash (1973) *The Impact of Drug Abuse Treatment Upon Criminality: A Look at 19 Programs.* Montclair State College, Upper Montclair, NJ.

[49]J. C. Ball and C. D. Chambers, eds. (1970) *The Epidemiology of Opiate Addiction in the United States.* Thomas, Springfield, IL.

[50]B. Crowther (1974) The college opiate user. *Int. J. Addict.* **9,** 241–253.

[51]H. Blumberg, S. D. Cohen, B. E. Dronfield, E. A. Mordecai, J. C. Roberts, and D. Hawks (1974) British opiate users I: People approaching London treatment centres. *Int. J. Addict.* **9,** 1–23.

[52]M. Rosenbaum (1981a) Sex roles among deviants. *Int. J. Addict.* **16,** 859–877.

[53]M. Rosenbaum (1981b) When drugs come in the picture, love flies out the window: Women addicts' love relationships. *Int. J. Addict.* **16,** 1197–1206.

[54]R. A. Steer, J. J. Platt, W. F. Ranieri, and D. S. Metzger (1989) Relationships of SCL-90 profiles to methadone patients' psychosocial characteristics and treatment response. *Multivariate Exp. Clin. Res.* **9,** 45–54.

[55]P. B. Sutker, R. P. Archer, and A. N. Allain (1980) Psychopathology of drug abusers: Sex and ethnic considerations. *Int. J. Addict.* **15,** 605–613.

[56]H. E. Hill, C. A. Haertzen, and R. Glaser (1960) Personality characteristics of narcotic addicts as indicated by the MMPI. *J. Gen. Psychiatry* **62,** 127–139.

[57]C. Sheppard, J. Fracchia, E. Ricca, and S. Merlis (1972) Indications of psychopathology in male narcotic abusers, their effects and relation to treatment effectiveness. *J. Psychiatry* **81,** 351–360.

[58]P. B. Sutker (1971) Personality differences and sociopathy in heroin addicts and non-addict prisoners. *J. Abnorm. Psychiatry* **78,** 247–251.

[59]P. B. Sutker and C. E. Moan (1972) Personality characteristics of socially deviant women: Incarcerated heroin addicts, street addicts, and non-addict prisoners, in *Drug Addiction: Clinical and Socio-Legal Aspects*, vol. 2. J. M. Singh, L. Miller, and H. Lal, eds. Futura, Mount Kisco, NY, pp. 107–114.

[60]J. W. Shaffer, T. W. Kinlock, and D. N. Nurco (1982) Factor structure of the MMPI-168 in male narcotic addicts. *J. Clin. Psychiatry* **38,** 656–661.

[61]P. B. Sutker, R. P. Archer, and A. N. Allain (1979) Volunteerism and self-reported psychopathology among opiate addicts. *J. Consult. Clin. Psychiatry* **88,** 59–67.

[62]J. J. Platt (1986) *Heroin Addiction: Theory, Research, and Treatment*, 2nd ed. Krieger, Malabar, FL.

[63]D. J. Baer and J. Corrado (1974) Heroin addict relationships with parents during childhood and early adolescent years. *J. Gen. Psychiatry* **124,** 99–103.

[64]C. D. Chambers, R. K. Hinesley, and M. Moldestad (1970) Narcotic addiction in females: A race comparison. *Int. J. Addict.* **5,** 257–278.

[65]A. E. Raynes, C. Climent, V. D. Patch, and F. Ervin (1974) Factors related to imprisonment in female heroin addicts. *Int. J. Addict.* **9,** 145–150.

[66]W. S. Aron (1975) Family background and personal trauma among drug addicts in the United States: Implication for treatment. *Br. J. Addict.* **70,** 295–305.

[67]S. F. Bucky (1971) The relationship between past background and drug use. Report no. 1135. Naval Aerospace Medical Research Lab, Pensacola, FL.

[68]S. F. Bucky (1973) The relationship between background and extent of heroin use. *Am. J. Psychiatry* **130,** 709–710.

[69]H. D. Beckett and K. J. Lodge (1971) Aspects of social relationships in heroin addicts admitted for treatment. *Bull. Narc.* **23,** 29–36.

[70]B. M. Goldsmith, W. C. Capel, K. J. Waddell, and G. T. Stewart (1972) Demographic and sociological implications of addiction in New Orleans: Implication for consideration of treatment modalities, in *Drug Addiction: Clinical and Sociological Aspects*, vol. 2. J. M. Singh, L. Mill, and H. Lal, eds. Futura, Mount Kisco, NY, pp. 137–152.

[71]J. Carr (1975) Drug patterns among drug-addicted mothers: Incidence, variance in use, and effects on children. *Pediatr. Ann.* **4,** 408–417.

[72]N. R. Lief (1981) Parenting and child services for drug dependent women, in *Treatment Services for Drug Dependent Women*, vol I. G. M. Beschner, G. B. G. Reed, and J. Mondanaro, eds. NIDA, Rockville, MD, pp. 455–498.

[73]J. T. Ungerleider (1973) The business of drugs, in *Drug Abuse in Industry*. J. M. Scher, ed. Thomas, Springfield, IL, pp. 45–48.

[74]S. M. Hall, P. Loeb, P. LeVois, and J. Cooper (1981) Increasing employment in ex-heroin addicts II: Methadone maintenance sample. *Behav. Med.* **12,** 453–460.

[75]J. J. Platt and D. S. Metzger (1985) The role of employment in the rehabilitation of heroin addicts, in *Progress in the Development of Cost-Effective Treatment for Drug Abusers*. R. S. Ashery, ed. NIDA, Rockville, MD, pp. 111–121.

[76]M. D. Anglin, M. W. Booth, T. M. Ryan, and Y.-I. Hser (1988) Ethnic differences in narcotics addition II: Chicano and Anglo addiction career patterns. *Int. J. Addict.* **23,** 1011–1027.

Cannabis Use in the General Population

Male/Female Differences?

Hilde Pape, Torild Hammer, and Per Vaglum

Introduction

Cannabis* was not extensively used in the industrialized world until the late 1960s. Its introduction initiated a new trend in the use of illicit drugs, as a large proportion of the users were young, and they had a relatively high standard of living.[1-5] Cannabis also soon became an important ingredient of the hippie movement, signalizing a nonconformist lifestyle, a fight against oppression, and an increase in value of personal freedom. In general, the "cannabis culture" in the late 1960s and the 1970s appeared to promote an orientation toward the gentler and perhaps more "feminine" values of society. This may have had a special appeal to women. Also, as some of the initial values and attitudes related to cannabis involvement have remained relatively unchanged,[6-9] this may still be the case.

However, other factors probably discourage cannabis use in women. First, the norms regulating substance use tend to be generally more restric-

---

*Hashish, the concentrate of the resin of the cannabis plant, is stronger than marijuana, the herbal form. However, in this chapter the words marijuana and cannabis will be used interchangeably.

From: *Drug and Alcohol Abuse Reviews, Vol. 5: Addictive Behaviors in Women*
Ed.: R. R. Watson ©1994 Humana Press Inc., Totowa, NJ

tive for females than for males.[10,11] Furthermore, the sex role of women appears to be incompatible with an involvement in criminal activities, and cannabis was introduced to the industrialized world as an illicit drug. It is true that the legislation concerning cannabis use has been liberalized, but in most cases it has not been totally legalized.[12–15] Irrespective of this, other changes may have weakened the barriers against female cannabis involvement. According to the so-called convergence hypothesis, the patterns of male and female deviance will become increasingly similar as the social position of women approximates that of men.[16] In line with this reasoning, it is possible that male and female rates of cannabis use have converged during the last two decades.

Comparative research on male and female cannabis use may shed light on general aspects of sex distinctions and sex roles. Studies in this field can presumably reveal whether the convergence hypothesis applies to male and female rates of cannabis use. Research on predisposing factors, reasons for use, consequences of use, and factors promoting cessation, may also disclose whether traditional sex differences still predominate. Furthermore, such studies may establish whether the same deviance theories are equally applicable to both sexes when explaining cannabis involvement.

Data on male and female cannabis use are also of interest in a preventive perspective. Thus, cannabis has been found to be a so-called "gateway drug," i.e., a drug that greatly increases the probability of subsequent use of other illicit drugs.[1,17–20] As more males than females get involved with illicit substances other than cannabis,[21] it is of interest to clarify whether priority should be given to the implementation of gender-specific strategies to prevent cannabis initiation. If so, it is of importance to identify factors that can enhance the effect of the preventive efforts in males.

On this background, we have reviewed the recent literature on sex differences in cannabis use. In the following, a description of the sources used to identify this literature is given, some of the weaknesses and limitations of the research in this field are mentioned, and studies that shed light on the questions outlined above are presented. Preference is given to longitudinal studies, because of their methodological advantages.

Materials and Methods

This review is limited to studies of the general population published after 1980. Data from patient populations or samples of addicted persons have systematically been omitted.

In the search for literature, the following data bases have been used: *Medline, Psychological Abstracts, Sociological Abstract*, and *Social Cita-*

tion Index. However, many publications of interest have not been registered with key words indicating that they report comparative data on male and female cannabis use. This problem has also been reported in a previous review on sex differences in alcohol and drug problems.[22] In order to avoid missing relevant contributions, the content of the last 12 volumes of important international journals in the drug use area (i.e., *Addictive Behavior, Advances in Alcohol and Substance Abuse, British Journal of Addiction, Bulletin on Narcotics, Drug and Alcohol Dependence, The International Journal of the Addictions, Journal of Drug Education*, and *Journal of Drug Issues*) have been carefully examined. Quite a few publications have also been identified by using the references of other authors. It is hoped that the most important findings are included in this presentation.

Weaknesses and Limitations in the Research on Sex Differences in Cannabis Use

Relatively few researchers on drug use seem to have been interested in exploring sex differences in cannabis involvement. Thus, several studies of potential interest have merged the samples of males and females,[23-26] or they have not included females at all.[27] In other cases, cannabis has not been analyzed separately from other illicit drugs.[28-30]

Although the recent literature on sex differences in cannabis use is of limited extent, some relevant studies have in fact been published. The majority of these studies have been carried out in the United States.* However, as Americans seem to have the highest rates of cannabis use of the populations in the industrialized world,[31] the findings may not apply to other nations. Furthermore, most studies are limited to youth samples. This is supposedly owing to the fact that adolescence is the major risk period for the onset of cannabis involvement.[20,32,33] A different kind of problem is the failure to distinguish between different degrees of cannabis involvement. This omission is highly regrettable, as the predisposing factors and psychosocial correlates of various stages of use (i.e., initiation, continuation, abuse, cessation, and relapse) appear to be different.[34-37] Another serious weakness is the absence of statistical testing for sex differences in many of the studies. Thus, some variables have been found to be related to cannabis involvement in only one of the sexes, but it has not been reported whether the correlations are significantly different in males and females. Such findings remain uncertain as they may be owing to sex differences in the variability of the variables included in the analyses.

---

*Unless other information is explicitly given, the studies that are reviewed have been carried out in the United States.

Finally, it should be pointed out that some important questions concerning male and female cannabis use do not appear to have been subject to research at all. Thus, comparative studies on the effects of liberalization of the laws regulating cannabis use seem to be nonexistent. Considering the fact that women tend to be more law-abiding than men, data on this topic would have been highly interesting. Furthermore, there seems to be a lack of research on possible sex differences in the physiological aspects of cannabis use.

Despite the limitations, some interesting studies on various aspects of sex differences in cannabis use do exist. These studies will be reviewed in different sections under the following main themes: prevalence and patterns of use, personality predictors, behavioral correlates, deviance theories and their relative applicability in explaining male and female cannabis involvement, subjective reasons for use, consequences of use, and finally, cessation.

Prevalence and Patterns
of Cannabis Use in Males and Females

As outlined in the introduction, some factors may promote cannabis involvement in females, whereas others probably function as barriers. However, the traditional barriers against illegal drug use in women may have become less influential during the last decades. If so, data on prevalence and patterns of cannabis use would be expected to be in agreement with the hypothesized convergence in male and female rates of deviance.[16]

In agreement with data from nations outside the industrialized world,[38] the majority of the studies from both the United States[1,21,39–43] and different European countries[6,37,44–48] have revealed that males are more involved with cannabis than females. This finding is in agreement with data on sex differences in the consumption of most other substances.[21] Furthermore, it agrees with the general distinctions between males and females regarding involvement in illegal activities.

However, there are also some empirical indications that the sex differences in cannabis use are becoming smaller. In a former review of the literature, it was found that studies carried out prior to the 1970s were somewhat more likely than later studies to find that more men than women used marijuana.[49] Recent documentation provides additional evidence for this trend. Comparable data from the nationwide Household Surveys in 1982 and 1988 showed that the prevalence of marijuana use in the United States was becoming increasingly similar in men and women.[39,42] This convergence was far more pronounced among youth and young adults than in older age groups. Interestingly, this change has taken place at the same time as the overall use

of cannabis was declining.[21,40,50,51] However, in general
siderably more men than women in the high-consump

The findings from the United States agree with tl
nations. Thus, data from annual representative surveys ...
region of the capital of Norway have also revealed a general decline, and
convergence of male and female rates of cannabis use, during the recent
years.[52] However, a persistence of traditional sex differences in the high-
consumption groups has also been found.[6] Studies of random national
samples of youth in Australia provide additional evidence for a downward
trend in cannabis use during the 1980s.[53] Nonetheless, young Australian
females increased their rate of cannabis use from 1985 to 1988, whereas the
corresponding rates for males declined. In contrast, there was a steady decline
in both sexes during the 1980s in the United States, but more so in males.

Summarizing, data from the United States, Australia, and Norway
reveal that there has been a convergence in male and female rates of cannabis use during the last decade. However, there are still more men than
women in the high-consumption groups, implying that it is premature to
conclude that recent research on cannabis use unambiguously supports the
convergence hypothesis.[16] Furthermore, because of the lack of trend data
from other nations, it remains unclear whether there have been similar
changes in the rates of cannabis use elsewhere.

Personality Predictors
of Male and Female Cannabis Use

Traditionally, the explanations of men's and women's deviant behavior have varied. Females who engage in deviant acts have been interpreted
in terms of intrapersonal factors, such as individual maladjustment or personality deviance. In contrast, corresponding behavior among men has been
understood as a consequence of external influences, for example, subcultural norms, environmental strains, and the like.[10,54] According to such gender-specific interpretations, personality factors would be expected to have
a stronger predictive effect on cannabis involvement in females than in males.

To date, only two prospective studies have examined the predictive
power of childhood personality characteristics on adolescent cannabis use:
a study from the San Francisco area,[55] and the so-called Woodlawn study.[56]

In the former study, childhood indications of antisocial tendencies and
several measures of ego under-control and emotional instability were significantly related to adolescent marijuana involvement in both sexes. However, the early signs of antisocial traits in boys were manifested in terms of

pulsiveness, aggression, lack of shyness, and acting-out. In contrast, an inability to empathize with others and insufficient social skills to form good relationships appeared to be the typical manifestation in girls.

In the Woodlawn study, it was also found that childhood aggressiveness and lack of shyness were significantly related to adolescent marijuana use in boys but not in girls. It was also shown that boys who had been classified as both shy and aggressive became the heaviest users of alcohol, marijuana, and cigarets in adolescence.

There are some important methodological differences between the studies on childhood precursors of cannabis use. The sample in the San Francisco study was relatively heterogenous, with respect to social class and ethnicity, but the majority were White and belonged to the middle or upper class.[57] The study originally consisted of 130 3-yr-old nursery school children, and information on cannabis involvement was gathered from 105 (81%) of these subjects at the age of 14. Thus, the dependent variable was actually early onset of cannabis use, and not cannabis involvement *per se*. The other study was initially based on a sample of the first graders in Woodlawn, a poor Black ghetto in Chicago.[56] The participants were assessed at the age of 6–7, and reassessed 10 yr later. At follow-up, the sample consisted of 705 subjects, and included 57% of the original participants. Unfortunately, statistical testing for the reported sex differences was not performed in either of these two studies, implying that these particular results are somewhat uncertain.

There is one more study in which personality predictors of male and female cannabis use have been analyzed. This study was limited to 16- to 18-yr-old pupils, and the aim was to explore the predictive power of Zuckerman's[58] sensation-seeking scale.[6] The sample, which consisted of adolescents living close to the capital of Norway, was followed over a period of almost 2 yr, and assessed twice. A total of 593 respondents participated in both assessments, corresponding to 93% of the subjects in the target sample.

Experience seeking, i.e., the nonconformist "hippie" subscale of the sensation-seeking inventory, was found to be significantly related to cannabis use during the following year, but only in males. Thus, it is possible that the anti-establishment component of cannabis use applies more to boys than to girls. The disinhibition subscale, which involves traditional norm violation, such as heavy drinking, gambling, and sexual experimentation, had an equally strong effect on cannabis involvement in both sexes. Interestingly, this subscale has been found to be closely related to the diagnostic construct of sociopathy.[58] This result thus seems to agree with the reviewed findings of the study from San Francisco[55] regarding the predictive power of antisocial tendencies on adolescent marijuana involvement.

Altogether, recent research on precursors of cannabis involvement does not suggest that this kind of deviance is more closely related to personality factors in females than in males. Few sex differences were identified, and those revealed indicate that early shyness and aggressiveness predict later cannabis involvement in boys but not in girls. However, this finding is somewhat uncertain, and may partly result from a lack of variability of these variables in girls. Antisocial characteristics were about equally important in predicting cannabis involvement in both sexes, but the early manifestations of these characteristics were different in girls and boys.

Other Types of Problem Behavior in Male and Female Cannabis Users

If cannabis use in females is socially defined as a more serious norm violation than similar behavior in males, female users might be expected to be more behaviorally deviant than their male counterparts in other areas too. Two different processes might account for this hypothesized sex difference. First, females who start using cannabis might initially be more rebellious and non-normative than males who do the same. Second, stigmatization might primarily affect cannabis-using females, leading to a more deviant career in them than in cannabis-using males.

However, longitudinal data from the study of Jessor and Jessor[59] revealed that the predictive power of problem behavior (e.g., heavy alcohol consumption and precocious sexual activity) and deviant activities (lying, stealing, vandalism, and the like) on adolescent cannabis involvement was invariant across sex. Furthermore, cross-sectional findings from the sixth wave of data collection disclosed a persistency in the high correlations between frequent marijuana use and engagement in problem behavior among adults in their middle and late 20s.[60] Apart from some indications that marijuana use was more strongly associated with a recent history of drunkenness in males than in females, no systematic sex differences were detected.

A major methodological limitation in the Jessors' research project is the low initial response rate. Only 53% of the subjects in their original random sample of high school students in a small Colorado city responded, whereas the response rate in a corresponding sample of college students was 60%. However, an absence of substantial sex differences in the association between cannabis involvement and other problem behavior is not limited to the study carried out by the Jessors. Similar results have been found in a study of high school students in Los Angeles,[61] and in the sample of adolescents in a large scale nationwide American survey.[60] Studies of youth from Norway[37] and Canada[62] provide additional evidence.

Whereas there is considerable documentation that cannabis involvement is strongly and equally related to other nonnormative behavior in both sexes, some studies have found indications of sex differences in this pattern. Thus, in a Household Survey of young adults in Baltimore, misbehavior and engagement in minor delinquency before the age of 18 were significantly related to last month's frequency of marijuana use in females but not in males.[63] Cross-sectional data from the previously reviewed study from San Francisco[55] also revealed that marijuana involvement at the age of 14 was somewhat more closely related to consumption of other substances in girls than in boys. Furthermore, in a study of 12- to 16-yr-old junior high school students in an urban district in the United States, the relative risk of coital experience was more than twice as high among girls who had used marijuana compared with boys in the same category.[64] Finally, retrospective data of a nationally representative sample of young American adults revealed that the linkages between early sexual activity and subsequent initiation of marijuana use were stronger in girls than in boys.[65]

To some extent, the reported sex differences may reflect the fact that biological maturation occurs at an earlier age in girls than in boys. It has been shown that girls who mature early are considerably more likely to use cannabis, get drunk, and to engage in other norm violations than girls who mature late.[66] This effect of biological age has been found to be mediated by the association with older peer groups. However, to our knowledge, no study has explored the interaction effects between gender, biological age, and engagement in different types of problem behavior.

To summarize, recent empirical evidence demonstrates that cannabis involvement is closely related to problem behavior and antisocial activities in both sexes. This finding agrees with the research on the predictive power of antisocial personality precursors.[6,55] Many studies failed to identify any substantial sex differences, whereas the results of others indicate that early or frequent cannabis use is somewhat more closely related to behavioral deviance in females than in males.

Are the Same Deviance Theories Equally Applicable in Explaining Male and Female Cannabis Use?

The major theoretical contributions on deviant behavior were originally constructed by men in order to explain male deviance. According to recent criticism, these theories apply primarily to men's involvement with deviant activities.[54] In line with this reasoning, important deviance theories would be of limited use in understanding any kind of deviant behavior among women, including cannabis use.

In order to examine the empirical tenability of traditional deviance theories in explaining male and female cannabis use, Smith and Paternoster[54] carried out a study of a large sample ($N = 1383$) of 16- to 17-yr-old high school students from an urban southeastern area in the United States. At the initial data collection, 13 predictor variables derived from four different deviance theories (i.e., social control theory, differential association, strain theory, and deterrence theory) were assessed. In the second year of the study, the respondents were asked to report their frequency of marijuana use in the previous year.

The results revealed that only 2 of the 13 predictor variables were differently related to prevalence (i.e., the use/nonuse dichotomy) of marijuana use in males and females. Moral objections to marijuana use predicted nonuse in both sexes, but the effect was significantly stronger in females. This may reflect the fact that marijuana use is illegal, implying that the barriers against use are probably regarded as more unalterable by females than by males. Furthermore, having marijuana-using peers increased the propensity to use marijuana in both sexes, but more so in males. No significant sex differences were identified at all with regard to frequency of marijuana use (nonusers excluded). In both sexes, the prevalence as well as the frequency of marijuana use were strongly related to the social support it receives from friends. This variable is one of the key elements in the differential association theory.[67]

Certain reservations should be made in interpreting the results of this study because the initial level of cannabis involvement was not taken into account. As males tend to start using this substance at an earlier age than females,[42] the findings may not be directly comparable across gender. Thus, the predictor variables might primarily be related to initiation of cannabis use in girls and to continuation in boys.

In any case, some cross-sectional studies have also failed to identify major sex differences in the explanatory power of traditional deviance theories on cannabis involvement.[68,69] Furthermore, in agreement with the findings of Smith and Paternoster,[54] peer influences have repeatedly been found to have a particularly strong effect on substance use in adolescents.[8,31,70,71] Interestingly, the somewhat stronger effect of exposure to peer modeling in males compared with females has also been reported by others. The results of a representative Norwegian survey of youth showed that in subgroups with high exposure to cannabis, more females than males remained nonusers.[72]

The findings of other studies do not agree with the results reported by Smith and Paternoster.[54] Cross-sectional data from the Woodlawn study[56] revealed sex differences in the effect of variables derived from the social control theory* on cannabis involvement. Thus, strong attachment to peers was significantly associated with heavy marijuana use in adolescent males, but not in females. Furthermore, for females, but not for males, stronger family bonds were related to less heavy marijuana use. The latter finding agrees with the results reported by Block et al.[55] In their study, family affairs and the parents' childrearing practices had significantly stronger effects on cannabis involvement in females than males.

Summing up, recent empirical evidence indicates that the traditional deviance theories are about equally applicable in explaining male and female cannabis involvement. However, as males seem to be somewhat more influenced by the exposure to cannabis-using friends than females, certain elements of the differential association theory apply more to males than to females. This may mean that acceptance and support from the peer group are more important to boys than to girls. Compared with young males, young females are more apt to be emotionally attached to a few close friends,[73] and such friendships are likely to weaken the effect of external group pressure. Sex differences regarding the importance of significant others may also explain why family characteristics and closeness to parents appear to be more strongly related to cannabis involvement in females than in males.

Subjective Reasons for Cannabis Use in Males and Females

From a sex role perspective, the subjective reasons for substance use might be assumed to be different in men and women. As using illicit drugs seems to be less sex-role-appropriate for females than for males, females might feel that they need a better justification for doing so. Self-medication might thus be expected to be a frequently reported subjective reason for cannabis use in females, but not in males.

The Monitoring the Future project, which involves annual surveys of large representative samples of American high school seniors, has collected some interesting data on self-reported reasons for cannabis use.[74] In 1983 and 1984, questionnaires dealing with this topic were distributed to one-fifth of the respondents ($N \approx 7000$). Analyses of these data revealed that the reasons for cannabis involvement were unrelated to sex, but only among the experimental and the occasional users. Among heavier users (i.e., those with a lifetime frequency of more than 10 times), a significantly higher proportion of the males than of the females reported that they used can-

*According to social control theory, deviant behavior is a result of insufficient bonds with conventional social groups or institutions, such as families and schools.[72]

nabis to "increase the effects of other drugs". Furthermore, women with daily use (a subgroup of the heavier users) were more likely to state that they used cannabis "because of anger and frustration" than their male counterparts. This finding agrees with data from a survey of 6th- to 12th-grade students in Oklahoma, which showed that frequency of marijuana use was related to coping reasons (e.g., to relieve nervousness or because of depression) in females but not in males.[75]

Newcomb et al.[76] have also examined sex differences in adolescents' subjective motivations for marijuana use. Information on this topic was gathered in the third data collection of their prospective study of high school students in Los Angeles ($N = 1068$). Analyses of the data structure resulted in the following four-factor solution: to enhance positive affect and creativity; to reduce negative affect; social cohesion (i.e., because of perceived peer pressure and to increase the feelings of social competence); and addiction (i.e., to feel better and to be able to get through the day). All the factors were related to frequency of marijuana use in both sexes, but the effect of social cohesion was significantly stronger in males than in females. This finding agrees with the previously reviewed indications that boys are more influenced by the drug use habits of their peers than girls are.[54,72] However, an examination of the predictive power of the motivation factors on cannabis involvement 1 yr later revealed an opposite sex difference to that in the cross-sectional analyses. Thus, when controlling for earlier cannabis use, the long-term effect of social cohesion was stronger in females than in males. This contradictory finding is not explained by the authors.

Altogether, recent evidence indicates that males and females who use cannabis infrequently have roughly the same subjective reasons for doing so. In contrast, some sex differences have been identified among the heavier users. Thus, high-consuming males report that they use cannabis for instrumental reasons (i.e., to enhance the effects of other drugs) more often than their female counterparts. Furthermore, frequent cannabis use seems to be more closely related to coping motivation and self-medication reasons in females than in males. This finding is in agreement with the expectation that females, in contrast to males, may feel that they need a solid justification for using an illicit drug.

Consequences of Cannabis Use in Males and Females

Robbins has specified three theoretical perspectives of interest with regard to the consequences of cannabis use in males and females.[77] One moment of concern is the hypothesized generalized female vulnerability to adverse implications of substance use. This hypothesis is grounded on the differences between the sexes concerning social control, stigmatization, and the physical vulnerability to certain substances. Another perspective focuses on distinctions between male and female styles of psychopathology. According to this approach, women are apt to experience harmful intrapsychic consequences of their substance use, whereas men are vulnerable to unfavorable behavioral and interpersonal effects. The third perspective is derived from the convergence hypothesis. An implication of this hypothesis is that the consequences of substance use might be expected to become more similar in men and women. In order to evaluate the empirical tenability of the various hypotheses, the nationwide sample of 12- to 34-yr-old Americans from the 1985 National Household Survey of Drug Abuse was examined.[77] The respondents in this study had been given a check list of problem items, together with questions on which particular substance the problem was considered to have resulted from.

Analyses of the data turned out to be most consistent with the perspective that emphasized sex differences in style and content of harmful effects. Thus, frequency of marijuana use was more closely related to an index of adverse social and behavioral consequences in males than in females. In contrast, the corresponding correlation with an index of harmful psychological consequences was comparatively stronger in females, although not significantly so. An examination of the interaction effects between sex and marijuana consumption on single problem items revealed several significant differences between males and females in agreement with this pattern. However, men used marijuana more frequently than women, and this was found to account for a substantial part of the sex difference in the reported social/behavioral problems. On the other hand, this implies that the increased vulnerability of women as regards experiencing harmful psychological consequences persists, despite the fact they are less involved with marijuana than men.

Instead of assessing subjective beliefs, Yamaguchi and Kandel[78] analyzed the temporal relationships between cannabis use and various life-events, in order to explore the consequences of use of this substance. Their hypothesis was that marijuana involvement is incompatible with conventional adult roles, and that conflicts in this respect may be solved by a postponement of marriage or parenthood, or by divorce. The analyses were based on retrospective data from 1325 adults in their middle 20s. These respondents had been included in the target sample of a representative survey of high school students in New York State 9 yr earlier. The completion rate was high (81%).

The results revealed that irrespective of age and other background variables, marijuana use postponed the timing of marriage in both sexes.

Furthermore, when marijuana use was retained after marriage, the propensity of getting separated or divorced was considerably increased. This effect was somewhat stronger in males than in females, but this apparent sex difference was not statistically tested. Marijuana use was also associated with a postponement of pregnancy in married women. In contrast, the timing of parenthood in married men was found to be unrelated to marijuana involvement, and this sex difference was significant.

In summary, cannabis use appears to have implications on the life situation of both males and females. It leads to a postponement of marriage and to an increased risk of marital break-up in both sexes. Some interesting sex differences have also been reported. First, females appear to experience comparatively more intrapsychic problems as a result of their cannabis involvement, whereas males are more apt to report impaired social functioning. This finding is highly contradictory to the convergence hypothesis,[16] and seems to reflect a persistence of traditional sex differences in this kind of deviance. Second, the effect of cannabis involvement on postponement of parenthood has been found to be limited to females. According to Yamaguchi and Kandel,[78] this finding may demonstrate a concern among marijuana-using women about anticipated harmful impacts of drug use on the fetus. However, it is also possible that females perceive their parental role as less compatible with marijuana involvement than males do. Furthermore, the results may indicate that the aversive effects of marijuana involvement on the reproductive system* affect females more than males.

Cessation of Cannabis Use
in Males and Females

Considering the fact that females tend to use cannabis less frequently than males, it seems likely that they stop using this substance at a comparatively earlier age. Females are presumably also comparatively less likely to relapse. Moreover, factors promoting cessation may be assumed to reflect some general differences between men and women. In agreement with Yamaguchi and Kandel's[78] study on the consequences of marijuana use, parenthood might be expected to have a stronger effect on cessation in females than in males.

Recent research seems to confirm these expectations. Additional results reported by Yamaguchi and Kandel showed that among nonexperimental

---

*There are some studies indicating that cannabis use affects the reproductive system of both males and females.[17,79]

marijuana-users (i.e., those with a lifetime frequency of more than 10 times), more females than males had become abstainers at the age of 25.[78] Females were also found to be less inclined to relapse than males. Similar sex differences were identified in a follow-up of this sample 4 yr later.[33]

Furthermore, it has been revealed that parenthood has a stronger effect on cessation in women than in men. Thus, in contrast to males, females tend to terminate their marijuana involvement 1 yr prior to the birth of the first child.[78] In addition, being a parent at the age of 24–25 predicts cessation in 28- to 29-yr-old females, but not in their male counterparts.[33] On the other hand, entry into marriage after the age of 24–25 has been found to have a significant and unique predictive power on later discontinuation of marijuana use in both sexes.

In a nationwide representative survey of 19- to 22-yr-old Norwegians, it was also revealed that cessation of cannabis use was more closely related to parenthood in females than in males.[37] Furthermore, high aspirations with regard to future careers had a stronger predictive power on cessation in males than in females, but this difference was not statistically significant.

In conclusion, recent studies show that parenthood has a stronger effect on cessation of cannabis use in females than in males. This finding seems to illustrate that becoming a parent has a greater impact on the life situation of women than of men. However, irrespective of parental status, it seems to be easier for females than for males to discontinue their cannabis involvement. Thus, females stop using this substance at an earlier age than males, and they are less likely to relapse. To some extent, this is probably owing to the fact that females do not use cannabis as often as males, implying that they are comparatively less likely to be addicted.

Discussion

The foregoing review of the literature revealed that the rate of cannabis use in females has approximated that of males during the last decade. But heavy use, which is generally considered deviant,[80] continues to be a male domain. Other indications of a persistence of traditional gender distinctions were also found, but these findings were few and the differences relatively small. Certain childhood characteristics, such as early aggressiveness in boys, and an absence of basic social skills in girls, predicted adolescent cannabis use. Furthermore, strong family bonds and parenthood were more closely related to nonuse in females than in males, indicating that close interpersonal relationships and family membership still affect the sexes differently. Females were also found to use cannabis for self-medication reasons more often than males. The consequences of cannabis use were also found to be related to gender. Males were apt to experience adverse social effects, whereas females were more likely to experience psychological problems.

Interestingly, the sex differences tended to be more pronounced among the early* and the heavy users than in other user groups. In the terminology of the theory on diffusion of innovation,[81] the more deviant cannabis-using groups may be later adopters of the recent changes in the sex roles. This, may in turn, be a result of differential selection processes. Thus, persons with unconventional values, including an opposition to traditional sex roles, may prefer using cannabis infrequently. These characteristics may not be shared by those who develop an extensive pattern of use. However, it has been revealed that an anti-establishment orientation characterizes both groups.[7] But the heavier users seem to have considerably poorer mental health, more family problems, and weaker ties to community organizations than the less frequent users. This provides reason to speculate whether the opposition to the establishment is comparatively more important to those using cannabis infrequently. Furthermore, it is possible that they tend to be politically engaged and to sympathize with radical movements, whereas the opposition of heavy users may be manifested in terms of norm violation and antisocial activities. Interestingly, such deviance has been found to be associated with traditional sex role characteristics in females. More specifically, the sex role of teenage girls who belong to delinquent juvenile groups tends to be conventional,[82] and the same is true for heroin-addicted women.[83]

Although certain interesting sex differences in cannabis use were detected, the absence of such differences in many important respects was conspicuous. In particular, the studies on personality predictors and the empirical testing of different deviance theories provided evidence for this trend. To some extent, this may reflect some of the peculiarities of the cannabis culture. Thus, ever since the late 1960s, the "feminine" characteristics of this culture may have had a special appeal to persons whose sex roles are indistinct or unconventional. These characteristics may in particular have attracted males with few typical masculine traits. On the other hand, it is also possible that the reported findings reflect the recent loosening of the traditional sex role pattern in the general population.

Irrespective of the reason, the limited number of sex differences in cannabis use clearly indicates that preventive efforts do not necessarily have to be gender-specific. However, some findings still suggest that it may be

---

*It should be mentioned that early cannabis use strongly predicts escalation into heavy use.[80]

particularly useful to teach boys to resist peer pressure, and to guide girls on how they can cope with their personal problems in other ways than by using cannabis.

The reported results and the conclusions that have been drawn from this review of the literature may be subject to several limitations.

First, the findings from the United States may not apply to other nations. Thus, Americans appear to be more involved with cannabis than the populations in other parts of the industrialized world, and when the consumption of a certain substance becomes widespread, the stigma associated with its use tends to decrease.[84] This provides a reason to speculate whether the sex differences in cannabis use are less pronounced in the United States than in other countries.

Characteristics of the samples and other methodological factors should also be considered. The majority of the recently published studies included only adolescents, and owing to age or cohort effects, the sex differences in cannabis use may be less pronounced in such samples than in corresponding samples of adults. In studies of student populations, additional biasing factors are likely to make the findings questionable. Thus, school dropouts tend to have considerably higher rates of drug use, and there are some indications that they are more likely to be males than females.[84] Differential rates of absenteeism may also result in a higher underrepresentation of drug-using males than drug-using females. The same problem is likely to exist in Household Surveys as well, because the homeless, and those living in prisons, hospitals, dormitories, and military installations are excluded. These selection processes may have distorted the results of the general population studies on cannabis use in two different ways. Thus, disproportionately few heavy cannabis users have probably been included, and the sex differences were found to be generally more pronounced in such user groups than among the experimental users. Furthermore, the sex differences may have been reduced as a result of a higher loss of high-consuming males than of their female counterparts.

Differential attrition rates in longitudinal studies may have similar effects. Thus, in the study of the Kandel group, it was found that the reinterview rates were unrelated or negatively related to earlier drug consumption and deviant activities in young adult males.[85] In contrast, the reinterviewed females reported engagement in minor delinquency more often than the noninterviewed, and they had higher initial levels of marijuana and alcohol consumption. Kandel et al. suggested that this finding may reflect a negative effect of deviance on the likelihood of getting married, implying that the more conforming females are harder to locate because of their name changes.[85] In any case, when a disproportional number of the nondeviant females are lost, the sex differences in cannabis use are likely to appear smaller than they really are.

In addition to the limitations and sources of error outlined, the possible omission of nonsignificant results or negative evidence should be considered. If negative findings are less likely to be reported than positive, the absence of sex differences in cannabis use may be even more pronounced than the available literature indicates. Unfortunately, it is hardly possible to find out to what extent the literature is biased in this way. According to Ashmore, the trend, at least in psychological research, was characterized by a maximizing of sex differences in the 1980s.[86] However, some factors may also have favored the publication of negative findings during the previous decade. As certain theories on human behavior were accused of being gender-specific, it was in the interest of the proponents of those theories to demonstrate that they applied equally well to both sexes. In particular, this assumption may apply to the studies of the explanatory power of traditional deviance theories on male and female cannabis involvement.

References

[1]D. I. Macdonald (1987) Patterns of alcohol and drug use among adolescents. *Pediatr. Clin. North Am.* **34,** 275–288.

[2]J. Auld (1981) *Marijuana Use and Social Control.* Academic, London.

[3]E. A. Suchman (1968) The "hang-loose" ethic and the spirit of drug use. *J. Health Soc. Behav.* **9,** 146–155.

[4]S. K. Schonberg and S. H. Schnoll (1986) Drugs and their effect on adolescent users, in *Teen Drug Use.* G. Beschner and A. S. Friedman, eds. Lexington Books, Lexington, MA, pp. 43–62.

[5]J. Mandel and H. W. Feldman (1986) The social history of teenage drug users, in *Teen Drug Use.* G. Beschner and A. S. Friedman, eds. Lexington Books, Lexington, MA, pp. 19–42.

[6]W. Pedersen (1991) Mental health, sensation seeking and drug use patterns: A longitudinal study. *Br. J. Addict.* **86,** 195–204.

[7]W. Pedersen (1990) Adolescents initiating cannabis use: Cultural opposition or poor mental health? *J. Adolesc.* **13,** 327–339.

[8]D. B. Kandel (1984) Marijuana users in young adulthood. *Arch. Gen. Psychiatry* **41,** 200–209.

[9]B. R. Carlson and W. H. Edwards (1990) Human values and marijuana use. *Int. J. Addict.* **25,** 1393–1401.

[10]R. A. Cloward and F. F. Piven (1979) Hidden protest: The channeling of female innovation and resistance. *J. Women Culture Soc.* **4,** 651–669.

[11]E. S. Gomberg (1982) Historical and political perspective: Women and drug use. *J. Soc. Issues* **38,** 9–23.

[12]E. W. Single (1989) The impact of marijuana decriminalization: An update. *J. Public Health Policy* **10,** 456–466.

[13]E. L. Engelsman (1989) Dutch policy on the management of drug-related problems. *Br. J. Addict.* **84,** 211–218.

[14]R. G. Schlaadt and R. T. Shannon (1990) *Drugs.* Prentice-Hall, Englewood Cliffs, NJ.

[15]D. McVay (1991) Marijuana legalization: the time is now, in *The Drug Legalization Debate, Studies in Crime, Law and Justice*, vol. 7. J. A. Inciardi, ed. Sage, Newbury Park, CA, pp. 147–160.

[16]F. Adler (1975) *Sisters in Crime*. Waveland, Prospect Heights, IL.

[17]M. S. Gold (1989) Marijuana. *Drugs of Abuse: A Comprehensive Series for Clinicans*, vol. 1: *Marijuana*. Plenum, New York.

[18]K. Yamaguchi and D. B. Kandel (1984) Patterns of drug use from adolescence to young adulthood: II. Sequences of progression. *Am. J. Public Health* **74,** 668–672.

[19]K. Yamaguchi and D. B. Kandel (1984) Patterns of drug use from adolescence to young adulthood: III. Predictors of progression. *Am. J. Public Health* **74,** 673–681.

[20]D. B. Kandel and J. A. Logan (1984) Patterns of drug use from adolescence to young adulthood: I. Periods of risk for initiation, continued use and discontinuation. *Am. J. Public Health* **74,** 660–666.

[21]D. B. Kandel (1991) The social demography of drug use. *Milbank Q.* **69,** 365–414.

[22]O. J. Kalant (1980) Sex differences in alcohol and drug problems—some highlights, in *Alcohol and Drug Problems in Women*, vol 5. O. J. Kalant, ed. Plenum, New York, pp. 1–24.

[23]M. A. Sheppard, M. S. Goodstadt, and M. M. Willett (1987) Peer or parents: Who has the most influence on cannabis use? *J. Drug Educ.* **17,** 123–128.

[24]J. Shelder and J. Block (1990) Adolescent drug use and psychological health. A longitudinal inquiry. *Am. Psychol.* **45,** 612–630.

[25]R. M. Jones and B. Hartmann (1988) Ego identity: Developmental differences and experimental substance use among adolescents. *J. Adolesc.* **11,** 347–360.

[26]P. R. Clifford, E. W. Edmunson, W. R. Koch, and B. G. Dodd (1991) Drug use and life satisfaction among college students. *Int. J. Addict.* **26,** 45–53.

[27]M. F. Sieber and J. Angst (1990) Alcohol, tobacco and cannabis: 12-year longitudinal associations with antecedent social context and personality. *Drug Alcohol Depend.* **25,** 281–292.

[28]M. D. Krohn and J. L. Massey (1980) Social control and delinquent behavior: An examination of the elements of the social bond. *Sociol. Q.* **21,** 529–543.

[29]E. W. Labouvie and C. R. McGee (1986) Relation of personality to alcohol and drug use in adolescence. *J. Consult. Clin. Psychol.* **54,** 289–293.

[30]D. F. Peck and M. A. Plant (1986) Unemployment and illegal drug use: Concordant evidence from a prospective study and national trends. *Br. Med. J.* **293,** 929–932.

[31]M. D. Newcomb and P. M. Bentler (1989) Substance use and abuse among children and teenagers. *Am. Psychol.* **44,** 242–248.

[32]V. H. Raveis and D. B. Kandel (1987) Changes in drug behavior from the middle to the late twenties: Initiation, persistence, and cessation of use. *Am. J. Public Health* **77,** 607–611.

[33]D. B. Kandel and V. H. Raveis (1989) Cessation of illicit drug use in young adulthood. *Arch. Gen. Psychiatry* **46,** 109–116.

[34]T. M. Kimlica and J. H. Cross (1978) A comparison of chronic versus casual users on personal values and behavioral orientations. *Int. J. Addict.* **13,** 1145–1156.

[35]W. L. Lucas (1978) Predicting initial use of marijuana from correlates of marijuana use: Assessment of panel and cross-sectional data: 1969–1976. *Int. J. Addict.* **13,** 1035–1047.

[36]R. M. Weinstein (1978) The avowal of motives for marijuana behavior. *Int. J. Addict.* **13,** 887–910.

[37]T. Hammer and P. Vaglum (1990) Initiation, continuation or discontinuation of cannabis use in the general population. *Br. J. Addict.* **85,** 899–909.

[38]M. Dreher (1984) Marijuana use among women: An antropological view. *Adv. Alcohol Subst. Abuse* **3,** 51–65.

[39]B. W. Lex (1991) Some gender differences in alcohol and polysubstance users. *Health Psychol.* **10,** 121–132.

[40]J. G. Bachman, J. M. Wallace, P. M. O'Malley, L. D. Johnson, C. L. Kurth, and H. W. Neighbours (1991) Racial/ethnic differences in smoking, drinking and illicit drug use among American high school seniors, 1976–89. *Am. J. Public Health* **81,** 372–377.

[41]D. M. Murray, C. L. Perry, C. O'Connell, and L. Schmid (1987) Seventh-grade cigarette, alcohol, and marijuana use: distribution in a north central US metropolitan population. *Int. J. Addict.* **22,** 357–376.

[42]R. R. Clayton, H. L. Voss, C. Robbins, and W. F. Skinner (1986) Gender differences in drug use: an epidemiological perspective. *NIDA Res. Monogr.* **65,** 80–99.

[43]National Institute on Drug Abuse (1989) *National Household Survey on Drug Abuse: Population Estimates 1988.* DHHS Publication No. ADM 89-1636. U.S. Government Printing Office, Washington, DC.

[44]G. Sylbing and J. M. G. Peerson (1985) Cannabis use among youth in the Netherlands. *Bull. Narc.* **37,** 51–60.

[45]J. Mott (1985) Self-reported cannabis use in Great Britain in 1981. *Br. J. Addict.* **80,** 37–43.

[46]M. E. Rodriguez and J. Cami (1986) Substance use among medical students in Barcelona. A comparison with previous studies. *Drug Alcohol Depend.* **18,** 311–318.

[47]D. Queipo, F. J. Alvarez, and A. Velasco (1988) Drug consumption among university students in Spain. *Br. J. Addict.* **83,** 91–98.

[48]K. Kaas Ibsen and K. Juel (1984) Employment of hashish by young people. A nationwide investigation among 3500 young Danes. *Ugeskr. Laeger* **146,** 3773–3775.

[49]J. E. Prather and L. S. Fidell (1978) Drug use and abuse among women: An overview. *Int. J. Addict.* **13,** 863–885.

[50]P. M. O'Malley, J. G. Bachman, and L. D. Johnston (1988) Period, age and cohort effects on substance use among young Americans: A decade of change, 1976–86. *Am. J. Public Health* **78,** 1315–1321.

[51]E. R. Oetting and F. Beauvais (1990) Adolescent drug use: Findings from national and local surveys. *J. Consult. Clin. Psychol.* **58,** 385–394.

[52]O. Irgens-Jensen (1988) *Trends in the Use of Drugs Among Norwegian Youth.* Report no. 1, National Institute of Drug and Alcohol Research, Oslo, Norway.

[53]I. McAllister and T. Makkai (1991) Whatever happened to marijuana? Patterns of marijuana use in Australia, 1985–88. *Int. J. Addict.* **26,** 491–504.

[54]D. A. Smith and R. Paternoster (1987) The gender gap in theories of deviance: Issues and evidence. *J. Res. Crime Delinquency* **24,** 140–172.

[55]J. Block, J. H. Block, and S. Keyes (1988) Longitudinal foretelling drug usage in adolescence: Early childhood personality and environmental precursors. *Child Dev.* **59,** 336–355.

[56]M. E. Ensminger, C. H. Brown, and S. G. Kellam (1982) Sex differences in the antecedents of substance use among adolescents. *J. Soc. Issues* **38,** 25–42.

[57]J. Block and J. H. Block (1980) The role of ego control and ego resiliency in the organization of behavior, in *Minnesota Symposium on Child Psychology*, vol. 13. W. A. Collins, ed. Erlbaum, Hillsdale, NJ, pp. 39–101.

[58]M. Zuckerman (1979) *Sensation Seeking. Beyond the Optimal Level of Arousal.* Erlbaum, Hillsdale, NJ.

[59]R. Jessor and S. L. Jessor (1977) *Problem Behavior and Psychosocial Development. A Longitudinal Study of Youth.* Academic, NY.

[60]J. E. Donovan and R. Jessor (1985) Structure of problem behavior in adolescence and young adulthood. *J. Consult. Clin. Psychol.* **53**, 890–904.

[61]M. D. Newcomb, E. Maddahian, and P. M. Bentler (1986) Risk factors for drug use among adolescents: Concurrent and longitudinal analyses. *Am. J. Public Health* **76**, 525–531.

[62]J. D. Hundleby (1987) Adolescent drug use in a behavioral matrix: Confirmation and comparision of the sexes. *Addict. Behav.* **12**, 103–112.

[63]J. C. Anthony (1984) Young adult marijuana use in relation to antecedent misbehaviors. *NIDA Res. Monogr.* **55**, 238–244.

[64]D. P. Orr, M. Beiter, and G. Ingersoll (1991) Premature sexual activity as an indicator of psychosocial risk. *Pediatrics* **87**, 141–147.

[65]F. L. Mott and R. J. Haurin (1988) Linkages between sexual activity and alcohol and drug use among American adolescents. *Fam. Plann. Perspect.* **20**, 128–136.

[66]D. Magnusson, H. Stattin, and V. L. Allen (1985) Biological maturation and social development: A longitudinal study of some adjustment processes from mid-adolescence to adulthood. *J. Youth Adolesc.* **14**, 267–283.

[67]E. H. Sutherland and D. R. Cressey (1978) *Criminology.* Lippincott, Philadelphia.

[68]H. R. White, V. Johnson, and A. Horwitz (1986) An application of three deviance theories to adolescent substance use. *Int. J. Addict.* **21**, 347–366.

[69]R. E. Johnson (1988) Correlates of adolescent drug use by gender and geographical location. *Am. J. Drug Alcohol Abuse* **14**, 51–63.

[70]M. Penning and G. E. Barnes (1982) Adolescent marijuana use: A review. *Int. J. Addict.* **17**, 749–791.

[71]L. Chassin (1984) Adolescent substance use and abuse, in *Adolescent Behavior Disorders. Advances in Child Behavior Analysis and Therapy*, vol. 3. P. Karoly and J. Steffen, eds. Lexington Books, Lexington, MA, pp. 99–152.

[72]T. Hammer and P. Vaglum (1991) Users and nonusers within a high risk milieu of cannabis use. A general population study. *Int. J. Addict.* **26**, 595–604.

[73]S. M. Dornbusch (1989) The sociology of adolescence. *Ann. Rev. Sociol.* **15**, 233–259.

[74]L. D. Johnston and P. M. O'Malley (1986) Why do the nation's students use drugs and alcohol? Self-reported reasons from nine national surveys. *J. Drug Issues* **16**, 29–66.

[75]J. Novacek, R. Raskin, and R. Hogan (1990) Why do adolescents use drugs? Age, sex and user differences. *J. Youth Adolesc.* **20**, 475–492.

[76]M. D. Newcomb, C. Chou, P. M. Bentler, and G. J. Huba (1988) Cognitive motivations for drug use among adolescents: Longitudinal tests of gender differences and predictors of change in drug use. *J. Counseling Psychol.* **35**, 426–438.

[77]S. Robbins (1989) Sex differences in psychosocial consequences of alcohol and drug abuse. *J. Health Soc. Behav.* **30**, 117–130.

[78]K. Yamaguchi and D. B. Kandel (1985) On the resolution of role incompatibility: A life event history analysis of family roles and marijuana use. *Am. J. Sociol.* **90**, 1284–1325.

[79]P. Mann (1985) *Marijuana Alert.* McGraw-Hill, New York.

[80]H. B. Kaplan, S. S. Martin, and R. J. Johnson (1986) Escalation of marijuana use: Application of a general theory of deviant behavior. *J. Health Soc. Behav.* **27,** 41–61.

[81]E. M. Rogers (1983) *Diffusion of Innovation.* Free, New York.

[82]A. Snare (1989) Women and control, in *Women, Alcohol and Drugs.* E. Haavio-Mannila, ed. NAD-Publication no. 16, Nordic Council for Alcohol and Drug Research, Helsinki, pp. 133–152.

[83]M. Rosenbaum (1981) Sex roles among deviants: The woman addict. *Int. J. Addict.* **16,** 859–877.

[84]R. G. Ferrence and P. C. Whitehead (1980) Sex differences in psychoactive drug use, in *Research Advances in Alcohol and Drug Problems,* vol. 5: *Alcohol and Drug Problems in Women.* O. J. Kalant, ed. Plenum, New York, pp. 125–152.

[85]D. B. Kandel, V. Raveis, and J. Logan (1983) Sex differences in characteristics of members lost to a longitudinal panel: A speculative research note. *Public Opinion Q.* **47,** 567–575.

[86]R. D. Ashmore (1990) Sex, gender and the individual, in *Handbook of Personality: Theory and Research.* L. A. Pervin, ed. Guilford, New York, pp. 487–526.

Effects
of Chemical Dependency
in Parenting Women

Shoni Davis

Introduction

The concept of chemical dependency in women of childbearing age has gained national attention over the past two decades. For women who are dependent on drugs, the effects are far-reaching. Not only are their own lives affected in areas of physical, social, and interpersonal functioning, but also, and maybe even more devastating, is the effect and outcome on the growth and normal development of their children.

The problems and issues that the treatment of chemically dependent women must address are related more to their being women than to their being drug dependent.[1] This chapter will attempt to integrate current findings regarding issues pertinent to perinatal chemical dependency and its effect on parenting outcome. Throughout this chapter the terms drug user, drug dependent, chemically dependent, and drug addicted are used interchangeably to describe women who abuse drugs. This chapter will focus on illicit substances, including heroin, cocaine, amphetamines, and PCP. Less is known about women who abuse prescription or over-the-counter drugs. Although alcohol dependency is known to have severely negative effects on the abuser and the family, the focus on alcohol is not included in this chapter. The following topics will be reviewed:

From: *Drug and Alcohol Abuse Reviews, Vol. 5: Addictive Behaviors in Women*
Ed.: R. R. Watson ©1994 Humana Press Inc., Totowa, NJ

1. Profile of chemically dependent women;
2. Attributes associated with effective parenting;
3. Parenting characteristics of chemically dependent women;
4. The effects to children raised by chemically dependent women; and
5. Parent–child treatment needs of chemically dependent women.

Since the 1970s, there has been a growing interest in women's issues, including an examination of the stereotypes attributed to chemically dependent women and the resulting effect her addiction has on her children, both prenatally and throughout the child's development. It has become apparent that the needs and issues of chemically dependent women are unique to their gender. Evidence across the nation reveals that treatment programs have been slow to incorporate the necessary changes needed to effectively treat chemically dependent women. Many of the issues that drug treatment programs must address in relation to their female clients have to do more with issues related to women in general than to the chemical dependency. Issues, such as mother–child interaction, coping skills, female related medical complications, passivity, learned helplessness, and a lack of vocational training, are as common to chemically dependent women as they are to women in general. Many treatment programs fail to address these issues. Consequently, treatment outcomes for chemically dependent women are frequently evaluated through invalid measures, and chemically dependent women often complete treatment requirements without having internalized attitudes and lifestyle changes necessary to maintain abstinence and to cope effectively in their social environment. As a result, the children of these women are at risk to suffer the results of ineffective parenting.

In order for researchers and clinicians to overcome these deficiencies, it is necessary to establish a conceptual framework from which to view chemical dependency. One existing theory on drug addiction is that it is a maladaptive response to both internal and external stressors. Alexander claimed that faulty upbringing, defective social support, and genetic unfitness comprise a causal relationship that results in the chemically dependent individual making maladaptive responses in the areas of interpersonal roles, awareness of self needs, development of self-worth, and competency in adult roles.[2] The addiction becomes a substitute way of adapting by providing the individual a false sense of stability and a compensation of needs.

Chemically dependent women of childbearing age are a special population who demand scientific attention because of the far-reaching effect their maladaptive lifestyles have on the four lifestyle areas identified by Alexander.[2] Multiple stressors have been identified that commonly impact chemically dependent women. Dysfunctional interpersonal skills, poverty, social isolation, low self-esteem and feelings of worthlessness, inadequate education, and insufficient job skills, are but a few of the stressors that prevail among this population. Because of poor coping abilities, chemically dependent women are unable to handle this bombardment of stressors effectively. Their attempt to do so through drug use results in maladaptive lifestyles, which influence all areas of their lives. Their addictions often result in their continued drug use throughout their pregnancies and while they are parenting their children. One of the most serious consequences of drug addiction is the negative parenting techniques that chemically dependent women have been shown to demonstrate.

Often, the initial abuse a chemically dependent woman subjects her child to is prenatal drug exposure. As many as 400,000–700,000 babies/yr are born exposed to illicit drugs. These figures do not take into account babies born exposed to alcohol.[3] Although findings are somewhat limited, there is evidence that shows infants exposed prenatally to drugs, such as cocaine, amphetamines, PCP, or heroin, to be at high risk for multiple problems, including sudden infant death syndrome (SIDS), susceptibility to infections, developmental delays, speech pathologies, and central nervous system insults, which are manifested in behavioral disorders, extreme irritability, and hypersensitivity to environmental stimuli.

Although long-term outcomes are still being determined, the negative effects these infants display may not always disappear as the child matures. Instead, long-term problems may develop among children who were exposed to drugs prenatally. Significant findings reveal attention deficit disorders, learning disabilities, and aggressive behavioral tendencies among these children.[4,5]

Caring for a child who has been prenatally exposed to drugs and/or who displays the immediate long-term effects of *in utero* drug exposure is a challenging task for even the most well-adapted parent. Studies by Chasnoff indicate the degree of special handling, patience, and enhanced environmental conditions these children require if they are to overcome the obstacles that would impede a healthy developmental and emotional maturity.[6]

According to adaptational theorists, individuals dependent on drugs have never achieved an integrated sense of emotional maturity.[2] As a result, chemically dependent women are ill prepared to effectively parent the children they are producing. Their children become the innocent victims of a dysfunctional family system, which has been shown to repeat itself from generation to generation.

These children often end up requiring long-term foster care or institutional placement as a result of abandonment, neglect, or abuse by their mothers and extended family members. Because of the physical and psychological problems these children frequently possess, they are often labeled as being "hard to place" for either foster or adoptive homes. Chemically dependent women who are the mothers of these children are often negatively stereotyped as not caring about the welfare of their children. A close examination of the profile of these women reveals situational and psychological variables that help explain why the chemically dependent mother relies on the use of drugs as an adaptational mechanism, even though she is aware of the negative impact her drug addiction has on her children.

Profile of Chemically Dependent Women

The psychological profile of chemically dependent women reveals characteristics that have been shown to negatively effect parenting success. In order to develop treatment programs and intervention strategies for chemically dependent women that enhance their parenting effectiveness, it is necessary to understand general patterns they maintain. It can be said that drug-abusing women possess many similar characteristics.

Psychological Issues

Family History

It is in their families of origin that chemically dependent women are first introduced to the ineffective parenting techniques that they may later rely on in raising their own children. These women, like all those who are chemically dependent, tend to grow up in emotionally deprived family environments, and become victims of society as they grow older. Being set up for failure by the time they reach adulthood, they learn that drugs not only relieve psychological pain but allow for a sense of spontaneity otherwise missing.

The role of family and childhood trauma is widely recognized in the geneses of drug addiction. Parental death and/or desertion, divorce, marital disharmony, poor parental role modeling, parental substance abuse, and high rates of physical and sexual abuse have been identified as characteristics of the family histories of drug addicts.[6,7]

Black has done extensive work in the area of adult children of alcoholics, and emphasized the emotional destruction that occurs in children raised in dysfunctional, chaotic family systems.[8] Her findings have indicated that these children grow up to be as equally dysfunctional in adulthood as their parents, and frequently turn to substance abuse as a way of coping.

There appears to be little gender difference in family background of male and female drug users. A study was conducted in which the families of drug-addicted men displayed significantly more dysfunctional patterns and disturbances than control families of nonusing men.[9] For the few drug-dependent women included in this study ($N = 20$), there was no control group, but their families appeared similar to those of the drug-addicted men. It could be speculated that their families displayed a higher incidence of dysfunctional characteristics than the families of nonaddicted women. Findings from Binion dispute this speculation by finding only minor differences in family backgrounds between addicted women entering treatment and a control group from the same geographical area.[10]

Evidence supporting the notion that chemically dependent women come from dysfunctional family backgrounds is provided in a study by Anglin and Hser.[11] Utilizing a sample of 328 Anglo and Chicano drug-using women, the authors examined the relationship between women's narcotic use and crime. The results from an extensive interviewing procedure revealed that 43% of the Anglo and 36% of the Chicano subjects admitted to having poor adolescent relationships with their parents. Thirty-nine percent of the Anglo and 60% of the Chicano subjects reported coming from disrupted family environments, which included parental separation or divorce before the age of 16.

Criminal behavior has been shown to correlate with drug addiction, and often gets its start when the individual is young and living at home with their family of origin. Criminal behavior is usually associated with male addicts. However, Anglin and Hser disputed criminal differences between men and women addicts.[11] They pointed out that, according to the Federal Bureau of Investigation's uniform crime reports, women accounted for 16.6% of the total arrests in 1983, and made up 14% of the arrests for drug abuse violations.

Childhood sexual victimization appears to be highly correlated as a contributing factor in the etiology of adult drug addiction. Benward and Densen-Gerber found that 44% of their sample of female addicts had been sexually molested as children.[12] A more recent study by Rohsenow et al. revealed that 77% of the female drug users in their study admitted to childhood sexual abuse after the question was routinely asked of them while in treatment.[13]

This author's experience in talking to chemically dependent women is that those who were sexually molested as children are more likely to have been sexually assaulted in adulthood. Many chemically dependent women view sexual victimization as something they deserve and are unable to avoid.

Social Support

Overall, chemically dependent individuals tend to be socially isolated. Their deviant lifestyles cause them to withdraw from family and friends owing to feelings of shame and disgrace. In time they are rejected by those they are close to. Hawkins and Fraser pointed out that over time, drug users become isolated from people from conventional domains, such as work, school, organizations, and clubs.[14] Most drug users are not connected with the type of associates or friends who could replace the peers who make up their drug-using network. These authors found that drug users become enmeshed in a subculture that rewards drug abuse and often endures through residential treatment. They found that drug users report close, sharing, intimate relationships with people from a variety of sources from within their support network. However, when availability of conventional support networks do exist, drug users are less likely to sustain relationships with other drug users. An important aspect of rehabilitation, according to these authors, should involve helping the drug user connect with a support network who functions as positive role models.

This may be of particular importance for chemically dependent women. In a comparison study of Anglo and Chicano male and female drug users, it was found that 51% of the female subjects claimed that they were initially introduced to drugs by a husband or boyfriend.[15] The study concluded that the kind of support received from their partners might affect the rehabilitative outcome of chemically dependent women. On one hand, the rehabilitation of chemically dependent women may involve severing relations with addicted men. On the other hand, the authors claimed that rehabilitation may be improved as a result of an encouraging mate. In another study, Tracy et al. claimed that men do not usually stay with addicted women unless they themselves are also addicted.[16] Therefore, chemically dependent women usually have no valid male support. From this, Tracy claimed that chemically dependent women are as isolated in the drug culture as they are in society in general.

To add to their dilemma, chemically dependent women tend to have problems relating to others, and, as a result, may be less likely than nonaddicted women to utilize social support systems to cope with emotional turmoil and interpersonal problems.[17,18] Tucker pointed out that, even when available, support networks are not necessarily activated.[17] It appears that utilization of support as a coping mode depends on the individual's activation of the system, which in turn depends on individual coping preference. Tucker also explored the extent to which a lack of social support is associated with dysfunctional coping strategies. Her findings reveal that in the absence of social support, women, but not men, tended to use nonsocial, dysfunctional strategies to handle stress. These strategies included the use of withdrawal, avoidance, substance use, and taking frustration out on their kids. From this it can be postulated that to enhance parenting effectiveness of chemically dependent women, treatment programs must help the client establish positive social support networks.

Self-Esteem

It is a general consensus that chemically dependent individuals exhibit lower levels of self-esteem than drug-free individuals, and that female addicts tend to score lower on self-esteem than male addicts.[19] A study by Wheeler et al. is unique to the study of self-esteem among drug users in that, rather than focus on self-esteem at a single point during treatment, this study traced changes in self-esteem between men and women as treatment progressed.[20] Findings revealed that women addicts scored lower on "acceptance by family" and high on "neuroticism" at the beginning of treatment, and lower on "acceptance by family," "achievement of self-standards," and "acceptance by peers" toward the end of treatment. The authors interpreted these findings as implying that the scores of "family acceptance" and "neuroticism" at the beginning of treatment supports evidence that chemically dependent women are more disturbed than chemically dependent men prior to treatment. The drop in scores of women subjects at the end of treatment in "acceptance by family," "achievement of self-standards," and "acceptance by peers" are interpreted by the authors as implying that chemically dependent women preparing to return to society may have a more difficult time than men, as they consider their worth in society.

Female drug users tend to exhibit external and stable attributional patterns for failure, which also tend to improve with treatment.[21,22] It is not surprising that chemically dependent women tend to score high on the psychological factor known as externality.[23] This suggests the belief that their lives and fates are controlled by forces outside of themselves and that they have no control over what happens to them in their lives. Strict sex role stereotyping is another predominant theme that chemically dependent women often learn from their families of origin. As a result, chemically dependent women tend to display learned helplessness, which is a result of being taught as a child to be passive, dependent, and yielding, rather than competitive and self-sufficient.[24] Physical and emotional battering, which chemically dependent women are prone to experience while growing up, enhance the symptoms of learned helplessness over time.

Affective States

Although few studies have been conducted that focus specifically on the affective moods of chemically dependent women, it has been repeatedly noted that female addicts are more depressed than both nonaddicted women and addicted men.[25,26] Other negative affective states, such as a sense of worthlessness, feelings of hostility, failure, and anger, have also been documented as representing these women.[7,27,28] Drug-abusing women have been shown to doubt their effectiveness as parents.[29]

Whether negative affective states, such as depression, is a result of stress or a means of coping with stress is controversial. Rhoads, who studied the relationship of life stress and social support among drug abusers, found that the chemically dependent women in her sample reacted to stressful life events by becoming depressed.[30] Males in the study were found to exhibit greater tendencies toward anxiety resulting from stress.

In another study of social support and coping among chemically dependent women, it was found that in the absence of social support, drug-using women often rely on maladaptive, dysfunctional methods of behavior to relieve feelings of depression and anger, which result in additional stress.[31] The study pointed out that even though drug abuse may cause and maintain depressive bouts in chemically dependent women, these women do not necessarily relate the cause of their depression to their drug use. More likely, they will use drugs to counteract their depressed state. Regardless of their cause, negative affective states, such as depression, anger, and anxiety, can interfere with the ability to parent one's children effectively.

Socioeconomics Issues

Statistics available on drug-abusing women show that 60–70% of women entering drug treatment programs have dependent children.[32,33] However, these women very often lack the social and trade skills necessary to enter the work force. Treasure and Liao claimed that chemically dependent women are more likely than chemically dependent men to be unemployed, dependent on others for support, or receiving welfare.[34] These authors also added that chemically dependent women often lack the problem-solving and interpersonal skills necessary for independent functioning. The rate of unemployment has been shown to as high as 96% among this population.[35] This situation adds to the chemically dependent woman's feelings of helplessness, and makes it hard for her to get on her feet and leave her deviant lifestyle. Many chemically dependent women prostitute to support themselves, their dependents, and their drug habit.

Medical Complications

It has been reported that chemically dependent women tend to have more medical complications than do their male counterparts.[36] Many of these women self-medicate with continued drug use as a way of coping with prevailing medical complications and illness. The existence of medical conditions and continued drug use not only work at keeping chemically dependent women out of treatment programs, but also interferes with their ability to tend effectively to their children's physical and psychological needs.

These women tend to present in treatment with multiple medical problems including anemia, infections, hepatitis, venereal disease, and AIDS. Histories of obstetrical complications, premature deliveries, C-sections, and frequent abortions also prevail.[37]

Pregnancy Issues

A study by Bean noted that approx 70% of chemically dependent women receive no prenatal care during pregnancy, and do not understand that drugs are harmful to the fetus.[37] This author concluded that the lifestyle of female addicts is not conducive to good general health. Mondanaro, on the other hand, claimed that the female addict is very much aware that she is harming her fetus through the use of drugs, but is unable to stop because of her addiction, as well as her painful psychological status.[27]

Chemically dependent women have been known to define themselves as impotent to cope with life situations, deserving of rejection, and forced to be dependent on men whom they frequently feel ambivalence toward.[38] As is typical with adult children from dysfunctional families, chemically dependent women tend to choose mates who, like themselves, maintain low self-esteem, feelings of worthlessness, inadequate coping skills, and maladaptive lifestyles. To overcome their feeling of powerlessness, these men may victimize those who are weaker than themselves, which is often their spouses and children. The abuse and badgering that the chemically dependent woman grew up with as a child often becomes a part of her adult lifestyle.

Inevitably, many drug-addicted women become pregnant. Although usually unintentional, their pregnancies bring valued secondary gains. For perhaps the first time in these women's lives, they receive positive attention and displays of concern for their well-being. Many chemically dependent women claim that, during their pregnancies, they had a closer relationship with their mothers than ever before. They begin to idealize the situation and believe that their babies will somehow make their lives better. In spite of all this, many chemically dependent women continue their drug use throughout their pregnancies.[39,40] The result is that a drug-exposed baby is born who is often sick, nonresponsive to maternal caregiving, and difficult to bond with. The idealizations that the chemically dependent woman counted on during her pregnancy are replaced by harsh reality.

Because chemically dependent women have poor ego functioning, they often personalize the neonatal abstinence syndromes that their newborns may be experiencing as personal rejection. Instead of their babies making their lives better, these chemically dependent women feel more guilt, shame, and failure than ever before in their lives. They feel inadequate in their most basic role, that of motherhood.

Their feelings toward their babies are often ambivalent, ranging from love to resentment. With ambivalence comes added guilt. To cope with this added stress, chemically dependent women will often turn to even more intense drug use in an effort to adapt.

Summary

Overall, the available findings indicate that chemically dependent women are emotionally deprived, have low self-esteem, live deviant lifestyles, and often display inadequate parenting techniques. It is becoming a political as well as a moral issue, as to whether or not chemically dependent women should have custody of their children, or whether these children will fare better in placement. The picture becomes clear, however, that with the typical psychological profile that most chemically dependent women maintain, it would be difficult, if not impossible, without comprehensive treatment, for these women to be positive parental role models (Table 1). An examination of the attributes that have been shown to correlate with effective childrearing and successful psychological development of the child will reveal the discrepancies between the chemically dependent woman and the emotionally mature, well-adapted parent.

Attributes Associated with Effective Parenting

Parental Self-Concept

Parental self-concept has been identified as a critical component in effective parenting. It is described as a psychological process that develops throughout the phase of parenthood, and is a combination from past childhood and current childcaring experiences.

According to Partridge, not only do contemporary thoughts, feelings, and experiences of childcaring influence the development of parental self-concept, but so do the experiences from the past, of how the parent was cared for as a child by his/her own parents. Parental self-concept is a mixture of present and past experiences.[41] Not only do the parent's actual encounters with the child, and the subsequent feelings the parent derives from these encounters, influence the development of parental self-concept, but so do memories about how the parent was treated as a child by his/her own parents.

Chodorow claimed that motherhood is more of a psychological role than a sociological one.[42] Being an adequate parent requires the capacity and sense of self as maternal. This sense of self as maternal is, in turn, derived from the woman's identification with and internalization of her own mother's qualities.

Table 1
Profile of the Chemically Dependent Woman

Family history
    Dysfunctional family of origin
    Poor parental role modeling and availability
    Physical abuse
    Sexual victimization

Psychological characteristics
    Social isolation
    Poor self-esteem
    Depression and other negative affective states

Socioeconomic issues
    Unemployed
    Uneducated
    Poor problem-solving and interpersonal skills

Medical issues
    Multiple medical problems
    History of obstetrical complications
    Lifestyles nonconducive to good health
    Self-medicate with illicit drugs

Pregnancy issues
    Idealization of motherhood
    Rationalization of continued drug use throughout the pregnancy
    Guilt and shame resulting from a drug-exposed newborn
    Ambivalence and resentment toward childrearing

Benedek supported the claim that motherliness is a "result of positive identification with the mother" (p. 114).[43] Benedek claimed that this identification can be burdened by unresolved psychosexual conflicts originating from childhood, as well as difficulties in the actual tasks of motherhood. Benedek also claimed that the origin of a negative parental self-concept develops as a result of the parent, both consciously and unconsciously, reliving his/her own developmental experiences while parenting and caring for the child. As the child moves through successive developmental stages, the parent recalls his/her own past. If psychological traumas, such as battering, incest, abandonment, or neglect, have not been worked through and resolved, they can resurface in the parent's life, and interfere with parental ability. These unresolved issues lead to the maternal self-concept developing as a parental reward and punishment system. If the child thrives and responds positively to the mother, the mother feels like a "good" mother; if the child responds negatively through crying and being nonresponsive, the mother feels like a "bad" mother. Thus Benedek postulated that past experiences, as well as current, are primary factors in the development of parental role functioning.

Fraiberg et al. referred to this concept of unresolved childhood traumas as "parental ghosts."[44] They believed that unresolved childhood conflicts can resurface and return to haunt the parent. Until the parent gains better self-understanding through the process of therapeutic resolution, healthy mature involvement with the child will be hindered.

Maternal Attitude

Another concept that has been used to discuss parental effectiveness is maternal attitude. Cohler, the "father of maternal attitude theory," defined this concept as "the attitudes a mother has toward childrearing which permit her to appraise and interpret transactions involving herself and the child" (p. 8).[45]

According to this theory, how well the mother is able to adapt effectively to crises that arise during the child's developmental process depends on her attitude. If the mother's appraisal and interpretation of the transactions between herself and her child are incongruent with the needs of her child, her attitude for that particular transaction is considered to be maladaptive. For example, if a mother has unresolved feelings of rejection from her own childhood, she may interpret her child's individuation issues as personal rejection, and attempt to compensate by developing an enmeshed relationship with the child. Cohler claimed that maladaptive maternal attitudes will not only damage the mother–child relationship, but will negatively affect the child's own developmental progress.

Parental Attributes

Specific parental attitudes, such as frustration intolerance, have been shown to correlate with child-abusing behaviors. It has been shown that child-abusing behaviors increase in the absence of frustration tolerance, and that as frustration tolerance increases, so do attitudes of objective parenting. Thompson demonstrated that if parents perceived their own parents as being loving and accepting, they tended to display a higher level of frustration tolerance and a decreased incidence of child-abusing behaviors.[46] From this it could be postulated that those parents most likely to abuse their children are those who have not acquired a sense of objectivity from their own experiences in being parented.

Newberger also identified specific variables that nonabusing parents maintain and that abusing parents do not.[47] By using a classification system to differentiate levels of parental cognitive moral development, Newberger found that parents in the highest classification were attuned to the importance of expressing feelings, and of the necessity to consider the psychological needs of both child and parent. These parents had more fluid boundaries, and were less rigid about designating right and wrong. The more able Newberger's parents were to identify the emotional cues of their children, the less likely they were to rely on child-abusing techniques.

Studies, such as the one by Newberger, reveal that parental awareness, insight, and self-understanding are central to the effectiveness of the parental role. A relationship between the degree of mother's understanding of the complex nature of the parent–child relationship and the provision of adequate maternal care has been determined. Mothers least likely to abuse and neglect their children are those who are most able to understand parental ambivalence, identify their own psychological needs, as well as those of their children, and balance the needs of self and child. Mothers identified as most effective are those who are able to integrate childrearing experiences into their overall life experiences and sense of self.

Bonding

Bonding is another attribute that is considered by some to be an important element in determining the quality of the mother–child relationship. Coppolillo hypothesized that there is a specific developmental phase, occurring shortly after birth, that is critical for the "successful symbiosis" of the mother with her child.[48] In order for this symbiosis to occur, the mother and child must have access to each other. He claimed that a disrupted bonding process can set an infant up for child abuse, abandonment, or failure to thrive. On the other hand, Lamb and Hwang claimed that early contact and mother–infant bonding are not supported by empirical evidence.[49] According to their findings, early mother–infant contact has no lasting social or psychological influence on the mother–infant relationship.

Summary

In summary, models of parenting maintained by the parent are associated with models developed by the child. A parent who is struggling with a negative parental self-concept is more apt to repeat dysfunctional parenting techniques and maintain maladaptive attitudes that originated form childhood experiences. When this occurs, the parent is less apt to accurately read all the cues and respond to the child's emotional needs (Table 2).

Chemically dependent women frequently maintain negative self-concepts, poor frustration tolerance, and maladaptive attitudes, and have often experienced maltreatment as children from their own parents. In addition,

Table 2
Attributes Associated with Effective Parenting

Parental self-concept

Thoughts, feelings, and experiences of caring for one's child, as well as experiences from the past of how the parent was cared for as a child by his/her own parents influence parental self-concept.[41]

To feel maternal, a woman must identify and internalize her own mother's maternal qualities.[42]

Unresolved psychological conflicts originating in childhood can resurface and interfere with one's own parenting effort.[43]

Unresolved traumatic childhood experiences resurface as "parental ghosts," which interfere with effective parenting.[44]

Maternal attitude

Maternal attitude determines how the mother perceives and interprets her child's needs.[45]

Parental attributes and child abuse

Child-abusing behaviors increase when parental attitudes are nonobjective and frustration tolerance is low.[46]

Ability to identify the emotional cues of children results in less abusive parental techniques.[47]

Bonding

Immediate access of mother and child following birth is necessary for successive symbiosis to occur.[48]

Early mother–infant interaction has no distinct effect on the mother–child relationship.[49]

---

the initial period following birth is often characterized by interruption between the chemically dependent women and her newborn owing to complications of neonatal abstinence syndrome or uninvolvement of a drug-induced mother. From this it can be concluded that parental self-concept in these women has developed as a negative identification, which affects their capacity to adequately parent their children.

This helps explain the ineffective parenting and ambivalence about motherhood that chemically dependent women tend to display. These women tend to neglect or abandon their children at a higher rate than nonaddicted women, and child abuse tends to be prevalent among this group. A closer look at the parenting characteristics of chemically dependent women will help reveal where these women fail in their parenting efforts and the types of parenting behaviors they display.

Parenting Characteristics
of Chemically Dependent Women

The findings on the effectiveness of chemically dependent women as parents tends to paint a somewhat gloomy picture. Even though these mothers claim to have children for the same reasons that other women do, and reveal expectations about their parenting experiences that are similar to those of nonaddicted women, they are basically ineffective in meeting their children's physical, psychological, and social needs. The literature reveals that chemically dependent women display ineffective parenting skills and practices in many different areas of childrearing (Table 3).

Fetal Abuse and Neglect

During pregnancy, chemically dependent women often display the first signs of poor judgment as parents, by continuing to use drugs. As a result, the number of babies being born drug-exposed has increased sharply over the past decade. Reports from the 1980s reveal that in some metropolitan areas the incidence of babies being born drug-exposed has increased by 453%.[50] As early as 1977, it was estimated that 10% or more of all babies being born in metropolitan cities are at risk of *in utero* addiction.[39]

Drug-dependent women, especially those addicted to opiates, often believe in the false assumption that drug use results in infertility and the inability to become pregnant. In reality, the birthrate for chemically dependent women is equal to nonaddicted women. The outcome of this erroneous thinking is that the drug-dependent woman may be 3 or 4 mo pregnant before she realizes she is, and mistakes "morning sickness" for drug withdrawal. Oftentimes she will self-medicate with her drug of choice to overcome the discomforts caused from the pregnancy.

Unfortunately, a large majority of chemically dependent women find excuses to continue their drug use throughout their pregnancies. A study by Rosenbaum revealed that opiate-addicted women showed contempt for addicts who did not "clean up" during their pregnancies, but all except two women in the study continued to use heroin while they were pregnant.[40] Their rationale was that they did not find out they were pregnant until they were 4 or 5 mo along, and therefore determined that any damage to the developing fetus was already done. Others rationalized that going through withdrawal late in pregnancy is more dangerous to the fetus than continued use. Some rationalize that they did not know the abused drug would harm their unborn babies.

Mondanaro claimed that the women who show the worst prognosis as parents are those who deny that their continued drug use during pregnancy

Table 3
Parenting Characteristics of Chemically Dependent Women

Fetal Abuse and Neglect

Use of defense mechanisms to justify continued drug use throughout
pregnancy:
Denial
Rationalization
Minimization

Bonding difficulties

Drug use prevents maternal response
Neonatal Abstinence Syndrome results in lethargic neonate

Child abandonment

Predicted by:
No involvement in drug treatment
No prenatal care
No legal income
No stable residence
Uninvolvement in the neonate's hospitalization
Chemically dependent women who relinquish parental rights are
characterized by:
Long-standing drug addiction
Personal demoralization
Multiple jail sentences

Attitudes and behaviors

Typical patterns of parenting behaviors:
Impulsiveness
Irresponsibility
Immaturity
Egocentrism
Difficult to engage in planning activities
Often do not visit children in placement
Demonstrate similar parental attitudes as other categories of parents
Feel powerless in influencing their children's lives

Child-abusing characteristics

Frequent episodes of physical and sexual abuse:
Medical needs are often neglected
Physical injuries
School absences
Psychological needs are often neglected
More chemically dependent parents exhibit the potential for abuse than
actually abuse their children

---

is affecting their baby.[27] The author claimed that these women often maintain a position of total denial following the delivery of their baby, in order to handle their overwhelming guilt of seeing their sick infants. Mondanaro also claimed that these women will blame overt signs of neonatal withdrawal symptoms on reasons such as colic or "fussiness." The result is that the drug-addicted mother may have a difficult time in getting close to her newborn. She claims her baby is either unmanageable, or she is doing a poor job as a mother. Both these rationalizations interfere with the development of satisfactory bonding between mother and child. Some researchers believe that it is this interference in bonding that sets the children of drug-addicted women up to be abandoned, neglected, and/or abused.

Bonding Difficulties

In the case of maternal addiction and/or neonatal abstinence syndrome, initial bonding is often interrupted for several reasons. According to researchers, because the mother is often in a drug-induced state, the infant is unable to elicit a maternal response.[51] At other times, the mother may be ready to respond to her infant but the infant, as a result of symptoms and complications of neonatal abstinence, is too lethargic to stimulate her. When compared with infants of nonaddicted mothers, babies born to addicted mothers appear less available for interaction, more easily upset, and less able to be soothed. At the same time, addicted mothers display the inability to provide the quality of stimulation for their infants as nonaddicted mothers. The result of this missed interaction between mother and baby often precipitates self-doubt in the chemically dependent mother.

Coppolillo emphasized that the chemically dependent woman, owing to the lack of motherliness she received from her own mother, seeks only material gratification from relationships.[48] As a result, she therefore gleans little gratification from viewing, fondling, or holding her baby because her materialistic orientation and egocentrism is not satisfied in the process. Mondanaro supported this claim, but adds that the drug-dependent mother may begin to feel rejected by her irritable, inconsolable child.[27] In reaction, she may begin to withhold her love, and mother coldly, indifferently, and distantly. The result is the baby becoming more irritable, and the mother feeling more and more inadequate. According to Mondanaro, it is this process that drives the woman further into her use of drugs.

Child Abandonment

Child abandonment by chemically dependent women occurs frequently. Risk factors have been identified that predict child abandonment by these women. No involvement in drug treatment, no prenatal care, not caring for previous children, no legal income, no stable residence, and uninvolvement in the neonate's hospitalization have been found to characterize those chemically dependent women who abandon their children.[28]

Prolonged hospitalization, which is a result of neonatal drug exposure, is a time when many chemically dependent women avoid maternal involvement. Even though these women may make little or no contact with hospital personnel during their babies' stays, they very rarely will agree to surrender their parental rights. This uncooperativeness during the infant's hospitalization has been used as a predictive measure of how a chemically dependent woman will care for her child overall. Lawson and Wilson claimed that maternal indifference during the infant's hospitalization sets the child up for abandonment to another caregiver within the first 6 mo.[28]

Statistics on abandonment of children by chemically dependent women has been provided through research. It has been shown that addicted women who relinquish parental rights tend to be characterized by severe long-standing drug abuse, personal demoralization, and multiple jail sentences. Children of chemically dependent women who enter placement tend to be younger than other foster-care children coming into the system. This suggests that addicted women display ineffective parenting skills earlier than mothers whose children are placed for other reasons. In addition, children of chemically dependent women who are in placement, remain in placement longer than children of nonaddicted parents. Fewer children of addicted mothers are returned to the mother, on being released from foster care. It appears that many of these children are placed in the care of extended family members, or are adopted by other families. Studies have also found that children of addicted mothers are the least visited of all groups of children in foster care. Chemically dependent mothers, overall, have been described as the most damaged of all categories of parents.[4,52]

Nictern collected statistical data on 95 New York children, of whom one or both parents were identified as being heroin addicts.[4] The author found differences in abandonment circumstances between younger and older children. The younger children in the study were often abandoned because their addicted mothers were unable to care for them. The older children coming into placement as a result of their mother's drug addiction tended to display physical and psychological disturbances commonly seen in children from dysfunctional social environments.

Nictern also found that children of chemically dependent women are frequently reared without the presence of the natural father, as a result of his abandoning both mother and child. If the father is drug addicted, he tends to abandon the children when they are very young. Overall, the children of chemically dependent women commonly suffer from the absence of a parental figure during their formative years.

Attitudes and Behaviors

Chemically dependent women tend to display typical patterns of behaviors when parenting their children. Broken appointments, loss of contact, ambivalence about their children's outcome, and resentment toward surrogate caregivers are characteristics of these women. Bauman and Dougherty compared the profile of chemically dependent mothers with nonaddicted mothers.[53] Although there were no differences between the two groups for parenting attitudes (i.e., both groups tended to have similar expectations regarding parenthood), the authors found that the drug-addicted mothers performed less adaptively on measures of personality and parenting behavior.

Personality characteristics common to chemically dependent women have been cited as creating childrearing difficulties for these women. Impulsiveness, irresponsibility, immaturity, and egocentrism, all of which chemically dependent women tend to display, make it difficult for these mothers to discipline themselves. Some researchers postulate that this lack of self-discipline, along with a lack of achievement orientation they tend to reveal, makes it difficult for addicted mothers to provide a structured environment for their children.[52]

A study by Fanshel assessed 624 children from 467 New York families, in which one or both of the parents were drug addicted.[52] Parental information gathered revealed significant findings about the characteristics of drug-abusing mothers. Fanshel found them to be extremely difficult to engage in meaningful planning activities involving their children. Their behavior patterns were typified by broken appointments, loss of contact, and ambivalence about their children's outcome. They were measured as visiting their children in placement less than other parents whose children were in placement for other reasons. In fact, Fanshel found the drug-abusing mothers to rate significantly more negatively than mothers who had suffered mental illness, those whose children had entered foster care because of child behavioral problems, and those who had suffered illness and hospitalization. The profile of these mothers tended to be similar to those whose children were in placement because of neglect, abuse, abandonment, or severe family dysfunction. Even though the drug-addicted mothers in Fanshel's study displayed the worst visiting behavior of their children of all mothers that were studied, they showed strong negative feelings about releasing their children for adoption. Many of these mothers displayed marked apathy toward foster family care as a resource for their children, and often exhibited negative feelings toward the foster parent.

Colten conducted a study of the mothering attitudes, experiences, and self-perceptions of drug-addicted and drug-free mothers.[25] Colten found that overall, drug-addicted women tend to have children for the same reasons that other women do. The addicted women revealed similar expectations about their parenting experiences than drug-free women. They did, however, differ significantly from the nonaddicted mothers in their fears of being an inadequate or "bad" mother. The drug-addicted women in Colten's study also reported that they believed they had little influence or control over their children and voiced fears of their children turning out to be like them.

A study by Burns and Burns tested the hypotheses that chemically dependent women, who experience both "emotional instability" and a "negative heritage," will demonstrate dysfunctional parenting techniques.[54] These authors claimed that "a mother who has been abused by her own parent, is more likely to experience personal instability in her own emotional development and to become a dysfunctional parent as a direct result of the social trauma and personal maladjustment" (p. 169).[54] In addition, these authors felt that social support deficits and parenting a high-risk infant can effect parenting outcome. Because these mothers often feel isolated, they may resort to child-abusing behaviors. Using a causal pathway model, these authors found a direct and cumulative effect from these factors, when applied to chemically dependent women.

Child-Abusing Characteristics

Black and Mayer investigated the adequacy of childcare in families of chemically dependent parents.[55] These authors estimated that, in addition to having difficulties disciplining their children, 23% of the drug-addicted mothers they studied physically and/or sexually abused their children. These authors demonstrated that the chemically dependent women in their study who relied on abusive techniques lack the ability to meet the physical and psychological needs of their children, in accordance with any regular schedule. In the case of severe addiction, the women in Black and Mayer's study were known to sometimes neglect their children's medical care, even in emergency situations. Physical injuries and frequent school absences, which these authors documented, are believed to be a result of inadequate parental supervision.

The study by Black and Mayer revealed that chemically dependent women who physically abuse their children have been shown to display low frustration tolerance, dependency, severe depression, difficulty in experiencing pleasure, and misperception of the needs and abilities of their children.[55] As tension and anxieties in these women mount, physically abusive behaviors increase.

Studies such as that by Black and Mayer, illustrate that chemically dependent women are more likely to neglect rather than physically harm their children.[55] After identifying the characteristics of child abusers, these authors found that the number of chemically dependent parents who exhibited potential for abuse was more than twice the number who actually abused their children. These findings may help to dispel the negative stereotype that all chemically addicted parents are physically abusive.

The fact still remains that children raised by chemically dependent parents tend to suffer negative consequences as a result of their parents' ineffective parenting techniques. Overall, studies that examine these issues are scarce. Those that do exist reveal that the children of drug-addicted parents may manifest a variety of behavior patterns and/or symptoms. The following section discusses the profile these children may exhibit.

Effects to Children
Raised by Chemically Dependent Parents

Adjustment and Interaction

In a study by Nictern of 95 children of drug-addicted parents from the Jewish Child Care Association of New York, it was found that nearly all of the children could be viewed as neglected.[4] The children in Nictern's study appeared withdrawn, lacking in animation, and generally inhibited in their responses. The older children in the study were diagnosed as suffering from behavior disorders.

In addition, the children in Nictern's study tended to demonstrate problems with their capacity for human relatedness.[4] Nictern's assessment included descriptions of excessive anxiety in adult and peer interactions, poor socialization, and withdrawal as a technique of handling stressful situations. Nictern attributed this to the fact that these children tend to be raised by many adults, coupled by the fact that their involvement with their natural mother was inconsistent, and in most incidences their father was absent.

A study by Fanshel of 624 foster-care children of drug-abusing mothers is unique in that the author was able to follow these children while they were in placement and after they returned home.[52] Fanshel explored the issue of whether a child's remaining in prolonged placement is associated with social adjustment and cognitive deterioration. His findings reveal that children of drug-abusing mothers tend to be locked into foster care at a disproportionately high rate. They also suffer greater replacement from one setting to another, while in care. In lieu of these findings, their adjustment, as measured over time, appeared no less problematic than that of children who were separated from their families because of other factors.

Clinical assessments revealed little significant difference among Fanshel's sample as compared with other children. Unlike Nictern,[4] Fanshel found these children to rate positively in the area of personal adjustment.[52]

He found them to be less withdrawn, more agreeable, and less tense than children who were in placement because of behavior problems. Their personal adjustments were found to be equal to children who were in placement for other reasons.

A study by Wilson et al. compared developmental characteristics of children born exposed to drugs and living with a mother who had a history of chemical dependency, with a control group of nondrug-exposed children whose mothers had no drug-abusing history.[56] Parents of the drug-exposed children rated these children as having greater difficulty adjusting in areas of personal, social, and physical requirements. The findings revealed that the drug-exposed children tended to display uncontrollable tempers, impulsiveness, poor self-confidence, aggressiveness, and difficulty in making and keeping friends. Whether these findings are a result of prenatal drug-exposure or the home environment was not differentiated.

Developmental Maturity

In the previously described study by Nictern, developmental lags were revealed in the study children, which were evidenced by histories of poor bowel and bladder control and delayed speech.[4] Temper tantrums were reported as occurring frequently among these children. Additionally Nictern's study revealed that these children showed marked deficits in their adaptive responses at all developmental stages.[4] Overall, they appeared withdrawn, irritable, but with little or no crying. As a result, these children tended to function below their potential, and continued to do so in spite of many supportive efforts including remedial and psychotherapeutic help. Even considering that children in placement for other reasons tend to display these characteristics, Nictern found the clinical configuration of these children of drug-addicted mothers to be specifically distinctive.

Fanshel found the children of drug-abusing mothers to fall in the middle range with respect to emotional maturity and fears.[52] Like Nictern,[4] Fanshel's most symptomatic behavior was found to relate to bowel and bladder control and psychosomatic reactions. The least symptomatic behavior in Fanshel's study was found in relation to aggressiveness. It should be noted that these findings from Fanshel's study did not show statistical significance.

Cognitive Ability

Learning problems have also been noted in children raised by chemically dependent mothers. Nictern found the older children in his study to demonstrate a variety of learning problems, as well as academic discrepancies, between their mental ages and their achievement levels.[4] Likewise, the study by Wilson et al. revealed that the drug-exposed children whose mothers had no drug-abusing history, performed poorer than the comparison group in areas of cognitive and perceptual abilities, as well as in quantitative and memory functioning.[56] Parental perception of the child's cognitive functioning did not differ among groups. Fanshel disputed these findings of cognitive deficiencies.[52] His study revealed that children of drug-abusing mothers were essentially undifferentiated from other children in their IQs and cognitive functioning.

Neglect and Abuse

Negative social environments have been shown to have adverse effects on childrearing outcomes. Children raised by chemically dependent women exemplify this. These children tend to show symptoms of neglect and, many times, physical abuse. Of the 95 children from drug-addicted parents that Nictern studied, nearly all showed obvious signs of neglect and many were suffering from physical abuse.[4] It has been documented that these children frequently tell authorities, when questioned, of having been routinely left without adult supervision, even at very young ages. Many of these children can describe their parent's drug activities in detail.[4]

Black and Mayer asserted that 26% of children in chemically dependent homes have been victims of incest.[55] Thus, according to these authors, as many as three to four million children in this country may be living in homes that are both chemically dependent and incestuous. The findings presented here, although varied, lend support to the belief that children raised by chemically dependent parents tend to suffer negative results in the areas of behavioral, social, and psychological functioning (Table 4). Most researchers agree that comprehensive treatment programs must be developed that address the serious problems that exist between chemically dependent women and their children. Without successful treatment programs, the outcome for these women and children remains dismal.

Parent–Child Treatment Needs of Chemically Dependent Women

Lack of Women-Sensitive Programs

In order to impact the needs of chemically dependent women and their children, comprehensive treatment programs must be developed that address the gender-specific needs of these women. There is currently a national trend to develop comprehensive programs, in an attempt to improve the lives of chemically dependent women and their dependents. However, the problem still exists that most treatment programs are based on the needs of

Table 4
Effects to Children Raised by Chemically Dependent Parents

Adjustment and interaction

  Controversial findings:
    Withdrawn
    Lacking in animation
    Inhibited in responses
    Anxiety in adult and peer responses
    Agreeable
    Complacent
    Uncontrollable tempers

Developmental maturity

  Developmental lags
    Evidenced by histories of bowel and bladder control and delayed
      speech
  Poor adaptive response at all developmental stages

Cognitive ability

  Learning problems
  Academic discrepancies between their mental ages and achievement
    level
  Cognitive and perceptual deficits
  Quantitative and memory functioning impairment

Neglect and abuse

  Children are left without supervision, even at very young ages
  Can describe their parents drug use behaviors in detail
  Show signs of neglect and/or abuse
  High incidence of incest

---

male addicts, and often intimidate and sexually incriminate against women. In the last decade, it was documented that a small portion of treatment programs maintained a 1:1 gender ratio, but the large majority continued with a 2:1 to 10:1 imbalance of men to women.[1] These statistics support the fact that more men than women addicts enter treatment facilities, which may be owing to the insensitivity women receive to their specific issues. A report by the Foster Care Police Board to the Los Angeles Board of Supervisors in 1985 indicated that one in every three referrals to a drug-treatment program is a young woman of childbearing age.[57] Less than one in five of these women actually enter treatment.

Women-Specific Treatment Needs

Medical Issues

In order to serve chemically dependent women more effectively, a broader scope of services than is typically available within drug-treatment programs must be made available. In order for chemically dependent women to improve in their parenting effectiveness, services must be available that address their social, psychological, and physical needs. One service that is often missing in treatment programs is medical services. Studies have shown that chemically dependent women, more often than men, enter treatment because of medical complaints. Once in treatment, these medical conditions often go undiagnosed and, if diagnosed, many times go untreated.[36,58]

Medical problems tend to play a major role in the treatment outcome of chemically dependent women. It has been noted that between 27 and 69% of chemically dependent women cite drug-related medical problems as the reason for entering and/or dropping out of treatment programs.[36,59,50] In another study, it was found that 56% of the chemically dependent women studied developed medical problems while in treatment, but only 36% were treated.[36] Stryker found that between 62 and 81% of all pregnant addicts studied developed complications during treatment.[61]

Medical complications, illnesses, and related physical discomforts that are common to female addicts may impede participation in treatment and successful rehabilitation. Health promotion and health education has been demonstrated to be effective in reducing anxiety and stress, helping individuals to become healthier and stronger, and in establishing a sense of well being. The relationship between health practice and habits, and physical and psychological wellness, is documented in the literature.[62,63] Therefore, if sexuality issues and health awareness are offered as part of treatment, addicted women may not only be less susceptible to illness, but might be helped to be less dependent on drugs.

Dependency Issues

Dependency is another issue that must be addressed in treatment programs for chemically dependent women. Treasure and Liao claimed that, for many female addicts, drug use is simply a manifestation of "socially encouraged dependence."[34] Since dependency means powerlessness for most, it makes sense that dependency interferes with developing a sense of worth and self-identify, both of which can result in negative parental self-concepts.

It has been suggested that survival skills that focus on problem solving, independent functioning, and interpersonal skills be offered to chemically dependent women at the beginning and throughout treatment. Without these skills, chemically dependent women are unable to function independently and meet their own and their childrens' needs. Assertiveness training has been shown to be one way of enhancing survival skills for chemically dependent women.[64] Learning to be assertive helps improve the self-esteem and self-concept of these women, by helping them become aware of how they interact with others, and by teaching them interpersonal and communication skills. Assertiveness training allows these women to feel that they have internal control over their lives, and that they have the power to get their needs met without abandoning their rights or stepping on the rights of others.

Family Issues

Liles and Childs recommended that education about healthy family patterns is another essential feature of treatment for chemically dependent women.[65] As a result of the intergenerational links to incest and substance abuse, which often occurred within their families of origin, and the distortion of what constitutes appropriate interpersonal boundaries, chemically dependent women often feel confused and unaware of what constitutes normal child and family development. Issues regarding sexuality and intimacy need to be addressed in drug-treatment programs, in an effort to help these women break the pattern of dysfunctional relationships, which often involve spousal abuse and battering. Communication techniques and effective expression of feelings and needs are important to teach these women as well as their children.

The incidence of child abuse and neglect in families of drug-abusing parents emphasizes the need for including parenting education skills as a crucial component of drug-treatment programs. Black and Mayer claimed that not only do parenting skills need to be a part of treatment, but provisions of social and economic support for chemically dependent parents who are recovering may prove to be even more effective.[61]

Effective Treatment Modalities

It is imperative that comprehensive treatment modalities be developed that meet the specific needs of chemically dependent women and their children. It is a general consensus, by those involved in examining the issues related to chemical dependency in women, that without a successful treatment outcome, the prognosis for these women is poor. Failure in treatment not only can lead to relapse and sustained addiction, but children raised by chemically dependent parents experience a higher incidence of abandonment, neglect, and abuse, as well as long-term psychosocial, interpersonal, and learning deficits, than children raised by nonaddicted parents.[1,52,66]

Mother–Child Coordinated Services

Colten claimed that the first step of any drug-treatment program for women is to focus on the needs of mother and child together.[25] Eldred et al. noted that drug-dependent women and their children could better be viewed as parts of a single interaction process.[67] According to these authors, they claimed that it is possible to have integrated treatment that address both the mother's and child's needs, since these needs are so closely tied together.

Many chemically dependent women enter treatment programs out of fear of losing custody of their children. Treatment staff need to recognize that the role of "mother" is likely to be very important to chemically dependent women, even though they may feel they are inept and ineffective as a parent. Colten claimed that if the program staff take the approach that addicted mothers have inherent, psychological deficits that prevent them from being adequate mothers, it could become a self-fulfilling prophecy, and be reflected in the treatment outcome of these women.[25]

Childcare

It has been advocated that childcare facilities be included as part of treatment programs for chemically dependent women. According to Mondanaro, coordination efforts should exist, between day-care facilities and treatment programs, that allow chemically dependent women to work at the childcare facility, so that they might learn effective parenting skills and develop maternal confidence.[27]

A study by Harris supported this belief.[68] Harris found that only 3 of the 49 programs he assessed offered childcare facilities, but that the women in these three programs were more available for treatment and demonstrated better childrearing techniques than did the women in programs where this service was not offered.

Coordination of Treatment and Social Services

Fanshel advocated that more money be diverted into the development of intensive treatment programs for drug-dependent women, in lieu of the high investment of funds required to sustain the children of these women in foster care.[52] Even though Fanshel has found that the adjustment of these foster-care children appears no less problematic than that of children who are separated from their families because of other situational factors, these children tend to be locked into placement for a much longer time as a result of the parent's ambivalence and the child welfare system's reluctance to terminate parental rights.

Fanshel suggested that there is a need for a closer working relationship between agencies offering foster-care services and those offering drug-treatment services.[58] Fanshel advocated that early and more reliable estimates of the treatability of a mother's drug-abuse problem, as provided by those who have expertise in the field, offer the child welfare agencies a more sound rationale for dispositional planning when such children enter the foster-care system.

Summary

Studies have shown that chemically dependent women who remain in and complete treatment programs demonstrate improved lifestyles. One such study revealed that chemically dependent women who remain in treatment for the duration of the program requirements are less likely to return to drug use and criminal involvement and more likely to become employed and earn money legally.[26] Other studies have shown that length of stay in a program is associated with the development of more appropriate parental attitudes, which include increased acceptance and a decrease in overprotection, overindulgence, and rejection. In addition, children of chemically dependent women who remain in and complete treatment have been tested and found that their developmental profiles are only slightly below those of children from drug-free mothers.[53] From this, it can be assumed that treatment programs that focus on the special needs of this population improve the overall lifestyle of chemically dependent women and their children (Table 5).

Conclusion

The alarming increase in the number of babies being born drug-exposed, as well as the developing knowledge of the detrimental effects to children being raised by drug-addicted mothers, emphasizes the need for early, planned intervention in order to prevent the development of a new generation of individuals with serious biopsychosocial problems.

When a comprehensive view is taken of the problems impacting drug-dependent women, it becomes clear that, without effective treatment programs that focus on their gender specific needs, these women will not be prepared to parent their children to their fullest potential. As a result, we will be facing a new generation of children with severe biopsychosocial problems. With these children will come an additional stress to our family systems and to the structure of our entire social environment.

Before anything can be done to intercept this growing problem, the characteristics of chemically dependent women must be identified and understood. Relationships between the psychological profile of these women and the parenting styles they utilize need to be identified in order to interrupt the cycle of family dysfunction, which commonly prevails among this population.

Table 5
Parent–Child Treatment Needs of Chemically Dependent Women

Lack of women-sensitive programs

Treatment programs based on the needs of men:
Often intimidate and sexually incriminate against women
2:1 to 10:1 imbalance of men to women in treatment programs
Less than 1 in 5 female referrals actually enter treatment

Women-specific treatment needs

Medical issues:
Health promotion and education reduce anxiety and stress
Dependency issues:
Problem-solving skills
Interpersonal skills
Assertiveness training
Family Issues
Sexuality and intimacy needs
Education regarding healthy family patterns
Parent education training

Effective treatment modalities

Mother–child coordinated services
Childcare
Coordination of treatment and social services

The traumatic childhood experiences that many chemically dependent women have experienced must be addressed and resolved before they will be capable of replacing dysfunctional coping strategies with better adapted lifestyles. Until they become aware of the negative impact their own experiences of being parented had on them, they will not be able to provide effective role modeling for their own children.

Treatment programs must be developed that incorporate the physical, psychological, and social needs of chemically dependent women. Treatment staff must be trained to be sensitive to the specific needs of these women. Although recovery involves gaining a positive self-concept and a sense of independence, it must not be forgotten that motherhood is often the most important role in these women's lives. Therefore, developing the program around the needs of mother and child together is beneficial.

Perhaps most importantly, treatment approaches for chemically dependent women must be developed that emphasize reparenting these women, in an attempt to resolve their own unmet childhood needs. That program must be followed by a second phase, which teaches them effective parenting techniques by which to parent their own children.

References

[1]B. G. Reed (1987) Developing women-sensitive drug dependence treatment services: why so difficult? *J. Psychoactive Drugs* **19**, 151–164.

[2]B. K. Alexander (1982) The disease and adaptive model of addiction: a framework evaluation, in *Visions of Addiction*. S. Peele, ed. Health, Lexington, MA, pp. 17–28.

[3]March of Dimes. (1989) Community needs assessment paper. Orange County Chapter, CA. Unpublished.

[4]S. Nictern (1973) The children of drug users. *J. Am. Acad. Child Psychiatry* **12**, 24–31.

[5]I. J. Chasnoff, ed. (1986) *Drug Use in Pregnancy*. MTP, Norwell, MA.

[6]K. A. Brown and J. Sunshine (1982) Group treatment of children from alcoholic families, in *Social Work With Groups*. M. Altman and R. Crocker, eds. Hawthorne, New York, pp. 65–72.

[7]A. E. Raynes, C. Clement, V. D. Patch, and F. Ervin (1974) Factors related to imprisonment in female heroin addicts. *Int. J. Addict.* **9**, 145–150.

[8]C. Black (1978) *It Will Never Happen to Me*. Hawthorne, Denver, CO.

[9]I. Chein, D. L. Gerard, R. S. Lee, and E. Rosenfeld (1964) *The Road to H*. Basic Books, New York.

[10]V. J. Binion (1979) A descriptive comparison of the families of origin of women heroin users and nonusers, in *Addicted Women: Family Dynamics, Self Perception, and Support Systems*. DHEW Pub. No. (ADM) 80-762, Service Research Branch, Division of Resource Development. National Institute of Drug Abuse, Rockville, MD, pp. 77–130.

[11]M. D. Anglin and Y. Hser (1987) Addicted women and crime. *Criminology* **25**, 359–397.

[12]J. Benward and J. Densen-Gerber (1975) Incest as a causative factor in anti-social behavior: an exploratory study. Paper presented at the meeting of the American Academy of Forensic Science, Chicago, IL.

[13]D. J. Rosenhow, R. Corbett, and D. Devine (1988) Molested as children: a hidden contribution to substance abuse? *J. Subst. Abuse Treatment* **5**, 13–18.

[14]J. D. Hawkins and M. W. Frasier (1985) Social networks of street drug users: a comparison of two theories. *Soc. Work Res. Abstracts* **21**, 3–12.

[15]J. I. Hser, M. D. Anglin, and M. W. Booth (1987) Sex differences in addict careers, 3. addiction. *Am. J. Drug Alcohol Abuse* **13**, 531–538.

[16]C. Tracy D. Talbut, and J. Steinschneider (1990) *Women, Babies and Drugs: Family Centered Treatment Options*. National Conference of State Legislatures, Washington, DC, p. 33.

[17]B. M. Tucker (1979) A description and comparative analysis of the social support structure of heroin-addicted women, in *Addicted Women: Family Dynamics, Self Perceptions and Support Systems*. DHEW Pub. No. (ADM) 80-762, Service Research Branch, Division of Resource Development. National Institute on Drug Abuse, Rockville, MD, 37–76.

[18]M. L. Griffin, R. D. Weiss, and S. M. Mirin (1989) A comparison of male and female cocaine abusers. *Arch. Gen. Psychiatry* **46**, 122–126.

[19]M. R. Gossop (1976) Drug dependence and self-esteem. *Int. J. Addict.* **11**, 741–753.

[20]B. L. Wheeler, D. V. Biase, and A. P. Sullivan (1986) Changes in self-concept during therapeutic community treatment: a comparison of male and female drug abusers. *J. Drug Addict.* **16**, 191–196.

[21]S. E. Gutierres and J. W. Reich (1988) Attributional analysis of drug abuse and gender: effects of treatment and relationship of rehabilitation. *J. Soc. Clin. Psychol.* **7**, 176–191.

[22]J. C. Marsh and N. A. Miller (1985) Female clients in substance abuse treatment. *Int. J. Addict.* **20**, 995–1019.

[23]J. H. Walsh (1991) The substance-abusing family: consideration for nursing research. *J. Pediatr. Nurs.* **6**, 49–56.

[24]K. Minkoff, E. Bergman, and A. Beck (1973) Hopelessness, depression and attempted suicide. *Am. J. Psychiatry* **130**, 455–460.

[25]M. E. Colten (1982) Attitudes, experiences and self perception of heroin addicted mothers. *J. Soc. Issues* **38**, 77–92.

[26]C. Dackis and M. Gold (1984) Depression in opiate addicts, in *Substance Abuse and Psychopathology*. M. Mirin, ed. American Psychiatric, Washington, DC, pp. 19–40.

[27]J. E. Mondanaro (1989) *Chemically Dependent Women.* Lexington, Lexington, MA.

[28]M. S. Lawson and G. S. Wilson (1979) Addiction and pregnancy: two lives in crisis. *Soc. Work Health Care* **4**, 445–455.

[29]K. Fiks, H. Johnson, and T. Rosen (1985) Methadone maintained mothers: a 3-year follow-up of parental functioning. *Int. J. Addict.* **20**, 651–660.

[30]D. L. Rhoads (1983) A longitudinal study of life stress and social support among drug abusers. *Int. J. Addict.* **18**, 195–222.

[31]B. M. Tucker (1983) Social support and coping: applications for the study of female drug abuse. *J. Soc. Issues* **38**, 117–137.

[32]B. Reed (1981) Intervention strategies for drug dependent women: an introduction, in *Treatment Services for Drug Dependent Women*, vol. 1. G. M. Beschner, B. G. Reed, and J. Mondanaro, eds. DHHS Publication No. (ADM) 85-1177. National Institute on Drug Abuse, Rockville, MD, pp. 1–24.

[33]C. Wasnick, B. Schaffer, and M. Bencivengo (1980) The sex histories of fifty female drug clients. Paper presented at the National Alcohol and Drug Coalition, Washington, DC.

[34]K. G. Treasure and H. Liao (1982) Survival skills training for drug dependent women, in *Treatment Services for Drug Dependent Women*, vol. 2. B. G. Reed, G. M. Beschner, and J. Mondanaro, eds. DHHS Pub. No (ADM) 82-1219. National Institute of Drug Abuse, Rockville, MD, pp. 137–212

[35]F. Suffet and R. Brotman (1976) Female drug use: some observations. *Int. J. Addict.* **11**, 19–33.

[36]L. P. Finnegan and R. J. Wapner (1984) Drug abuse in pregnancy. *J. Practical Nurs.* **34**, 14–23.

[37]X. Bean (1985) Summary of transcripts of proceedings on "drug babies." Data presented to Los Angeles Board of Supervisors. Foster Care Policy Board, Children's Research Institute of California, Los Angeles.

[38]D. K. Wellisch and M. R. Steinberg (1980) Parenting attitudes of addict mothers. *Int. J. Addict.* **15**, 809–819.

[39]J. N. Carr (1975) Drug patterns among drug-addicted mothers. *Pediatr. Ann.* **July,** 408–417.

[40]M. Rosenbaum (1979) Difficulties in taking care of business: women addicts as mothers. *Am. J. Drug Alcohol Abuse* **6,** 431–446.

[41]S. E. Partridge (1988) The parental self-concept: a theoretical exploration and practical application. *Am. J. Orthopsychiatry* **58,** 281–287.

[42]N. Chodorow (1978) *The Reproduction of Mothering: Psychoanalysis and Sociology of Gender.* University of California, Berkeley, CA.

[43]T. Benedek (1970) The family as a psychologic field, in *Parenthood: Psychology and Psychopathology.* E. J. Anthony and T. Benedek, eds. Little, Brown, Boston, pp. 109–136.

[44]S. Fraiberg, E. Adelson, and V. Shapiro (1975) Ghosts in the nursery: a psychoanalytic approach to the problems of impaired infant-mother relationships. *J. Am. Acad. Child Psychiatry* **14,** 387–421.

[45]B. J. Cohler, J. L. Weiss, and H. U. Greenbaum (1970) Child-care attitudes and emotional disturbance among mothers of young children. *Genet. Psychol. Monogr.* **82,** 3–47.

[46]J. W. Thompson (1977) Frustration tolerance, parenting attitudes and perceptions of parenting behavior as factors in the incidence of child abuse. *Dissertation Abstracts Int.* **38,** 5598-B.

[47]C. Newberger (1980) The cognitive structure of parenthood: designing a descriptive measure. *New Dir. Child Dev.* **7,** 41–67.

[48]H. P. Coppolillo (1975) Drug impediments to mothering behavior. *Addict. Dis. Int. J.* **2,** 201–208.

[49]M. E. Lamb and C. P. Hwang (1982) Maternal attachment and mother-neonate bonding: a critical review, in *Advances in Developmental Psychology*, vol. 2. M. E. Brown and A. L. Brown, eds. Erlbaum, Hillsdale, NJ, pp. 1–39.

[50]J. McIntosh (1985) Summary of transcript of proceedings on "drug babies." Data presented to Los Angeles Board of Supervisors. Foster Care Policy Board, Children's Research Institute of California, Los Angeles.

[51]J. C. B. Householder (1980) An investigation of mother-infant interaction in a narcotic addicted population. *Dissertation Abstract Int.* **6,** 2516.

[52]D. Fanshel (1975) Parental failure and consequences for children: the drug abusing mother whose children are in foster care. *Am. J. Pub. Health* **65,** 604–612.

[53]P. S. Bauman and F. E. Dougherty (1983) Drug-addicted mothers' parenting and their children's development. *Int. J. Addict.* **18,** 291–302.

[54]W. J. Burns and K. A. Burns (1988) Parenting dysfunction in chemically dependent women, in *Drugs, Alcohol, Pregnancy and Parenting.* I. J. Chasnoff, ed. Kluwer, Dordrecht, Netherlands, pp. 159–172.

[55]R. Black and J. Mayer (1980) Parents with special problems: alcoholism and opiate addiction. *Child Abuse Neglect* **4,** 45—54.

[56]G. S. Wilson, R. McCreary, J. Kean, and J. C. Baxter (1979) The development of preschool children of heroin-addicted mothers: a controlled study. *Pediatrics* **63,** 135–141.

[57]R. Snyder (1985) Summary of transcript of proceedings on "drug babies." Data presented to Los Angeles Board of Supervisors. Foster Care Policy Board, Children's Research Institute of California, Los Angeles.

[58]G. Beschner and P. Thompson (1982) Women and drug abuse treatment: needs and services. *Focus Women J. Addict Health* **3,** 152–170.

[59]B. S. Brown, S. K. Gauvey, M. B. Meyers, and S. D. Stark (1971) In their own words: addicts reasons for initiating and withdrawing from heroin. *Int. J. Addict.* **6**, 635–645.

[60]E. W. Flaherty, M. Bencivengo, and K. Olson (1978) *The Causes of Demand Reduction: An Exploratory Study*. Philadelphia Health Management Corporation, Philadelphia, PA.

[61]J. C. Stryker (1979) Physical health for the women who abuse substances. Report No. H81 DA 1855 submitted to the National Institute on Drug Abuse. Rockville, MD.

[62]N. B. Belloc (1973) Relationship of health practices and mortality. *Prev. Med.* **2**, 67–81.

[63]L. Breslow and J. E. Enstrom (1980) Persistence of health habits and their relationship to mortality. *Prev. Med.* **9**, 469–483.

[64]K. M. Doyle (1982) Assertiveness training for the drug dependent woman, in *Treatment Services for Drug Dependent Women*, vol. 2. B. G. Reed, G. M. Beschner, and J. Mondanaro, eds. DHHS Pub. No. (ADM) 82-1219, National Institute on Drug Abuse, Rockville, MD, pp. 213–246.

[65]R. E. Liles and D. Childs (1986) Similarities in family dynamics of incest and alcohol abuse; issues for clinicians. *Alcohol Health Res. World* **2**, 66–69.

[66]M. A. Naegle (1988) Substance abuse among women: prevalence, patterns, and treatment issues. *Issues Ment. Health Nurs.* **9**, 127–137.

[67]C. A. Elred, V. V. Grier, and N. Berlinger (1974) Comprehensive treatment for heroin addicted mothers. *Soc. Casework* **55**, 1450–1477.

[68]S. Harris (1975) Mothers in methadone programs need day care, in *Development in the Field of Drug Abuse*. E. Senay, V. Shorty, and H. Alksne, eds. Schenksman, Cambridge, MA, pp. 415–417.

Women and Health-Related Behaviors

Interrelations Among Substance Use, Sexual Behaviors, and Acquired Immunodeficiency Syndrome (AIDS)

Michael Windle, Pamela Carlisle-Frank, Limor Azizy, and Rebecca C. Windle

Introduction

Acquired immunodeficiency syndrome (AIDS) continues to be a major public health problem, as AIDS has been diagnosed in over 196,000 Americans,[1] with cumulative projections of 390,000–480,000 AIDS cases by the end of 1993.[2] Furthermore, the spread of AIDS is becoming more pervasive, with about 2000 children under 13 yr of age diagnosed with AIDS,[3] and with increases in the prevalence of human immunodeficiency virus (HIV) infection and AIDS among heterosexuals and women.[4]

Two major risk factors for contracting HIV are unsafe sexual practices (e.g., vaginal or anal intercourse without the use of condoms) and intravenous drug use (specifically, the sharing of injection equipment, whether injection is intravenous, under the skin, intramuscular, and so forth). As such, much of the existing research on HIV infection and AIDS in the

From: *Drug and Alcohol Abuse Reviews, Vol. 5: Addictive Behaviors in Women*
Ed.: R. R. Watson ©1994 Humana Press Inc., Totowa, NJ

United States has focused on the behaviors of homosexual/bisexual men and injecting drug users (IDUs). However, the changing prevalence of AIDS cases among different portions of the populace (e.g., heterosexuals, adolescents, women, pediatric AIDS cases) has stimulated a broader public health interest in potential risk factors for HIV contraction, as well as an expanded emphasis on prevention to subpopulations (e.g., IDUs, homosexual/bisexual men, adolescents).[5] There has also been an emerging literature focused on psychological factors (e.g., alcohol expectancies, health locus of control), lifestyle habits (e.g., sexual activities), and possible cofactors (e.g., alcohol use) that may increase exposure and susceptibility to HIV, and influence the duration of the disease process from HIV infection to full-blown AIDS.[6,7]

In this chapter, we focus on the prevalence of HIV/AIDS among women, on special problems and issues of women with (or at risk for) AIDS, and on the specific influences that alcohol and drug use may play in contracting HIV. We also focus principally on women because of the rapid increases in HIV/AIDS among women and pediatric AIDS cases.[3,8] The chapter provides somewhat more coverage to the influences of alcohol, because its potential etiological significance often has been either absent or minimized in prior reviews, in large part because of its perceived ancillary role. However, we attempt to provide data suggestive of the multiple influences (direct and, especially, indirect) of alcohol use on high-risk behaviors for contracting HIV.

The chapter is divided into six sections. First, epidemiological data on HIV/AIDS among women are presented to specify the scope of the problem, to identify high-risk subgroups, and to note recent changes in the prevalence and projections of AIDS cases. Second, issues and problems that are unique to women with AIDS or at risk for AIDS are presented. Third, a concise description of the immunological basis of HIV infection and AIDS is provided. Fourth, empirical studies are presented with regard to substance use, risky sexual behaviors, and contraction of HIV and other sexually transmitted diseases (STDs). Although many of the empirical studies reviewed are not specific to women, their findings are relevant to the special needs associated with women and HIV infection (e.g., the relationship between alcohol use and gynecological complications that may increase a woman's susceptibility to contraction of HIV or other STDs; the interrelations among malnutrition, depression, poverty, and immune system compromise). Fifth, a dynamic, ecological model of epidemiological risk is presented along with a description of an ongoing research study designed to evaluate features of the ecological model. Finally, a chapter summary is provided along with suggestions for future research.

We have attempted to provide concise, but not necessarily comprehensive, coverage to salient issues and studies concerning alcohol use and risk for HIV and AIDS among women. There exists an expanding literature that includes men and has focused on other high-risk groups (e.g., homosexuals) and on the significance of specific substance use practices (e.g., IDUs).[9,10]

Epidemiology of HIV/AIDS Among Women

The number of AIDS cases in the United States as of November, 1991, was 195,718. The cumulative number of AIDS deaths was over 126,100.[11] As of January, 1989, women comprised 9% of the total adult AIDS cases in the United States. A large majority of these women are in their childbearing years, with 79% between ages 13 and 39 yr.[8] Fifty-two percent of women with AIDS are Black, and 19% are Hispanic. AIDS cases have occurred 14 times more frequently among Black women, and 9 times more frequently among Hispanic women, relative to White women.[12] Chu et al.[13] reported that AIDS was the leading cause of death among Black women between the ages of 15 and 44 in New York and New Jersey.

The major transmission category for women with AIDS is injecting drugs.[12] Fifty-two percent of female AIDS cases fall into this category, which has been the major route of transmission for women since the onset of the disease. The proportion of women with AIDS in the heterosexual transmission category has increased annually in the last 6 yr such that heterosexual contact with an HIV-infected male is the second largest transmission category for women, with 30% of female AIDS cases falling into this category. Female IDUs and female sexual partners of male IDUs constitute the largest number of HIV-infected women of childbearing age. As discussed later, this fact has had major implications for the rise of pediatric AIDS cases. Transmission from blood transfusions comprises 11% of female cases. The final transmission category for women is a residual one in which no specific risk is identified. Seven percent of female cases fall into this undetermined risk category.[12]

Heterosexual women in the United States are at greater risk of becoming infected with HIV through sexual intercourse than are heterosexual men. There are two major reasons for this finding. First, there are a greater percentage of men than women infected with HIV; as such, on a probability basis, heterosexual women are more likely than heterosexual men to encounter an infected partner.[14] Second, HIV is more easily transmitted from men to women.[15] Cohen et al. reported that in 1987 approx 4% of the total number of AIDS cases were attributable to probable, or definite, heterosexual transmission.[4] However, among women with AIDS, heterosexual transmission was associated with 29% of AIDS cases; more than 50% of these female AIDS cases were non-iv drug-using partners of male IDUs. Moreover, heterosexual transmission of AIDS among women varies considerably by racial/ethnic group, with 53% of the cases being Black, and 22% of the cases being Hispanic.[16]

Special Problems and Issues of Women with (or at Risk for) AIDS

The majority of female sex partners of male IDUs do not use drugs and may not be aware of the risk that they confront through sexual relations with their partners.[17] Of those women who are aware of the risk, several factors may affect their ability to insist on the use of condoms. First, a woman's emotional or economic dependence on her male partner and the threat of physical coercion from the partner may play a critical role in a woman's level of control to protect herself.[18] Second, condom use is a particularly sensitive issue among male members of some minority groups, who view this use as a threat to their sense of masculinity,[19] and women often defer to male sexual partners who object to condom use.[20] Finally, the position of the Catholic church on the use of condoms has influenced some minority group members' views, and condom use may be interpreted by some minorities as having genocidal implications.[21]

Women with AIDS have most of the same symptom manifestations and illnesses as men except that Kaposi's sarcoma is infrequent among women. Women with AIDS most frequently contract pneumonia or other opportunistic infections.[22] Although rapid loss of health, frequent loss of employment, reduced finances, and health insurance costs are problems for both sexes with AIDS, women often have additional problems and concerns.[12,14] Women with AIDS are usually more financially disadvantaged than men with AIDS, and women with HIV infection have been reported to have high rates of gynecological and obstetrical disorders.[23] Pregnancy in HIV-infected women may accelerate the progression of HIV infection.[24]

Additionally, AIDS presents complex fertility and reproductive decisions for women. Many infected women do not know that they are infected when they become pregnant, so difficult decisions may have to be made regarding abortion.[12] Furthermore, amniocentesis cannot determine if a fetus is infected with HIV. Childbearing for some women is often linked to strong cultural expectations, so much so that they may decide that a 25–50% chance of having an infected child may be acceptable odds.

Women IDUs are a population of special concern, given that they comprise over one-half of all women reported to have AIDS in the United States. Despite the finding that women IDUs represent the majority of symptomatic AIDS cases in women seen by clinicians, a large portion are, neverthe-less, the most difficult to reach since their lifestyles are often transient, unstable, and impoverished.[12] High rates of pregnancy have been documented in women IDUs, in part owing to a lack of options regarding birth control methods.[25] A recent study of contraceptive practices among female heroin addicts found that only 3% used condoms with their sexual partners.[26]

Female IDUs more often develop lethal opportunistic infections than do other patient groups, and thus have a shorter life expectancy.[27] They frequently have other complicating conditions, such as hepatitis or cirrho-sis, and their immune systems are often extremely suppressed.[28] Female IDUs are also more likely to have young children and to be the sole sup-porters of these children.[29] These women have fewer friendships, less edu-cation, and fewer employment opportunities than men.[30] Therefore, HIV-infected women IDUs and their family members confront consider-able difficulties in coping with AIDS. Complicating this situation is the fact that fewer drug treatment programs exist for women IDUs than for men. Furthermore, most of these programs are highly limited for women, in that they often contain male-oriented approaches to problem identification and treatment, and therefore may not necessarily serve the needs of chemically dependent women.[14] Additionally, most treatment centers will not house women who are pregnant or who have children.[29]

Pediatric AIDS

The number of pediatric AIDS cases is increasing dramatically. The majority of such cases (78%) result from perinatal transmission from high-risk mothers.[31,32] The first cases of pediatric AIDS in the United States were reported in 1979. More recently, the Centers for Disease Control reported a total of approx 2000 pediatric AIDS cases (diagnosed between birth and 12 yr of age).[3] Pediatric AIDS cases constitute <2% of the total reported AIDS cases in the United States; however, there has been a 10-fold increase in the number of pediatric cases from 1986 to 1991.[33]

Women with AIDS are disproportionately represented in minority groups (infected primarily through injecting drugs or being the sexual part-ner of an IDU); thus, infants with HIV are disproportionately of Black or Hispanic background. Blacks constitute 53% of pediatric AIDS cases, and Hispanics 23%. The clinical situation is complicated greatly by social fac-tors (e.g., poverty, lack of adequate healthcare, and minimal or no health insurance) that impede optimal mother/infant care.[34] Most children with HIV infection are currently under 5 yr of age.[33]

The frequency of transmission from an infected mother to her fetus or newborn infant ranges from 25–50%.[12,35] The stage of pregnancy at which infection can occur is still uncertain. Caesarian deliveries have failed to prevent fetal infection. The virus has also been found to be present in breast milk.[34] Three cases of HIV transmission from mother to infant through breast milk have been reported.[36] There has been no systematic pattern of perinatal transmission of HIV to infants from seropositive mothers. That is, the subsequent offspring of an HIV-infected mother may be seropositive or seronegative, even if the mother's initial offspring was seropositive.

The actual rate of perinatal transmission is difficult to determine, and there are, as yet, no laboratory tests that can reliably establish HIV infection perinatally or in newborns.[12] HIV serostatus in infants cannot be accurately determined using current technological methods until the child is 15–18 mo of age, when maternal antibodies have been filtered from the child's blood.

Perinatal acquisition of HIV by infants of infected mothers is associated with a high probability of infant morbidity and mortality.[12] There is a high rate of disease progression in perinatally infected children during the first year of life.[36] Various neurological symptoms have been found in as many as 60–70% of pediatric AIDS patients.[37] Some children are symptomatic at birth, some become symptomatically ill shortly after birth, and still others seem to grow and develop normally for several months before exhibiting symptoms of HIV infection.[38] The infections accompanying pediatric AIDS cases may include those opportunistic infections (e.g., pneumonia) seen in adult AIDS patients.[34]

Immunology and Pathogenesis of HIV/AIDS

The immune system is most easily described as a defense system that responds to infectious agents that enter the organism. Most immune responses are mediated by T- and B-lymphocytes (or more simply B- and T-cells). B-cells originate in the bone marrow, and are involved principally in attacking and destroying infectious agents that cause damage outside the cells, including bacterial agents. T-cells originate in the thymus gland, and are involved principally in attacking and destroying infectious agents that invade cells, including viruses, parasites, and fungi. There are three types of T-cells: natural killer cells, T-helper (or T4) cells, and T-suppressor (or T8) cells. T-helper cells are integrally involved in antibody production for both T-cells and B-cells, and therefore are of the utmost importance to immune system functioning. These T-helper cells are referred to as T4-cells because their expression may be detected by the phenotypic surface marker CD4.

The focus of the HIV assault on the human organism is centered on the vitally important T4-cells. It has been proposed that HIV binds to the CD4 surface molecule, thus permitting it to enter the T4-cell.[39] HIV is a retrovirus, and once it enters the cell, viral ribonucleic acid (RNA) is transcribed to deoxyribonucleic acid (DNA), and then integrated into the host cell's chromosomal DNA.[39,40] The integrated (host) DNA is then capable of producing additional RNA viruses to attack other T4-cells, and, through reproduction and proliferation, T4-cells are progressively destroyed, leaving the organism susceptible to opportunistic infections or illnesses. Furthermore, as mentioned previously, T4-cells are not only involved in antibody production associated with T-cell functioning, but also B-cell functioning; therefore, the impact of HIV on T4-cell functioning is especially undermining to immune system functioning.

There is substantial variation with regard to the interval between HIV infection and full-blown AIDS. A number of factors contribute to this variation, including the number and quality of T4-cells in the body, nutritional status, the existence of other diseases, environmental stress, and lifestyle habits, including alcohol and drug use.[40,41] In subsequent sections we discuss the roles of some of these factors (e.g., alcohol use, sexually transmitted diseases) as they may influence both susceptibility to HIV infection and the progression to full-blown AIDS.

Empirical Associations: Alcohol Use, Sexual Behaviors, and Health-Related Indexes

Alcohol Use and Sexual Behavior

The association of alcohol use with unsafe sexual activity (e.g., unprotected sex) has been indicated in a number of studies.[10,42–44] Furthermore, these associations have been robust across diverse populations, including the general population,[45] homosexual men,[46] and adolescents.[42] With a Scottish sample, Robertson and Plant reported a high correlation between increased alcohol consumption and unsafe sexual practices among 18- to 25-yr-olds.[44] Leigh reported that correlations between unsafe sexual behavior and the use of alcohol and other drugs during sex were strong and consistent—the more often a person consumed alcohol or used drugs during sex, the more risky his/her behavior was overall.[43]

Alcohol and drug use may reduce the likelihood of condom use. Research by Hingson et al. indicated that adolescents who consumed five or more drinks daily and those who used marijuana in the past month were 2.8 and 1.9 times, respectively, less likely to use condoms during penetrative sex.[42] Sixteen percent of the adolescent drinkers or drug users reported less frequent use of condoms after drinking than when not drinking. Cooper and Pierce studied the relationships between alcohol use and several specific risk behaviors among adolescents.[47] The results indicated that respondents who drank prior to or during first intercourse were significantly less likely to use a condom (32 vs 49%), were less likely to have discussed AIDS-related risk issues with their partners, and were significantly more likely to have had a casual partner. Anecdotal reports from bartenders in the Association of Bartenders against AIDS have noted unsafe sexual behaviors among customers who, when sober, are known advocates of safe sex.[48]

A number of explanations have been promulgated regarding the association between alcohol use and risky sexual behaviors (for a review, *see* ref. 49). Some explanations have focused on disinhibition associated with the pharmacological properties of ethanol, whereas others have focused on disinhibition associated with folk beliefs[50] or alcohol expectancies.[49] George and Norris concluded that the relationship between alcohol and sexuality is highly complex, and that alcohol use indeed may influence sexual behaviors, but that numerous qualifying conditions (e.g., dosage, gender) must be specified to more adequately account for the observed relations.[51]

Alcohol Use and Immune System Functioning

Significant associations between heavy alcohol use and medical illnesses frequently have been reported.[52-54] Excessive, prolonged consumption of alcohol, as well as alcoholic liver disease, lead to altered immune functioning, which, in turn, is proposed to contribute to increased susceptibility to HIV infection.[55-58] Molgaard et al. provided a succinct review of the literature supporting alcohol-immune system relations, and suggested that alcoholics have a reduced number of total lymphocytes and decreased levels of circulating T-cells, including T4-cells that are basic to the functioning of B- and T-cells.[57] Alcoholic liver disease tends to exacerbate the indicators of immunosuppression. Acute alcohol consumption also has been implicated experimentally in the impairment of both cellular and humoral immunity.[53,54] Pillai and Watson have suggested that alcohol can serve as a cofactor in the development of HIV/AIDS:

1. By indirectly reducing immune functioning in combination with other drugs;
2. As a consequence of nutritional and emotional modifications of the neuroendocrine system;
3. By directly suppressing the host's immune response against HIV and other pathogens (e.g., STDs); and/or
4. By creating conditions favoring the increased proliferation and development of the virus.[58]

Other factors that are prevalent in alcoholics may further compromise the immune system and increase risk of HIV infection and disease. Malnutrition is an important factor suppressing various components of the immune system.[56] Immune system suppression is also associated with high life stress, poverty, poor coping skills, and depression, all of which are highly prevalent among a large subset of alcoholics.[59] Cigaret use and polysubstance use are also highly prevalent among alcoholics,[28] and the use of these substances is associated with immune suppression. These lifestyle factors may further exacerbate HIV risk, opportunistic disease manifestations, and progression to full-blown AIDS.[40]

Although the data are relatively consistent in suggesting that prolonged heavy alcohol use may alter immune system functioning, there is controversy regarding its purported role in influencing the progression from HIV to full-blown AIDS.[7,60] Westerberg reported on three studies that investigated the relation between alcohol consumption and progression to AIDS, and indicated that none of these studies supported the association. For example, he reported on findings from the Multicenter AIDS Cohort Study by Kaslow et al., in which level of drinking was not predictive of HIV serostatus.[61] In addition, among a subsample of seropositive men with low CD4+ cell counts, there was no overall significant relation between alcohol consumption and progression to AIDS. Kaslow et al. did, nevertheless, suggest that although their findings were not supportive of alcohol as a cofactor in the progression of HIV to AIDS, alcohol may still be instrumental in risk behaviors leading to HIV infection.

Given the limited number of studies that have been conducted on the possible role of alcohol as a cofactor in the progression from HIV to AIDS, we would argue that it is premature to suggest that alcohol is not a cofactor for at least some subgroups. None of the studies reported by Westerberg[60] contained a sample of alcoholics, and carefully monitored longitudinal designs are required to adequately assess alcohol, or any other factor, as a cofactor in the temporal progression from HIV infection to AIDS. Because of the host of possible confounding variables (e.g., nutritional status, other drug use), in vitro methods and murine models may also facilitate the investigation of alcohol as a cofactor in the progression from HIV to AIDS.[58,62]

Sexually Transmitted Diseases

Numerous epidemiological studies have shown associations among alcohol and drug use, sexual behaviors, and STDs.[45,63–65] Number of sex partners has also been associated with higher rates of gonorrhea, chlamydia, genital herpes infections, and human papillomavirus infections, as well as with increased risk for cervical and other genital cancers.[66] During the 1980s, rates of heterosexually acquired syphilis, gonorrhea, and chancroid began to increase—especially among Blacks and Hispanics.[31,67,68] Trends in crack and chronic cocaine use have been paralleled by trends for syphilis, gonorrhea, chancroid, and HIV infection, both temporally and with respect to the groups most affected (Black/White ratio = 3.2:1; Hispanic/White ratio = 2.8:1 in the number of AIDS cases).[65]

Research has indicated high HIV seroprevalence rates among persons with STDs.[41] The biological susceptibility linkage here is that STDs, such as gonorrhea or chlamydia, among women, for example, may contribute to inflammation that reduces the integrated functioning of vaginal and urethral mucosa, which, in turn, may increase access by viruses (such as HIV) to the bloodstream. Alcohol and drug use may contribute to STDs in several ways. Molgaard et al. suggested that alcohol and drug use may contribute to indiscriminate choice of sex partners (possibly including partners with HIV or STDs), to prostitution to purchase drugs, and to a reduced likelihood of using condoms.[57] Ericksen and Trocki reported that frequent bar-going, drunkenness episodes, high volume drinking, and feeling disinhibited while drinking and taking drugs increased risk for STDs via their effects on rate of sex partner change.[45]

The prevention, early diagnosis, and treatment of STDs among women are important not only to reduce risk of HIV infection, but also because of possible severe consequences with regard to pelvic inflammatory disease (PID), ectopic pregnancy, and infertility.[69] PID, which may result from untreated chlamydia infection and gonorrhea, can lead to infertility, tubal pregnancy, fetal wastage, and congenital infections in the offspring of infected mothers.[70] It should also be noted that STDs, similar to HIV, are more easily transmitted from men to women than from women to men.[15,69,71] Women who abuse alcohol or drugs are often subject to increased risk for STDs and HIV for numerous reasons (e.g., prostitution to obtain drugs, HIV- or STD-infected partners). Furthermore, for those alcoholic and drug-abusing women who are financially disadvantaged, healthcare facilities may not be easily accessible or provide adequate services. In short, financially disadvantaged alcoholic and drug-abusing women generally are both at highest risk for contracting STDs or HIV, and healthcare services may be the least accessible.[41]

Neuropsychiatric Impairment

In addition to its impact on the immune system, prolonged alcohol use may adversely effect the central nervous system (CNS), and pose diagnostic problems in relation to the manifestations of AIDS.[40,72] Navia et al. reported that 25% of 121 AIDS cases exhibited CNS manifestations that accompanied or preceded other AIDS symptoms, whereas 10% exhibited CNS manifestations as the presenting sign of AIDS.[73] Diagnostic clarity is clouded with alcohol abusers who may manifest temporary, or permanent, neuropsychiatric impairment as a result of prolonged alcohol use. In addition to focal syndromes (e.g., Wernicke-Korsakoff's syndrome), alcohol abuse can cause diffuse brain dysfunction that may persist for months, years, or indefinitely—even after withdrawal of the substance. Cognitive impairment has been shown in 70–90% of alcoholics after detoxification.[74] Symptoms of alcoholic organic brain syndrome, such as loss of intellectual abilities, memory deficits, and personality change, may be difficult to differentiate from early HIV-associated cognitive impairment. However, in alcoholics, the impairment is usually mild, and can be stabilized or reversed by abstinence. In the AIDS patient, impairment is progressive and is severe by the terminal phase. Alcoholics who develop AIDS may suffer from both drug- and infection-related cognitive impairment.[40] Future research needs to focus on methods to distinguish alcohol-related and AIDS-related cognitive impairment, as well as to investigate any possible linkages that may, for example, contribute synergistically to more pervasive and rapid mental decline for dually diagnosed AIDS and substance-abusing patients.

Prevalence of AIDS Among Alcoholics in Treatment Settings

Substance abusers and their partners are the fastest growing segment of the HIV-infected population. For IDUs, HIV prevalence is estimated to range from 50–60% in some urban centers.[75] In order to determine HIV status among outpatients at an inner-city alcohol treatment center in Newark, NJ, Schleifer et al.[76] anonymously screened 99 patients (76 men, 92% Black, age range from 30–50 yr). Clinical intake interviews rendered results with approx 50% of the subjects reporting exclusive use of alcohol, and 50% reporting the use of other substances in addition to alcohol. Twenty-seven percent indicated current or past iv drug use. HIV-positive serostatus was found in 4.5% of those who abused alcohol exclusively. In contrast, 48.1% of those reporting the abuse of alcohol and other drugs were found to be seropositive for HIV. HIV seropositivity appeared highest in male alcoholics with a history of injecting drugs (57.9%), and was considerably lower in female IDUs (25%). The relatively low incidence of seropositivity among alcoholics without a history of injecting drugs (4.5%) suggests that non-iv drug-using alcoholics are a relatively distinct group from their alcohol/drug-injecting counterparts. However, these results must be tempered in that 100% of those subjects who reported that they were sexually active indicated that they always used alcohol before or during sex, and acknowledged the role that alcohol played in facilitating unsafe sexual practices.[76] As such, these individuals are engaging in risky behaviors that increase risk for HIV/AIDS.

Jacobson et al.[77] assessed the HIV serostatus of 143 consecutive in- and outpatient male alcoholics at the Bronx VA Medical Center. All patients had annual incomes <$15,000, and the racial composition of the sample was 58% Black, 26% White, and 16% Hispanic. Thirteen percent ($n = 19$) of the alcoholics were HIV seropositive, and 42% of these seropositive alcoholics were also iv drug users. There were no race differences in the distribution of seropositive cases. The most frequent risk behaviors associated with HIV acquisition were iv drug use and sexual contact with an iv drug user. Similar to the findings of Schleifer et al.,[76] these findings suggest relative distinct groups of non-iv drug-using alcoholics and a group of iv drug-using alcoholics who manifest differential risk behaviors for HIV infection.

Windle studied the prevalence of high-risk behaviors for AIDS among 51 alcoholic inpatients in western New York (34 men, 65% White, 29% Black, mean age = 34.2 yr).[78] The study had three objectives:

1. To assess the frequency of commonly identified AIDS-risk behaviors (e.g., iv drug use, unsafe sexual practices) among alcoholics;
2. To investigate interrelations between specific risk factors and non-iv drug using activities (e.g., use of drugs during sexual activities); and
3. To examine possible differences in illicit drug use and non-iv drug use activities for subjects categorized according to sexual-risk status.

The findings indicated that a significant subset of heterosexual alcoholics were engaging in behaviors (beyond unprotected vaginal intercourse with a primary partner) that increase risk for the transmission of HIV. Twenty percent of the sample reported iv drug usage in the last 6 mo, and over 40% reported three or more sexual partners in the last 6 mo. Unprotected vaginal intercourse was highly frequent, along with a high frequency of using drugs during sexual activities. The overall rate of high-risk behaviors did not differ according to gender. The results suggest that a significant portion of male and female alcoholics are engaging in behaviors that increase risk for HIV infection for themselves as well as their partners.

The three studies by Schleifer et al.,[76] Jacobson et al.,[77] and Windle[78] suggest that the seroprevalence rate of HIV infection and high-risk behaviors among alcoholics are considerably higher than the general population. These rates are also higher than those reported in studies of inpatients in psychiatric hospitals, where HIV seroprevalence rates are about 5.5–6.0%.[79,80] Those alcoholics who are also injecting drugs are at risk for AIDS at a rate equivalent to IDUs; non-iv drug-using alcoholics still may be at increased risk as a result of other high-risk behaviors (e.g., unprotected sex, promiscuity). The population of alcoholics is, of course, not limited to patients seen at alcohol treatment centers, and the heavy use of alcohol (if not clinically diagnosed alcoholism) has been associated with HIV and AIDS in other special populations, such as prison inmates, the homeless, and runaway adolescents. An HIV seroprevalence study of runaway and homeless adolescents at the Covenant House in New York yielded a 5.3% seropositive rate (males = 6%; females 4.2%). The seropositivity rate was 1.3% for 15-yr-olds and 8.6% for 20-yr-olds.[81] Alcohol was used by 80% of the total sample of adolescents, although the HIV seropositivity was associated most highly with iv drug use, male homosexual/bisexual behaviors, prostitution, and a history of an additional sexually transmitted disease.

Conceptual Model

Much of the information presented thus far in the chapter has focused on "parts of the puzzle" linking alcohol and drug use to HIV/AIDS. At this juncture, we present a provisional conceptual model to facilitate the integration of material presented in this chapter, as well as to serve a heuristic function in future research. This conceptual model is presented in Fig. 1. The model has been influenced globally by general systems perspectives,[82,83] and specifically by perspectives that emphasize person–environment relations with health promotion implications.[84-87] In addition, the model has been influenced by the "epidemiological triangle" conceptualization that has focused on the dynamic relations between agent, host, and environment domains.[41] We have modified the epidemiological triangle model for several reasons to be enumerated subsequently. We believe that the revised model provides added clarity to person–environment relations, and facilitates envisioning targeted prevention and intervention strategies.

The conceptual model is referred to as a dynamic, ecological model of epidemiological risk for the following reasons. By dynamic, reference is made both to the multivariate nature of the phenomena to be studied and the crosstemporal stabilities and changes in individual characteristics and coherent, co- or multivariable interrelations or assemblages. That is, individual characteristics and coherent patterns function in a coordinated and integrated fashion, even though in all systems there are periods of both stability and change across time. Furthermore, transitions of individual characteristics or coherent assemblages may be temporally asynchronous, i.e., manifesting differential rates of change. For example, emotion-laden cognitive appraisals may be occurring at a much faster rate than associated physiological indexes of emotional arousal (e.g., changes in heart rate). By ecological, reference is made to the concept of multilayered, embedded systems that serve as mediums of exchange for material and information. As such, different systems and subsystems (e.g., cells, organs, persons, cul-

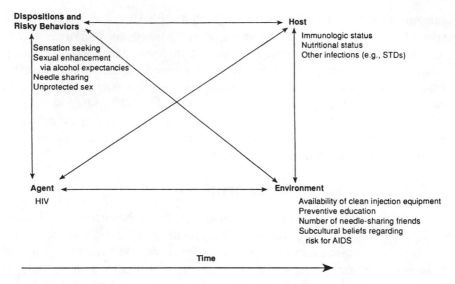

Fig. 1. Dynamic, ecological model of epidemiological risk for HIV/AIDS.

tures, and so forth) are embedded in contexts that constrain as well as facilitate the expression of specific beliefs, attitudes, and behaviors.

A further defining feature of the model is that dispositions and risky behaviors have been decoupled from host (susceptibility) factors in the epidemiological triangle conceptualization. This seemed useful to us for three interrelated reasons. First, we conceive of dispositions and risky behaviors within an active agent framework[84,88,89] in which individual differences, influenced by genetic and environmental sources, increase or decrease exposure to infectious and toxic agents, including HIV. Second, we conceive of host factors as biological status factors that reflect features of disease susceptibility, but that are viewed more as consequences of activities in other components of the conceptual model (e.g., substance abuse, eating practices). This also enables us to separate possible genetic influences of the host, which at times have been used erroneously to suggest increased risk for AIDS among Blacks,[41] from possible genetic influences on dispositions and risky behaviors that may directly, or indirectly, increase risk for AIDS. For example, heritability estimates for the personality trait of sensation seeking are about .58, and sensation seeking has been associated with higher levels of alcohol and substance use and sexual activity.[90] To the extent that sensation seeking is associated with high-risk behaviors and the selection of high-risk environments (e.g., having friends who are risk takers or injecting drug users), genetic and environmental factors conjointly influence risk exposure. Third, the conceptual model may be used to identify specific targets for prevention and intervention. Some dispositions and risky behaviors may be more amenable to psychological-based approaches (e.g., cognitive–behavioral therapy to modify attitudes or beliefs), whereas host deficiencies may be more amenable to pharmacological or nutritional supplement interventions.

Finally, it should be observed in Fig. 1 that the lines with two-headed arrows imply that the direction of effects among the identified components are bidirectional, or reciprocal.[84,88] For example, injecting drug users not only engage in high-risk behaviors, but they also may be more highly involved in social networks where they have a number of needle-sharing friends and socially constructed subcultural belief systems (e.g., nonhomosexuals do not get AIDS) regarding drug injection as a highly valued activity that may perpetuate the identified high-risk behavior (e.g., sharing needles). Whereas the conceptual model in Fig. 1 implies reciprocal relations among components, the relations themselves may be symmetrical or asymmetrical. That is, reciprocity of effects does not imply equality of effects. For instance, the agent (HIV) presumably has a more potent effect on the host (e.g., immunological status) than the converse; however, pharmacological interventions (e.g., AZT) may (temporarily) slow the replication of the human immunodeficiency retrovirus (i.e., slow down the reverse transcriptase process), and thus impact on the magnitude of the agent (at least for some parameters, e.g., the rapidity of the spread of the virus and the associated reduction of T4-cells). Based on this conceptualization, two major research agendas arise. First, how potent and symmetrical/asymmetrical are the interrelations among the components of the model? Second, how do the interrelations among components change across time, and how do targeted preventions/interventions influence the system of interrelations?

Behavioral Risk Study (BRS)

A current project being conducted by the first author of this chapter focuses on several aspects of the model presented in Fig. 1. Data are being collected from 750 alcohol treatment center inpatients with regard to:

1. Dispositions and risky behaviors (e.g., alcohol expectancies for sexual enhancement, childhood conduct problems, needle sharing, unprotected sex);
2. Host features (e.g., STDs, reproductive dysfunction);
3. Environmental characteristics (e.g., number of drinking and needle-sharing friends, homeless status); and
4. HIV status via self-report or patient record data (with informed consent).

Five alcohol treatment centers are participating in the study, three in New York City and two in western New York. The sampling design includes an oversampling of women and two minority groups (Blacks and Hispanics). Of particular interest are the potential differences in risky behaviors between gender and racial/ethnic groups, as well as possible differences among these subgroups (e.g., Black males) between regional environmental settings (i.e., New York City vs western New York). Differential risk for HIV is being investigated according to three different categorical approaches:

1. Alcoholic iv drug users vs alcoholic non-iv drug users;
2. Coexisting psychiatric disordered subgroups (e.g., antisocial alcoholics, depressive alcoholics); and
3. Family history of alcoholism and criminality.

Consistent with Fig. 1, it is proposed that dispositions and risky behaviors will be associated with host characteristics (e.g., STDs), environmental features (e.g., number of sexual partners, friendships with IDUs), and a higher rate of HIV infection.

The principal goal of the BRS is to investigate behavioral risk factors and associated person and environment variables that may moderate (or exacerbate) the incidence and prevalence of HIV/AIDS among alcoholic inpatients. The study seeks to identify alcoholic subtypes at high risk for contracting AIDS because of higher levels of engagement in high-risk behaviors. Based on prior research,[76,77] we propose that a substantial subset of alcohol treatment center populations may be at high risk for AIDS. It is hypothesized that person variables (such as age, gender, racial/ethnic group, childhood behavior problems, psychiatric disorders, attitudes and knowledge about AIDS, alcohol expectancies of sexual enhancement, and perceived consequences of drinking behavior), in combination with socioenvironmental conditions (such as geographical/regional area, socioeconomic status, and social and physical drinking contexts), may influence some individuals to engage in higher levels of alcohol consumption and illicit substance use, to frequent more high-risk drinking contexts (e.g., bars), to have a more deviant peer group, and to engage in a wider range of sexual activity and with more sexual partners.

Summary and Future Research Directions

The changing prevalence of AIDS cases and the current projections indicate that an alarming number of women and their offspring are either infected or at high risk for HIV infection. Among women, the two groups at greatest risk for HIV infection are IDUs and females engaging in high-risk sexual behaviors (e.g., sex without condoms) with infected male partners. As mentioned earlier, women IDUs have high pregnancy rates, are often impoverished, and lack access to quality healthcare (both in medical and chemical treatment settings). Because of lifestyle patterns, these women may also have compromised immune system functioning, and thus have increased susceptibility to HIV infection and other STDs. As such, women IDUs are a subgroup that must be the target of additional outreach efforts, have access to more supportive healthcare, and have easy accessibility to clean injection equipment.

Heterosexual women with HIV-infected male partners are also at risk for HIV transmission for a number of reasons. First, more men than women are infected with HIV, and the probability that a heterosexual woman will have sexual contact with an HIV-infected partner is thus greater. Second, STDs and HIV are more easily transmitted from men to women than from women to men. Third, women may find themselves in a relationship in which they lack the power to insist that their partners use a condom. Assertiveness training with regard to practicing safe sex may be useful for some women. However, for financially dependent women, assertiveness regarding protective devices may result in adverse consequences (e.g., physical abuse, partner departing). Alternative contraceptive methods may be the only viable option for these women, and yet the efficacy of these methods for the prevention of HIV is still unknown.[69]

STDs pose particular problems for women, given that these diseases have been related to a number of health complications, including the development of cervical/genital cancers, pelvic inflammatory disease, ectopic pregnancy, and infertility. A relationship has also been found between STDs and HIV seroprevalence rates. This relationship may be accounted for, in part, by the fact that gynecological problems and STDs may yield the vaginal walls less resistant to infectious agents such as HIV, and reduce overall immunocompetence. As such, careful and systematic medical attention to obstetrical and gynecological problems, as well as STDs, is advised so as to minimize susceptibility to infectious diseases.

The use of alcohol and drugs among women poses additional risks for the contraction of STDs and HIV. Heavier alcohol use has been found to be associated with higher rates of sexually risky activities (e.g., less condom use, more sexual partners). Women who are consuming higher amounts of alcohol may be more vulnerable to infection because they may be more likely to engage in sexual activity with an infected partner, less able to insist on the use of condoms, or simply more forgetful with regard to protection. Women IDUs may resort to prostitution in order to support their drug habits. Although men may also engage in these types of behaviors while using alcohol or drugs, for reasons outlined earlier, women are especially susceptible to contracting HIV and STDs (e.g., vulnerability as a result of gynecological problems).

We presented a dynamic, ecological model of epidemiological risk for HIV/AIDS and the outline of a research project that will evaluate some aspects of the model. The model is useful for generating future questions about differences among groups (e.g., men and women, Blacks and Whites), with implications for targeted prevention and intervention strategies. For example, prevention and intervention strategies could focus on one (e.g., subcultural beliefs) or multiple components of this model, contingent on perceptions (or knowledge) of the prevalence of the risk behaviors. In financially disadvantaged neighborhoods and/or areas where there are a number of shooting galleries, a focus on reducing sexual enhancement is likely to be a quite limited prevention/intervention strategy; however, for some college students or young, heavy drinking adults, a focus on sexual enhancement via nonalcohol alternatives may be plausible. Given that there is no known pharmaceutical agent on the horizon to "cure" AIDS, behaviors must be changed to reduce AIDS cases. It is necessary to have some knowledge of the co-ocurrence and interrelatedness of behaviors in order to optimize prevention and intervention strategies. The dynamic, ecological model facilitates this effort by highlighting the complexity of the interrelations, yet it retains the flexibility to be adapted to a wide range of high-risk behaviors for HIV and AIDS. Future research may benefit from models that incorporate the diversity and complexity that we know to characterize human behavior.

Acknowledgments

This chapter was supported in part by grant number 08051 from the National Institute on Alcohol Abuse and Alcoholism awarded to Michael Windle.

References

[1]Centers for Disease Control (1991) *HIV/AIDS Surveillance.* December, Center for Infectious Disease Control, Atlanta, GA, pp. 1–18.

[2]Centers for Disease Control (1992) *Voice Informational System.* January 27, Center for Infectious Disease Control, Atlanta, GA.

[3]Centers for Disease Control (1990) *HIV/AIDS Surveillance Report: Year-End Edition.* Center for Infectious Disease Control, Atlanta, GA, pp. 1–22.

[4]J. B. Cohen, L. B. Hauer, and C. B. Wofsky (1989) Women and IV drugs: Parenteral and heterosexual transmission of human immunodeficiency virus. *J. Drug Issues* **19**, 39–56.

[5]J. D. Fisher and W. A. Fisher (1992) Changing AIDS risk behavior. *Psychol. Bull.* **11**, 455–474.

[6]J. A. Kelly, J. S. St. Lawrence, T. L. Brasfield, A. Lemke, T. Amidei, R. E. Roffman, H. V. Hood, J. E. Smith, H. Kilgore, and C. McNeill Jr. (1990) Psychological factors

that predict AIDS high-risk versus AIDS precautionary behavior. *J. Consult. Clin. Psychol.* **58,** 117–120.

[7]M. Plant (1990) Alcohol, sex and AIDS. *Alcohol Alcohol.* **25,** 293–301.

[8]M. E. Guinan and E. Hardy (1987) Epidemiology of AIDS in women in the United States 1981–1986. *JAMA* **257,** 2039–2042.

[9]D. Des Jarlais, S. Friedman, and R. Stoneburner (1988) HIV infection and intravenous drug use: Critical issues in transmission dynamics, infection outcomes, and prevention. *Rev. Infect. Dis.* **10,** 151–158.

[10]R. Stall and D. Ostrow (1989) Intravenous drug use, the combination of drugs and sexual activity and HIV infection among gay and bisexual men: The San Francisco men's health study. *J. Drug Issues* **19,** 57–73.

[11]S. Weinstein, P. DeMaria, and M. Rosenthal (1992) AIDS and alcohol: Concerns for the physician. *Hospital Pract.* **27,** 98–105.

[12]C. Campbell (1990) Women and AIDS. *Soc. Sci. Med.* **30,** 407–415.

[13]S. Y. Chu, J. W. Buehler, and R. L. Berkelman (1990) Impact of the human immunodeficiency virus epidemic on mortality in women of reproductive age, United States. *JAMA* **264,** 225–229.

[14]D. B. V. Wells and J. F. Jackson (1992) HIV and chemically dependent women: Recommendations for appropriate healthcare and drug treatment services. *Int. J. Addict.* **27,** 571–585.

[15]N. S. Padian, S. C. Shiboski, and N. P. Jewell (1991) Female-to-male transmission of human immunodeficiency virus. *JAMA* **266,** 1664–1667.

[16]V. M. Mays (1989) AIDS prevention in black populations: Methods of a safer kind, in *Primary Prevention of AIDS.* V. M. Mays, G. W. Albee, and S. F. Schneider, eds. Sage, Newbury Park, CA, pp. 264–279.

[17]D. Des Jarlais (1984) Heterosexual partners: A risk group for AIDS. *Lancet* **2,** 1346–1347.

[18]J. Peterson and R. Bakeman (1989) AIDS and IV drug use among ethnic minorities. *J. Drug Issues* **19,** 27–37.

[19]J. Gross (1987) The bleak and lonely lives of women who carry AIDS. *The New York Times,* August 27, pp. A1, B5.

[20]D. Worth and R. Rodriquez (1987) Latina women and AIDS. *SIECUS Rep.* **15,** 5–7.

[21]P. Stephens (1989) U.S. women and HIV infection, in *The AIDS Epidemic.* P. O'Malley, ed. Beacon, Boston, MA, pp. 381–401.

[22]Centers for Disease Control (1987) Human immunodeficiency virus infection in the U.S.: A review of current knowledge. *Morbidity Mortality Weekly Rep.* **36,** 1–48.

[23]R. Kapila, A. Grigoriu, and P. Kloser (1986) Women with AIDS/ARC. Paper presented at Second International Conference on AIDS, Paris, June 23–25.

[24]H. Minkoff, R. de Regt, S. Landesman, and R. Schwarz (1986) Pneumocystis Carinii Pneumonia associated with acquired immunodeficiency syndrome in pregnancy: A report of three maternal deaths. *Obstet. Gynecol.* **67,** 284–287.

[25]S. Deren (1986) Parents in methadone treatment and their children. *New York State Division of Substance Abuse Services Treatment Issue* (Report 50).

[26]D. Mackintosh, L. Mundey, G. Fischer, and E. Morgan (1986) Condom usage by IV drug users. *Am. J. Pub. Health* **76,** 1460.

[27]P. Porter (1989) Minorities and HIV infection, in *The AIDS Epidemic.* P. O'Malley, ed. Beacon, Boston, MA, pp. 371–379.

[28]R. R. Watson (ed.) (1990) *Drugs of Abuse and Immune Function*. CRC, Boca Raton, FL.

[29]N. Shaw and L. Paleo (1986) Women and AIDS, in *What to do About AIDS*. L. McKusick, ed. University of California Press, Berkeley, CA, pp. 150–151.

[30]M. Rosenbaum (1981) *Women on Heroin*. Rutgers University Press, New Brunswick, NJ.

[31]Centers for Disease Control (1988) AIDS profile update. *AIDS Rec.* **2**, 11.

[32]R. A. Olson, H. C. Huszti, P. J. Mason, and J. M. Seibert (1989) Pediatric AIDS/HIV infection: An emerging challenge to pediatric psychology. *J. Pediatric Psychol.* **14**, 1–21.

[33]Task Force on Pediatric AIDS-American Psychological Association (1989) Pediatric AIDS and human immunodeficiency virus infection. *Am. Psychol.* **44**, 258–264.

[34]J. Osborn (1988) The AIDS epidemic: Six years. *Ann. Rev. Pub. Health* **9**, 551–583.

[35]A. Semprini, A. Vucetich, G. Pardi, and M. Cossu (1987) HIV-infection and AIDS in new born babies of mothers positive for HIV antibody. *Br. Med. J.* **294**, 610.

[36]J. Curran, H. Jaffe, A. Hardy, W. Morgan, R. Selik, and T. Dondero (1988) Epidemiology of HIV infection and AIDS in the U.S. *Science* **239**, 610–616.

[37]R. Price, B. Brew, J. Sidtis, M. Rosenblum, A. Scheck, and P. Cleary (1988) The brain in AIDS: Central nervous system, HIV-1 infection and AIDS determine complex. *Science* **239**, 586–592.

[38]K. Martin, B. Katz, and B. Miller (1987) AIDS and antibodies to human immunodeficiency virus (HIV) in children and their families. *J. Infect. Dis.* **252**, 54–63.

[39]A. S. Fauci (1988) The human immunodeficiency virus: Infectivity and mechanisms of pathogenesis. *Science* **239**, 617–622.

[40]S. Schleifer, B. Delaney, S. Tross, and S. Keller (1991) AIDS and addictions, in *Clinical Textbook of Addictive Disorders*. R. Frances and S. Miller, eds. Guilford, New York, pp. 299–319.

[41]S. Duh (1991) *Blacks and AIDS: Causes and Origins*. Sage, Newbury Park, CA.

[42]R. Hingson, L. Strunin, B. Berlin, and T. Heeren (1990) Beliefs about AIDS, use of alcohol and drugs, and unprotected sex among Massachusetts adolescents. *Am. J. Pub. Health* **80**, 295–299.

[43]B. Leigh (1990) The relationship of substance use during sex to high-risk sexual behavior. *J. Sex Res.* **27**, 199–213.

[44]J. A. Robertson and M. A. Plant (1988) Alcohol, sex and risks of HIV infection. *Drug Alcohol Depend.* **22**, 75–78.

[45]K. P. Ericksen and K. F. Trocki (1992) Behavioral risk factors for sexually transmitted diseases in American households. *Soc. Sci. Med.* **34**, 843–853.

[46]R. Stall (1988) The prevention of HIV infection associated with drug and alcohol use during sexual activity. *Adv. Alcohol Subst. Abuse* **7**, 73–88.

[47]M. L. Cooper and R. Pierce (1991) Sex Differences in Alcohol Use and Sexual Risk-Taking. Paper presented at annual meeting of the American Psychological Association, San Francisco, CA, August 16–20.

[48]D. Flavin and R. Frances (1987) Risk-taking behavior, substance abuse disorders, and the acquired immune deficiency syndrome. *Adv. Alcohol Subst. Abuse* **6**, 23–32.

[49]L. C. Crowe and W. H. George (1989) Alcohol and human sexuality: Review and integration. *Psychol. Bull.* **105**, 265–272.

[50]R. Room and G. Collins (eds.) (1983) *Alcohol and Disinhibition and Meaning of the Link, NIAAA Research Monograph 12*. U.S. Department of Health and Human Services, Washington, DC.

[51]W. H. George and J. Norris (1991) Alcohol, disinhibition, sexual arousal, and deviant sexual behavior. *Alcohol Health Res. World* **15**, 133–138.

[52]H. Adams and C. Jordan (1984) Infections in the alcoholic. *Med. Clin. North Am.* **68**, 179–200.

[53]R. R. MacGregor (1986) Alcohol and immune defense. *JAMA* **256**, 1474–1479.

[54]F. Smith and D. Palmer (1976) Alcoholism, infection and altered host defenses: A review of clinical and experimental observations. *J. Chronic Dis.* **29**, 35–49.

[55]M. Gafoor (1990) Alcohol is a co-factor in HIV-transmission and hastens the onset of AIDS. *Nurs. Times* **86**, 14.

[56]R. R. MacGregor (1988) Alcohol and drugs as co-factors for AIDS. *Adv. Alcohol Subst. Abuse* **7**, 47–71.

[57]C. A. Molgaard, C. Nakamura, M. Hovell, and J. P. Elder (1988) Assessing alcoholism as a risk factor for acquired immunodeficiency syndrome (AIDS). *Soc. Sci. Med.* **27**, 1147–1152.

[58]R. Pillai and R. Watson (1990) Letter to Editor: Response to "Alcohol, sex, and AIDS". *Alcohol Alcohol.* **25**, 711–713.

[59]J. Jaffe and D. Ciraulo (1986) Alcoholism and depression, in *Psychopathology and Addictive Disorders*. R. E. Meyer, ed. Guilford, New York, pp. 293–320.

[60]V. S. Westerberg (1992) Alcohol measuring scales may influence conclusions about the role of alcohol in human immunodeficiency virus (HIV) risk and progression to acquired immunodeficiency syndrome. *Am. J. Epidemiol.* **135**, 719–725.

[61]R. A. Kaslow, W. C. Blackwelder, D. G. Ostrow, J. Yerg, J. Palenicek, A. H. Coulson, and R. O. Valdiserri (1989) No evidence for a role of alcohol or other psychoactive drugs in accelerating immunodeficiency in HIV-1-positive individuals. A report from the Multicenter AIDS Cohort Study. *JAMA* **261**, 3424–3429.

[62]R. R. Watson (1989) Murine models for acquired immune deficiency syndrome. *Life Sci.* **44**, i–xiii.

[63]R. S. Ernst and P. S. Houts (1985) Characteristics of gay persons with sexually transmitted diseases. *Sex. Transm. Dis.* **12**, 59–63.

[64]B. Hoegsberg, T. Dotson, and O. Abulafia (1989) Social, sexual and drug use profile of HIV+ and HIV− women with PID. Paper presented at Fifth International Conference on AIDS, Montreal, June 4–9.

[65]R. Marx, S. Aral, R. Rolfs, C. Sterk, and J. Kahn (1990) Crack, sex and STD. *Sex. Transm. Dis.* **18**, 92–101.

[66]S. O. Aral, V. Soskoline, R. M. Joesoef, and K. R. O'Reilly (1991) Sex partner recruitment as a risk factor for STD: Clustering of risky males. *Sex. Transm. Dis.* **18**, 10–17.

[67]R. Rolfs and W. Cates (1989) The perpetual lessons of syphilis. *Arch. Dermatol.* **125**, 107–109.

[68]H. Handsfield, R. Rice, M. Roberts, and K. Holmes (1989) Localized outbreak of penicillinase-producing gonorrhea. *JAMA* **261**, 2357–2361.

[69]M. J. Rosenberg, A. J. Davidson, J. H. Chen, F. N. Judson, and J. M. Douglas (1992) Barrier contraceptives and sexually transmitted diseases in women: A comparison of female-dependent methods and condoms. *Am. J. Pub. Health* **82**, 669–674.

[70]W. L. Yarber and A. V. Parrillo (1992) Adolescents and sexually transmitted diseases. *J. School Health* **62,** 331–338.

[71]K. K. Holmes, D. W. Johnson, and H. J. Trostle (1970) An estimate of the risk of men acquiring gonorrhea by sexual contact with infected females. *Am. J. Epidemiol.* **91,** 17–24.

[72]S. Lunn, M. Skudsbjerg, H. Schulsinger, J. Parnas, C. Pedersen, and L. A. Mathiesen (1991) A preliminary report on the neuropsychologic sequelae of human immunodeficiency virus. *Arch. Gen. Psychiatry* **48,** 139–142.

[73]B. A. Navia, B. D. Jordan, and R. W. Price (1986) The AIDS dementia complex: I. Clinical features. *Ann. Neurol.* **19,** 517–524.

[74]M. Pohl (1988) Neurocognitive impairment in alcoholics: Review and comparison with cognitive impairment due to AIDS. *Adv. Alcohol Subst. Abuse* **7,** 107–116.

[75]D. Des Jarlais, S. Friedman, and D. Novick (1989) HIV-1 infection among intravenous drug users in Manhattan, New York City, from 1977 through 1987. *JAMA* **261,** 1008–1012.

[76]S. Schleifer, S. Keller, J. Franklin, S. LaFarge, and S. Miller (1990) HIV seropositivity in inner-city alcoholics. *Hospital Community Psychiatry* **41,** 248–254.

[77]J. M. Jacobson, T. M. Worner, H. S. Sacks, and C. S. Lieber (1992) Human immunodeficiency virus and hepatitis B virus infections in a New York City alcoholic population. *J. Stud. Alcohol* **53,** 76–79.

[78]M. Windle (1989) High-risk behaviors for AIDS among heterosexual alcoholics: A pilot study. *J. Stud. Alcohol* **50,** 503-507.

[79]F. Cournos, M. Empfield, E. Howarth, K. McKinnon, I. Meyer, H. Schrage, C. Currie, and B. Agosin (1991) HIV seroprevalence among admissions at two psychiatric hospitals. *Am. J. Psychiatry* **148,** 1225–1230.

[80]J. Volavka, A. Convit, J. O'Donnell, R. Douyon, C. Evangelista, and P. Czobor (1992) Assessment of risk behaviors for HIV infection among psychiatric inpatients. *Hospital Community Psychiatry* **43,** 482–485.

[81]R. L. Stricof, J. T. Kennedy, T. C. Nattell, I. B. Weisfuse, and L. F. Novick (1991) HIV seroprevalence in a facility for runaway and homeless adolescents. *Am. J. Pub. Health* **81(suppl.),** 50–53.

[82]L. von Bertalanffy (1968) *General Systems Theory.* Braziller, New York.

[83]J. Miller (1978) *Living Systems.* McGraw-Hill, New York.

[84]A. Bandura (1978) The self-system in reciprocal determinism. *Am. Psychol.* **33,** 344–358.

[85]U. Bronfenbrenner (1979) *The Ecology of Human Development. Experiments by Nature and Design.* Harvard University Press, Cambridge, MA.

[86]R. Moos (1979) Social ecological perspectives on health, in *Health Psychology: A Handbook.* G. Stone, F. Cohen, and N. Adler, eds. Jossey-Bass, San Francisco, CA, pp. 523–547.

[87]D. Stokols (1992) Establishing and maintaining healthy environments: Toward a social ecology of health promotion. *Am. Psychol.* **47,** 6–22.

[88]R. M. Lerner (1984) *On the Nature of Human Plasticity.* Cambridge University Press, New York.

[89]R. Plomin (1986) *Development, Genetics and Psychology.* Erlbaum, Hillsdale, NJ.

[90]M. Zuckerman (1991) *Psychobiology of Personality.* Cambridge University Press, New York.

Effects
of Drugs of Abuse
on Reproductive Function
in Women and Pregnancy

Siew K. Teoh, Nancy K. Mello,
and Jack H. Mendelson

Introduction

In the United States, the prevalence of substance use and abuse in women has been increasing over the last 20 yr. According to a 1984 survey in three major metropolitan areas sponsored by the National Institute on Mental Health (NIMH), alcohol abuse and dependence ranked fourth among psychiatric disorders in women aged 18–24, and drug abuse and/or dependence was the second most common psychiatric disorder among women aged 18–24.[1,2] In a National Household Survey conducted in 1991, more than half (57.8 and 52.8%, respectively) of all women ages 18–25 and 26–34 yr reported that they had used alcohol during the previous month, and more than 1 in 10 women surveyed in these age groups (13.4 and 11.2%, respectively) had used some illicit drug during the same interval.[3] Prevalence estimates for alcohol, marijuana, cocaine, and heroin use are presented in Fig. 1. However, these figures may be underrepresented as this was a household survey and the prevalence of substance abuse may indeed be higher in women who have comprised socioeconomic status.

From: *Drug and Alcohol Abuse Reviews, Vol. 5: Addictive Behaviors in Women*
Ed.: R. R. Watson ©1994 Humana Press Inc., Totowa, NJ

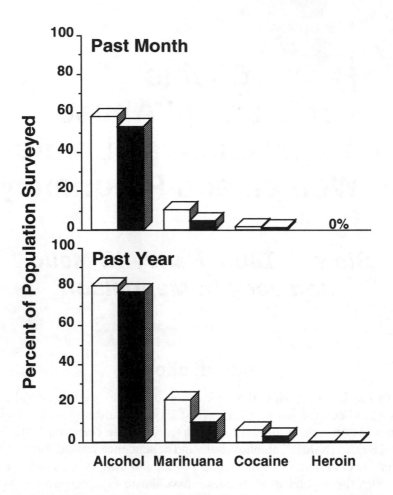

Fig. 1. Prevalence estimates for alcohol, marijuana, cocaine, and heroin use by women. (□) Age 18–25, n = 14,553,121. (■) Age 26–34, n = 19,658,929. Source: ref. 3.

It is increasingly recognized that substance abuse is associated with deleterious effects on reproductive function in both men and women. The adverse consequences of maternal drug abuse for the developing fetus have been documented repeatedly (*see* ref. 4 for review). Drugs of abuse may disrupt reproductive function by direct toxic effects on the hypothalamus, pituitary, or gonads, or all in combination, but these pathophysiological processes are poorly understood. The degree of reproductive toxicity of substance abuse may depend on frequency and duration of drug use. The extent to which the reproductive system develops tolerance to the disruptive effects of drug abuse is unclear, and the time-course and prospects for recovery are unknown.

There has been relatively little research on substance abuse and reproductive function in women until recently.[5,6] Interpretation of clinical studies is often complicated by the fact that many drug abusers do not use only one drug but, rather, may use several drugs in various combinations. Cocaine abusers often use alcohol as well as opiates and marijuana to modulate the cocaine "high" and "crash."[7,8] Alcohol abusers may also use marijuana, tobacco, opiates, and cocaine. Since polydrug abuse appears to be an increasingly prevalent drug use pattern, it is difficult to categorize women by use or abuse of a single drug. Moreover, the medical consequences of the combined effects of several drugs may be more severe than use of a single drug alone.[9,10] It is likely that polydrug abuse also increases risk for derangements of reproductive system function. A higher incidence of sexual dysfunction (62%) has been reported in men who abuse both cocaine and alcohol.[7] Poor nutritional status and inadequate medical care may augment disruptive effects on reproductive function, and it may be difficult to document associations of reproductive disorders and drug use practices.

Ethical concerns prohibit administration of drugs of abuse to women with no prior experience with the drug or to women who are seeking treatment for substance abuse. Thus, most clinical research has been limited to retrospective epidemiological studies and case reports. Consequently, many studies of drug abuse and reproductive dysfunction have been conducted in animal models (*see* refs. 5 and 11 for review). Studies in animal models offer several important advantages:

1. There are no confounding effects of unreported polydrug use;
2. The drug history of the subject is known;
3. Nutritional status may be controlled.

Since alcohol is the most frequently abused substance in women, this review will mainly focus on recent studies of alcohol effects on neuroendocrine function in women of reproductive age as well as on pregnancy and outcome. Effects of marijuana, cocaine, and opiates on reproductive function in women and pregnancy will also be reviewed briefly.

Alcohol

The impact of excessive alcohol use in women has been incompletely explored. It has long been known that alcoholism is associated with severe disruption of reproductive function in men. Testicular atrophy, low testosterone levels, gynecomastia, impotence, and diminished sexual interest are consistently reported.[12-15] Clinical reports indicate that alcoholism in women can result in derangements of menstrual cycle function such as amenorrhea, anovulation, luteal phase dysfunction, and, in some instances, early menopause.[5,11,16–20]

A higher incidence of uterine curettages and higher variability of menstrual cycles (abnormal duration and/or menstrual flow) was found in 51 chronic alcoholic women than in age-matched controls.[21] In the general population, there is evidence that heavy alcohol consumption is associated with menstrual cycle disorders as well as high rates of gynecological and obstetrical surgery.[22] There also is emerging evidence that reproductive disorders and sexual dysfunction may be a risk factor for development of heavy drinking.[23,24]

However, the mechanisms of alcohol's toxic effects on female reproductive function are unknown[13,25] (*see* refs. 5 and 11 for review). Alcoholic women often have other medical problems, such as liver disease, pancreatitis, and malnutrition, that could cause menstrual cycle disturbances independently of alcohol. But recent replications of these reproductive disorders in animal models under controlled conditions[26–30] and in healthy social drinkers[31] indicate the generality of observations on alcoholic women with other medical complications.

Pathogenesis of Alcohol-Related Reproductive Dysfunction

Neuroendocrine control of the human menstrual cycle is complex, with variation of pulsatile hormonal secretion during the follicular, ovulatory, and luteal phases. Thus, the menstrual cycle phase during which alcohol intoxication occurs may determine the type of menstrual cycle dysfunction. However, it is not known whether the toxic effects of chronic alcohol dependence occur primarily at the level of the hypothalamus, pituitary, or ovaries, or if alcohol simultaneously disrupts each component of the hypothalamic–pituitary–gonadal axis. In contrast, acute alcohol administration has little effect on pituitary or gonadal hormone secretion in normal women.[32–34]

Alcoholic women frequently report amenorrhea, or complete cessation of menses.[18–20,35] The clinical literature on endocrine concomitants of alcohol-related amenorrhea is very limited. Twenty-two women admitted for treatment of liver disease or pancreatitis were studied in Finland ($n = 9$) and in Paris ($n = 13$).[18,20] Twenty-three women admitted for treatment of alcoholism were studied in Japan.[36–38] Of these 23 Japanese women, 10 patients were diagnosed as having alcoholic hepatitis and 13 patients had fatty liver.[36–38] Normal estrogen levels were measured in 8 of the 22 European alcoholic amenorrheic women, and there was a positive estradiol response to stimulation with clomiphene or human chorionic gonadotropin (hCG).[18] However, 14 of the European women showed low levels of estrogen and high levels of LH and FSH compared to controls. The amenorrheic alcoholic Japanese women also had low estrogen levels and high FSH levels.[36-38]

Pituitary function as evaluated with 100 µg of synthetic luteinizing-hormone-releasing hormone (LHRH) in the European alcoholic amenorrheic women showed no significant difference in LH and FSH response compared to normal controls. However, the magnitude of LHRH-stimulated (100 µg) increase in gonadotropins was significantly higher in the Japanese women with less severe amenorrhea.[36-38] Hence, the normal gonadotropin response to LHRH stimulation suggested that the pituitary may not be the primary site of alcohol's toxic effects in amenorrheic alcoholic women.

It is possible that alcohol-induced amenorrhea may be due to aberrant gonadotropin secretory patterns. Recent clinical data suggest that primary amenorrhea and secondary hypothalamic amenorrhea are associated with suppression of gonadotropin secretory activity.[39-42] Normal ovulatory function can be restored in amenorrheic patients by pulsatile infusion of synthetic LHRH.[40-43] However, there has been no systematic evaluation of gonadotropin secretory pattern in alcoholic amenorrheic women. In normal men, alcohol (1.5 g/kg) administered over 3 h did not reduce LH and FSH pulse frequency or amplitude[45] although increased pulse amplitude of LH and FSH has been reported in generally healthy alcoholic men after cessation of alcohol ingestion.[45]

Another possibility is that alcohol may stimulate corticotropin-releasing-factor (CRF), ACTH, and cortisol, and disrupt menstrual cycle function through the hypothalamic–pituitary–adrenal axis.[46-48] Administration of synthetic CRF inhibited pulsatile release of LH and FSH in ovariectomized rhesus females,[49] but administration of ACTH and cortisol did not. Their data suggest that CRF-induced suppression of LH and FSH is a central effect mediated through the hypothalamic-pituitary axis rather than through adrenal action.[50] Synthetic CRF administration also suppressed endogenous LHRH in rat portal blood.[51] Thus, alcohol-induced amenorrhea may be due to CRF-induced suppression of gonadotropin secretory activity at the hypothalamic–pituitary axis.

Anovulation (failure to ovulate) and luteal phase dysfunction (inadequate progesterone levels during the luteal phase) may occur in alcoholic women who continue to menstruate[18,19,52] (*see* ref. 11 for review). The mechanisms for alcohol-related anovulation and luteal phase dysfunction in alcoholic women are poorly understood. Hugues and coworkers evaluated four alcoholic women with anovulatory cycles, three of whom had chronic pancreatitis and one had cirrhosis.[18] Clomiphene induced a significant rise of plasma LH and estradiol. Six alcoholic women with luteal phase inad-

equacy were also studied.[18] Of these six women, four had chronic pancreatitis and two had cirrhosis, but their gonadotropin response to LHRH was
adequate and hCG stimulation during the second part of the cycle induced a
progesterone rise of >10 ng/mL in three of the six women.

Hormonal imbalance during the follicular phase of the menstrual cycle
may result in abnormal folliculogenesis and subsequent anovulation and
luteal phase dysfunction.[53-55] Studies on the primate ovarian cycle indicate
that recruitment of follicles occur during d 1–4 of the menstrual cycle; one
follicle is selected during d 5–7 and achieves dominance during d 8–12.[53,55]
The process of folliculogenesis is associated with increased levels of FSH.
Suppression of FSH during the follicular phase may delay follicle maturation and ovulation.[53-55]

There is evidence that alcohol prevents stimulation of FSH by synthetic LHRH during the follicular phase of the menstrual cycle in normal
female rhesus monkeys.[57] However, acute alcohol administration did not
suppress LHRH-stimulated FSH during the follicular phase of the menstrual cycle in normal women.[56] The lack of acute alcohol effects on LHRH-
stimulated FSH in normal women[56] is at variance with data reported in the
rhesus monkey.[57] In part, this may result from different experimental designs.
In the female rhesus monkey study, much higher blood alcohol levels of
184–276 mg/dL were achieved when LHRH administration failed to stimulate FSH,[57] and LHRH was administered when blood alcohol levels were
approaching peak levels.[57] However, in the clinical study, a peak alcohol
level of 113.3 ± 7.5 mg/dL was achieved, and LHRH was administered at
initiation of alcohol ingestion.[56]

Recent data show that an increase in estradiol (E_2) levels during the
early follicular phase suppresses FSH, inhibits pre-ovulatory follicular
growth, and prolongs the follicular phase.[58,59] Luteal phase defects were
consistently observed after 6, 12, and 24 h of exposure to estradiol during
the follicular phase (d 6 or 7 of the menstrual cycle).[58] Increases in estradiol
(E_2) levels have been observed within 25 min after initiation of alcohol
(0.695 g/kg) ingestion in normal women during the follicular phase of the
menstrual cycle under basal (nonstimulated) conditions.[31] Concurrent administration of alcohol and LHRH also produced a significant increase in plasma
estradiol during the follicular and luteal phases of the menstrual cycle.[57]
The mechanism for increases in estradiol levels following alcohol consumption may be due to increased E_2 production and/or decreased E_2 metabolism. Hepatic oxidative metabolism of steroids may become rate-limiting
at times of alcohol metabolism when relatively low blood alcohol concentrations (45 mg/dL) may saturate alcohol dehydrogenase and decrease the

NAD to NADH ratio.[60-63] This could, in turn, decrease the rate of oxidation of estradiol to estrone and result in increased plasma estradiol levels.

It has also been reported that a midcycle surge in progesterone is critical for induction of ovulation in normal women.[64] Administration of a progesterone antagonist (RU 486) delayed midcycle gonadotropin surge (2–5 d) and ovulation in normal women, despite rising estradiol levels and normal follicle development.[64] These data suggest that progesterone may play a critical role in the induction of ovulation. Administration of alcohol (0.694 g/kg) 1 h after 50 mg of naltrexone orally resulted in decreased progesterone levels.[65] It was postulated that intrahepatic alcohol metabolism reduced NAD availability for oxidation of pregnenolone to progesterone, resulting in decreased plasma progesterone levels.[65] It is possible that alcohol-induced anovulatory cycles may be due to suppression of the midcycle progesterone surge, but as yet, there are no confirmatory data.

Hyperprolactinemia, defined as prolactin levels above 20 ng/mL, is commonly reported for alcohol-dependent women.[36-38,52,66] Hyperprolactinemia associated with pituitary adenomas may cause amenorrhea and other disruptions of menstrual cycle function.[67-69]

Twenty-three women (ages 20–40) admitted for alcoholism treatment were studied in Japan. The maximum drinking history was 18 yr and the average period of problem drinking was 7.2 ± 4.2 yr.[37] All women were diagnosed as having alcoholic hepatitis or fatty liver, but none had cirrhosis. All patients had normal body weight, and none were undernourished. Of the 23 Japanese women, 6 women had prolactin levels >100 ng/mL (115–184 ng/mL); 10 women had prolactin levels >50 ng/mL (59–97 ng/mL); 6 women had elevated prolactin levels ranging from 27 and 38 ng/mL and 1 woman had a normal prolactin level (11 ng/mL).[36-38] All women had amenorrhea ($n = 21$) or oligomenorrhea ($n = 2$). Following treatment and alcohol abstinence, all women had prolactin levels <30 ng/mL and normal liver function tests. Of these 23 patients, a follow-up study was possible for 8 on an outpatient basis, of whom 7 experienced spontaneous recurrence of menstruation but endocrine profiles were not mentioned. It was concluded that hyperprolactinemia occurred with a high frequency in alcoholic women in association with disrupted menstrual cycle function. However, hyperprolactinemia without amenorrhea has also been reported in alcoholic women (ages 18–46) during abstinence.[52] Conversely, Välimäki and coworkers reported normal prolactin levels in nine amenorrheic alcoholic women with liver disease.[20]

One clinical study examined the effects of chronic alcohol intake on menstrual cycle function and hormonal status in 26 healthy women with a history of regular drinking under controlled clinical research ward conditions.[70] After a 7-d alcohol-free baseline period, these women could self-administer alcohol for 21 consecutive days. Access to alcohol was contingent on performance of a simple operant task. Acquisition of one drink required 30 min of operant performance on an F1 1-s (FR 300) reinforcement schedule. An Intoximeter III was used for measurement of alcohol levels. Blood samples were collected on alternate days for subsequent measurements of LH, prolactin, progesterone, and estradiol. Following 3 wk of alcohol availability, women remained on the clinical research ward for an additional 7 d prior to discharge.

The 26 women were classified as heavy, moderate, or occasional alcohol users on the basis of the actual number of drinks acquired while on the clinical research ward. Heavy users drank an average of 7.81 ± 0.69 drinks/d. Moderate users drank an average of 3.84 ± 0.19 drinks/d, and occasional users drank an average of 1.22 ± 0.21 drinks/d during the 21-d period of alcohol availability. No evidence of menstrual cycle dysfunction or abnormality in reproductive hormone levels was found in the occasional drinkers or in two of the moderate drinkers who consumed less than an average of three drinks/d.[70] In contrast, 50% of the moderate drinkers who consumed more than three drinks/d and 60% of the heavy drinkers had significant derangements of menstrual cycle and reproductive hormone function. Three of the five heavy drinkers had persistent hyperprolactinemia. However, the woman who consumed the most alcohol (10 ± 0.69 drinks/d) did not have abnormal menstrual cycles or hyperprolactinemia.

In an animal model, Mello and coworkers reported that during chronic high-dose alcohol self administration (3.4 g/kg/d), one amenorrheic alcohol-dependent macaque monkey had prolactin levels ranging from 16.5–63 ng/mL, and immunocytochemical examination of the anterior pituitary showed apparent hyperplasia of the lactotrophs.[28] Hyperprolactinemia may contribute to alcohol-induced amenorrhea but this hypothesis was not confirmed in subsequent studies.[29] Prolactin levels were intermittently elevated above 20 ng/mL during four amenorrheic cycles (85–194 d), but did not differ significantly from prolactin levels during normal ovulatory menstrual cycles when no alcohol was available.[29]

Acute alcohol effects on basal levels of prolactin in normal human subjects have yielded conflicting findings. Decreased plasma prolactin levels have been observed over 4 h following acute alcohol administration to normal women during the midluteal phase of the menstrual cycle.[34] Another study of normal women during the luteal phase of the menstrual cycle reported increases in plasma prolactin levels for 3 h following 1.2 g/kg of alcohol, when blood alcohol levels averaged 100 mg/dL.[38] However, acute alcohol administration during the midfollicular phase had no effect on basal prolactin levels when blood alcohol levels averaged 88 mg/dL.[33]

Alcohol and Pregnancy

It is important to emphasize that chronic alcohol intake may not be invariably associated with menstrual cycle disorders. This can be inferred from the fact that alcohol abusing and alcohol-dependent women do become pregnant; and their children may be afflicted with physical abnormalities (*see* ref. 71 for review) and biobehavioral disorders range from hyperactivity to mental retardation.[72,73] One major unresolved question concerns the range of alcohol doses that are likely to produce adverse consequences for the fetus. Since alcohol diffuses freely across the placental barrier, the fetus is exposed to the same effective dose of alcohol as the mother. One drink/d has been associated with fetal dysmorphologies in a prospective study.[74]

The fetal alcohol syndrome (FAS) was first recognized as a syndrome in 1973.[75] In the general population, it is estimated that 1–3 of every 1000 live births is afflicted with some variant of alcohol-related impairment.[76,77] Among alcoholic women, the prevalence of the fetal alcohol syndrome has been estimated at 21–29%/1000 live births.[76] The fetal alcohol syndrome is a clinically defined entity,[78] and the principal features of FAS include:

1. Adverse central nervous system effects, marked by microcephaly and mild to moderate mental retardation;
2. Prenatal and postnatal growth retardation;
3. Typical dysmorphological features, particularly of the midfacial and mandibular area, such as short palpebral fissures, hypoplastic upper lip with thinned vermilion, a diminished to absent philtrum.

The severity of anomalies associated with the fetal alcohol syndrome may vary in different individuals.

A prospective study of 263 women examined the effects of maternal alcohol use during pregnancy and infant birth weight.[79] Alcohol consumption was estimated for 6 mo before pregnancy, in early pregnancy (first 4 mo), and late pregnancy (mo 5–8). Using regression analysis which adjusted for maternal age, height, parity, daily cigarets, gestational age, and sex of child, it was found that ingestion of an average of 1 oz of absolute alcohol daily before pregnancy was associated with an average decrease in birth weight of 91 g; the same amount ingested in late pregnancy was associated with a decrease of 160 g.[79] There is also evidence that drinking prior to pregnancy may have residual effects on subsequent prenatal growth.[80] Other studies confirmed that intrauterine growth retardation was estimated to be increased by 2.4-fold in association with alcohol abuse alone, 1.8-fold with smoking alone, and 3.9-fold with these risks together,[81] independent of demographic factors, medical care, or nutritional status of the alcohol-abusing patients. Another prospective study of 633 women reported that infants born to heavy drinkers had twice the risk of abnormality than those born to abstinent or moderate drinkers.[82] Thirty-two percent of infants born to heavy drinkers demonstrated congenital anomalies, as compared to 9% in the abstinent and 14% in the moderate group.[82]

The pathogenesis of fetal alcohol syndrome (FAS) is unknown. It is reasonable to assume that alteration of maternal hormonal homeostasis subsequent to alcohol intake may affect fetal growth and outcome. However, there is very little information on alcohol's effects on the endocrine system during pregnancy.[83] Halmesmäki and coworkers evaluated hormonal levels of estradiol, estriol, progesterone, prolactin, and hCG in 40 pregnant women who chronically abused alcohol and in 20 abstinent pregnant women at 4-wk intervals.[84] None of the alcohol users had liver damage as assessed by serum aminotransferase activities. Sixteen alcohol users (40%) gave birth to infants with fetal alcohol syndrome, whereas the remaining 24 infants born to alcohol users and abstinent women were healthy. The women who gave birth to infants with FAS had decreased estradiol and estriol levels throughout pregnancy, and progesterone levels tended to be low. In contrast, the alcohol users had increased prolactin levels during the gestational wk 16–24 compared with those in the abstinent women, but the rise was not related to FAS. Levels of hCG fluctuated widely, without any consistent difference between alcohol users and abstinent women.[84]

In another study, serum total and free testosterone, androstenedione, dehydroepiandrosterone sulfate (DHEAS), and sex-hormone-binding globulin were measured in 40 pregnant alcohol users and 20 abstainers.[85] Drinking leading to fetal alcohol effects was associated with lowered concentrations of sex-hormone-binding globulin throughout pregnancy and lowered total testosterone and higher free testosterone levels between wk 16 and 20 of gestation. Maternal drinking leading to fetal alcohol effects was also accompanied by lowered concentrations of DHEAS between wk 16 and 32 of gestation, whereas androstenedione levels tended to be high throughout pregnancy. The physiological role of androgens in the regulation of maternal physiology and fetal growth and development are poorly understood.[86] Whether these hormonal changes contribute to the development of FAS is not known.

Alcohol's effects on maternal hormones during early pregnancy have not been explored adequately. The omission is significant, as confirmation of pregnancy often does not occur until midway into the first trimester, and the developing fetus is especially prone to drug-induced malformations during this period of organogenesis.[76,87] Recent data from a prospective study of 650 nonalcoholic women indicates that alcohol exposure (0.84–1.28 drinks/d) during the first and second month of the first trimester was associated with several morphological abnormalities in the newborn.[74]

Since it is not ethically feasible to give alcohol to pregnant women, administration of hCG is an established method for simulating maternal hormonal conditions during the first trimester of pregnancy.[88,89] We examined alcohol's effects on ovarian steroids following hCG stimulation during the midluteal phase of the menstrual cycle.[90] Following concurrent administration of hCG (5000 IU im) and alcohol (0.7 g/kg), there was a significant increase in plasma estradiol levels; this was not observed after hCG and placebo administration.[90] The magnitude of alcohol-related augmentation of hCG-stimulated E_2 was 55–91 pg/mL within 10 min of alcohol ingestion, and E_2 remained elevated for 240 min. As discussed earlier, these alcohol-related increases in estradiol could be due to decreased estradiol metabolism or increased estradiol production.

Administration of exogenous estrogens may have adverse effects on sexual differentiation in male and female fetuses.[91–94] Our finding of alcohol-related augmentation of estradiol under hCG stimulation suggests a possible mechanism for alcohol-related congenital anomalies in infants born to women who continue to consume alcohol during early pregnancy when chorionic gonadotropin levels are high.

Alcohol use during pregnancy also increases the risk of spontaneous abortion.[95,96] A prospective survey of 32,019 women at their first prenatal visit showed that women who consumed more than one drink/d had significant increased risks for spontaneous abortions during the second trimester (gestational wk 15–27), independent of age, parity, race, marital status, smoking, or the number of previous spontaneous or induced abortions.[95] Similar conclusions concerning associations between spontaneous abortion and moderate drinking were also observed by other investigators.[96] It was estimated that about 25% of pregnant women who drank more than twice a week were more likely to abort compared with 14% among women who drank less frequently.[96] In contrast to these findings, Halmesmäki and coworkers did not find increases in risk for spontaneous abortions in women who consumed one or two drinks (13 g of alcohol) per week.[97]

Although the mechanism for alcohol-related spontaneous abortion is unknown, it is known that progesterone is essential for maintenance of pregnancy. Administration of a competitive progesterone antagonist within 24 d after conception usually results in abortion.[98] We have previously reported a lack of progesterone response following hCG stimulation and alcohol administration.[90] During nonalcohol placebo administration, hCG stimulated a significant increase in progesterone. If alcohol also suppresses progesterone levels while chorionic gonadotropin levels are high, this may be a possible mechanism for alcohol-induced abortion. Halmesmäki and coworkers reported low progesterone levels in alcoholic women who gave birth to fetal alcohol syndrome children during gestational wk 16–24.[16–24]

Marijuana

Marijuana is prepared from the plant *Cannabis sativa*, and tetrahydrocannabinol (Δ^9-THC) appears to be the principal psychoactive component. The Δ^9-THC concentration in typical marijuana cigarets may vary between 5 and 20 mg. Marijuana is a commonly abused drug among women of reproductive age, and approx 10% of women between the ages of 18 and 25 and 26 and 35 yr responding to the National Household Survey in 1991 reported that they had used marijuana during the previous month.[3]

Effects of marijuana use on human reproductive function, especially in women of childbearing age, have caused considerable concern. Disruption of normal hormonal function may adversely affect pregnancy, fetal growth, and outcome. Until recently, there was relatively little information. Although most endocrine studies in experimental animals have consistently shown that the female reproductive system is very sensitive to cannabis effects, there are apparent inconsistencies in the findings. Neuroendocrine consequences of marijuana use on reproductive system in females have been reviewed previously (*see* refs. 6, 99–102 for review). Conflicting results also were reported for chronic marijuana use on pregnancy and its teratogenic effects on the fetus.[103] Studies of marijuana effects on male reproductive hormones have yielded inconsistent findings. Kolodny and coworkers[104] reported decrements in plasma testosterone levels in chronic male marijuana users compared to age- matched controls, but this finding was not confirmed by subsequent studies.[105–109]

Marijuana-Related
Reproductive Dysfunction

Most studies of marijuana's effects on female endocrine function have been conducted in the rhesus monkeys. Female rhesus monkeys offer the advantage that neuroendocrine regulation of menstrual cycle is very similar to that of human females.[100,111] The administration of Δ^9-THC to ovariectomized rhesus monkeys has been shown to suppress LH secretion over 12–24 h.[112] These studies have been confirmed and extended in a series of well-controlled studies, which showed that in ovariectomized monkeys the degree of LH suppression was not correlated with Δ^9-THC dose, but the duration of LH suppression was dose-dependent and LH was reversed within 48 h after Δ^9-THC administration.[113]

Acute effects of marijuana during different phases of the menstrual cycle in the rhesus monkeys have also been examined.[114,115] During the follicular phase of the menstrual cycle, monkeys were treated with 2.5 mg/kg of Δ^9-THC from d 1–18 of the cycle;[115] the blood concentrations of Δ^9-THC were similar to those found in heavy marijuana users. The Δ^9-THC-treated animals presented with anovulation and cycles of abnormal length (range 59–145 d) with lack of temporal estrogen rise and midcycle LH surge. There was no luteal elevation of progesterone, but prolactin concentrations were within the normal range.[115] In monkeys treated with simultaneous administration of Δ^9-THC and exogenous hMG and hCG, ovulation occurred between d 9–10 of the cycle and the monkeys had normal luteal function, as evidenced by serum progesterone concentrations and luteal phase lengths. These data suggested that the antiovulatory effect of Δ^9-THC did not occur primarily at the ovarian or pituitary level but rather at the hypothalamic level.

In another study, Δ^9-THC (2.5 mg/kg) was administered to rhesus monkeys during the luteal phase of normal ovulatory cycles.[114] THC- treated monkeys demonstrated progesterone levels and luteal phase lengths that were not different from those in untreated controls. In addition, Δ^9-THC did not impair the normal pattern of response of the corpus luteum to increasing doses of hCG as measured by serum progesterone concentrations and luteal phase lengths.[114] However, THC-treated monkeys exhibited abnormal menstrual cycles after Δ^9-THC treatment during the luteal phase.[99] The mechanism for prolonged disruption of the menstrual cycle after discontinuation of short-term Δ^9-THC treatment is unknown. However, the lack of Δ^9-THC effects on hCG-stimulated corpus luteum function is of particular importance as the experimental condition mimics progesterone secretion in early pregnancy.

One clinical study reported the effects of marijuana on reproductive hormones in women at different phases of the menstrual cycle.[116] Eight women were studied during the follicular phase and eight women were studied during the luteal phase of the menstrual cycle. Each woman served as her own control, and the effects of a 1-g marijuana cigaret containing 1.8% Δ^9-THC or a 1-g marijuana placebo cigaret on LH, estradiol, and progesterone were examined. Placebo cigarets caused no change in plasma LH, but Δ^9-THC induced a 30% suppression of plasma LH during the luteal phase of the menstrual cycle. There were no significant changes in estradiol or progesterone levels after marijuana or placebo smoking during either the follicular or luteal phases of the menstrual cycle.[116] These data are consistent with findings in experimental animals that Δ^9-THC actively suppresses LH levels.[113,114]

Tolerance to marijuana-induced suppression of reproductive hormones in primates has been reported.[117] Treatment of female rhesus monkeys with Δ^9-THC injections three times per week at doses of 2.5 or 1.5 mg/kg resulted in disruption of menstrual cycles for several months, with absence of ovulation and decreased basal concentrations of gonadotropin and sex steroids in the plasma. The duration of drug effects (days until next normal menstruation) was 70–135 d depending on the dose of the drug, but with chronic drug treatment, menstrual cycles were re-established with normal hormonal concentrations. Prolactin levels appeared to decrease during the period of disruption, but there were no significant effects of drug treatment. The mechanisms for tolerance are not known, but pharmacokinetic data in the study showed that there was no increase in drug metabolism or clearance that could have accounted for the tolerance produced. Thus, it was inferred that tolerance to reproductive effects of Δ^9-THC was probably caused by adaptation of neural mechanisms in the hypothalamus.[117]

The extent to which marijuana tolerance develops in human females is unknown. Twenty-six women who reported using marijuana at least four times/wk were compared with 16 age-matched controls who stated that they had never used marijuana.[118] Marijuana users had shorter menstrual cycles and shorter luteal phases than nonmarijuana smokers, but documentation of marijuana use relied solely on subjects' self reports.

Another clinical study examined effects of chronic marijuana use on reproductive hormones and cortisol in 56 women between the ages 18 and 42.[105] Hormone values were compared among groups of subjects stratified according to frequency of marijuana use; women who were on oral contraceptives were analyzed separately from those who were not. It was reported that chronic marijuana use showed no significant effects on plasma LH, FSH, prolactin, and cortisol levels. However, these data were based on single blood samples, results were not analyzed according to menstrual cycle phases, and subjects reported use of other drugs in addition to marijuana during the previous month.

Effects of Marijuana on Prolactin

Studies of the effects of Δ^9-THC on prolactin have yielded inconsistent results. Administration of Δ^9-THC produced a significant but brief suppression of prolactin levels in males and ovariectomized female rhesus monkeys.[114] However, Δ^9-THC inhibition of prolactin secretion was reversed by thyrotropin-releasing hormone, which directly stimulates prolactin secretion from the pituitary.[114] These data suggest that Δ^9-THC inhibition of prolactin secretion may be due to effects of the drug at hypothalamic sites. Marijuana-related suppression of plasma prolactin levels has also been reported in men (*see* refs. 102, 104, 119 for review).

One clinical study measured plasma prolactin levels in 16 healthy adult females before and after smoking a marijuana cigaret containing 1.83% Δ^9-THC and a placebo cigaret.[120] Acute marijuana smoking did not produce any significant changes in plasma prolactin levels during the follicular phase of the menstrual cycle. However, plasma prolactin levels were significantly lower after marijuana smoking during the luteal phase of the menstrual cycle.[120]

Another study of 26 women who reported using marijuana at least four times/wk showed that prolactin levels were significantly lower, compared to age-matched controls who had never used marijuana.[118] However, Block and coworkers did not report any significant differences in plasma prolactin levels subsequent to chronic marijuana use.[105]

Marijuana and Pregnancy

Marijuana is a commonly used illicit substance and, after alcohol and tobacco, the most commonly used drug during pregnancy, but its effects on pregnancy and outcome are still unclear. Following marijuana cigaret smoking, Δ^9-THC is rapidly absorbed from the lungs and then sequestered from blood into body tissues. Δ^9-THC is metabolized chiefly in the liver, but clearance of the cannabinoids is slow, indicating potential for prolonged fetal exposure in regular marijuana users.

Most women decrease marijuana use during pregnancy. The decrease in marijuana use was greatest after the recognition of pregnancy, during the first trimester.[103] Women who used marijuana heavily during the first trimester of pregnancy were not different from women who abstained throughout pregnancy in terms of age and education. However, women who continued to smoke were more likely to be Black, unmarried, of a lower socioeconomic status, and were more likely to use other drugs during pregnancy.[121] Similar patterns were found for women who used marijuana heavily during the second and the third trimester when compared to women who abstained throughout pregnancy.[121]

The effects of prenatal marijuana exposure on gestational length and fetal growth have yielded conflicting results. In a prospective study of 583 women who delivered single live infants, Fried and coworkers reported that use of marijuana six or more times/wk during pregnancy was associated with a statistically significant reduction of 0.8 wk in the gestational length, but there were no effects on infant birth weight.[122] Similar findings were also reported in another prospective study of 3857 pregnancies ending in single live births.[123] It was found that regular marijuana use (2–3 times/mo) was related to preterm delivery (gestational age <37 wk from last menstrual period) and an increased risk of delivering a low birth weight (<2400 g) infant in White women but not in non-White women. A significant effect of marijuana use during pregnancy on birth weight and length at birth was also reported by Zuckerman and coworkers.[124]

Offspring of women who tested positive for urine assays of marijuana had a 79 g decrease in birth weight and a 0.5 cm decrement in length compared to women who had negative urine screens. However, in a longitudinal study of 510 women conducted by Day and coworkers, there were no significant effects of prenatal marijuana exposure on gestational length and prematurity, adjusting for maternal age, gravidity, weight gained during pregnancy, maternal height, and use of alcohol, tobacco, and other illicit drugs.[103] In the same study, there was a small but significant negative effect between marijuana use during the first 2 mo of pregnancy and birth length, and a positive effect between marijuana use during the third trimester and birth weight.[103]

In general, there appears to be no association between prenatal marijuana exposure and major physical anomalies at birth.[103,125] Only one study reported that women who used marijuana during pregnancy were five times more likely to deliver infants with features considered compatible with the fetal alcohol syndrome when confounding variables were controlled.[126]

The pathogenesis of impaired fetal growth associated with prenatal marijuana use is unknown. Marijuana smoking is associated with a nearly fivefold increment in the blood carboxyhemoglobin level compared with tobacco smoking, attributed to larger puff volumes, greater depth of inhalation, and longer breath-holding time.[127] Thus fetal oxygenation may be impaired indirectly with resultant impaired fetal growth.

Little is known about the effects of prenatal exposure to Δ^9-THC on hormonal milieu during different periods of gestation. The effects of Δ^9-THC have been studied in the pregnant rhesus monkeys.[128] Δ^9-THC (2.5 mg/kg/d) or vehicle was administered during different gestational periods, and the effects of pregnancy outcome and concentrations of estradiol, progesterone, macaque chorionic gonadotropin (mCG) and prolactin levels during pregnancy were studied. The most significant finding was that pregnancy loss was observed in four out of five pregnancies when Δ^9-THC was administered during early pregnancy (i.e., from day of diagnosis of pregnancy). Spontaneous abortions were observed in three animals soon after initiation of drug administration, and a stillbirth occurred in one animal at 140 d of gestation. One pregnancy resulted in live birth of an infant of normal size and appearance at 157 d. In the three monkeys who aborted,

Δ^9-THC administration began before the normal, physiological decline in mCG. Marked decreases in mCG concentration were observed after the onset of Δ^9-THC treatment and were followed by a subsequent fall in progesterone concentration to nondetectable levels. By chance, drug administration began after the onset of the physiological decline in mCG concentration in the two monkeys who continued to term. Estradiol concentrations were higher in these animals compared to vehicle-treated controls, but no changes were observed in concentrations of mCG, prolactin, or progesterone. Daily Δ^9-THC treatment during the middle or third portion of gestation resulted in a lower pregnancy loss with no significant effects on serum concentrations of prolactin, mCG, or progesterone. These data implied that there was a critical interval for inhibition of chorionic gonadotropin by Δ^9-THC and alterations of hormonal milieu that may affect pregnancy outcome.[128]

In a clinical study, Braunstein and coworkers observed no significant differences in human chorionic gonadotropin concentrations or pregnancy outcome in 13 women who smoked marijuana regularly throughout pregnancy compared to controls.[129] However, endocrine profiles were not reported in these women.

In summary, marijuana use is prevalent among women of childbearing age. Marijuana smoking produces significant changes in female reproductive hormone function. In addition, impaired fetal growth and decreased length of gestation have been reported, but results to date are equivocal and further research is needed to address these issues.

Cocaine

During the past decade, cocaine abuse and dependence have reached epidemic proportions in the United States.[130] Although men and women report that acute cocaine self-administration enhances libidinal drive,[131] chronic cocaine abuse is associated with significant decrements in libidinal and reproductive function.[132] Impotence and gynecomastia have been observed in male cocaine users, and these abnormalities have persisted for long periods of time after cocaine abstinence.[133] Amenorrhea, dysmenorrhea, and infertility have been reported in women who abuse cocaine.[132–134] Cocaine use during pregnancy may be associated with increased risk for spontaneous abortion and abruptio placentae,[135] as well as fetal malformation and impaired neurobehavioral development,[136,137] However, the mechanisms underlying cocaine's toxic effects on reproductive function are unknown, and there have been few systematic studies of cocaine effects on reproductive function.

Cocaine's Effects on Prolactin

Regulation of prolactin secretion is complex and appears to involve both neuroendocrine and paracrine mechanisms.[138,139] It is known that dopaminergic systems are important modulators of prolactin secretion.[138,139] Acute and chronic cocaine exposure appear to have opposite effects on prolactin. Gawin and Kleber measured plasma prolactin levels in 15 males and 6 females who abused cocaine for an average of 3.4 yr.[140] Plasma prolactin levels for females were within the normal range, but plasma prolactin levels were decreased in male cocaine abusers when compared with healthy age-matched control subjects. Although the mean plasma prolactin levels for the males who abused cocaine was 5.3 ng/mL and within the range of normal prolactin levels for healthy adult males, 5 of the 14 males who abused cocaine had abnormally low prolactin levels. In contrast, recent clinical studies indicate that both cocaine abuse and cocaine withdrawal are associated with elevated prolactin levels.[133,141–143] Hyperprolactinemia with galactorrhea was reported in a female cocaine abuser 18 d after cocaine withdrawal.[133] We recently reported that male cocaine abusers with hyperprolactinemia had significantly higher peak prolactin pulses and higher mean valley levels than normal controls or cocaine abusers with normal prolactin levels, but prolactin pulse frequency was equivalent in each group.[142] Pulse frequency analysis of LH, testosterone, and cortisol showed no significant differences between cocaine users and controls.[142]

Lee and coworkers measured plasma prolactin in 16 male patients meeting DSM-III-R criteria for cocaine dependence (8 cocaine users, 8 cocaine plus alcohol users, and 8 normal controls).[144] Plasma prolactin concentrations were also measured following administration of a dopamine agonist, apomorphine (0.01 mL/kg, sc), or saline. Three of the cocaine patients had basal plasma prolactin levels of 12.0, 22.0, and 18.1 ng/mL, which were more than 2.5. SD than that of the normal controls. However, there were no differences in plasma prolactin responses to apomorphine challenges between the cocaine patients and normal controls. It was concluded from the data that cocaine did not produce consistent abnormalities in dopaminergic function at the pituitary or hypothalamus.

One limitation of most clinical studies is that samples from prolactin analyses have been collected after a period of self-reported cocaine abuse, and the dose and duration of cocaine use has been difficult to verify. The possible confounding effects of antecedent polydrug abuse are also difficult to rule out in this clinical population. Studies with rhesus monkeys reveal that acute administration of cocaine intravenously (0.4 or 0.8 mg/kg, iv) during the follicular phase of the menstrual cycle caused a fall in plasma prolactin levels and a subsequent rebound hyperprolactinemia 80 min following injection, which corresponded to the half life of cocaine in plasma.[145] Acute cocaine treatment also decreased PRL levels in midluteal phase female rhesus monkey.[146]

Dissociation between acute and chronic effects of cocaine on prolactin is consistent with the hypothesis that cocaine may block dopamine reuptake.[147] Acute cocaine administration increases brain dopamine and thus suppression on prolactin levels, as prolactin is under dopaminergic control.[138,139] However, chronic cocaine administration may deplete dopamine. Protracted dopamine depletion is consistent with clinical observations of hyperprolactinemia during and after chronic cocaine abuse.[138,139] It is possible that a disruption of dopaminergic inhibition regulation of prolactin may anticipate the reproductive system dysfunctions observed in chronic cocaine users.

Cocaine's Effects on Plasma Luteinizing Hormone

A number of clinical observations have emphasized that both men and women report that cocaine self-administration enhances libidinal drive,[131,148] and LH increases appear to be associated with reports of sexual arousal.[149] Acute cocaine administration (0.4 and 0.8 mg/kg, iv) during the follicular phase stimulated an increase in plasma LH levels with a concomitant suppression of plasma prolactin levels in female rhesus monkeys.[145] Acute cocaine treatment also increased LH levels in the midluteal-phase female rhesus monkey.[146] Cocaine augmentation of LH secretion following concurrent administration of synthetic LHRH has been observed in female rhesus monkeys.[150] In cocaine-dependent men, acute cocaine administration (30 mg, iv) induced an increase in plasma LH levels 15 min following iv drug administration,[151] but LH levels were normal before cocaine administration. Pulsatile secretion of LH between cocaine users and control subjects showed minimal differences in pulse frequency analysis of LH parameters.[142]

The mechanism underlying cocaine-induced stimulation of plasma LH levels is unclear. LH release is modulated by several neurotransmitter systems in brain including epinephrine, serotonin, and endogenous opioid peptides, as well as by gonadal steroid feedback effects[152,153] (*see* ref. 138 for review). A cocaine-induced increase in dopamine in the hypothalamus would be expected to inhibit LH secretions in humans.[139,154,155] Intravenous (peripheral) dopamine (DA) administration decreased LH secretion.[156] Since DA cannot pass the blood–brain barrier,[157] the inhibitory effect of DA on LH may be mediated through the anterior pituitary and/or the median eminence.

Cocaine can easily pass the blood–brain barriers and binds to specific cocaine recognition sites located, among others, in different parts of the hypothalamus, especially in the zona incerta and preoptic area,[158] which are critically involved in LHRH and subsequent LH secretions.[159] Central infusion of DA and D_1 dopamine agonists into the zona incerta stimulate LH secretion in rats.[160] It seems possible that the stimulatory action of cocaine on LH is mediated through central (hypothalamic) mechanisms.

Cocaine's Effects on the Hypothalamic–Pituitary–Adrenal Axis

Several experimental animal studies have shown that cocaine stimulates adrenocorticotropic hormone (ACTH) secretion.[161,162] Rivier and Vale found that cocaine-induced stimulation of plasma ACTH levels was completely suppressed following pretreatment with corticotropin-releasing factor (CRF) antiserum.[163] This investigation provided evidence that cocaine produces a rapid activation of release of CRF in brain. However, activation of the HPA axis in rats is dependent on the mode and frequency in which cocaine is administered.[164] Continuous exposure to cocaine does not appear to activate the HPA axis, whereas intermittent injections of the drug induce repeated increases in plasma ACTH and cortisol serum levels.[164] Further studies have shown that cocaine stimulation of ACTH secretion may occur during rapid systemic increases in drug concentrations, and a critical threshold of cocaine plasma concentrations is necessary for activation of the hypothalamic–pituitary–adrenal axis.[165]

We recently reported increased plasma ACTH levels in men following acute cocaine (30 mg) administration intravenously.[151,166] Cocaine-induced increases in plasma ACTH levels may be due to its effects on dopaminergic systems, which modulate CRF release in brain.[167] It has been shown that synthetic CRF administration suppressed endogenous LHRH in rat portal blood.[51] Administration of synthetic CRF also inhibited pulsatile release of LH and FSH in ovariectomized rhesus females.[49] It is possible that cocaine's effects on the hypothalamic–pituitary–adrenal axis may modify menstrual cycle function. CRF may inhibit LH and FSH secretion through an endogenous opiate-mediated mechanism.[168]

Most studies of cocaine's effects on reproductive hormones have been conducted in men. It is important to extend these analyses to women as the majority of women who abuse cocaine are of childbearing age.[169] Acute cocaine stimulation of LH and disruption of dopaminergic inhibitory regulation of prolactin may anticipate the reproductive system dysfunctions and hyperprolactinemia often associated with chronic cocaine abuse. The adverse effects of cocaine on the hypothalamic–pituitary–adrenal axis may also result in abnormalities of reproductive function.

Cocaine and Pregnancy

Cocaine abuse during pregnancy is associated with obstetrical complications including spontaneous abortion and abruptio placentae.[135,170–173] In addition, maternal cocaine abuse increases mortality of the newborn[174] as well as fetal malformation and impaired neurobehavioral development.[135,136,175–177] Decreased and low birth weight was a common finding among cocaine-exposed infants when compared to nonexposed infants.[171,175,178,179] Occurrence of sudden infant death syndrome (SIDS) was reported in 15% of cocaine-exposed infants.[180] However, in subsequent studies, the incidence of SIDS in cocaine-exposed infants was between 0.5 and 0.9%.[178,181,182] Teratogenic effects of cocaine on neurologic development, including microcephaly, cerebral infarction, and intracranial hemorrhage have been reviewed previously.[183]

The mechanism by which cocaine exerts its toxic effects during pregnancy is unclear. Cocaine readily crosses the placenta.[184] Following iv cocaine injection, cocaine rapidly appeared in the fetal circulation, was approx 15% of maternal concentration by 5 min, and was undetectable in both circulations by 60 min.[184] Experimental iv administration of cocaine to pregnant ewes produced dose-dependent increases in maternal heart rate and blood pressure and dose-dependent decreases in uterine blood flow. It is possible that impaired fetal growth is a result of fetal hypoxemia subsequent to decreased placental perfusion.

The effects of cocaine on reproductive hormones during pregnancy have not been studied. Administration of cocaine to the pregnant ewes (125–137 d gestation) resulted in increases in maternal and fetal adrenocorticotropin and cortisol levels.[185,186] However, maternal plasma ACTH and cortisol levels were not affected by fetal administration of cocaine,[185,186] although there was a tendency for fetal plasma ACTH and cortisol to rise after cocaine administration, but this was not statistically significant.

Patterns of cocaine use during pregnancy may vary widely from patient to patient.[179] It has been found consistently that cocaine users are less likely to receive prenatal care than nonusers.[124,175,187,188] Streissguth and coworkers reported that cocaine users were more likely to be Black, single/separated/divorced, and had less than a high school education.[73] Effects of cocaine on pregnancy have been reviewed previously.[176,189–192] However, methodological issues prevent conclusive definition of a direct causal relation.[189,193,194] The possibility and extent of birth defects relative to cocaine use will continue to be difficult to assess because of problems inherent in studying drug abuse during pregnancy. Because cocaine use is correlated with many potential risk factors (poor medical care, malnutrition, other illicit drug use), large sample sizes and multivariate statistical techniques are needed to determine whether cocaine use during pregnancy poses an independent risk for adverse neonatal outcomes.

Opiates

Endogenous opioids are found throughout the central nervous system (CNS), and they have profound effects on neuroendocrine functions.[195] It is beyond the scope of this review to discuss the many diverse pharmacological actions of opioids on the CNS. Rather, the actions of opioids (morphine or morphine-like drugs) on the female reproductive system will be discussed.

Opiate addiction is frequently associated with altered sexual activities. Effects of opioids on sexual behavior have been reviewed previously.[196,197] In men, heroin and methadone both increased the frequency of impotence and retarded ejaculation.[198,199] In women, menstrual irregularities such as amenorrhea, anovulatory cycles, and infertility have been reported.[200,201] Women who abuse heroin may abuse other illicit drugs, smoke cigarets, have poor nutritional status, and be at increased risk for sexually transmitted diseases and human immunodeficiency virus infections. These confounding variables may affect the reproductive system *per se*. In addition, drug histories of addicts are notoriously unreliable with respect to dosages and purity of the agent.

The adverse effects of chronic heroin abuse on the hypothalamic–pituitary–gonadal axis may cause derangements of sexual and reproductive function.[202] Impaired secondary sex-organ and testicular function and lower testosterone levels have been reported in heroin users and methadone clients.[203] Suppression of plasma luteinizing hormone and testosterone levels occur following acute iv administration of heroin to opiate dependent men.[204] A decrease in plasma LH levels was also observed in heroin-dependent men who chronically self-administered the drug when they were 14–20 yr of age.[205] Similar findings were observed in laboratory animals.[206–208] The effects of narcotics on serum LH appear to be mediated via specific opioid receptors in the hypothalamic–pituitary–LH axis, probably by inhibiting the secretion of luteinizing hormone releasing hormone (LHRH) from the hypothalamus. In support of this, administration of naloxone, an opiate receptor blocker, markedly increased serum LH levels. Adolescent morphine exposure in male rats resulted in decreased serum testosterone and LH levels as well as reduced weights of testes and seminal vesicles.[209] Breeding morphine- and placebo-implanted male rats with drug-naive females resulted in smaller litters from morphine-treated fathers when compared to controls, but development of the offspring of the two groups was equivalent.[209] Age-related differences in the sensitivity of opiate-induced perturbations of the hypothalamic-pituitary-gonadal axis in male rats have also been demonstrated.[210]

Acute doses of morphine have been shown to block ovulation in laboratory animals.[211] Menstrual cycle irregularity and infertility have been reported in female heroin addicts.[200,201,212] A clinical study of 76 former female heroin addicts receiving daily methadone maintenance revealed that more than one-half of these women had experienced menstrual abnormalities while taking heroin or methadone.[212] Endocrinological studies were carried out in seven of these patients who complained of amenorrhea or irregular menses while receiving methadone. Four of these seven women manifested abnormalities of gonadotropin secretion, as evidenced by absence of increased levels of follicular phase FSH, midcycle gonadotropin peaks, or luteal phase progesterone increments.[212] The data suggested that opiates produced disruptions in female reproductive function by altering the hypothalamic mechanisms controlling gonadotropin secretion, although tolerance to these effects may develop after chronic ingestion.

Opiates and Pregnancy

Illicit heroin is the most widely used opioid, and the treatment of choice in the United States for heroin abuse has been methadone maintenance. Pregnancies in opioid-dependent women are often complicated by inadequate prenatal care, transmission of infection such as syphilis or human immunodeficiency virus. Infants born to opioid-dependent women frequently have low birth weights,[187,213–215] although birth weight may be higher in infants born to methadone-maintained women.[213] Reduced head circumference has also been consistently reported.[216,217]

The mechanism by which opiates compromise fetal development is unclear. It is not known whether opiates have direct effects on the fetus or impair fetal development through disruption of maternal health and/or maternal hormonal balance. We are unaware of any neuroendocrine studies of opioid-dependent women during pregnancy. Studies in laboratory animals show that exposure to morphine during pregnancy attenuated prolactin response to sucking stimulus[218] and may alter response of hypothalamic-pituitary axis to gonadal steroids in the offspring[218] and affect development of feminine sexual behavior.[219]

Neonatal abstinence syndrome is characterized by CNS hyperirritability, high-pitched cry, tremors, increased muscle tone, gastrointestinal dysfunction, and respiratory distress.[215] This may be severe and persist as for long as 3 mo. Infants born to mothers on methadone maintenance may have more severe withdrawal symptoms than newborns of heroin-addicted

Table 1
Derangements of Reproductive Function Reported
in Alcohol, Marijuana, Cocaine, and Opiate Abusers

	Alcohol	Marijuana	Cocaine	Opiate
Amenorrhea	X	X	X	X
Anovulation	X	X	X	X
Luteal phase dysfunction	X	X	X	X
Hyperprolactinemia	X		X	X
Spontaneous abortion	X	X	X	X

mothers, although the frequency of the abstinence syndrome is equivalent in both groups. It appears that the occurrence of withdrawal signs in infants is correlated with the length and duration of maternal addiction.[220] An increase of maternal heroin intake was associated with increased incidence of neonatal withdrawal; and the closer to delivery the last dose of heroin was taken, the higher and earlier was the occurrence of withdrawal signs in the neonate.[220] The incidence of SIDS in infants of mothers on methadone maintenance is reported to be higher than that in the general population.[217,221] It is thought that infants born to opiate-abusing mothers have decreased ventilatory response to carbon dioxide.[221] Longitudinal studies are necessary to examine the neurobehavioral consequences of prenatal exposure to heroin and methadone[89] (*see* refs. 222 and 223 for review). Because of the many social problems encountered by opioid drug-using women, a multivariate systems approach is recommended to promote effective addiction treatment and facilitate the best possible outcomes for both mothers and infants.[224]

Summary

The adverse consequences of substance abuse on female reproductive functions are summarized in Table 1.

Interpretation of clinical data is often complicated by the fact that many subjects do not use only one drug, but rather may use several drugs in various combinations.[10] Polydrug abuse appears to be an increasingly prevalent drug-use pattern. Thus, it is difficult to attribute teratogenic effects of intrauterine exposure to any one drug. These women may come from a socially impoverished environment and may be at increased risk for malnutrition and sexually transmitted diseases. Behavioral symptoms consequent to intrauterine drug exposure may continue through infancy and early childhood.

References

[1]J. K. Myers, M. M. Weissman, G. L. Tischler, C. E. Holzer, P. J. Leaf, H. Orvaschel, J. C. Anthony, J. H. Boyd, J. D. Burke, M. Krammer, and R. Stoltzman (1984) Six month prevalence of psychiatric disorders in three communities. *Arch. Gen. Psychiatry* **41**, 959–967.

[2]L. N. Robins, J. E. Helzer, M. M. Weissman, H. Orvaschel, E. Gruenberg, J. D. Burke Jr., and D. A. Reiger (1984) Lifetime prevalence of specific psychiatric disorders in three sites. *Arch. Gen. Psychiatry* **41**, 949–958.

[3]National Institute on Drug Abuse (1992) *National Household Survey on Drug Abuse: Population Estimates 1991.* U.S. Government Printing Office, Washington, DC.

[4]D. E. Hutchings, ed. (1989) *Prenatal Abuse of Licit and Illicit Drugs.* N. Academy of Sciences, New York.

[5]N. K. Mello, J. H. Mendelson, and S. K. Teoh (1992) Alcohol and neuroendocrine function in women of reproductive age, in *Medical Diagnosis and Treatment of Alcoholism.* J. H. Mendelson and N. K. Mello, eds. McGraw-Hill, New York, pp. 575–621.

[6]C. G. Smith and M. T. Smith (1990) Substance abuse and reproduction, in *Seminars in Reproductive Endocrinolology.* Thieme, New York, pp. 55–64.

[7]J. A. Cocores, N. S. Miller, A. C. Pottash, and M. S. Gold (1988) Sexual dysfunction in abusers of cocaine and alcohol. *Am. J. Drug Alcohol Abuse* **14**, 169–173.

[8]C. Van Dyke and R. Byck (1983) Cocaine use in man, in *Advances in Substance Abuse, Behavioral and Biological Research.* vol. 3. N. K. Mello, ed. JAI, Greenwich, CT, pp. 1–24.

[9]M. Kreek (1987) Multiple drug abuse patterns and medical consequences, in *Psychopharmacology, The Third Generation of Progress.* H. Meltzer, ed. Raven, New York, pp. 1597–1604.

[10]M. J. Kreek (1991) Multiple drug abuse patterns: Recent trends and associated medical consequences, in *Advances in Substance Abuse, Behavioral and Biological Research,* vol. 4. N. K. Mello, ed. Jessica Kingsley, London, pp. 91–112.

[11]N. K. Mello, J. H. Mendelson, and S. K. Teoh (1989) Neuroendocrine consequences of alcohol abuse in women, in *Prenatal Abuse of Licit and Ilicit Drugs.* D. E. Hutchings, ed. Annals of the New York Academy of Sciences, New York, pp. 211–240.

[12]T. W. Boyden and R. W. Pamenter (1983) Effects of ethanol on the male hypothalamic-pituitary-gonadal axis. *Endocrinol. Rev.* **4**, 389–395.

[13]T. J. Cicero (1980) Common mechanisms underlying the effects of ethanol and the narcotics on neuroendocrine function., in *Advances in Substance Abuse, Behavioral and Biological Research.* vol. I. N. K. Mello, ed. JAI, Greenwich, CT, pp. 201–254.

[14]J. H. Mendelson and N. K. Mello (1979) Biologic concomitants of alcoholism. *N. Engl. J. Med.* **301,**912–921.

[15]R. H. Noth and R. M. J. Walter (1984) The effects of alcohol on the endocrine system. *Med. Clin. N. Am.* **68**, 133–146.

[16]J. S. Gavaler (1985) Effects of alcohol on endocrine function in post-menopausal women: A review. *J. Stud. Alcohol* **46**, 495–516.

[17]J. S. Gavaler (1992) Alcohol effects in postmenopausal women: Alcohol and estrogens, in *Medical Diagnosis and Treatment of Alcoholism.* J. H. Mendelson and N. K. Mello, eds., McGraw-Hill, New York, pp. 623–638.

[18]J. N. Hugues, T. Coste, G. Perret, M. F. Jayle, J. Sebaoun, and E. Modigliani (1980) Hypothalamo-pituitary ovarian function in thirty-one women with chronic alcoholism. *Clin. Endocrinol.* **12,** 543–551.

[19]S. Moskovic (1975) Effect of chronic alcohol intoxication on ovarian dysfunction. *Srp. Arh. Celok. Lck.* **103,** 751–758.

[20]M. Välimäki, R. Pelkonen, M. Salaspuro, M. Harkonen, E. Hirvonen, and R. Ylikahri (1984) Sex hormones in amenorrheic women with alcoholic liver disease. *J. Clin. Endocrinol. Metab.* **59,** 133–138.

[21]U. Becker, H. Tonnesen, N. Kaas-Claesson, and C. Gluud (1989) Menstrual disturbances and fertility in chronic alcoholic women. *Drug Alcohol Depend.* **24,** 75–82.

[22]S. C. Wilsnack, A. D. Klassen, and R. W. Wilsnack (1984) Drinking and reproductive dysfunction among women in a 1981 national survey. *Alcohol Clin. Exp. Res.* **89,** 451–458.

[23]R. W. Wilsnack, A. D. Klassen, and S. C. Wilsnack (1986) Retrospective analysis of lifetime changes in women's drinking behavior. *Adv. Alcohol Subst. Abuse* **5,** 7–28.

[24]S. C. Wilsnack, A. D. Klassen, B. L. Schur, and R. W. Wilsnack (1991) Predicting onset and chronicity of women's problem drinking: A five year longitudinal analysis. *Am. J. Public Health* **81,** 305–317.

[25]N. K. Mello (1988) Effects of alcohol abuse on reproductive function in women, in *Recent Developments in Alcoholism.* M. Galanter, ed. Plenum, New York, pp. 253–276.

[26]R. L. Eskay, R. S. Ryback, M. Goldman, and E. Majchrowicz (1981) Effect of chronic ethanol administration on plasma levels of LH and the estrous cycle in the female rat. *Alcohol: Clin. Exp. Res.* **5,** 204–206.

[27]J. S. Gavaler, D. H. Van Thiel, and R. Lester (1980) Ethanol: A gonadal toxin in the mature rat of both sexes. *Alcohol. Clin. Exp. Res.* **4,** 271–276.

[28]N. K. Mello, M. P. Bree, J. H. Mendelson, J. Ellingboe, N. W. King, and P. K. Sehgal (1983) Alcohol self-administration disrupts reproductive function in female macaque monkeys. *Science* **221,** 677–679.

[29]N. K. Mello, J. H. Mendelson, N. W. King, M. P. Bree, A. Skupny, and J. Ellingboe (1988) Alcohol self-administration by female rhesus monkey: A model for study of alcohol dependence, hyperprolactinemia and amenorrhea. *J. Stud. Alcohol* **49,** 551–560.

[30]D. H. Van Thiel, J. S. Gavaler, and R. Lester (1978) Alcohol-induced ovarian failure in the rat. *J. Clin. Invest.* **61,** 624–632.

[31]J. H. Mendelson, S. E. Lukas, N. K. Mello, L. Amass, J. Ellingboe, and A. Skupny (1988) Acute alcohol effects on plasma estradiol levels in women. *Psychopharmacology* **94,** 464–467.

[32]B. McNamee, J. Grant, J. Ratcliffe, W. Ratcliffe, and J. Oliver (1979) Lack of effect of alcohol on pituitary-gonadal hormones in women. *Br. J. Addict.* **74,** 316–317.

[33]J. H. Mendelson, N. K. Mello, and J. Ellingboe (1981) Acute alcohol intake and pituitary gonadal hormones in normal human females. *J. Pharmacol. Exp. Ther.* **218,** 23–26.

[34]M. Välimäki, M. Harkonen, and R. Ylikahri (1983) Acute effects of alcohol on female sex hormones. *Alcohol: Clin. Exp. Res.* **7,** 289–293.

[35]R. S. Ryback (1977) Chronic alcohol consumption and menstruation. *JAMA* **238,** 2143.

[36]M. Seki (1988) A physiopathological study on ovarian dysfunction in female patients with alcoholism. *Fukuoka Acta Med.* **79,** 738–748.

[37]M. Seki, K. Yoshida, and Y. Okamura (1991) Hormones in amenorrheic women with alcoholics. *Jpn. J. Fertil. Steril.* **36,** 630–635.

[38]M. Seki, K. Yoshida, and Y. Okamura (1991) A study on hyperprolactinemia in female patients with alcoholics. *Jpn. J. Alcohol Drug Depend.* **26,** 49–59.

[39]S. L. Berga, J. F. Mortola, L. Girton, B. Suh, G. Laughlin, P. Pham, and S. S. C. Yen (1989) Neuroendocrine aberrations in women with functional hypothalamic amenorrhea. *J. Clin. Endocrinol. Metabol.* **68,** 301–308.

[40]P. M. Conn and W. F. J. Crowley (1991) Gonadotropin-releasing hormone and its analogues. *N. Engl. J. Med.* **324,** 93–103.

[41]W. F. Crowley Jr., M. Filicori, D. I. Spratt, and N. F. Santoro (1985) The physiology of gonadotropin-releasing hormone (GnRH) secretion in men and women. *Rec. Prog. Horm. Res.* **41,** 473–526.

[42]N. Santoro, M. Filicori, and J. Crowley (1986) Hypogonadotropic disorders in men and women: Diagnosis and therapy with pulsatile gonadotropin-releasing hormone. *Endocrine Rev.* **7,** 11–23.

[43]N. Santoro, M. E. Wierman, M. Filicori, J. Waldstreicher, and W. F. Crowley Jr. (1986) Intravenous administration of pulsatile gonadotropin-releasing hormone in hypothalamic amenorrhea: Effects of dosage. *J. Clin. Endocrinol. Metab.* **62,** 109–116.

[44]M. Välimäki, V. Tuominen, I. Huhtaniemi, and R. Yilkahri (1990) The pulsatile secretion of gonadotropins and growth hormone, and the biological activity of luteinizing hormone in men acutely intoxicated with ethanol. *Alcohol: Clin. Exp. Res.* **14,** 928–931.

[45]A. Iranmanesh, J. D. Veldhuis, E. Samojlik, A. D. Rogol, M. L. Johnson, and G. Lizarralde (1988) Alterations in the pulsatile properties of gonadotropin secretion in alcohol men. *J. Andrology* **9,** 207–214.

[46]E. Redei, B. J. Branch, and A. N. Taylor (1986) Direct effect of ethanol on adrenocorticotropin (ACTH) release in vitro. *J. Pharmacol. Exp. Ther.* **237,** 59–64.

[47]C. Rivier, J. Rivier, and W. Vale (1986) Stress-induced inhibition of reproductive functions: Role of endogenous corticotropin-releasing factor. *Science* **31,** 607–609.

[48]C. Rivier and W. Vale (1984) Influence of corticotropin-releasing factor (CRF) on reproductive functions in the rat. *Endocrinology* **114,** 914–919.

[49]D. H. Olster and M. Ferin (1987). Corticotropin-releasing hormone inhibits gonadotropin secretion in the ovariectomized rhesus monkey. *J. Clin. Endocrinol. Metab.* **65,** 262–267.

[50]E. Xiao and M. Ferin (1988) The inhibitory action of corticotropin-releasing hormone and gonadotropin-releasing secretion in the ovariectomized rhesus monkey is not mediated by adrenocorticotropic hormone. *Biol. Reprod.* **38,** 763–767.

[51]F. Petraglia, S. Sutton, W. Vale, and P. Plotsky (1987) Corticotropin-releasing factor decreases plasma LH levels in female rats by inhibiting gonadotropin-releasing hormone release into hypophysial-portal circulation. *Endocrinology* **120,** 1083–1088.

[52]M. Välimäki, R. Pelkonen, M. Harkonen, P. Tuomala, P. Koistinen, R. Roine, and R. Ylikahri (1990) Pituitary-gonadal hormones and adrenal androgens in non-cirrhotic female alcoholics after cessation of alcohol intake. *Eur. J. Clin. Invest.* **20,** 177–181.

[53]G. S. diZerega and G. D. Hodgen (1981) Luteal phase dysfunction infertility: A sequel to aberrant folliculogenesis. *Fertil. Steril.* **35,** 489–499.

[54]G. S. diZerega and J. W. Wilks (1984).Inhibition of the primate ovarian cycle by a porcine follicular fluid protein(s). *Fertil. Steril.* **41,** 1094–1100.

[55]A. L. Goodman and G. D. Hodgen (1983) The ovarian triad of the primate menstrual cycle. *Rec. Prog. Horm. Res.* **39,** 1–67.

[56]J. H. Mendelson, N. K. Mello, S. K. Teoh, and J. Ellingboe (1989) Alcohol effects on luteinizing hormone-releasing hormone-stimulated anterior pituitary and gonadal hormones in women. *J. Pharmacol. Exp. Ther.* **250,** 902–909.

[57]N. K. Mello, J. H. Mendelson, M. P. Bree, and A. S. T. Skupny (1986) Alcohol effects on LHRH stimulated LH and FSH in female rhesus monkeys. *J. Pharmacol. Exp. Ther.* **236,** 590–595.

[58]D. J. Dierschke, R. J. Hutz, and R. C. Wolf (1985) Induced follicular atresia in rhesus monkeys: Strength-duration relationships of the estrogen stimulus. *Endocrinology* **117,** 1397–1403.

[59]A. J. Zeleznek (1981) Premature elevation of systemic estradiol reduces serum levels of FSH and lengthens the follicular phase of the menstrual cycle in rhesus monkeys. *Endocrinology* **109,** 352–355.

[60]T. Cronholm and J. Sjovall (1968) Effect of ethanol on the concentrations of solvolyzable plasma steroids. *Biochem. Biophys. Acta* **152,** 233–236.

[61]T. Cronholm, J. Sjovall, and K. Sjovall (1969) Ethanol induced increase of the ratio between hydroxy- and ketosteroids in human pregnancy plasma. *Steroids* **13,** 671–678.

[62]E. P. Murono and V. Fisher-Simpson (1984) Ethanol directly increases dihydrotestosterone conversion to 5-androstan-3 , 17-diol and 5-androstan-3, 17-diol in rat leydig cells. *Biochem. Biophys. Res. Commun.* **121,** 558–565.

[63]E. P. Murono and V. Fisher-Simpson (1985) Ethanol directly stimulates dihydrotestosterone conversion to 5-androstan-3, 17-diol and 5-androstan-3, 17-diol in rat liver. *Life Sci.* **36,** 1117–1124.

[64]M. C. Batista, T. P. Cartledge, A. W. Zellmer, L. K. Nieman, G. R. Merriam, and D. L. Loriaux (1992) Evidence for a critical role of progesterone in the regulation of the midcycle gonadotropin surge and ovulation. *J. Clin. Endocrinol. Metab.* **74,** 565–570.

[65]S. K. Teoh, J. H. Mendelson, N. K. Mello, and A. Skupny (1988) Alcohol effects on naltrexone-induced stimulation of pituitary, adrenal and gonadal hormones during the early follicular phase of the menstrual cycle. *J. Clin. Endocrinol. Metab.* **66,** 1181–1186.

[66]S. K. Teoh, B. W. Lex, J. H. Mendelson, N. K. Mello, and J. Cochin (1992) Hyperprolactinemia and macrocytosis in women with alcohol and polysubstance dependence. *J. Stud. Alcohol* **53,** 176–182.

[67]G. C. Buchanan and D. R. Tredway (1979) Hyperprolactinemia and ovulatory dysfunction, in *Human Ovulation.* E. S. E. Hafez, ed. Elsevier, Amsterdam, pp. 255–277.

[68]J. B. Martin and S. Reichlin, eds. (1987) *Clinical Neuroendocrinology,* 2nd ed. F. A. Davis, Philadelphia.

[69]G. Tolis (1980) Prolactin: Physiology and pathology, in *Neuroendocrinology: Interrelationships of the Body's Two Major Integrative Systems in Normal Physiology and in Clinical Disease .* D. T. Krieger and J. C. Hughes, eds. Sinauer, Sunderland, MA, pp. 321–328.

[70]J. H. Mendelson and N. K. Mello (1988) Chronic alcohol effects on anterior pituitary and ovarian hormones in healthy women. *J. Pharmacol. Exp. Ther.* **245,** 407–412.

[71]J. H. Hannigan, R. A. Welch, and R. J. Sokol (1992) Recognition of fetal alcohol syndrome and alcohol-related birth defects, in *Medical Diagnosis and Treatment of Alcoholism.* J. H. Mendelson and N. K. Mello, eds. McGraw-Hill, New York, pp. 639–667.

[72]A. P. Streissguth, H. M. Barr, and P. D. Sampson (1986) Attention, distraction and reaction time at age 7 years and prenatal alcohol exposure. *Neurobehav. Toxicol. Teratol.* **8,** 717–725.

[73]A. P. Streissguth, T. M. Grant, H. M. Barr, Z. A. Brown, J. C. Martin, D. E. Mayock, S. L. Ramey, and L. Moore (1991) Cocaine and the use of alcohol and other drugs during pregnancy. *Am. J. Obstet. Gynecol.* **164,** 1239–1243.

[74]N. Day, D. Jasperse, and G. Richardson (1989) Prenatal exposure to alcohol: Effect on infant growth and morphologic characteristics. *Pediatrics* **84,** 536–541.

[75]K. L. Jones, D. W. Smith, C. N. Ulleland, and A. P. Streissguth (1973) Pattern of malformation in offspring of chronic alcoholic mothers. *Lancet* **1,** 1267–1271.

[76]E. L. Abel and R. J. Sokol (1987) Incidence of fetal alcohol syndrome and economic impact of FAS-related anomalies. *Drug Alcohol Depend.* **19,** 51–70.

[77]Department of Health and Human Services (1990) *Seventh Special Report to the U.S. Congress on Alcohol and Health,* No. DHHS (ADM) 90-1956.U.S. Government Printing Office, Washington, DC.

[78]S. K. Clarren and D. W. Smith (1978) The fetal alcohol syndrome. *N. Engl. J. Med.* **298,** 1063–1067.

[79]R. E. Little (1977) Moderate alcohol use during pregnancy and decreased infant birth weight. *Am. J. Public Health* **67,** 1154–1156.

[80]R. E. Little, A. P. Streissguth, H. M. Barr, and C. S. Herman (1980) Decreased birth weight in infants of alcoholic women who abstained during pregnancy. *J. Pediatrics* **96,** 974.

[81]R. J. Sokol, S. I. Miller, and G. Reed (1980) Alcohol abuse during pregnancy: An epidemiologic study. *Alcohol Clin. Exp. Res.* **4,** 135–145.

[82]E. M. Ouellette, H. L. Rosett, N. P. Rosman, and L. Weiner (1977) Adverse effects on offspring of maternal alcohol abuse during pregnancy. *N. Engl. J. Med.* **297,** 528–530.

[83]R. A. Anderson (1981) Endocrine balance as a factor in the etiology of the fetal alcohol syndrome. *Neurobehav. Toxicol. Teratol.* **3,** 89–104.

[84]E. Halmesmäki, I. Autti, M.-L. Granström, U.-H. Stenman, and O. Ylikorkala (1987) Estradiol, progesterone, prolactin, and human chorionic gonadotropin in pregnant women with alcohol abuse. *J. Clin. Endocrinol. Metabol.* **64,** 153–156.

[85]O. Ylikorkala, U.-H. Stenman, and E. Halmesmäki (1988) Testosterone, androstenedione, dehydroepiandrosterone sulfate, and sex-hormone-binding globulin in pregnant alcohol abusers. *Obstet. Gynecol.* **71,** 731–735.

[86]H. M. Gandy (1977) Androgens, in *Endocrinology of Pregnancy*. F. Fuchs and A. Klopper, eds. Harper and Row, New York, pp. 123–156.

[87]L. Beeley (1986) Adverse effects of drugs in the first trimester of pregnancy. *Clinics Obstet. Gynecol.* **13,** 177–195.

[88]J. S. Ottobre and R. L. Stouffer (1984) Persistent versus transient stimulation of the Macaque corpus luteum during prolonged exposure to human chorionic gonadotropin: A function of age of the corpus luteum. *Endocrinology* **114,** 2175–2182.

[89]J. W. Wilks and A. S. Noble (1983) Steroidogenic responsiveness of the monkey corpus luteum to exogenous chorionic gonadotropin. *Endocrinology* **113,** 1256–1266.

[90]S. K. Teoh, J. H. Mendelson, N. K. Mello, A. Skupny, and J. Ellingboe (1990) Alcohol effects on hCG-stimulated gonadal hormones in women. *J. Pharmacol. Exp. Ther.* **254,** 407–411.

[91]O. P. Heinonen, D. Slone, R. R. Monson, E. B. Hook, and S. Shapiro (1977) Cardiovascular birth defects and antenatal exposure to female sex hormones. *N. Engl. J. Med.* **296,** 67–70.

[92]N. M. Kaplan (1959) Male pseudohermaphrodism: Report of a case, with observations on pathogenesis. *N. Engl. J. Med.* **261,** 641–644.

[93]J. J. Nora, A. H. Nora, A. G. Perinchief, J. W. Ingram, A. K. Fountain, and M. J. Peterson (1976) Congenital abnormalities and first-trimester exposure to progestogen/ oestrogen. *Lancet* **1,** 313–314.

[94]J. L. Schardein (1980) Congenital abnormalities and hormones during pregnancy: A clinical review. *Teratology* **22,** 251–270.

[95]S. Harlap and P. H. Shiono (1980) Alcohol, smoking, and incidence of spontaneous abortions in the first and second trimester. *Lancet* **2,** 173–176.

[96]J. Kline, Z. Stein, P. Shrout, M. Susser, and D. Warburton (1980) Drinking during pregnancy and spontaneous abortion. *Lancet* **2,** 176–180.

[97]E. Halmesmäki, M. Valimaki, R. Roine, R. Ylikahri, and O. Ylikorkala (1989) Maternal and paternal alcohol consumption and miscarriage. *Br. J. Obstet. Gynaecol.* **96,** 188–191.

[98]J. Itskovitz and J. D. Hodgen (1988) Endocrine basis for the initiation, maintenance and termination of pregnancy in humans. *Psychoneuroendocrinology* **13,** 155–170.

[99]C. G. Smith (1980) Effects of marijuana on neuroendocrine function, in *Marijuana Research Findings: 1980*. R.C. Petersen, ed. U.S. Government Printing Office, Washington, DC, pp. 120–136.

[100]C. G. Smith and R. H. Asch (1984) Acute, short-term, and chronic effects of marijuana on the female primate reproductive function, in *Marijuana Effects on the Endocrine and Reproductive Systems*. M. C. Braude and J. P. Ludford, eds. U.S. Government Printing Office, Washington, DC, pp. 82–96.

[101]C. G. Smith and R. H. Asch (1987) Drug abuse and reproduction. *Fertil. Steril* **3,** 355–373.

[102]J. H. Mendelson and N. K. Mello (1984) Effects of marijuana on neuroendocrine hormones in human males and females, in *Marijuana Effects on the Endocrine and Reproductive Systems. A RAUS Review Report* . M. C. Braude and J. P. Ludford, eds. U.S. Government Printing Office, Washington, DC, pp. 97–114.

[103]N. L. Day and G. A. Richardson (1991) Prenatal marijuana use: Epidemiology, methodologic issues, and infant outcome. *Chem. Depend. Preg.* **18,** 77–91.

[104]R. C. Kolodny, W. H. Masters, R. M. Lolodner, and G. Toro (1974) Depression of plasma testosterone levels after chronic intensive marihuana use. *N. Engl. J. Med.* **290,** 872–874.

[105]R. I. Block, R. Farinpour, and J. A. Schlechte (1991) Effects of chronic marijuana use on testosterone, lutenizing hormone, follicle stimulating hormone, prolactin and cortisol in men and women. *Drug Alcohol Depend.* **28,** 121–128.

[106]P. Cushman (1975) Plasma testosterone levels in healthy male marijuana smokers. *Am. J. Drug Alcohol Abuse* **2,** 269–276.

[107]J. H. Mendelson, J. Ellingboe, J. C. Kuehnle, and N. K. Mello (1978) Effects of chronic marihuana use on integrated plasma testosterone and luteinizing hormone levels. *J. Pharmacol. Exp. Ther.* **207,** 611–617.

[108]J. H. Mendelson, J. Kuehnle, J. Ellingboe, and T. F. Babor (1974) Plasma testosterone levels before, during and after chronic marihuana smoking. *N. Engl. J. Med.* **291,** 1051–1055.

[109]J. H. Mendelson, J. Kuehnle, J. Ellingboe, and T. F. Babor (1975) Effects of marihuana on plasma testosterone, in *Marihuana and Health Hazards: Methodological Issues in Current Research.* J. R. Tinklenberg, ed. Academic, New York, pp. 83–93.

[110]E. Knobil (1974) On the control of gonadotropin secretion in the rhesus monkey. *Rec. Prog. Horm. Res.* **30**, 1–46.

[111]E. Knobil (1980) The neuroendocrine control of the menstrual cycle. *Rec. Prog. Horm. Res.* **36**, 53–88.

[112]N. R. Besch, C. G. Smith, P. K. Besch, and R. H. Kaufman (1977) The effect of marihuana (delta-9-tetracannabinol) on the secretion of luteinizing hormone in the ovariectomized rhesus monkey. *Am. J. Obstet. Gynecol.* **128**, 635–642.

[113]C. G. Smith, R. G. Besch, R. G. Smith, and P. K. Besch (1979) Effects of tetrahydrocannabinol on the hypothalamic-pituitary axis in the ovariectomized rhesus monkey. *Fertil. Steril.* **31**, 335–339.

[114]R. Asch, C. Smith, T. Siler-Khodr, and C. Pauerstein (1979) Effects of delta-9-tetrahydrocannabinol administration on gonadal steroidogenic activity in vivo. *Fertil. Steril.* **32**, 576.

[115]R. H. Asch, C. G. Smith, T. M. Siler-Khodr, and C. J. Pauerstein (1981) Effects of delta-9-tetrahydrocanabinol during the follicular phase of the rhesus monkey (Macaca mulatta). *J. Clin. Endocrinol. Metabol.* **52**, 50–55.

[116]J. H. Mendelson, N. K. Mello, J. Ellingboe, A. S. T. Skupny, B. W. Lex, and M. Griffin (1986) Marihuana smoking suppresses luteinizing hormone in women. *J. Pharmacol. Exp. Ther.* **237**, 862–866.

[117]C. G. Smith, R. G. Almirez, and J. Barenberg (1983) Tolerance develops to the disruptive effects of delta 9 tetrahydrocannbinol on the primate menstrual cycle. *Science* **219**, 1453–1455.

[118]J. E. Bauman, R. C. Kolodny, R. L. Dornbush, and S. K. Webster (1979) Effectos endocrinos del uso cronico de la mariguana en mujeres, in *Cuadernos Cientificos CEMESAM* . D. F. Julio, ed. Centro Mexicano de Estudios en Salud Mental, p. 85.

[119]L. Lemberger, R. Crabtree, H. Rowe, and J. Clemens (1973) Tetrahydrocannabinoids and serum prolactin levels in man. *Life Sci.* **16**, 1339–1343.

[120]J. H. Mendelson, N. K. Mello, and J. Ellingboe (1985) Acute effects of marihuana smoking on prolactin levels in human females. *J. Pharmacol. Exp. Ther.* **232**, 220–222.

[121]N. Day, U. Sambamoorthi, P. Taylor, G. Richardson, N. Robles, Y. Jhon, M. Scher, D. Stoffer, M. Cornelius, and D. Jasperse (1990) Prenatal marijuana use and neonatal outcome. *Neurotoxicol. Teratol.* **13**, 329–334.

[122]P. A. Fried, B. Watkinson, and A. Willan (1984) Marijuana use during pregnancy and decreased length of gestation. *Am. J. Obstet. Gynecol.* **150**, 23–27.

[123]E. E. Hatch and M. B. Bracken (1986) Effect of marijuana use in pregnancy on fetal growth. *Am. J. Epidemiol.* **124**, 986–993.

[124]B. Zuckerman, D. A. Frank, R. Hingson, A. Hortensia, S. M. Levenson, H. Kayne, S. Parker, R. Vinci, K. Aboagye, L. E. Fried, H. Cabral, R. Timperi, and H. Bauchner (1989) Effects of maternal marijuana and cocaine use on fetal growth. *N. Engl. J. Med.* **320**, 762–768.

[125]P. A. Fried (1991) Marijuana use during pregnancy: Consequences for the offspring. *Semin. Perinatol.* **15**, 280-287.

[126]R. Hingson, J. J. Alpert, N. Day, E. Dooling, H. Kayne, S. Morelock, E. Oppenheimer, and B. Zuckerman (1982) Effects of maternal drinkiing and marijuana use on fetal growth and development. *Pediatrics* **70**, 539–546.

¹²⁷T.-C. Wu, D. P. Tashkin, B. Djahed, and J. E. Rose (1988) Pulmonary hazards of smoking marijuana as compared with tobacco. *N. Engl. J. Med.* **318,** 347–351.

¹²⁸R. H. Asch and C. G. Smith (1986) Effects of delta-9-THC, the principal psychoactive component of marijuana, during pregnancy in the rhesus monkey. *J. Reprod. Med.* **31,** 1071–1081.

¹²⁹G. D. Braunstein, J. E. Buster, J. R. Soares, and S. J. Gross (1983) Pregnancy hormone concentrations in marijuana users. *Life Sci.* **33,** 195–199.

¹³⁰N. J. Kozel and E. H. Adams (1986) Epidemiology of drug abuse: An overview. *Science* **234,** 970–974.

¹³¹R. K. Siegel (1984) Changing patterns of cocaine use: Longitudinal observations, consequences and treatment, in *Cocaine: Pharmacology, Effects, and Treatment of Abuse.* J. Grabowski, ed. U.S. Government Printing Office, Washington, DC, pp. 92–110.

¹³²R. K. Siegel (1982) Cocaine smoking. *J. Psychoactive Drugs* **14,** 277–359.

¹³³J. A. Cocores, C. A. Dackis, and M. S. Gold (1986) Sexual dysfunction secondary to cocaine abuse in two patients. *J. Clin. Psychiatry* **47,** 384–385.

¹³⁴D. E. Smith, D. R. Wesson, and M. Apter-Marsh (1984) Cocaine- and alcohol-induced sexual dysfunction in patients with addictive disease. *J. Psychoactive Drugs* **16,** 359–361.

¹³⁵I. J. Chasnoff, W. J. Burns, S. H. Schnoll, and K. A. Burns (1985) Cocaine use in pregnancy. *N. Engl. J. Med.* **313,** 666–669.

¹³⁶I. J. Chasnoff and D. R. Griffith (1989) Cocaine: Clinical studies of pregnancy and the newborn, in *Prenatal Abuse of Licit and Illicit Drugs*. D. E. Hutchings, ed. The New York Academy of Sciences, New York, pp. 260–266.

¹³⁷L. L. Cregler and H. Mark (1986) Medical complications of cocaine abuse. *N. Engl. J. Med.* **315,** 1495–1500.

¹³⁸S. S. C. Yen (1986) Neuroendocrine control of hypophyseal function, in *Reproductive Endocrinology.* S. S. C. Yen and R. B. Jaffe, eds. Saunders, Philadelphia, pp. 33–74.

¹³⁹S. S. C. Yen (1986) Prolactin in human reproduction, in *Reproductive Endocrinology.* S. S. C. Yen and R. B. Jaffe, eds. Saunders, Philadelphia, pp. 178–263.

¹⁴⁰F. H. Gawin and H. D. Kleber (1985) Neuroendocrine findings in chronic cocaine abusers: A preliminary report. *Br. J. Psychiatry* **147,** 569–573.

¹⁴¹C. A. Dackis and M. S. Gold (1985) Pharmacological approaches to cocaine addiction. *J. Subst. Abuse Treatment* **2,** 139–145.

¹⁴²J. H. Mendelson, N. K. Mello, S. K. Teoh, J. Ellingboe, and J. Cochin (1989) Cocaine effects on pusatile secretion of anterior pituitary, gonadal, and adrenal hormones. *J. Clin. Endocrinol. Metab.* **69,** 1256–1260.

¹⁴³J. H. Mendelson, S. K. Teoh, U. Lange, N. K. Mello, R. Weiss, and A. S. T. Skupny (1988) Hyperprolactinemia during cocaine withdrawal, in *Problems of Drug Dependence 1987.* L. S. Harris, ed. U.S. Government Printing Office, Washington, DC, pp. 67–73.

¹⁴⁴M. A. Lee, M. M. Bowers, J. F. Nash, and H. Y. Meltzer (1990). Neuroendocrine measures of dopaminergic function in chronic cocaine users. *Psychiatry Res.* **33,** 151–159.

¹⁴⁵N. K. Mello, J. H. Mendelson, J. Drieze, and M. Kelly (1990) Acute effects of cocaine on prolactin and gonadotropins in female rhesus monkey during the follicular phase of the menstrual cycle. *J. Pharmacol. Exp. Ther.* **254,** 815–823.

[146]N. K. Mello, Z. Sarnyai, J.H. Mendelson, J. Drieze, and M. Kelly (1993) Acute effects on anterior pituitary hormones in male and female rhesus monkey. *J. Pharmacol. Exp. Ther.* in press.

[147]M. C. Ritz, R. J. Lamb, S. R. Goldberg, and M. J. Kuhar (1987) Cocaine receptors on dopamine transporters are related to self-administration of cocaine. *Science* **237,** 1219–1223.

[148]F. Gawin and E. H. Ellinwood (1988) Cocaine and other stimulants: Actions, abuse and treatment. *N. Engl. J. Med.* **318,** 1173–1182.

[149]J. J. LaFerla, D. L. Anderson, and D. S. Schalch (1978) Psychoendocrine response to sexual arousal in human males. *Psychosom. Med.* **40,** 166–172.

[150]N. K. Mello, J. H. Mendelson, J. Drieze, and M. Kelly (1990) Cocaine effects on luteinizing hormone-releasing hormone-stimulated anterior pituitary hormones in female rhesus monkey. *J. Clin. Endocrinol. Metab.* **71,** 1434–1441.

[151]J. H. Mendelson, S. K. Teoh, N. K. Mello, J. Ellingboe, and E. Rhoades (1992) Acute effects of cocaine on plasma ACTH, luteinizing hormone and prolactin levels in cocaine-dependent men. *J. Pharm. Exp. Ther.* **263,** 505–509.

[152]M. E. Freeman (1988) The ovarian cycle of the rat, in *The Physiology of Reproduction.* E. Knobil, J. Neill, L. L. Ewing, G. S. Greenwald, C. L. Markert, and D. W. Pfaff, eds. Raven, New York, pp. 1893–1928.

[153]E. Knobil and J. Hotchkiss (1988) The menstrual cycle and its neuroendocrine control, in *The Physiology of Reproduction.* E. Knobil, J. Neill, L. L. Ewing, G. S. Greenwald, C. L. Markert, and D. W. Pfaff, eds. Raven, New York, pp. 1971–1994.

[154]S. Judd, J. Rakoff, and S. S. C. Yen (1978) Inhibition of gonadotrophin and prolactin release by dopamine: Effect of endogenous estradiol levels. *J. Clin. Endocrinol. Metab.* **47,** 494–498.

[155]J. F. Ropert, M. E. Quigley, and S. S. C. Yen (1984) The dopaminergic inhibition of LH secretion during the menstrual cycle. *Life Sci.* **34,** 2067–2073.

[156]H. LeBlanc, G. C. Lachelin, S. Abu-Fadil, and S. S. C. Yen (1976) Effects of dopamine infusion on pituitary hormone secretion in humans. *J. Clin. End. Metab.* **43,** 668–674.

[157]W. H. Oldendorf (1971) Brain uptake of radiolabelled amino-acids, amines and hexoses after arterial injection. *Am. J. Physiol.* **221,** 1629–1639.

[158]M. J. Kaufman, R. D. Spealman, and B. K. Madras (1991) Distribution of cocaine recognition sites in monkey brain. I. In vitro autoradiography with [^{3}H] CFT. *Synapse* **9,** 177–187.

[159]F. J. MacKenzie, A. J. Hunter, C. Daly, and C. A. Wilson (1986) Evidence that the dopaminergic incertohypothalamic tract has a stimulatatory effect of ovulation and gonadotropin release. *Neuroendocrincolgy* **39,** 289–295.

[160]M. D. James, F. J. MacKenzie, P. A. Touhy-Jones, and C. A. Wilson (1987) Dopaminergic neurones in the sona incerta exert a stimulatory control on gonadotropin release via D1 dopamine receptors. *Neuroendocrinology* **65,** 348–355.

[161]J. A. Kiritsy-Roy, S. M. Stnadish, R. D. Whitmore, M. Smith, J. B. Halter, and L. C. Terry (1988) Cocaine-induced cardiovascular (CV) and pituitary-adrenal stimulation: Role of dopamine (DA) and corticotropin releasing hormone (CRH). *Soc. Neurosci. Abstr.* **14,** 445.

[162]R. L. Moldow and A. J. Fischman (1987) Cocaine induced secretion of ACTH, beta-endorphin, and corticosterone. *Peptides* **8,** 819–822.

[163]C. Rivier and W. Vale (1987) Cocaine stimulates adrenocorticotropin (ACTH) secretion through a corticotropin-releasing factor (CRF)-mediated mechanism. *Brain Res.* **422,** 403–406.

[164]G. Torres and C. Rivier (1992) Differential effects of intermittent or continuous exposure to cocaine on the hypothalamic-pituitary-adrenal axis and c-fos expression. *Brain Res.* **571,** 204–211.

[165]G. Torres and C. Rivier (1992) Cocaine-induced ACTH secretion: Dependence of plasma levels of the drug and mode of exposure. *Brain Res. Bull.* **29,** 51–56.

[166]J. H. Mendelson, S. K. Teoh, N. K. Mello, and J. Ellingboe (1992) Buprenorphine attenuates the effects of cocaine on adrenocorticotropin (ACTH) secretion and mood states in man. *Neuropsychopharmacology* **7,** 157–162.

[167]B. Borowsky and C. M. Kuhn (1991) Monoamine mediation of cocaine-induced hypothalamo-pituitary-adrenal activation. *J. Pharmacol. Exp. Ther.* **256,** 204–210.

[168]P. R. Guidoff and M. Ferin (1987) Endogenous opioid peptides mediate the effect of corticotropin-releasing factor on gonadotropin release in the primate. *Endocrinology* **121,** 837–842.

[169]A. M. Washton, M. S. Gold, and A. C. Pottash (1985) The 800-cocaine helpline: survey of 500 callers, in *Problems of Drug Dependence 1984* . L. S. Harris, ed. U.S. Government Printing Office, Washington, DC, pp. 224–230.

[170]D. Acker, B. P. Sachs, K. J. Tracey, and W. E. Wise (1983) Abruptio placentae associated with cocaine use. *Am. J. Obstet Gynecol.* **146,** 220–221.

[171]N. Bingol, M. Fuchs, V. Diaz, R. K. Stone, and D. S. Gromisch (1987) Teratogenicity of cocaine in humans. *J. Pediatr.* **110,** 93–96.

[172]B. B. Little, L. M. Snell, M. K. Palmore, and L. I. Gilstrap (1988) Cocaine use in pregnant women in a large public hospital. *Am. J. Perinatol.* **5,** 206–207.

[173]R. R. Townsend, F. C. Laing, and R. B. Jeffrey (1988) Placental abruption associated with cocaine abuse. *Am. J. Roentgenol.* **150,** 1339–1340.

[174]L. Ryan, S. Ehrlich, and L. Finnegan (1987) Cocaine abuse in pregnancy: Effects on the fetus and newborn. *Neurotoxicol. Teratol.* **9,** 295–299.

[175]R. Cherukuri, H. Minkoff, J. Feldman, A. Parekh, and L. Glass (1988) A cohort study of alkaloidal cocaine ("Crack") in pregnancy. *Obstet. Gynecol.* **72,** 147–151.

[176]D. L. Dow-Edwards (1989) Long-term neurochemical and neurobehavioral consequences of cocaine use during pregnancy. *Ann. NY Acad. Sci.* **562,** 280–289.

[177]J. D. Madden, T. F. Payne, and S. Miller (1986) Maternal cocaine abuse and effect on the newborn. *Pediatrics* **77,** 209–211.

[178]H. Bauchner, B. Zuckerman, M. McClain, D. Frank, L. E. Fried, and H. Kayne (1988) Risk of sudden infant death syndrome among infants with in utero exposure to cocaine. *Pediatrics* **113,** 831–834.

[179]D. A. Frank, B. S. Zuckerman, H. Amaro, K. Aboagye, H. Bauchner, H. Cabral, L. Fried, R. Hingson, H. Kayne, S. M. Levenson, S. Parker, H. Reece, and R. Vinci (1988) Cocaine use during pregnancy: Prevalence and correlates. *Pediatrics* **82,** 888–895.

[180]I. J. Chasnoff, C. E. Hunt, R. Kletter, and D. Kaplan (1989) Prenatal cocaine exposure is associated with respiratory pattern abnormalities. *AJDC* **143,** 583–587.

[181]D. J. Durand, A. M. Espinoza, and B. G. Nickerson (1990) Association between prenatal cocaine exposure and sudden infant death syndrome. *J. Pediatr.* **117,** 909–911.

[182]S. L. Ward, D. Bautista, L. Chan, M. Derry, A. Lisbin, M. J. Durfee, K. S. C. Mills, and T. G. Keens (1990) Sudden infant death syndrome in infants of substance-abusing mothers. *J. Pediatrics* **117,** 876–881.

[183]J. J. Volpe (1992) Effect of cocaine use on the fetus. *N. Engl. J. Med.* **327**, 399–407.

[184]J. R. Woods Jr., M. A. Plessinger, and K. E. Clark (1987) Effect of cocaine on uterine blood flow and fetal oxygenation. *JAMA* **257**, 957–961.

[185]J. R. Owiny, M. T. Jones, D. Sadowsky, A. Massmann, X. Y. Ding and P. W. Nathanielsz (1991) Lack of Effect of fetal administration of cocaine on maternal and fetal plasma adrenocorticotropin, cortisol and lactate concentrations at 127–138 days gestational age. *Gynecol. Obstet. Inves.* **32**, 196–199.

[186]J. R. Owiny, M. T. Jones, D. Sadowsky, T. Myers, A. Masman, and P. W. Nathanielsz (1991) Cocaine in pregnancy: The effect of maternal administration of cocaine on the maternal and fetal pituitary-adrenal axes. *Am. J. Obstet. Gynecol.* **164**, 658–663.

[187]K. Kaye, L. Elkind, D. Goldberg, and A. Tyton (1989) Birth outcomes for infants of drug abusing mothers. *NY State J. Med.* **89**, 256–261.

[188]S. MacGregor, L. G. Keith, I. J. Chasnoff, M. A. Rosner, G. M. Chisum, P. Shaw, and J. P. Minogue (1987) Cocaine use during pregnancy: Adverse perinatal outcome. *Am. J. Obstet. Gyynecol.* **157**, 686–690.

[189]I. J. Chasnoff (1991) Cocaine and pregnancy: Clinical and methodologic issues. *Clin. Perinatol.* **18**, 113–123.

[190]M. E. James and C. D. Coles (1991) Cocaine abuse during pregnancy: Psychiatric considerations. *Gen. Hosp. Psychiatry* **13**, 399–409.

[191]S. R. Kandall (1991) Perinatal effects of cocaine and amphetamine use during pregnancy. *Bull. NY Acad. Med.* **67**, 240–255.

[192]C. S. Lindberg (1991) A review of the literature on cocaine abuse in pregnancy. *Nurs. Res.* **40**, 69–75.

[193]L. C. Mayes, R. H. Granger, M. H. Bornstein, and B. Zuckerman (1992) The problem of prenatal cocaine exposure. *JAMA* **267**, 406–408.

[194]B. Zuckerman and K. Bresnahan (1991) Development and behavioral consequences of prenatal drug and alcohol exposure. *Ped. Clin. N. Am.* **38**, 1387–1406.

[195]S. S. C. Yen (1984) Opiates and reproduction: Studies in women, in *Opioid Modulation of Endocrine Function* . G. Delitala, M. Motta, and M. Serio, eds. Raven, New York, pp. 191–209.

[196]J. G. Pfaus and B. B. Gorzalka (1986) Opioids and sexual behavior. *Neurosci. Biobehav. Rev.* **11**, 1–34.

[197]J. A. Thomas, K. S. Shahid-Salles, and M. P. Donovan (1977) Effects of narcotics on the reproductive system. *Adv. Sex. Horm. Res.* **3**, 169–195.

[198]P. Cushman Jr. (1972) Sexual behavior in heroin addiction and methadone maintenance. Correlation with plasma luteinizing hormone. *NY State J. Med.* **72**, 1261–1265.

[199]J. Mintz, K. O'Hare, C. P. O'Brien, and J. Goldschmidt (1974) Sexual problems of heroin addicts. *Arch. Gen. Psychiatry* **31**, 700–703.

[200]E. C. Gaulden, D. C. Littlefield, O. E. Putoff, and A. L. Seivert (1964) Menstrual abnormalities associated with heroin addiction. *Am. J. Obst. Gynecol.* **90**, 155–160.

[201]S. S. Stoffer (1968) A gynecologic study of drug addicts. *Am. J. Obstet. Gynecol.* **101**, 779–783.

[202]S. M. Mirin, R. E. Meyer, J. H. Mendelson, and J. Ellingboe (1980) Opiate use and sexual function. *Am. J. Psychiatry* **137**, 909–915.

[203]T. J. Cicero, R. D. Bell, W. G. Wiest, J. H. Allison, K. Polakoski, and E. Robins (1975) Function of the male sex organs in heroin and methadone users. *N. Engl. J. Med.* **292**, 882–887.

[204]S. M. Mirin, J. H. Mendelson, J. Ellingboe, and R. E. Meyer (1976) Acute effects of heroin and naltrexone on testosterone and gonadotropin secretion: A pilot study. *Psychoneuroendocrinology* **1,** 359–369.

[205]J. H. Mendelson, J. Ellingboe, N. K. Mello, and J. Kuehnle (1982) Buprenorphine effects on plasma luteinizing hormone and prolactin in male heroin addicts. *J. Pharmacol. Exp. Ther.* **220,** 252–255.

[206]T. J. Cicero, T. M. Badger, C. E. Wilcox, R. D. Bell, and E. R. Meyer (1977) Morphine decreases luteinizing hormone by an action on the hypothalamic-pituitary axis. *J. Pharmacol. Exp. Ther.* **203,** 548–555.

[207]T. J. Cicero, R. D. Bell, E. R. Meyer, and J. Schweitzer (1977) Narcotics and the hypothalamic-pituitary-gonadal axis: Acute effects on luteinizing hormone, testosterone and androgen-dependent systems. *J. Pharmacol. Exp. Ther.* **201,** 76–83.

[208]T. J. Cicero, C. E. Wilcox, R. D. Bell, and E. R. Meyer (1976) Acute reductions in serum testosterone levels by narcotics in the male rat: Stereospecificity, blockade by naloxone and tolerance. *J. Pharmacol. Exp. Ther.* **198,** 340–346.

[209]T. J. Cicero, M. L. Adams, A. Giordano, B. T. Miller, L. O'Connor, and B. Nock (1991) Influence of morphine exposure during adolescence on the sexual maturation of male rats and the development of their offspring. *J. Pharmacol. Exp. Ther.* **256,** 1086–1093.

[210]T. J. Cicero, L. O'Connor, B. Nock, M. L. Adams, B. T. Miller, R. D. Bell, and E. R. Meyer (1989) Age-related differences in the sensitivity to opiate-induced perturbations in reproductive endocrinology in the developing and adult male rat. *J. Pharmacol Exp. Ther.* **248,** 256–261.

[211]C. A. Barraclough and C. H. Sawyer (1955) Inhibition of the release of pituitary ovulatory hormone in the rat by morphine. *Endocrinology* **57,** 329–337.

[212]R. J. Santen, J. Sofsky, B. Nedjelko, and R. Lippert (1975) Mechanism of action of narcotics in the production of menstrual dysfunction in women. *Fertil. Steril.* **26,** 538–548.

[213]S. R. Kandall, S. Albin, E. Dreyer, M. Comstock, and J. Lowinson (1975) Differential effects of heroin and methadone on birth weights. *Addict. Dis.* **2,** 347–355.

[214]R. L. Naeye, W. Blanc, W. Leblanc, and M. A. Khatamee (1973) Fetal complications of maternal heroin addiction: Abnormal growth, infections, and episodes of stress. *Pediatrics* **83,** 1055–1061.

[215]C. Zelson, S. J. Lee, and M. Casalino (1973) Neonatal narcotic addiction: Comparative effects of maternal intake of heroin and methadone. *N. Engl. J. Med.* **289,** 1216–1223.

[216]R. Fulroth, B. Phillips, and D. J. Durand (1989) Perinatal outcome of infants exposed to cocaine and/or heroin in utero. *Am. J. Dis. Child.* **143,** 905–910.

[217]T. S. Rosen and H. L. Johnson (1988) Drug-addicted mothers, their infants, and SIDS. *Ann. NY Acad. Sci.* **533,** 89–95.

[218]W. J. Litto, J. P. Griffin, and J. Rabii (1983) Influence of morphine during pregnancy on neuroendocrine regulation of pituitary hormone secretion. *J. Endocrinol.* **98,** 289–295.

[219]I. U. Vathy, A. M. Etgen, J. Rabii, and R. J. Barfield (1983) Effects of prenatal exposure to morphine sulfate on reproductive function of female rate. *Pharmacol. Biochem. Behav.* **19,** 777–780.

[220]C. Zelson, E. Rubio, and E. Wasserman (1971) Neonatal narcotic addiction: 10 year observation. *Pediatrics* **48,** 178–189.

[221]S. D. Ward, S. Schuetz, V. Krishna, K. Bean, W. Wingert, L. Wachsman, and T. G. Keens (1986) Abnormal sleeping ventilatory pattern in infants of substance-abusing mothers. *Am. J. Dis. Child.* **140,** 1015–1020.

[222]S. L. Hans (1989) Developmental consequences of prenatal exposure to methadone, in *Prenatal Abuse of Licit and Illicit Drugs.* D. E. Hutchings, ed. The New York Academy of Sciences, New York, pp. 195–207.

[223]G. Wilson (1989) Clinical studies of infants and children exposed prenatally to heroin, in *Prenatal Abuse of Licit and Illicit Drugs* . D. E. Hutchings, ed. New York Academy of Sciences, New York, pp. 183–194.

[224]L. P. Finnegan, T. Hagan, and K. A. Kaltenbach (1991) Scientific foundation of clinical practice: Opiate use in pregnant women. *Bull. NY Acad. Med.* **67,** 223–239.

Sex Differences in Children of Substance-Abusing Parents

Sydney L. Hans

Introduction

In recent years, the American public has become increasingly concerned about the adverse effects parental substance abuse can have on the development of children. Issues surrounding "crack babies" and adult children of alcoholics have been widely discussed in the popular media, and have been addressed by lawmakers, educators, and health practitioners around the country. Although scientific evidence on this topic clearly lags behind public concern, a growing body of research data documents the ways parental substance abuse can reverberate throughout the lifespan of offspring. Until recently, most scientists have focused on the issue of whether parental substance abuse affects the development of children. They have asked questions about whether prenatal exposure to a particular drug is associated with a particular developmental problem: For example, is maternal crack use related to premature birth, does maternal alcoholism cause mental retardation, is maternal heroin abuse associated with attention deficits in school-age children, or are children raised by alcoholic parents likely to have drinking problems themselves? Although studies posing questions, such as these, have often found that prenatal exposure to drugs of abuse increases the likelihood that children will have developmental problems,

From: *Drug and Alcohol Abuse Reviews, Vol. 5: Addictive Behaviors in Women*
Ed.: R. R. Watson ©1994 Humana Press Inc., Totowa, NJ

the same studies have also documented the great variability in the outcome of children exposed to drugs before birth, or being raised by substance-abusing parents. Some children of substance-abusing parents fare very poorly; others do quite well.

Increasingly, scientists are trying to understand why some children with substance-abusing mothers do well and others do not. Researchers seek to understand why some children are protected from the risks associated with parental substance abuse and others are especially vulnerable. The focus of this chapter is to explore whether children's gender is related to developmental outcome in children from families in which a parent is a substance abuser. Specifically, this chapter will explore the issue of whether female gender protects children from the effects of family substance abuse and male gender places children at increased risk for developmental problems or different types of problems.

Before exploring this question, however, it is important to consider the multiple pathways through which parental substance abuse can affect the development of a child. At least three pathways are important. First, alcohol and drugs can have a direct teratological effect on the offspring. When a woman uses alcohol or psychoactive drugs during pregnancy, those substances cross the placenta and enter the system of the fetus. If the direct pharmacological action of the substance on the embryo or fetus disrupts normal development, the substance is said to have acted as a teratogen. A drug that is a teratogen can cause physical birth defects in a child or abnormalities of behavior. Alcohol provides the clearest example of how an abused substance can have a direct teratological effect on offspring. When exposed to large amounts of alcohol *in utero*, children may develop fetal alcohol syndrome—a distinct pattern of head and face anomalies, growth retardation, mental retardation, and attentional problems. Exposure to lower levels of alcohol may result in more subtle physical anomalies and behavior problems.[1,2]

The second mechanism through which parental substance abuse can affect children is genetics. Substance abusers often have other behavioral disorders, such as antisocial personality, depression, and attention deficit that coincide with, as well as precede, substance abuse.[3-6] Since many of these behavioral disorders are currently believed to have a genetic basis—including substance abuse itself—vulnerability to behavioral problems can be transmitted genetically from a substance-abusing parent to child regardless of whether the child has been exposed prenatally to alcohol or drugs and regardless of whether the parent is involved in rearing the child.

The third way in which parental substance abuse can also affect the lives of children is through the environment that a substance-abusing family provides the children. Many reports suggest that families in which a parent abuses alcohol[7,8] or drugs[9,10] provide less than optimal childrearing environments. It may be that behavioral problems in children are a direct result of poor parenting behavior or other characteristics of a family environment that is organized around a parent's substance abuse.

Finally, it is likely that complicated transactions occur among the various teratological, genetic, and environmental risk factors associated with parental substance abuse mediate child outcome.[11] For example, a drug-withdrawing infant or a hyperactive child may elicit a response from a substance-abusing parent that is more negative than that elicited by a more passive and malleable child,[12–14] particularly if the substance-abusing parent also has a personality disorder that makes him or her especially prone to inappropriate expression of anger.[15]

The remainder of this chapter will explore whether gender of offspring might moderate the teratological, genetic, and environmental effects of parental substance abuse. We are interested in whether boys and girls of substance-abusing parents have different developmental outcomes, and whether prenatal substance abuse affects boys and girls to a different extent or in a different manner. There is not a systematically gathered body of research on this topic. Virtually no investigator has conducted a study on offspring of substance-abusing parents that was designed specifically to explore hypotheses about differences between male and female children. In fact, most investigators studying offspring of substance-abusing parents have not even bothered to explore or report differences between boys and girls. Hence this chapter will report isolated findings gleaned from a variety of literatures—animal teratology studies, human studies of children exposed *in utero* to drugs and alcohol, human studies of children being raised by substance-abusing parents, and behavioral genetics studies of twins and adopted children. It is hoped that the resulting montage of information will provide some insight into the role of child's gender in families with substance-abusing parents, and additionally will serve to draw focus to this topic as one that deserves further attention by those interested in substance-abusing families.

Teratological Effects on Sexually Dimorphic Behavior

When considering the role of children's gender in moderating the effects of parental substance abuse, an obvious starting place are those domains of behavior that normally differ between males and females. In all mammalian species, there are normal gender-linked differences in patterns of behavior. Many sexually dimorphic behaviors are specific to mating behavior, whereas others have no obvious basis in reproduction. Even though the basis of many sexually dimorphic patterns of behavior—especially in humans—is social learning, there is substantial evidence that male and female brains differ in their basic structural organization.[16] A large animal literature has shown that these sex differences in brain structure and behavior are related to the early presence or absence of sex hormones—particularly the male hormones[17,18]—during the time at which basic sex differences in neural organization are established. Although data on human subjects are sparse—coming primarily from patients with abnormalities in endocrine functioning, prenatal sex steroids are believed also to play an important role in the process of psychosexual differentiation in humans.[19] It is conceivable that sex differences in early hormonal exposure and brain development affect even largely learned human sex differences, such as gender identity, since basic brain differences may influence the ease with which a child learns gender-appropriate behavior and thereby achieves clarity of gender identity.[20]

Because many common drugs of abuse have effects on the endocrine system, it is plausible that when used by pregnant women they might alter fetal sex-hormone levels, which in turn might be expected to cause alterations in the developing brain that would interfere with normal patterns of sexually dimorphic behavior. A substantial body of data from animal studies supports this hypothesis.

Take, for example, a study Hard and colleagues conducted of the effects of prenatal exposure to alcohol on adult sexual behavior in rats.[21] Female rats were given an ethanol solution as their sole liquid during pregnancy. At birth, the 41 pups were removed from their natural mothers and given to alcohol-free foster mothers for rearing, as were 48 pups whose mothers had not been given ethanol during pregnancy. When mature, at between the ages of 40 and 70 d, the male rats were placed with a sexually receptive female for observation of male-appropriate sexual behavior—mounting, penile intromission, and ejaculation. At 80 d of age, males were tested for lordotic behavior by placing them with a "sexually vigorous" male who was allowed to mount the test animal 10 different times. (Lordosis is the curvature of the back normally shown by females in preparation for being mounted by a study male.) Compared to male animals who were not exposed to alcohol *in utero*, prenatally exposed males showed no differences in masculine behavior, but showed an increase in feminine behavior. Forty-five percent of the ethanol-exposed males displayed lordosis in preparation for being mounted, compared to only 8% of the nonexposed males. Sexual maturity of female offspring was assessed through daily examination beginning at 30 d to determine when the vaginal opening was established, when evidence of estrous cycles was present, and when, on handling by examiner, the female responded with lordosis. There were no differences between ethanol-exposed and nonexposed rats in terms of onset of estrous cycles, although the onset of lordotic response was delayed in ethanol exposed females by approx 5 d.

Other studies of prenatal exposure to alcohol in rodents suggest that alcohol also disrupts nonreproductive sexually dimorphic behaviors in rats. For example, female rats normally show a clear preference for saccharin over tap water, and males do not; on maze learning tasks, males normally perform better than females. These normal sex differences are not observable in rats who were exposed prenatally to alcohol.[22] Findings of altered patterns of behavior related to prenatal alcohol exposure are supported by evidence that prenatal exposure to alcohol effects normal sexually dimorphic anatomical aspects of brain anatomy in male rats,[23] and results in lowered adult plasma testosterone levels in male rats.[24]

Similar types of studies have also been conducted with rodents exposed to other substances prenatally and soon after birth. Exposure to barbiturates has been related to demasculinization and/or feminization of males and defeminization and/or masculinization of females with respect to reproductive behavior (such as mounting and lordosis)[25–30] and sexually dimorphic nonreproductive behavior (such as maze learning).[31] Prenatal exposure to nicotine, opioids, and marijuana have also been shown to interfere with anatomical and behavioral differentiation of the sexes in rodents.[32–37] Recently, in a review of the many animal studies linking prenatal exposure to alcohol and drugs to abnormal sexually dimorphic behavior, Segarra and McEwen argued that across all the studies on this topic there is strong replicated evidence that males are either less masculine or more feminine than normal.[38] Evidence for females being either more masculine or less feminine than normal exists, but has been less clearly replicated.

Although there are few data on the effects of prenatal drug exposure on the sexually dimorphic behavior of humans, the studies to date are provocative. Sandberg et al. studied 30 children at ages 6–8 who had been exposed to methadone before birth.[39] Based on standardized questionnaires completed by children's caregivers, the investigators concluded that methadone-exposed boys showed more stereotypically feminine behavior than unexposed male control subjects. Their caregivers were more likely to indicate that the methadone-exposed males were "good at imitating females" and "dress in female clothing." They found no differences in reported behavior between exposed and unexposed girls. Similarly, Ward et al. assessed a sample of 48 opioid-exposed children 5- to 7-yr-old using two projective tests.[40] On the Draw-A-Person Test children are given the freedom to draw a person of their choice.[41] Compared to unexposed children, drug-exposed boys were more likely to draw a female figure. On the IT Scale for Children, children are given the opportunity to describe a neuter figure called "It."[42] Compared to unexposed children, drug-exposed boys were more likely to view the "It" figure as having feminine characteristics. In free play, opioid-exposed boys generally chose masculine toys, but were more likely to at least briefly play with feminine toys than other boys. The investigators reported that this tendency to play with feminine toys was unrelated to the presence of a father figure in the boys' lives. There were no differences in test behavior between opioid-exposed and unexposed girls.

In summary, a variety of abused substances appear to disrupt the development of normal sex-linked reproductive behavior and gender dimorphic nonreproductive behavior in rodents. This disruption may be greater in males than females. Although little work on this topic has been conducted in human samples, two provocative studies suggest that opioid exposure may disrupt normal sexually dimorphic behavior in male children.

Male Vulnerability to Teratological Effects

The studies of sexually dimorphic behavior suggest that perhaps males may be more vulnerable to the effects of prenatal substance exposure than females. Such a finding is consistent with the general view that the human male is more vulnerable than the female to a variety of biological insults, including those occurring prenatally.[43–46] A number of factors have been suggested to contribute to greater male vulnerability, including the lack of a second "protective" X-chromosome,[43,47,48] greater male immaturity during fetal development,[43,49] and immune system reactions between mothers and male fetuses.[50]

Although a variety of types of data have been cited as evidence for male vulnerability, the greater loss of male fetuses during pregnancy is key to the argument.[51,52] In the general population, 120 males are conceived for every 100 females (55% males). In the general population, by the time of birth there are 110 males delivered for every 100 females (52% males), and 106 live males delivered for every 100 females (51% males).[45,53] It is assumed that the greater loss of males is the result of greater vulnerability to fetal stressors.

If a drug has teratogenic effects, one might expect the loss of male fetuses in prenatally exposed samples to be greater than in unexposed samples. Martin reviewed all studies of fetally exposed animals and human infants for information on sex ratios at birth.[54,55] She found evidence, in multiple studies of both animals and humans, that the sex ratios at birth were altered, such that when the mother was receiving nicotine, alcohol, amphetamine, opiates, and barbiturates, less than half of the live births were male. For example, Abel combined data from 39 studies of fetal alcohol syndrome and found that only 47% of the births to alcoholic women were males.[56] The data reviewed by Martin came from both animal and human samples. The largest alterations of sex ratios at birth occurred in the human samples, although in the human studies it is not possible to rule out the possibility that the shift in the sex ratio is owing to paternal factors, including the possibility that paternal substance abuse alters the sperm in a manner that decreases the numbers of males conceived. Although there were inconsistencies across studies, taken as a whole, the data suggest that male embryos/fetuses are more vulnerable to the effects of exposure to drugs *in utero*, and are less likely to survive to the time of birth.

Speculating from these studies, one might also predict that males would be more vulnerable than females to nonlethal damage during fetal life. If so, one might also expect males to have more brain-based behavioral problems than females; and in fact, in the general population male children do have a higher incidence of neurological signs, learning problems, and attentional deficits.[57] It remains unclear, however, whether the specific stressor of prenatal substance exposure has a particularly adverse effect on male offspring—whether the difference between males and females is even larger in substance-exposed children than in children in general. Few studies of substance exposure in either human or animal populations have reported comparisons between male and female offspring, and more to the point, no study has examined whether the magnitude of sex differences is greater in substance-exposed children than in unexposed children.

Sex Differences in Vulnerability to Environmental Stressors

Just as it has been suggested that males are more vulnerable to biological stressors than females, it has also been argued that males are more vulnerable to environmental stressors, in particular, to the effects of nonoptimal rearing conditions or family disruption.[43]

Clearly, parental substance abuse is related to children experiencing less than optimal rearing environments. Parental alcoholism alters family life in many ways. Families with an alcoholic parent have a high incidence of divorce and separation, disruption of family rituals, increased family discord and violence, and impaired intrafamilial interaction in problem-solving situations.[3,7,8] Although there is less systematically gathered information available on drug-using families, it can be assumed that a family with a parent using illicit drugs would be characterized by many of the same qualities as families with alcoholic parents, and be further disrupted by the parents' engagement in illegal activities related to drug procurement.[58,59]

It is also reasonably clear that parental substance abuse places offspring at increased risk for behavioral problems of the sort related to high-risk rearing environments. Although the research on children of alcoholics is full of contradictions, numerous studies have suggested that individuals with alcoholic parents may be at increased risk for psychological impairment. For example, it has been suggested that children of alcoholics show lifelong difficulties in peer relationships, may have more conduct disorders, may showed increased incidence of emotional difficulties, and perhaps have more problems in academic achievement and intellectual functioning.[3,60–63] Although less is known about the children of drug-abusing parents, the available evidence suggests an increased incidence of problems during childhood.[64,65]

If males truly are more vulnerable to environmental stressors, one would hypothesize that, to the extent that behavioral and emotional difficulties are related to stressors in the environment, the difficulties would be more serious in male offspring of substance-abusing parents than in female offspring, and more severe in male offspring of substance abusers than in males without substance-abusing parents. At least one study offers direct support for this hypothesis. As part of a large longitudinal study of high-risk children, Werner followed 40 Hawaiian children with alcoholic parents from birth through age 18.[66] As a group, these children showed many academic and behavioral problems: By age 10, a third of them were in need of long-term remedial education; by age 18, a third of them had records of repeated or serious delinquencies, and a quarter of them had serious mental health problems. Altogether, 41% of the sample had either serious learning or behavioral problems by age 18. Comparing those with problems to the 59% who were without major problems, there was a significant sex difference between the problem and resilient groups. Nearly three-quarters of the resilient offspring were females; more than two-thirds of those who had developed problems were males.

Although data of this type support the hypothesis that males exposed to substances are at particularly high risk for environmental stressors, an alternative hypothesis is that males and females are vulnerable to different types of problems, or that problems develop with a different timetable.[67] Parents and teachers are particularly likely to notice and report to investigators disruptive behavior problems, and more likely to be unaware of or to minimize the severity of problems that are more related to children's internal states, such as anxiety and depression. In the general population, there are clear sex differences in the rates of specific forms of psychopathology, with males more vulnerable to personality disorders and substance abuse, and females to somatic and affective disorders. The types of disorders more common to females tend not only to be internalizing disorders, but also ones that develop later in life. Thus, it may be that female offspring of substance abusers are not less vulnerable, just vulnerable to different disorders—disorders that may be less obvious to observers, and particularly less obvious during childhood. Although very few studies of the development of behavioral problems in children of substance-abusing parents have looked for sex differences or have focused on female offspring, there are suggestions in the literature that female offspring of alcoholics may be particularly vulnerable to depression, eating disorders, and selection of alcoholics as marriage partners.[68,69]

If, in fact, male and female offspring of substance-abusing parents are at risk for different types of disorders, there still remain at least two hypotheses as to why such differences occur: (1) that males and females differ biologically in such a way that when exposed to nonoptimal rearing circumstances they tend to develop different disorders or (2) that males and females experience different rearing environments.

Gender Differences
in Genetic Susceptibility to Substance Abuse

The final area of research to be explored is whether gender of offspring moderates genetically transmitted risk from substance-abusing parents. A substantial research literature now documents that alcoholism and other types of substance abuse tend to run in families. For example, Goodwin reported that the prevalence of alcoholism among male relatives of alcoholics is approx 25%—compared to a prevalence of approx 5% in the general population.[70,71] The prevalence of alcoholism among female relatives of alcoholics, although considerably lower, also is greater than the prevalence of alcoholism in the general population. Although much remains to be learned about the mechanisms by which substance abuse is transmitted across generations, a large body of evidence has accumulated suggesting that such familial linkages are based at least to some extent on genetics.[72]

Perhaps the most convincing evidence for the genetic transmission of alcoholism comes from adoption studies. In the first major adoption study, Goodwin and colleagues took advantage of the detailed adoption and medical records available in Denmark to identify a group of 55 men who had been separated from their biological parents early in life and who had one biological parent (usually the father) with a history of hospitalization for alcoholism.[73] Seventy-eight adopted men were identified for two control groups: one in which the biological parents had no record of psychiatric hospitalization, and a second in which a biological parent had a record of psychiatric hospitalization for conditions other than alcoholism, most commonly depression or character disorder. The researchers found that 16% of the offspring of alcoholics had been treated for alcoholism compared to only 1% of the offspring from the control groups. Thirty-three percent of the offspring of alcoholics were considered to be alcoholics; only 6% of the comparison groups were considered to be alcoholics. Other adoption studies have reported similar increased risk of alcohol-related problems in individuals whose biological parents were alcoholics.[73–77]

Although these studies have clearly demonstrated the contribution of biological fathers' alcoholism to alcohol problems in the male offspring, the pattern of findings has not been as clear or strong for female offspring or offspring of female alcoholics. The apparent sex difference in genetic contribution to alcoholism prompted Cloninger and colleagues to suggest that there may be at least two types of alcoholism with different genetic and environmental causes.[74,78] Type 1—observed in both males and females—is relatively common, is associated with mild alcohol abuse in the biological parents, and is related to rearing environment in both male and female patients. Type 2—found only in men—is characterized by severe alcohol abuse, criminality, and extensive treatment history in the biological fathers of patients. This conclusion, however, must remain tentative since the most recent and most sophisticated study of the genetics of alcohol abuse in women—drawn from the Virginia Twin Registry[79]—suggests, unlike previous work, that genetic factors play a etiological role in alcoholism in women comparable to that in men.

Familial patterns of alcoholism have received far more research attention than familial patterns of drug abuse, although data also suggest an association between substance use in parents and drug abuse in offspring[80–82]— and perhaps some suggestion of a genetic basis. For example, in a study of Iowa adoptees, Cadoret et al. found that drug abuse was related to parental alcoholism and that parental alcoholism did not affect the drug abuse of male and female offspring differently.[83] Pickens and colleagues, in a study of substance abuse in twins, found that monozygotic twins were slightly more likely than dizygotic twins to be concordant for drug abuse, and that this effect was stronger in males than females.[84]

Summary

This chapter has presented studies from many different research arenas. Taken as a whole, they suggest that we have much to learn about the differences between male and female offspring of substance-abusing parents, but also that offspring gender may play a key role in gaining a full understanding of the effects of parental substance abuse.

A variety of kinds of evidence suggest that males may be more vulnerable to the effects of their parents' substance abuse: More male fetuses are lost during pregnancy; normally sexually dimorphic behavior, possibly including human gender identity, may be more disrupted in males; males may be at particularly high risk for learning problems and conduct disorders; and males may be particularly genetically vulnerable to alcoholism. Although not all of these findings have been replicated and studied with sufficient care, clearly male offspring of substance abusers are a group at high risk and a group in need of attention and preventive intervention.

It would be easy to conclude that females with substance-abusing parents are resilient. Such a conclusion is probably premature. The studies to date have primarily suggested that females are at less risk than males in substance-abusing families—not that they are at less risk than other females from nonsubstance-abusing families. It also remains unclear and of concern that females may be at risk for different problems than males—perhaps the sorts of problems that are experienced internally but which do not necessarily draw the attention of others. Such a pattern of sex differences in emotional problems has been found in studies of high-risk families that are not involved in substance abuse: Male children respond to stress with anger and difficult behavior, and female children by accepting the psychological responsibility for their families' problems.[85] Future studies on children in substance-abusing families, as well as other children at risk, should give increased focus to differences in developmental pathways and outcomes in girls and boys. In particular more attention needs to be given to possible differences in family dynamics involving male and female children, and to behavioral outcomes that may be typical of high-risk girls.

Acknowledgments

This chapter was prepared while the author was being supported by a grant from the National Institute on Drug Abuse (R01DA05396).

References

[1]E. L. Abel (1984) *Fetal Alcohol Syndrome and Fetal Alcohol Effects*. Plenum, New York.

[2]A. P. Streissguth, S. Landesman-Dwyer, J. C. Martin, and D. W. Smith (1980) Teratogenic effects of alcohol in humans and animals. *Science* **209,** 353–361.

[3]K. J. Sher (1991) Children of alcoholics: A Critical Appraisal of Theory and Research. University of Chicago Press, Chicago.

[4]B. J. Rounsaville, M. M. Weissman, H. D. Kleber, and C. H. Wilber (1982) The heterogeneity of psychiatric disorders in treated opiate addicts. *Arch. Gen. Psychiatry* **39,** 161–166.

[5]J. E. Helzer and T. R. Pryzbeck (1988) The co-occurrence of alcoholism with other psychiatric disorders in the general populations and its impact on treatment. *J. Stud. Alcohol* **49,** 219–224.

[6]S. S. Luthar, S. F. Anton, K. R. Merikangas, and B. J. Rounsaville (1992) Vulnerability to substance abuse and psychopathology among siblings of opioid abusers. *J. Nerv. Ment. Dis.* **180,** 153–161.

[7]P. Steinglass, L. A. Bennett, S. J. Wolin, and D. Reiss (1987) *The Alcoholic Family*. Basic, New York.

[8]R. A. Seilhamer and T. Jacob (1990) Family factors and adjustment of children of alcoholics, in *Children of Alcoholics: Critical Perspectives*. M. Windle and J. S. Searles, eds. Guilford, New York, pp. 168–186.

[9]M. S. Lawson, and G. W. Wilson (1980) Parenting among women addicted to narcotics. *Child Welfare* **59,** 67–79.

[10]K. B. Fiks, H. L. Johnson, and T. S. Rosen (1985). Methadone-maintained mothers: three-year follow-up of parental functioning. *Int. J. Addict.* **20,** 651–660.

[11]A. J. Sameroff and M. J. Chandler (1975) Reproductive risk and the continuum of caretaking casualty, in *Review of Child Development Research*, vol 4. F. D. Horowitz, E. M. Hetherington, S. Scarr-Salapatek and G. M. Sigel, eds. University of Chicago Press, Chicago, pp. 187–244.

[12]H. L. Johnson and T. S. Rosen (1990) Mother-infant interaction in a multirisk population, *Am. J. Orthopsychiatry* **60,** 281–288.

[13]K. Kaltenbach and L. P. Finnegan (1988) The influence of the neonatal abstinence syndrome on mother-infant interaction, in *The Child in His Family: Perilous Development: Child Raising and Identity Formation Under Stress*, vol. 8. E. J. Anthony and C. Chiland, eds. Wiley, New York, pp. 223–230.

[14]V. J. Bernstein, S. L. Hans, and C. Percansky (1991) Advocating for the young child in need through strengthening the parent-child relationship, *J. Clin. Child Psychol.* **20,** 28–41.

[15]S. L. Hans, V. B. Bernstein, and L. G. Henson (1990) Interaction between drug-using mothers and their toddlers [abstract]. *Infant Behav. Dev.* **13(Special),** 190.

[16]R. A. Gorski (1987) Sex differences in the rodent brain: Their nature and origin, in *Masculinity/Femininity: Basic Perspectives*. J. M. Reinisch, L. A. Rosenblum, and S. A. Sanders, eds. Oxford University Press, New York, pp. 37–67.

[17]R. W. Goy and B. S. McEwen (1980) *Sexual Differentiation of the Brain*. MIT Press, Cambridge, MA.

[18]H. H. Feder (1981) Perinatal hormones and their role in the development of sexually dimorphic behaviors, in *Neuroendocrinology of Reproduction*. N. T. Adler (ed.) Plenum, New York, pp. 127–157.

[19]A. A. Ehrhardt and H. F. L. Meyer-Bahlburg (1981) Effects of prenatal sex hormones on gender-related behavior. *Science* 211, 1312–1318.

[20]F. A. Beach (1987) Alternative interpretations of the development of G-I/R, in *Masculinity/Femininity: Basic Perspectives*. J. M. Reinisch, L. A. Rosenblum and S. A. Sanders, eds. Oxford University Press, New York, pp. 29–36.

[21]E. Hard, I. L. Dahlgren, J. Engel, K. Larsson, S. Lijequist, A.-S. Lindh, and B. Musi (1984) Development of sexual behavior in prenatally ethanol-exposed rats. *Drug Alcohol Dependence* 14, 51–61.

[22]R. F. McGivern, A. N. Clancy, M. A. Hill, and E. P. Noble (1984) Prenatal alcohol exposure alters adult expression of sexually dimorphic behavior in the rat. *Science* 224, 896–898.

[23]B. Zimmerberg, and J. M. Reuter (1989) Sexually dimorphic behavioral and brain asymmetries in neonatal rats: Effects of prenatal alcohol exposure. *Dev. Brain Res.* 46, 281–290.

[24]S. Parker, M. Udani, J. S. Gavaler, and D. H. Van Thiel (1984) Adverse effects of ethanol upon the adult sexual behavior of male rats exposed in utero. *Neurobehav. Toxicol. Teratol.* 6, 289–293.

[25]L. G. Clemens (1973) Neurohormonal control of male sexual behavior, in *Reproductive Behavior*. W. Montagna and W. A. Sadler, eds. Plenum, New York, pp. 23–53.

[26]L. G. Clemens, T. V. Popham, and P. H. Ruppert (1979) Neonatal treatment of hamsters with barbiturate alters adult sexual behavior. *Dev. Psychobiol.* 12, 49–59.

[27]C. Gupta, B. R. Sonawane, S. J. Yaffe, and B. H. Shapiro (1980) Phenobarbital exposure in utero: Alterations in female reproductive function in rats. *Science* 208, 508–510.

[28]C. Gupta, S. J. Yaffe, and B. H. Shapiro (1982) Prenatal exposure to phenobarbital permanently decreases testosterone and causes reproductive dysfunction. *Science* 216, 640–642.

[29]C. Gupta, B. H. Shapiro, and S. J. Yaffe (1980) Reproductive dysfunction in male rats following prenatal exposure to phenobarbital. *Pediatr. Pharmacol.* 1, 55–62.

[30]C. Gupta and S. J. Yaffe (1981) Reproductive dysfunction in female offspring after exposure to phenobarbital: Critical period of action. *Pediatr. Res.* 15, 1488–1491.

[31]J. M. Reinisch and S. A. Sanders (1982) Early barbiturate exposure: the brain, sexually dimorphic behavior and learning. *Neurosci. Biobehav. Rev.* 6, 311–319.

[32]W. Lichtensteiger and M. Schlumpf (1985) Prenatal nicotine affects fetal testosterone and sexual dimorphism of saccharin preference. *Pharmacol. Biochem. Behav.* 23, 439–444.

[33]O. B. Ward, T. M. Orth, and J. Weisz (1983) A possible role of opiates in modifying sexual differentiation, in *Monographs in Neural Sciences*, vol. 9. M. Schlumpf and W. Lichtensteiger, eds. Karger, Basel, pp. 194–200.

[34]I. U. Vathy, A. M. Etgen, J. Rabii, and R. J. Barfield (1983) Effects of prenatal exposure to morphine sulphate on reproductive function of female rats. *Pharmacol. Biochem. Behav.* 19, 777–780.

[35]I. U. Vathy, A. M. Etgen, and R. J. Barfield (1985) Effects of prenatal exposure to morphine on the development of sexual behavior in rats. *Pharmacol. Biochem. Behav.* 22, 227–232.

[36]S. Dalterio and A. Bartke (1979) Perinatal exposure to cannabinoids alters male reproductive function in mice. *Science* **205,** 1420–1422.

[37]P. A. Fried and A. T. Charlebois (1980) Cannabis administered during pregnancy: First- and second-generation effects on rats. *Physiol. Psychol.* **7,** 307–310.

[38]A. C. Segarra and B. S. McEwen (1992) Drug effects on sexual differentiation of the brain: Role of stress and hormones in drug actions, in *Maternal Substance Abuse and the Developing Nervous System.* I. S. Zagon and T. A. Slotkin, eds. Academic, San Diego, CA, pp. 323–367.

[39]D. E. Sandberg, H. F. L. Meyer-Bahlburg, T. S. Rosen, and H. L. Johnson (1990) Effects of prenatal methadone exposure on sex-dimorphic behavior in early school-age children. *Psychoneuroendocrinology* **15,** 77–82.

[40]O. B. Ward, D. M. Kopertowski, L. P. Finnegan, and D. E. Sandberg (1989) Gender-identify variations in boys prenatally exposed to opiates. *Ann. NY Acad. Sci.* **562,** 365–366.

[41]K. Machover (1949) *Personality Projection in the Drawing of the Human Figure: A Method of Personality Investigation.* Thomas, Springfield, IL.

[42]D. G. Brown (1957) Masculinity-femininity development in children. *J. Consult. Psychol.* **21,** 197–202.

[43]M. Rutter (1970) Sex differences in children's responses to family stress, in *The Child in His Family.* E. J. Anthony and C. Koupernik, eds. Wiley, New York, pp. 165–196.

[44]D. M. Potts (1970) Which is the weaker sex? *J. Biosoc. Sci.* **(suppl. 2),** 147–157.

[45]C. Hutt (1972) *Males and Females.* Penguin, Harmondsworth, Middlesex, England.

[46]C. N. Jacklin (1989) Female and male: Issues of gender *Am. Psychol.* **44,** 127–133.

[47]J. M. Reinisch, R. Gandelman, and F. S. Spiegel. (1979) Prenatal influences on cognitive abilities: Data from experimental animals and human genetic and endocrine syndromes, in *Sex-Related Differences in Cognitive Functioning.* M. A. Wittig and A. C. Petersen, eds. Academic, New York, pp. 215–239.

[48]C. Carter (1978) Sex differences in the distribution of physical illness in children. *Soc. Sci. Med.* **12B,** 163–166.

[49]D. P. Waber (1979). Cognitive abilities and sex-related variations in the maturation of cerebral cortical functions, in *Sex-Related Differences in Cognitive Functioning.* M. A. Wittig and A. C. Petersen, eds. Academic, New York, pp. 161–186.

[50]P. Toivanen and T. Hirvonen (1970) Sex ratio of newborns: Preponderance of males in toxemia of pregnancy. *Science* 170, 187–188.

[51]M. M. McMillen (1979) Differential mortality by sex in fetal and neonatal deaths. *Science* **204,** 89–91.

[52]R. L. Trivers and D. E. Willard (1973) Natural selection of parental ability to vary the sex ratio of offspring. *Science* **179,** 90–92.

[53]A. C. Stevenson (1966) Sex chromatin and the sex ratio in man, in *The Sex Chromatin.* K. L. Moore, ed. Saunders, Philadelphia, pp. 263–276.

[54]J. Martin (1985) Perinatal psychoactive drug use: Effects on gender, development, and function in offspring, in *Psychology and Gender.* T. Sonderegger, ed. University of Nebraska Press, Lincoln, NE, pp. 227–266

[55]J. Martin (1992) The effects of maternal use of tobacco products or amphetamines on offspring, in *Perinatal Substance Abuse: Research Findings and Clinical Implications.* T. B. Sonderegger, ed. Johns Hopkins University Press, Baltimore, MD, pp. 279–305.

[56]E. L. Abel (1979) Sex ratio in fetal alcohol syndrome. *Lancet* **2**, 105.

[57]American Psychiatric Association (1987) *Diagnostic and Statistical Manual of Mental Disorders*, 3rd ed., rev. ed. American Psychiatric Association, Washington, DC.

[58]S. J. Levy and E. Rutter (1992) *Children of Drug Abusers*. Lexington, New York.

[59]S. Deren (1986) Children of substance abusers: A review of the literature. *J. Subst. Abuse Treatment* **3**, 77–94.

[60]N. El Guebaly and D. R. Offord (1977) The offspring of alcoholics: A critical review. *Am. J. Psychiatry* **134**, 357–365.

[61]N. El Guebaly and D. R. Offord (1979) On being the offspring of an alcoholic: An update. *Alcohol. Clin. Exp. Res.* **3**, 148–157.

[62]M. Russell, C. Henderson, and S. Blume (1985) *Children of Alcoholics: A Review of the Literature*. Children of Alcoholics Foundation, New York.

[63]M. Windle (1990) Temperament and personality attributes among children of alcoholics, in *Children of Alcoholics: Critical Perspectives*. M. Windle and J. S. Searles, eds. Guilford, New York, pp. 129–167.

[64]B. J. Sowder and M. R. Burt (1980) *Children of Heroin Addicts: An Assessment of Health, Learning, Behavioral and Adjustment Problems*. Praeger, New York.

[65]S. L. Hans (1992) Maternal opioid drug use and child development, in *Maternal Substance Abuse and the Developing Nervous System*. I. S. Zagon and T. A. Slotkin, eds. Academic, New York, pp. 177–213.

[66]E. E. Werner (1986) Resilient offspring of alcoholics: A longitudinal study from birth to age 18. *J. Stud. Alcohol* **47**, 34–40.

[67]C. S. Widom (1984) *Sex Roles and Psychopathology*. Plenum, New York.

[68]J. Nici (1979) Wives of alcoholics as "repeaters." *J. Stud. Alcohol* **40**, 677–682.

[69]L. Silvia, G. Sorell, and N. Busch-Rossnagel (1988) Biopsychosocial discriminators of alcoholic and nonalcoholic women. *J. Subst. Abuse* **1**, 55–65.

[70]D. W. Goodwin (1976) *Is Alcoholism Hereditary?* Oxford University Press, New York.

[71]D. W. Goodwin (1985) Alcoholism and genetics: The sins of the fathers. *Arch. Gen. Psychiatry* **42**, 171–174.

[72]D. W. Goodwin (1988) *Is Alcoholism Hereditary?* Balantine, New York.

[73]D. W. Goodwin, F. Schulsinger, L. Hermansen, S. B. Guze, and G. Winokur (1973) Alcohol problems in adoptees raised apart from alcoholic biological parents. *Arch. Gen. Psychiatry* **28**, 238–243.

[74]C. R. Cloninger, M. Bohman, and S. Sigvardsson (1981) Inheritance of alcohol abuse: Cross-fostering analysis of adopted men. *Arch. Gen. Psychiatry* **38**, 861–868.

[75]R. J. Cadoret, C. A. Cain, and W. M. Grove (1980) Development of alcoholism in adoptees raised apart from alcoholic biologic relatives. *Arch. Gen. Psychiatry* **37**, 561–563.

[76]R. J. Cadoret, E. Troughton, and T. W. O'Gorman (1987) Genetic and environmental factors in alcohol abuse and antisocial personality. *J. Stud. Alcohol* **48**, 1–8.

[77]M. Bohman (1978) Some genetic aspects of alcoholism and criminality: A population of adoptees. *Arch. Gen. Psychiatry* **35**, 269–276.

[78]C. R. Cloninger (1987) Neurogenetic adaptive mechanisms in alcoholism. *Science* **236**, 410–416.

[79]K. S. Kendler, A. C. Heath, M. C. Neale, R. C. Kessler, and L. J. Eaves (1992) A population-based twin study of alcoholism in women. *JAMA* **268**, 1877–1882.

[80]E. W. Skiffington and P. M. Brown (1981) Personal, home, and school factors related to eleventh graders' drug attitudes. *Int. J. Addict.* **16,** 879–892.

[81]O. Simcha-Fagan, J. C. Gersten, and T. S. Langner (1986) Early precursors and concurrent correlates of patterns of illicit drug use in adolescence. *J. Drug Issues* **16,** 7–28.

[82]F. I. Fawzy, R. H. Coombs, and B. Gerber (1983) Generational continuity in the use of substances: The impact of parental substance use on adolescent substance use. *Addict. Behav.* **8,** 109–114.

[83]R. J. Cadoret, E. Troughton, T. W. O'Gorman, and E. Heywood (1986) An adoption study of genetic and environmental factors in drug abuse. *Arch. Gen. Psychiatry* **43,** 1131–1136.

[84]R. Pickens, D. Svikis, M. McGue, D. Lykken, M. Heston, and P. Clayton (1991) Heterogeneity in the inheritance of alcoholism: A study of male and female twins. *Arch. Gen. Psychiatry* **48,** 19–28.

[85]C. Zahn-Waxler, R. Iannotti, E. M. Cummings, and S. Denham (1990) Antecedents of problem behaviors in children of depressed mothers. *Dev. Psychopathol.* **2,** 271–292.

A Comparison
of Addictive Behaviors
Between Homeless
Men and Women

Myra Q. Elder, Aaron T. Hogue,
Thomas E. Shipley Jr.,
and Irving W. Shandler

Introduction

Homelessness has always existed in the United States, with upsurges and downswings strongly dependent on the state of the nation's economy. Before the 1980s, the last great surge of homelessness occurred during the 1930s, when the country was in the throes of the Great Depression. Depression-era estimates of the number of homeless people ranged from 200,000 to 1.5 million.[1] Apparently, getting a handle on just how many homeless people there are is a problem that plagued researchers then as well as now.

The United States' entry into World War II greatly reduced the number of homeless people in this country, as a result of their absorption into the armed forces and the war industries.[1] In the first two decades after the war, the skid rows that had existed before the war began to grow again. These skid rows were collections of cheap hotels, restaurants and bars, religious missions, and centers for recruitment of day-laborers.[1]

From: *Drug and Alcohol Abuse Reviews, Vol. 5: Addictive Behaviors in Women*
Ed.: R. R. Watson ©1994 Humana Press Inc., Totowa, NJ

In the 1950s, there was an increasing interest in the possibility of urban renewal for America's larger cities. This interest ignited a revival of social science research on skid row, which had its origins in the late 1800s.[2] This postwar research shifted attention to alcohol problems and their relationship to homelessness, and it laid the foundation of the work to be reviewed here.[3] Therefore, a quick overview of the major researchers and their findings is in order.

Groundbreaking studies were conducted on Minneapolis' Lower Loop by Caplow et al., on New York's Bowery by Bahr and Caplow, on Chicago's skid row by Bogue, and on Philadelphia by Blumberg et al.[4-7] These researchers reported similar findings: Skid row was populated largely by older, alcoholic White males living on a pension. In the study that provided the groundwork for Blumberg et al. (1973), Blumberg et al. (1960) interviewed 2249 skid row residents, which accounted for 79% of Philadelphia's estimated skid row population. Of this sample, almost 75% of the men were over 45 yr old, and the median age was 52. In terms of substance use, 29% were found to be "spree drinkers," meaning that they chronically lost control of their drinking. An additional 28% of the men drank on a daily basis. Better than 83% of these men were White, with <15% being Black. In terms of marital status, 46% of the men in the Philadelphia study had never been married. Approximately 45% of the men were subsisting on a nonwage income, usually public assistance or social security. These figures were consistent with the findings of the aforementioned researchers in other cities.[7,8]

In 1973, Garrett and Bahr warned that homeless women had been generally ignored by researchers up to that time. Garrett and Bahr further suggested that, not only did homeless women exist, they also had the same problems as their male counterparts, such as high rates of alcoholism and problem drinking, medical and psychiatric disorders, and chronic unemployment.[9] Blumberg et al. addressed the phenomenon of the "invisible skid row" in a follow-up analysis of their 15 yr of work with the Philadelphia skid row population. These researchers pointed out that White men had been thus far overrepresented in the research, so that both women and the people "hidden in the Black slum" (p. 124) were essentially ignored.[10] Before the turn of the century, W. E. B. DuBois had pointed out that Blacks were overrepresented among those arrested by Philadelphia's Vagrant Detectives.[11] In terms of the female population of skid row, Blumberg et al. suggested that women have always been associated with skid row, although evidence was sparse.[10] For instance, during their 1960 survey, Blumberg et al. were able to locate only 28 homeless women.[8] Generally, the studies conducted in the 1950s and 1960s reported that women made up <3% of the homeless population.[1]

Blumberg et al. predicted that the concept of skid row would expand from being conceptualized as a physical place to being seen as a human condition of homelessness, powerlessness, addiction, and disability that would include all races and ethnic groups and both genders.[10] This expansion has occurred, with the result being the transition from the "old" to the "new" homeless population.

This chapter examines the differences in the use of alcohol and illicit drugs between homeless men and women by reviewing research conducted since 1980. This review is divided into six sections: epidemiology (including the characteristics of the new homeless), correlates of drug and alcohol use, family issues, research problems and issues, treatment issues, and policy issues and recommendations. Where appropriate, we will first discuss research on the general homeless population, and then contrast those general findings with specific findings from the female homeless population. Within the treatment section, we will also discuss the findings of two studies that have been undertaken at the Diagnostic and Rehabilitation Center (DRC) in Philadelphia, one with homeless mothers that was recently completed, and one with homeless men that is currently underway.

Epidemiology

Characteristics of the New Homeless

Fischer and Breakey noted that because research on homelessness has been largely descriptive over the past decade, a great deal about sociodemographic characteristics of the homeless population is known. They suggested that the 1980s witnessed the growth of the new homeless, who were younger by an average of 13 yr, had a greater proportion of single women, and had an overrepresentation of minorities (especially Blacks and Hispanics), than traditional skid row populations.[12] A 1987 study by Wright and Weber (cited in ref. 1), conducted in a New York men's shelter, found that >75% of the men there were Black, a proportion that has been on the rise since 1980. Also, Rossi's 1989 Chicago study found that 54% of the sampled homeless population was Black (cited in ref. 1). Furthermore, compared to the traditional picture of the older, White homeless man, the new homeless slept in more public places, were more likely to use illicit drugs in addition to or in place of alcohol, exhibited more symptoms of mental illness, and were about 25% women.[1,13]

The prevalence estimates of the new homeless are as widely varied as the counts taken during the Great Depression. A 1984 report by the United States Department of Housing and Urban Development put the national figure at somewhere between 250,000 and 300,000. The Urban Institute recently estimated the count to be 500,000 homeless persons. This figure was based on direct counts in shelters and soup kitchens.[14] However, according to the Community for Creative Non-Violence, there are more than 3 million homeless persons, as of 1987. Rossi cited studies reviewed by the General Accounting Office during 1985 and 1988 that suggested an annual growth rate of the homeless population somewhere between 10 and 38%.[1]

Based on his review of the literature, Rossi asserted that homelessness today is much more a condition of housing deprivation, or *houselessness*, than before. Also, the new homeless suffer a greater degree of economic destitution than the old homeless. The homeless population of the past was perhaps able to rely more on Social Security pensions and day work than the present homeless population. Thus, Rossi concluded that the new homeless are poorer than the old homeless. However, he did not take into account the possible incomes derived from illegal activities, such as drug dealing and theft.[1]

Homeless Women Today

Sullivan and Damrosch observed that prior to 1976 there was little public interest in homeless women. Up to that time, most homeless women who came to public attention were older, widowed, and in ill health.[15] In the last decade, however, the new homeless have been found to be younger people whose roots of homelessness lay in general economic forces, such as lack of affordable housing, and individual factors. Homeless women also reflect the demographic changes seen across the general homeless population, and furthermore are part of the fastest-growing segment of this population. Since 1984 there has been a 180% increase in the number of homeless women, and the number of shelter families has quadrupled nationwide.[16]

Most homeless women today are mothers, are under 35 yr of age, are members of a minority group, have often not completed high school, and have usually suffered more than one experience of homelessness in their lifetimes.[17] Burt and Cohen reviewed 28 studies of homeless female populations conducted during the 1980s. They found that women comprised nearly 20% of the homeless, and half were with children and half without children. In total, women, including their children, accounted for about one-third of the total population of homeless individuals.[18]

Prevalence of Alcohol and Illicit Drug Use

Reviewing the literature concerning the prevalence of alcohol and illicit drug use among the current homeless population is complicated by several factors. These include: differences in each site's definition of homelessness, regional differences in the use of substances, different assessment instruments and research methodologies, and the lack of attention given to sub-groups of the population, such as women and ethnic minorities.[17,20] However, some recent reviews have taken these issues into account.[12,19,21]

Concerning the definition of homelessness, Fischer stated that conventional definitions are based on a lack of a permanent place to live. More broad definitions include marginally housed people and persons at risk for being homeless.[21] The majority of research cited in our review is based on samples found at shelters, clinics, and soup kitchens; and unless otherwise noted, for our review, being homeless in these studies means not having a permanent place to live.

Fischer, covering the period from 1980–1990, cited over 80 studies that used various sampling techniques and assessment methods, such as psychiatric examinations, self-report, records review, and standardized instruments. These studies provided an extremely wide range of prevalence estimates for the general homeless population: Thus alcohol problems ranged from 4–86%, and drug problems ranged from 1–70%. Not surprisingly, there were clear regional differences in these studies. Alcohol use was higher in the West, and other drug use was higher in the Northeast.[21] However, more research is needed to determine whether these trends are basically an artifact of sampling differences.

In trying to arrive at meaningful, general prevalence estimates of drug and alcohol use among the homeless population, Fischer computed the median of the prevalence estimates from what she considered to be technically sound studies and concluded that about one-third of the present homeless population (37% for males and 17% for females) suffers from an alcohol problem. Using this same procedure, she estimated that about one-quarter of the population (23% for males and 26% for females) suffers from an illicit drug problem.[21]

Fischer pointed to these differential rates for alcohol abuse across genders in order to emphasize the fallacy of lumping men and women together when considering the needs of the homeless population. She asserts that few studies have attempted to differentiate prevalence rates between genders, even though such breakdowns are vital for projecting and implementing an enlightened policy for the needs of homeless persons.[21] These and other policy issues will be discussed in a later section.

We get a somewhat different range of estimates from McCarty et al., who stated that alcohol and drug abuse appears to be highest in samples drawn from shelters, streets, and clinics. They added that data from the Health Care for the Homeless project show that 47% of homeless men and 16% of homeless women can be classified as problem drinkers, and drug abuse is as high as 11% for men and 9% for women.[13] Dockett et al. report in their review that alcohol problems affect between 3 and 36% of homeless women, and illicit drug problems affect between 3 and 26%. These researchers later made the medians of these ranges available.[19] Table 1, which presents data provided by Dockett based on her research, displays the median prevalence estimates of alcohol, drug, and mental health problems among homeless females and males.

Generally speaking, homeless men are more likely to use alcohol than homeless women. However, when it comes to illicit drug use, no significant differences can be found across genders; about the same proportion of homeless men and homeless women use drugs. In addition, Fischer and Breakey reported that illicit drug users are more likely to abuse alcohol in addition to drugs, whereas drinkers are less likely to abuse drugs in addition to alcohol.[12] It is also of some interest that McCarty et al. found a strong negative correlation between nonalcoholic drug use and age in the homeless population: The younger the person, the less likely he or she is to use alcohol exclusively as opposed to other illicit drugs.[13]

Alcohol and drug problems seem to have a more severe impact on the homeless population than on the general population. Robertson pointed out that studies have shown alcohol and drug use to be an important contributing factor to homelessness, and that alcohol and drug use is more prevalent among homeless populations than among the general population.[22] Fischer and Breakey suggested that alcohol is the most pervasive health problem of the homeless overall; homeless adults abuse alcohol at six or seven times the rate of the general population. Also, alcoholism in the homeless tends to be of a more severe nature, in that homeless people may have a greater duration, regularity, frequency, amount, and symptoms of alcohol dependence.[12]

Compared to homeless men, homeless women may exhibit signs of more severe substance abuse as expressed in more intensive polydrug use and more devastating physical and social consequences.[21] Also, Fischer and Breakey reported one study that found that female heads of homeless families were more than twice as likely to be alcohol abusers than a comparison group of housed, indigent women.[12] Table 2 illustrates the findings from four recent studies done specifically on homeless women. These studies represent a cross-section of current research efforts. From these four studies, it appears that the female homeless population has gotten younger over time, is comprised mostly of minorities, and now includes a significant number of women with children.

Significance of Gender Differences in Alcohol Use

The higher incidence of alcohol usage among homeless males reflects the same trend found in the general population: Men drink more than women. The gender differences are similar across ethnic groups, although the dif-

Table 1

Prevalence Estimates of Alcohol, Drug, and Mental Health Problems Among Homeless Female and Male Populations in the 1980s[a]

Gender	Alcohol		Drug		Mental Health	
	Number of samples	Median % prevalence	Number of samples	Median % prevalence	Number of samples	% Prevalence
Woman	24[b]	14.5	13	16.7	28	44.5
Men	14	37.5	7	22.0	15	30.5

[a]Provided by Kathleen Dockett upon request from the authors.
[b]Studies reporting combined alcohol and drug use, or use of prescribed and illicit drugs were excluded from this analysis.

Table 2
Major Demographic Characteristics from Four Recent Studies
Conducted with Homeless Women and Their Children

Researchers	N	Origin of sample	Mean age	Ethnicity	Children	Substance use	Psychiatric history
Bassuk et al.[28]	80	Family shelters	27	48% White 45% Black 6% Latino	66% under 5 yr old	Alcohol 8% Drug 9%	25% axis I diagnosis 71% axis II diagnosis
Mercier et al.[39]	158	Rehabilitation agency	31	95% White	33% in foster care	Alcohol 7% Drug 11.4%	33% previous psychiatric hospitalization
Sullivan and Damrosch[15]	105	Full-service center for homeless persons	28.4	59% minorities	40% had one or more dependent children	Substance abuse 50%	32% exhibited psychiatric symptoms
Chiacone and Anderson[16]	50	Shelter	30	100% Black	Median of 3 children per subejct, non-custodial mothers	36% using substances	18% history of mental illness

ference is smaller for Blacks than for Whites.[23] These differences appear to reflect societal attitudes toward the use of alcohol among men and women.

Compared to men, women are much less likely to have been exposed to alcohol during adolescence. Women seem to believe that drunkenness is more socially disapproved for themselves than for men. Furthermore, women's expectations about the effect alcohol will have on them may result in increased rather than decreased distress. For men, alcohol provides an accepted way for them to socialize. Garrett and Bahr noted that male alcoholics outnumbered females by five to one, social disapproval for alcohol intake was greater for females, and homeless men were believed to be more likely to drink in groups and to have more social contacts than homeless women.[9] Heavier drinking exemplifies an unconventional, risk-taking style that is not only accepted, but expected, in men.[23] More men than women report using alcohol to relieve tension, and this gender difference remains after accounting for the socioeconomic status of the respondents: 29 vs 16%; and men were more than twice as likely to use alcohol only: 16% of men vs 6% of women (Parry et al. 1974, cited in Biener, 1987).[23,24]

Correlates of Homelessness and Substance Abuse

Mental Health Problems

Researchers have discovered various prevalence rates for mental illness in the homeless population, ranging from 28–37%.[25] Fischer and Breakey added that homeless people showed signs of emotional distress between two and eight times more frequently than the general population across a number of studies.[12] Generally, research findings suggest that up to one-third of all homeless people have some type of severe mental illness.[21,25] In an analysis by gender, Fischer found that mental health problems affect about a quarter to a third of all homeless men and about a third to a half of all homeless women.[21]

Persons suffering from both a substance use problem and a psychiatric disorder are said to be dually diagnosed. Koegel and Burnam have found that homeless individuals in Los Angeles with alcohol problems cannot be neatly separated from those having other psychiatric disorders.[26] Nonetheless, several studies have presented a relatively high rate of dual diagnosis in the homeless population. Fischer and Breakey reviewed several studies and found that up to 28% of all homeless people have a dual diagnosis of alcohol or illicit drug use in combination with another mental health problem.[12] Drake et al. estimated that between 10 and 20% of the homeless population could be given a dual diagnosis. These authors stated that dually diagnosed homeless individuals are more likely to be older, male, and unemployed than are homeless adults with a single or no diagnosis.[27] This finding contrasts with research reported by Koegel and Burnam, who reported that older White males were the predominant members of a "pure" alcohol use group, who had no other diagnosis. Instead, dually diagnosed, alcohol-using clients in Koegel and Burnam's study were more likely to be younger and female. In this study, drug abuse or dependence was considered to be another psychiatric diagnosis.[26] The reasons for these different findings could be owing to a number of different factors: regional sampling differences, defining substance abuse itself as a psychiatric disorder, and/or counting the frequency of psychiatric hospitalizations to determine a person's psychiatric history. For example, older homeless individuals, who lived before the age of deinstitutionalization, might be more apt to be labeled mentally ill based on having been in an institution for their substance use problem.

With regard to dual diagnosis concerns specifically in homeless women, many studies report a higher rate of mental illness in homeless women than in homeless men. In studies conducted over the past decade, up to 71% of women (and up to 52% of men) have been diagnosed with some form of mental health problem.[12] In addition, evidence for a true gender difference in mental illness is limited so far, and any difference may be disorder-specific.[12] For example, one study reviewed by Fischer and Breakey found equivalent rates across gender for mental illness in general and unipolar depression in particular, but women showed twice as much schizophrenia and bipolar disorder (manic-depression) as men.[12] Such differences are, however, difficult to explain.

Two studies focusing exclusively on homeless women provide specific accounts of the instances of mental illness in their clients. Bassuk et al. studied 80 homeless women living in city shelters and found that 44% had contact with the mental health system at some point. However, perhaps unlike those populations who are homeless because of recent deinstitutionalization from psychiatric hospitals, only 8% were diagnosed as being schizophrenic or mentally retarded.[28] In their study of 50 noncustodial (no longer living with one or more of their children) homeless mothers, Chiacone and Anderson found that 18% had a history of mental illness, and 12% of these clients were also substance users.[16]

Compared to investigations of mental illness and alcoholism, little effort has been made to examine the relationship between mental illness and illicit drug use in the contemporary homeless population.[21] One possible reason for this apparent lack of effort could be that mental illness and substance use get studied by different agencies that do not engage in cooperative research efforts. In order to learn more about homeless persons diagnosed with an illicit drug use problem as well as a mental health problem, researchers need to differentiate substance use from other psychiatric disorders such as depression or psychosis.

We think that the foregoing information on dual diagnosis should be interpreted with caution for other reasons as well. Diagnostic labeling in general tends to exaggerate the degree of psychopathology and does not take into account the extremely stressful extrinsic variables faced by the homeless.[28] Also, Drake et al. listed three particularly difficult obstacles to assessing the mental health status of dually diagnosed homeless people: definition of the problem, appropriate assessment, and the heterogeneous nature of the population.[27]

Lastly, Bassuk et al. asserted that today's economic and political climate fosters the increasing trend of homeless shelters becoming permanent institutions with their own bureaucracy and vested self-interests. The authors cautioned us that these shelters may turn into mini-institutions that are more poorly staffed and provide less care than the old ones did. Unfortunately, it seems that today's homeless shelters have become "open asylums" (Bassuk et al., p. 1549) to replace the mental institutions of decades ago.[29]

Other Problems Associated with Homelessness and Substance Use

Ropers and Boyer considered the condition of homelessness itself to be a health risk; when substance use is added to this picture, the consequences are even more disconcerting.[30] In addition to mental illness, there are other significant health risks typically associated with substance-using homeless persons. With regard to medical concerns, homeless people who abuse alcohol or drugs are up to twice as likely as nonabusing homeless people to have medical problems such as liver disease, seizure disorders, pulmonary and arterial disease, and nutritional deficiencies.[13] Ropers and Boyer reported that the most common health problem faced by their homeless clients is hypertension. Homeless persons are also at increased risk for such problems as influenza, colds, bronchitis, and tuberculosis.[30]

Homeless alcohol and drug users are also disaffiliated to a greater degree than nonusing homeless individuals. Disaffiliation is a term used by Bahr to denote the fact that homeless people have fallen through the web of social relationships that connect most people with others.[31] Also, homeless substance users have been homeless for longer periods of time, are more likely to have arrest histories, and are victimized to a greater degree than homeless nonusers. Homeless drug users are more likely to report using the more damaging, or "hard," drugs like cocaine, crack, and heroin compared to nonhomeless users. Homeless drug users are much more likely to gain income from illegal activities compared to other homeless persons. They are also more transient and sleep "rougher" than do other homeless persons.[21] Also, homeless alcoholics tend to have fewer occupational skills than nonhomeless alcoholics.[12]

Homeless women face additional problems, such as suffering from more recent injuries and acute illnesses as compared to homeless men; and they also have more chronic health problems.[17] Fischer and Breakey have pointed out that the high levels of intravenous drug use and prostitution among homeless women are linked to various sexually transmitted diseases.[12]

With regard to violence and abuse, homeless women are much more likely than housed women to have experienced abuse (physical and sexual) or other traumatic events as children. Several different studies indicate that 22–66% of homeless women have been battered, 31–33% have been sexually molested as children, and perhaps over 40% have been or are being physically abused.[17]

Family Issues

The literature on homeless men does not really address any family issues in any depth, beyond giving demographic descriptions of the number of children fathered by homeless men. Therefore, in this section we will deal exclusively with research on homeless women. When considering the existing research on homeless women and their children, it is difficult to generalize across the wide variations that exist in samples and assessment methods. Despite the paucity of information available regarding homeless families, it is generally believed that young children, mostly minorities cared for in mother-only households, are the fastest growing element of the homeless population.[15,22]

Robertson concluded that there is insufficient empirical evidence available to generate a reliable prevalence estimate for alcohol and drug use among homeless women with children.[22] However, trends in the available findings suggest that homeless women with children use less alcohol and illicit drugs than do homeless men or homeless women without children. However, substance use among homeless women with children appears to be higher than among poor, housed women with children. Overall, Robertson believed that homeless women with dependent children are a distinctive subgroup among the homeless population, with lower rates of substance use and other related problems.[22]

Dockett et al. estimated that fewer homeless mothers have alcohol problems compared to homeless women without children (12 vs 31%), and fewer mothers suffer from mental illness than homeless women without children, although there appears to be no difference between these groups in drug use (10 vs 9%).[19] Furthermore, homeless women with children are less likely than those without children to have been homeless for a prolonged period of time.[17]

Additionally, substance use is associated with the following family-related risks for homeless women: increased sexual risk-taking and the possibility of sexually transmitted diseases (STD); prenatal drug and STD exposure and a lack of prenatal care; neglect, abandonment, and violence toward children related to the mother's depleted material resources and mood swings; and expulsion from social programs and service-providing agencies.[22]

Social and Family Support Networks

Homeless women have weaker social support networks in general than do housed women, and homeless women rarely have the support of a spouse: Between 78 and 98% of women in shelter samples have never been married.[17] Homeless women have more disruptions in their social support network than do homeless men. These disruptions include failed marriages and being raised in an institutional or foster-care setting.[17,32] Robertson added that losing custody of her children to foster care automatically decreased a homeless woman's support network as well as her financial resources (usually public assistance).[22]

Shinn et al. compared the social relationships of 495 poor, housed mothers with 677 recently homeless mothers in New York City.[32] The authors observed that the family networks of homeless women often provided considerable support and served as a safety net, although homeless women typically taxed their networks to the point of exhaustion. The authors concluded that homelessness generally derived from poverty and a lack of available housing rather than weak social ties, although weak social ties did create a vulnerability to becoming homeless.

Homeless Children

Although research on homeless women and their children is just beginning to emerge, even less is known about homeless children themselves. Although there is a growing interest in homeless children, little attention has been paid to them as a separate subgroup of the homeless population.[16]

Homeless pregnant women are among the groups at highest risk for low birthweight babies and infant mortality.[15] Homeless children may suffer significant impairment in cognitive and language development, as well as increased stress and depression.[16,33] Bassuk and her colleagues in Massachusetts have done much of the research in this area. One follow-up study conducted on homeless preschoolers found that approximately half of the 48 children in a Boston shelter exhibited at least one serious impairment in language, social skills, or motor development, as compared to 16% of the 75 low-income, housed preschoolers.[34] In another investigation with pre-school children, Bassuk and Rubin found that sleep problems, shyness, and aggression were more common in homeless children (3–5 yr old) than in a control group of emotionally disturbed children.[35]

Lastly, Chiacone and Anderson asked 50 noncustodial mothers in Washington, DC about their children being separated from them.[16] They found that 36% of the mothers were homeless with their children prior to being separated from them. Also, 82% said the separation was a voluntary choice (as opposed to foster care), 78% said that a lack of affordable hous-ing prevented them from being with their children, 28% listed a lack of income as the cause of their separation, and 18% listed substance abuse as the cause. Despite these separations, however, over half the mothers in the study managed to see their children at least once a month.

Research Problems and Issues

Barriers to Effective Research

We have already mentioned many of the obstacles that present them-selves when comparing the results of several different studies conducted on various subgroups of the homeless population. Now, we narrow our focus and examine the challenges that present themselves when conducting any *one* study on this population.

Although homeless alcoholics comprise no more than 5% of the entire alcoholic population, they have been the most studied subgroup of alcohol-ics over the last 50 yr.[36] Garrett has listed several reasons for this phenom-enon: The homeless alcoholic reflects an alcoholism in its most dramatic form, thus making this condition an obvious focus; skid row and its institutions have served as field laboratories in which sociologists can test their theo-ries; the homeless have been easily located for study; and the basic human and moral concern motivating the researchers of this subpopulation.[3]

However, despite the popularity of homeless substance users as research subjects, conducting productive, reliable research on homeless persons has proven to be difficult for many reasons. Dockett et al. lamented that although research in the previous decade had indeed reflected the growing socioeco-nomic diversity of the homeless population, most studies had been largely de-scriptive and lacking the scientific rigor needed to propel research forward.[19]

Fischer and Breakey outlined the methodological pitfalls associated with "fugitive" studies, which are regional surveys that sacrifice rigorous design on behalf of expedient assessment of the needs of the local homeless population.[12] Robertson listed these common problems in research on the substance use patterns of homeless persons: Cross-sectional studies over-represent those who have been homeless for longer periods of time, thereby overestimating the prevalence of alcohol and illicit drug problems; there is a lack of standardized instruments to measure alcohol and illicit drug use, and there is also a failure to distinguish among various kinds of drugs.[22] Koegel and Burnam further warned that researchers are often led astray by making intuitive modifications, rather than empirically based modifications, on standard measures of mental illness that are redesigned for study of homeless persons in particular.[37]

Nemes cautioned us about the systematic bias introduced by data derived from treatment centers, since these sites consistently underrepresent certain groups, such as women and Hispanics.[38] She warned that empirical research in the area of substance use is characterized by two significant flaws: Most of it has been conducted primarily with men and then generalized to women, and it generally takes the form of survey research that may omit certain groups, and lump other groups together that are potentially distinct along critical dimensions, such as gender, ethnicity, and religious values.[21,38]

Caution must also be used when attempting to generalize findings from a clinical, or treatment, sample to the larger population of homeless persons. Researchers must be cognizant of the differences implicit between these two groups: Why do some homeless substance users seek treatment and not others? It is very important that researchers make this distinction between purely epidemiological studies and research with homeless persons seeking specific services.

Follow-up studies on homeless substance users are notoriously difficult to execute because the client's condition often fluctuates so drastically in short periods of time that no "level of current functioning" variable adequately captures the many and subtle transitions experienced.[39] Furthermore, research assignment itself can be a precipitating factor in client attrition; random assignment restricts the ability of treatment programs to engage the clients fully in recovery, and the mandate of treatment programs to connect their clients with other social services poses threats to the internal validity of the research. Mercier et al. added that client attrition has made experimental and quasi-experimental designs almost impossible to use, so that most projects now utilize within-group controls or employ pre/post designs.[39]

Future Research Needs

Several investigators have voiced concern over the future direction of research with the homeless population, and the subgroups therein. With regard to general research needs, Fischer and Breakey pointed out that cross-sectional designs over the past decade have not permitted the examination of directional effects in the relationship between homelessness and alcohol, drug, and mental illness problems.[12] Dennis et al. recommended that future research with homeless persons proceed along two fronts: the establishment of longitudinal research designs with representative samples, and the development of designs that consider the needs and problems of women, ethnic and racial minorities, homeless families with children, and homeless adolescents.[25,38] Drake et al. added that future research must focus on assessment validity, quantitative methods, longitudinal studies, prevention, housing, client engagement, and assessing treatment implementation and utilization.[27] From these many voices, general themes begin to emerge: the pressing need for longitudinal research, movement beyond an epidemiological focus, and the need to study subgroups of the homeless population.

More specifically, Mercier et al. believed that studies assessing the effectiveness of substance abuse treatment for homeless persons should be less concerned with program objectives (such as sobriety) and more concerned with the conditions associated with attainment of those objectives (such as housing, services, and so forth).[39] They also recommended that treatment effectiveness studies carefully control for participation in the program, use living conditions as indicators of success, and consider how the service system changes to meet the needs of the community. In addition, Jones et al. stressed that more attention should be paid to the racial, cultural, and ethnic background of the participants when research programs are designed.[20]

Blasi pointed out that much additional research remains to be conducted on how images of homelessness are communicated through the mass media, on the determinants of attitudes of ordinary citizens and policy makers toward the homeless, and on the determinants of success or failure of organized advocacy.[40] He asserted that we have reached a plateau in terms of our epidemiological and demographic knowledge, and that we must adopt a broader focus, which examines the various levels of scorn many people feel for the poor—from the concern for families and the mentally ill, to disgust and rejection toward the single, unemployed male.

The female homeless population is a subgroup presenting unique barriers to effective research. Dockett et al. called attention to the need for studies that examine the patterns of substance use among homeless women and how these patterns differ for homeless men.[19] Additionally, most research studies of homeless females concentrate on women in shelters and therefore miss an important, growing section of the female homeless population that does not utilize the shelter system.[22] Milburn and D'Ercole observed that because many different treatment facilities do not accept homeless women with children, we know little about the effects of keeping children, or of being separated from children, during the recovery process.[17] They added that we lack subjective and objective measures of how homeless women appraise and cope with the many stressors in their lives, and that there are no studies examining how women cope with stress before and after they become homeless.

Treatment Issues

Although there is a considerable and growing body of literature on the prevalence of substance use and mental illness in the homeless population, relatively little has been written about the specific treatment strategies required to help homeless persons with addiction or mental illness. One of the more recent efforts to address the program needs of homeless families comes from Bassuk et al.[41] The reader is referred to their "Community Care of Homeless Families: A Program Design Manual," which gives an in-depth, descriptive account of how to design programs for several different subgroups of homeless persons.[41]

Breakey has identified several special issues to be considered when designing a treatment plan for homeless people, who often have a great distrust of authority and a disenchantment with service providers.[42] In many cases, they have had bad previous experiences with agencies or health services. Breakey asserted that working with this population is made more complex by the multiplicity of needs that they face, such as a need for medical care, housing, substance abuse treatment, psychological services, and vocational counseling. Also, homeless persons face extraordinary stigma and bias within the service community. Among health service providers, homeless people are generally not considered "good patients." Additionally, there is a general bias permeating our society regarding the "unworthiness" of poor people: Poverty is often attributed to a character flaw or to some moral or spiritual deficit. We will discuss this issue in more detail in the policy section.

Homeless people themselves are clear about their hierarchy of needs. Ball and Havassy listed the expressed needs of San Francisco homeless people diagnosed as mentally ill.[43] The rank-ordered perception of their needs included: affordable housing, financial entitlements, employment, and free-time activities. Interestingly, substance abuse treatment was far down on the list, ranked sixth out of ten expressed needs, immediately after food. Mental health services came next to last under "interpersonal skills," and after money management. This suggests that encouraging treatment in this group may be quite difficult.

Treating the Homeless Substance User

McLellan et al. have provided evidence for the effectiveness of traditional substance abuse treatment in facilitating measurable gains for their nonhomeless clients along several dimensions, including substance use, employment, and psychological functioning.[44,45] However, traditional treatment programs may not be effective for the homeless substance user because they typically do not actively recruit clients, provide continuity of care and support, or facilitate re-entry into the community.[13] Also, treatment facilities serving homeless persons concentrate on creating environments rather than instituting treatment.[27]

Shipley et al. made these observations regarding the treatment of homeless alcoholics: Any treatment is preferable to no treatment, although no consistently superior treatment model has been established; those researchers reporting the importance of individual differences for substance use treatment are generally pessimistic about the possibility of treating the homeless on an outpatient basis; many homeless alcoholics ride the "revolving door," leaving shortly after detoxification and returning later for more detoxification; long-term residential treatment, preferably at least 4 wk in length, is required for the homeless and socially deteriorated alcoholic; treatment success may be related to the quality and success of social relationships; and long-term, intensive treatment is feasible on an outpatient basis if the person's living conditions are stabilized and supportive of the treatment process.[46]

There has been some controversy around the question of whether inpatient alcoholism treatment is more effective than outpatient treatment. In their review of 26 controlled studies, Miller and Hester concluded that there was no overall advantage for residential over nonresidential treatment for those clients who had stable marriages and fewer years of problem drinking.[47] However, these researchers reported that the more severe and less socially stable alcoholics seemed to fare better in inpatient (or more intensive) treatment. To what degree these observations regarding homeless alcoholics also pertain to homeless drug users, or to the dually diagnosed, remains to be determined within future treatment and research projects.

Mercier et al. made these recommendations for planning programs for the treatment of homeless alcohol and illicit drug users, based on their 3-yr follow-up study of this clientele: facilities must provide essential relief (such as food and shelter) first and foremost; it is very difficult to modify one person's individual trend toward deterioration; and special support must be provided for caregivers and workers who are themselves supports in the lives of the clients.[39] Their findings suggest that longer stays in treatment, and more readmissions to treatment, were positive indicators of recovery at 1-yr follow-up.

Treating Homeless Women

Comfort et al. noted that women in particular have been seeking treatment for cocaine in increasing numbers over recent years.[48] In their study of 66 homeless, substance-using mothers, the authors found that almost every mother had at least one prior admission for alcohol and/or illicit drug treatment. They pointed to an urgent need for family-oriented treatment approaches that concurrently address cocaine addiction, homelessness, family relationships, parenting, and social support issues.

Additionally, homeless women with children have special programmatic needs that must be taken into account by shelters and treatment facilities, such as parenting skills training, nutritional education, budgeting, housekeeping, and vocational education.[13] Robertson cited these barriers to effective treatment for homeless, substance-using women who have children: inadequate number of alcohol and illicit drug treatment programs willing to treat women with their children; refusal of these programs to enroll pregnant women; treatment programs are not always prepared to handle the polysubstance abuse and dual-diagnosis problems that are more common to female homeless populations; and the lack of housing that makes it difficult to maintain outpatient treatment.[22]

Penn et al. outlined a model of treatment for homeless, substance-using mothers that focused on the utilization of the indigenous resources of communities and families.[49] They proposed this model because agencies have been slow in responding to the homelessness and substance use crisis. Their model consists of three steps: developing and nurturing within the recovering person a sense of hope; reintegrating the homeless client into her family and community of origin; and developing skills and coping strategies for long-term recovery.

Treatment for the Dually Diagnosed Homeless Person

The additional factor of psychiatric problems must also be taken into account when providing treatment for the homeless substance user. Sullivan and Damrosch conducted a study on 105 homeless women in a residential treatment center and found that 35% had previous inpatient treatment for psychiatric problems, whereas 14% had received previous outpatient help for psychiatric problems.[15] And Comfort et al. reported that 97% of their detoxification clients, 77% of their outpatient clients, and 87% of their residential clients reported having some combination of these psychiatric symptoms: depression, anxiety, hallucinations, and suicidal thoughts.[48]

Several authors have recognized the additional treatment burdens faced by homeless clients who are also dually diagnosed. Much more must be learned about effective treatment and management of the dually diagnosed homeless person.[13] Treatment providers must overcome community resistance to program sites, the difficulty in engaging clients in treatment, and the reluctance of staff and family members to accept the challenge of pursuing treatment for these clients.

Drake et al. looked at several projects funded by the National Institute of Mental Health (NIMH) over the past 5 yr to serve dually diagnosed homeless people.[27] The combined wisdom of these projects include these most important needs for dually diagnosed clients: All aspects of treatment (counseling, social services, placement services) must be thoroughly integrated; intense case management is required; group treatment has proven beneficial; the four phases of treatment are engagement, persuasion, active treatment, and relapse prevention; clients need substitute/alternative activities; cultural issues are extremely relevant; job training is crucial; and treatment for families, and family involvement in treatment, is becoming increasingly important. The authors concluded that programs that do not treat both the substance use and the mental illness may not be able to sufficiently treat either problem.

The DRC Studies

In this subsection, we will present some findings from our completed project with homeless, substance-using mothers and our current work with homeless men. We will discuss research as well as treatment issues within the framework of our experience with these two projects.

In Philadelphia, the Diagnostic and Rehabiliation Center (DRC) has conducted an investigation of homeless, substance-using mothers supported by the National Institute of Alcohol Abuse and Alcoholism (NIAAA). This project, dubbed FORM (Families of Recovering Mothers), was summarized in an early progress report and in a final technical report.[48,50] In this study, 198 homeless women seeking treatment for substance use were randomly divided into a residential (145 clients) or nonresidential (53) treatment group. The original research design called for between-group comparisons of residential vs nonresidential clients, but this proved to be impossible owing to the high percentage of homeless women who never completed the referral process once they discovered that housing would not be made available to them. Because of the high attrition rate of the nonresidential group, only findings related to the residential group will be addressed here.

The residential women fit the profile of the new homeless in that their average age was 26 yr and 95% were Black. The FORM residents had used an average of three drugs on a regular basis prior to treatment; a total of 78% of the women reported regular use of crack and 42% reported extended histories of cocaine use (other than crack). In addition, 32% also reported extended use of intoxicating amounts of alcohol.

The second investigation recently undertaken at the DRC, also funded by NIAAA, began with homeless men in April 1991. The two research populations are not directly comparable, however, owing to the fact that the women came to the DRC for substance use treatment, whereas the men are recruited into the research project when they arrive at one of the major homeless shelters in Philadelphia. Once recruited, they are assessed at a baseline interview and then randomly assigned to one of three treatment groups. These groups vary in degrees of structure and length of residential stay. As of May 1992, over 1400 men have been initially screened, and 550 of these men have received a baseline interview and have been randomized into one of the three treatment groups. Of the men randomized into treatment groups, the average age of these men is 33 yr, and 92% are Black. A total of 75% of participants reported a problem with cocaine or crack, and 18% reported having a problem with alcohol. We are also witnessing high attrition rates in our current work with homeless men in Philadelphia, although it is too early to draw conclusions here.

A large percentage of the female residents in the FORM study reported that they suffered a variety of psychiatric symptoms in their lifetimes as well as in the 30 d before the interview. Since these homeless mothers were in the research project to receive treatment for substance use, those reporting psychiatric problems would be dually diagnosable. In our current research with homeless men, we have gathered some preliminary figures on the incidence of psychiatric problems. These data are presented in Table 3, showing the prevalence of psychiatric symptoms by gender.

Our Philadelphia women's project encountered several problems related to the research design. The research design called for a follow-up interview for all clients 6 mo after leaving the residence. However, locating these women after their exit from the residence proved to be extremely difficult; letters and phone calls to the clients themselves or to other agencies also involved with the clients proved largely unsuccessful. Maintaining contact with an informed family member turned out to be the most effective way of keeping abreast of a client's whereabouts. We offer this advice, based on our experience with FORM, for following up clients in treatment outcome studies: Schedule interviews at neutral sites, rather than at the client's home in order to lessen the risk of stigmatization; begin follow-up procedures as soon as the clients first enter treatment; establish as much personal contact between clients and follow-up staff as possible; and understand that it probably takes several months to establish the trust and network of family communication typically required to maintain contact with this population.

Table 3

Lifetime and Recent Rates of Psychiatric Symptoms
for the Female and Male Homeless Populations Studied by the DRC

	Lifetime				Last 30 d			
	Depression	Anxiety	Nondrug-induced hallucinations	Suicide attempt	Depression	Anxiety	Nondrug-induced hallucinations	Suicide attempt
Women	67%	37%	26%	40%	50%	38%	7%	4%
Men	65%	62%	9%	14%	63%	58%	4%	3%

With regard to the DRC's experience in treating the 145 homeless women who were randomized into the residential treatment group in the NIAAA-funded study, 63% of these women did receive shelter and other services for at least a short period of time.[50] In the majority of cases the residence proved to be a temporary solution to the clients' homelessness. Only 9% of the 92 residential clients moved into their own homes or into cohabitation with their partners on exiting the residence, whereas 64% moved in with extended family and 15% moved into another homeless shelter.

The substance-use treatment component of the project appeared to be somewhat more successful.[50] Almost none of the women who were interviewed 6 mo after exiting the residence reported using alcohol or illicit drugs in the 30 d prior to the interview. However, these findings should be interpreted with caution owing to several factors, such as possible selection and social desirability biases, as well as the fact that 37% of the women had undergone further substance use treatment at some point during the 6 mo after leaving the residence.

Common themes emerged from the circumstances of female clients who did relapse, from which a list of important treatment issues can be culled: A larger and more established repertoire of social and emotional coping skills would have been invaluable to these clients for dealing with stressful circumstances that typically preceded relapse, and clients should be clearly told that professional services are available immediately and without reproach should relapse occur.[50]

Multiple regression analyses on the data from the DRC's project revealed that five factors measured within the initial weeks of placement in the residence significantly predicted the length of time that residents would remain in treatment at the shelter ($p = .0003$): lifetime cocaine use, lifetime alcohol use, positive mood and negative mood at the time of interview, and the number of close friends reported.[51] Interestingly, a longer history of both cocaine and alcohol use predicted a longer stay in treatment; perhaps the deleterious effects of substance use gradually convince the women to remain committed to treatment, or perhaps long-term users simply run out of options and resources beyond the homeless shelter. Having a larger network of close friends predicted a significantly shorter stay in treatment. Also, both highly positive and highly negative moods were associated with shorter stays in treatment.

Finally, we would like to report briefly on those children ($N = 21$) born to mothers while in residence. Only 12 hospitals responded to requests for infant birth records. The average birth weight, head circumference, and length of these 12 newborns were almost at the 50th percentile on standardized growth charts.[52] None of the babies born to mothers in residence were categorized as high risk medically, and all of the 21 children were discharged from the hospital within 3 d after birth. We believe that this is an impressive record, and in view of the problems often found for the children of cocaine-addicted mothers may well have saved considerable sums of money for each day the infants did not spend in the intensive care unit. Clearly this experience warrants further exploration of this potentially important outcome.

Policy Issues and Recommendations

General Concerns

Owing to space considerations, we will only briefly touch on the thorny area of policy issues relevant to meeting the needs of male and female homeless substance users. Many of the recommendations discussed here have been given before.[10] Unfortunately, many of these recommendations have still not been put into effect, so that researchers and treatment planners continue to voice them.

The issue of community attitudes toward homeless people has received relatively little attention.[40] This issue has important implications for policy, because government representatives are obviously influenced by the attitudes of their constituents. A 1988 national opinion poll found that the public has a much more harsh response to homeless persons who use alcohol and illicit drugs than to those who do not.[53] Somehow, the members of the larger, housed community assume that they can accurately attribute responsibility for the plight of homeless individuals. However, a great deal of research consistently shows that problems of causality are extremely complicated, and accurate assignment of responsibility is obviously difficult to make.

As mentioned previously, the housed community's attitudes toward homeless single men are much less charitable than the attitudes toward women and families. Peter Marin, in an article in *The Nation*, made a compelling observation on this point:

> Imagine walking down a street and passing a group of homeless women. Do we not spontaneously see them as victims and wonder what has befallen them, how destiny has injured them? Do we not see them as unfortunate and deserving of help and want to help them?

> Now imagine a group of homeless men. Is our reaction the same? Is it as sympathetic? Or is it subtly different? Do we have the same impulse to help and protect? Or do we not wonder, instead of what befell them, how they have got themselves where they are? (p. 48)[54]

This disparity is unfortunate, because the majority of homeless persons are young minority males.

Dennis et al. highlighted the need for investigators to be sensitive to macrolevel forces, such as economic forces, lack of employment and housing, as well as individual-level forces that contribute to client homelessness.[25] Shore and Cohen further suggested that the mental health authority must become a producer of housing for the homeless.[55] Particularly in urban areas, there is a need for a central authority for the homeless mentally ill, since state hospitals no longer provide support. People with chronic mental illness, particularly schizophrenia, also have social disabilities that make it hard to maintain a home.

Sullivan and Damrosch described the general havoc created by the deinstitutionalization of the mentally ill, and the recent underinstitutionalization of those in need of psychiatric treatment, as major precipitants of homelessness.[15] In addition, they list these policy factors as being particularly relevant to homeless women: reproductive control and motherhood; sexual exploitation and violence; shortage of shelter space; incarceration in lieu of institutionalization for mental health problems; and social stigma. Robertson listed these policy concerns of special relevance to homeless mothers with children: the tension between women's rights and children's/fetal rights; criminalization vs treatment for substance users; and the lack of treatment programs tailored to the needs of homeless women with children.[22]

Our Observations and Recommendations

Until there are clear, workable policies at the federal, state, and local levels, the current problem of homelessness will continue to exist and probably get worse. In spite of the millions of dollars made available, there is no sense that the agencies theoretically responsible for such a complex problem really are geared toward developing workable solutions. This population does not represent, nor has it historically represented a high priority for government agencies; and the perception that the homeless or incipient homeless do not vote clearly reduces the problem to one of less than critical concern for government officials.

In terms of funding for programs, public dollars are available, but they are available on a competitive basis, which may or may not direct the money to where it is needed most. Therefore, this money is not problem-focused but limited to the particular area of concern projected by the funding agency. We end up having a reworking of the old tale of the three blind men and the elephant: a political blind man and the elephant of homelessness.

The skid row of the past tended to be geographically limited, so that documenting populations was comparatively easy. However, the lack of a specific and geographically limited skid row today makes counting the homeless difficult, which in turn makes for a lack of effective planning.

It is also evident that workable policies are needed at the national and local levels. At the national level the issues of race, economic development, evaluation, abortion, housing, mental health, and substance use are all component parts of addressing the issues that relate to homelessness. At this time there is no coordinated effort that is sensitive to the interrelationship of these diverse issues and therefore there is no real national policy.

At the local level in various parts of the country, efforts to respond to the issue of homelessness have been successful in only a small, limited way. What does it take with regard to policy to make local efforts work? The following is based on recommendations the DRC has made to the City of Philadelphia.

1. The local government must view the problem of homelessness as a high priority and want to do something about it. Without this obvious-sounding cornerstone, there is little chance of success.

2. Centralize authority and accountability. There is a need for a "czar" to give direction to and ensure cooperation among the city departments of Health, Human Services, and Housing. The responsibility would be a full-time job, if each city is to develop and implement a long-range plan to resolve the problem. The czar must be of sufficient stature to negotiate with key state and federal agencies on programs of expanded funding and other support.

3. Each city needs to convene a blue-ribbon task force to assist the czar. The task force should include the "movers and shakers" of each city and state—both public and private interests should be represented. The task force should be small enough to be workable and large enough to get things done.

4. Adopt new (or revise the old) state legislation on commitment. The current procedures for involuntary commitment of the mentally ill should be reviewed and made more workable. Procedures for the emergency involuntary commitment of the substance user should be developed. With appropriate safeguards, this process can help the individual. In addition, local police practices should be adopted that recognize there is no private right to reside on public streets.

5. Avoid making "temporary" housing permanent. Emergency shelters should be limited to providing bona fide emergency service. The boarding house game needs further investigation. The city of Philadelphia, for instance, buys a certain number of rooms, of which only a limited supply are available. Therefore, compromises are made. Operators of such marginal facilities lobby politically to lessen the possibility of vacancies in their operations. Overall, greatly increased provisions for affordable permanent housing are needed.

6. Utilize existing resources. Each city's public and private agencies should accept some responsibility for a difficult population that most agencies do not want as clients. The chronically mentally ill should be the responsibility

of the mental health system (which gets much public financial support), whereas the substance user should be treated by those agencies in the alcohol/drug field. Treatment and housing can and must be coordinated.

7. Recognize the racial and political issues. The problem of the "new" poor or homeless has strong racial and political overtones. This is the major new factor in the homelessness situation.
8. Cases must be managed as individuals. Although temporary and permanent housing are important, they are not the answer unless there is a plan, an enhanced system of case management, and service that will increase the probability that those housed will not return to the street. It takes greater time and financial and personnel resources to begin to turn the situation around. However, the alternative of not doing more than is now being done may, in time, be worse.

In Philadelphia and in other cities, there were public policies with regard to clearing skid rows. Because there was a policy that focused on the problem, action did take place. Although the rationale for clearing skid row and working with its inhabitants was primarily economic, programs were initiated and completed. Not every city had programs that served the best interests of the people who inhabited skid row, but those actions indicated the importance of a public policy in addressing the problem.

We can only hope that any public policy regarding the present homeless population will be rational and serve not only the community, but the various mix of people who make up this population.

Acknowledgments

The authors would like to thank Deborah Barron and Alan Fink for their technical assistance in preparing this chapter. Correspondence concerning this article should be addressed to Myra A. Elder, Department of Psychology, 6th Floor Weiss Hall, Temple University, 13th and Cecil B. Moore Ave., Philadelphia, PA 19122.

References

[1] P. H. Rossi (1990) The old homeless and the new homelessness in historical perspective. *Am. Psychol.* **45,** 954–959.

[2] L. Stark (1987) A century of alcohol and homelessness: Demographics and stereotypes. *Alcohol Health Res. World* **11,** 8–13.

[3] G. R. Garrett (1989) Once over lightly: An historical overview of research on alcohol problems and homelessness. Paper presented at the National Conference on Homelessness, Alcohol and Other Drugs, San Diego, CA.

[4] T. Caplow, K. Lovald, and S. Wallace (1958) *A General Report of the Problem of Relocating the Population of the Lower Loop Redevelopment Area.* The Minneapolis Housing and Redevelopment Authority, Minneapolis, MI.

⁵H. Bahr and T. Caplow (1974) *Old Men Drunk and Sober*. New York University Press, New York.

⁶D. Bogue (1963) *Skid Row in American Cities*. University of Chicago, Chicago.

⁷L. Blumberg, T. Shipley, and I. Shandler (1973) *Skid Row and Its Alternatives*. Temple University Press, Philadelphia.

⁸L. Blumberg, F. Hoffman, V. LoCicero, H. Niebuhr, J. Rooney, and T. Shipley (1960) *The Men on Skid Row: A Study of Philadelphia's Homeless Man Population*. Technical report authorized by The Greater Philadelphia Movement and the Redevelopment Authority of the City of Philadelphia.

⁹G. Garrett and H. Bahr (1973) Women on skid row. *Q. J. Stud. Alcohol* **34,** 1228–1243.

¹⁰L. U. Blumberg, T. E. Shipley, and S. F. Barsky (1978) *Liquor and Poverty: Skid Row as a Human Condition*. Rutgers Center of Alcohol Studies, New Brunswick, NJ.

¹¹W. E. B. DuBois (1967) *The Philadelphia Negro: A Social Study*. University of Pennsylvania Series in Political Economy and Public Law, Study No. 14, Schocken (reprint of 1899 ed.), New York.

¹²P. J. Fischer and W. R. Breakey (1991) The epidemiology of alcohol, drug, and mental disorders among homeless persons. *Am. Psychol.* **46,** 1115–1128.

¹³D. McCarty, M. Argeriou, R. Huebner, and B. Lubran (1991) Alcoholism, drug abuse, and the homeless. *Am. Psychol.* **46,** 1139–1148.

¹⁴M. R. Burt and B. E. Cohen (1988) *Feeding the Homeless: Does the Prepared Meals Provision Help?* The Urban Institute, Washington, DC.

¹⁵P. Sullivan and S. Damrosch (1987) Homeless women and children, in *The Homeless in Contemporary Society*. R. Bingham, R. Green, and S. While, eds. Sage, Newbury Park, CA, pp. 82–98.

¹⁶J. Chiacone and E. Anderson (1990) Homeless women in shelters who are separated from their children. Paper presented at a symposium of the Annual Conference of the National Council on Family Relations, Seattle, WA.

¹⁷N. Milburn and A. D'Ercole (1991) Homeless women: moving toward a comprehensive model. *Am. Psychol.* **46,** 1161–1169.

¹⁸M. R. Burt and B. E. Cohen (1989) Differences among homeless single women, women with children, and single men. *Soc. Problems,* **36,** 508–524.

¹⁹K. Dockett, A. Ashley, and J. Smith-Haynie (1990) Prevalence estimates of alcohol, drug, and mental health problems of homeless female populations in the 1980s: A review of the empirical literature. Paper presented at the annual convention of the American Psychological Association, Boston, MA.

²⁰J. Jones, I. Levine, and A. Rosenberg (1991) Homelessness research, services, and social policy. *Am. Psychol.* **46,** 1139–1148.

²¹P. J. Fischer (1991) *Alcohol, Drug Abuse and Mental Health Problems Among Homeless Persons: A Review of the Literature, 1980–1990*. Publication # (ADM) 91-1763A. United States Department of Health and Human Services, Rockville, MD.

²²M. Robertson (1991) Homeless women with children: The role of alcohol and other drug abuse. *Am. Psychol.* **46,** 1198–1204.

²³L. Biener (1987) Gender differences in the use of substances for coping, in *Gender and Stress*. R. Barnett, L. Biener, and G. Baruch, eds. Free, New York, pp. 330–349.

²⁴S. Timmer, J. Veroff, and M. Colten (1985) Life stress, helplessness, and the use of alcohol and drugs to cope: An analysis of national survey data, in *Coping and Substance Use*. S. Shiffman and T. Willis, eds. Academic, London, pp. 171–198.

[25]D. Dennis, J. Buckner, F. Lipton, and I. Levine (1991) A decade of research and services for homeless mentally ill persons: Where do we stand? *Am. Psychol.* **46,** 1129–1138.

[26]P. Koegel and A. Burnam (1987) Traditional and non-traditional homeless alcoholics. *Alcohol Health Res. World* **11,** 28–36.

[27]R. Drake, F. Osher, and M. Wallach (1991) Homelessness and dual diagnosis. *Am. Psychol.* **46,** 1149–1158.

[28]E. Bassuk, L. Rubin, and A. Lauriat (1986) Characteristics of sheltered homeless families. *Am. J. Publ. Health* **76,** 1097–1101.

[29]E. Bassuk, L. Rubin, and A. Lauriat (1984) Is homelessness a mental health problem? *Am. J. Psychiatry* **141,** 1546–1550.

[30]R. Ropers and R. Boyer (1987) Homelessness as a health risk. *Alcohol Health Res. World* **11,** 38–42.

[31]H. M. Bahr (1973) *Skid Row: An Introduction to Disaffiliation.* Oxford University Press, New York.

[32]M. Shinn, J. Knickerman, and B. Weitzman (1991) Social relationships and vulnerability to becoming homeless among poor families. *Am. Psychol.* **46,** 1180–1187.

[33]B. Whitman, P. Accardo, M. Boyert, and R. Kendagor (1990) Homelessness and cognitive performance in children: A possible link. *Soc. Work* **35,** 516–519.

[34]E. Bassuk and L. Rosenberg (1988) Why does family homelessness occur? A case-control study. *Am. J. Publ. Health* **78,** 783–788.

[35]E. Bassuk and L. Rubin (1987) Homeless children: A neglected population. *Am. J. Orthopsychiatry* **57,** 279–286.

[36]R. Schutt and G. Garrett (1992) The homeless alcoholic: Past and present, in *Homelessness: A National Perspective.* M. Roberston and G. Greenblatt, eds. Plenum, New York, pp. 177–186.

[37]P. Koegel and A. Burnam (1992) Problems in the assessment of mental illness among the homeless: An empirical approach, in *Homelessness: A National Perspective.* M. Roberston and G. Greenblatt, eds. Plenum, New York, pp. 77–99.

[38]S. Nemes (1991) Substance abuse: Ethnic and gender issues in the United States. Unpublished manuscript, Department of Psychology, Temple University, Philadelphia, PA.

[39]C. Mercier, L. Fournier, and N. Peladeau (1990) A three-year follow-up study of homeless women: Methodological and pragmatic issues. Paper presented at the American Evaluation Association Annual Meeting, Washington, D. C.

[40]G. L. Blasi (1990) Social policy and social science research on homelessness. *J. Soc. Issues* **46,** 207–219.

[41]E. Bassuk, R. Carman, L. Weinreb, and M. Herzig, eds. (1990) *Community Care for Homeless Families: A Program Design Manual.* Interagency Council on the Homeless, Washington, D. C.

[42]W. R. Breakey (1987) Treating the homeless. *Alcohol Health Res. World* **11,** 42–48.

[43]F. L. J. Ball and B. E. Havassy (1984) A survey of the problems and needs of homeless consumers of acute psychiatric services. *Hosp. Comm. Psychiatry* **35,** 917–921.

[44]A. McLellan, L. Luborsky, G. Woody, C. O'Brien, and R. Kron (1981) Are the "addiction-related" problems of substance users really related? *J. Nerv. Ment. Dis.* **169,** 232–239.

[45]A. McLellan, L. Luborsky, G. Woody, C. O'Brien, and K. Druley (1982) Is treatment for substance abuse effective? *JAMA* **247,** 1423–1428.

[46]T. Shipley, I. Shandler, and M. Penn (1989) Treatment and research with homeless alcoholics. *Contemp. Drug Problems* **Fall,** 505–526.

[47]W. R. Miller and R. K. Hester (1986) Inpatient alcoholism treatment: Who benefits? *Am. Psychol.* **41,** 794–805.

[48] M. Comfort, T. Shipley, K. White, E. Griffith, and I. Shandler (1990) Family treatment for homeless alcohol/drug-addicted women and their preschool children. *Alcohol. Treatment Q.* **7,** 129–147.

[49]M. Penn, G. Stahler, T. Shipley, M. Comfort, and A. Weinberg (1992) Returning home: Re-integration of substance abusing African-American mothers. *Contemp. Drug Problems*, in press.

[50]I. Shandler, T. Shipley, K. White, M. Comfort, A. Hogue, J. Poling, L. Richlin, and M. Callahan (1991) *Families of Recovering Mothers*. Report # 2R18AA0796602. Final technical report presented to the National Institute of Alcohol Abuse and Alcoholism, Rockville, MD.

[51]A. Hogue, T. Shipley, and M. Comfort (1991) The impact of substance use history and mood on length of stay in treatment. Unpublished manuscript, Department of Psychology, Temple University, Philadelphia, PA.

[52]F. Battaglia and L. Lubchenco (1967) A practical classification of newborn infants by weight and gestational age. *J. Pediatr.* **71,** 159–163.

[53] J. Wilhite (1992) Public policy and the homeless alcoholic: Rethinking our priorities for treatment programs, in *Homelessness: A National Perspective*. M. Roberston and M. Greenblatt, eds. Plenum, New York, pp. 187–196.

[54]P. Marin (1991, July 8) Why are the homeless mainly single men? *The Nation* pp. 46–51.

[55] M. Shore and M. Cohen (1992) Homelessness and the chronically mentally ill, in *Homelessness: A National Perspective*. M. Roberston and M. Greenblatt, eds. Plenum, New York, pp. 67–75.

Index

Marijuana, 300, 303, 306, 448, 452
  pregnancy, 451
Marital disruption, 311
Marital status, 351
MAST, 265
Maternal attitude, 392
Maturity, 402
Mean corpuscular volume, 135
Medical complications, 388
Medical issues, 405
Men's misperceptions, 111
Mental health, 499
Methadone, 331
Millon clinical multiaxial inventory
    (MCMI), 17, 22
Minnesota multiphasic personality
    inventory (MMPI), 7
MMPI and cocaine, 15
MMPI and drug abuse, 13
Mortality, 286

N

Narcission, 90
Needle use, 342, 348
Neglect, 395, 403
Neuropsychiatric, 424
NHANES I, 48
Nicorette, 56
Nicotine, 47, 53
Nicotine dependence, 46
NIDA high school senior survey,
    181
Norwood, 246
Novelty seeking, 4

O

Opiate, 285, 458
Opiate addicts, 301
Opiate use, 329
Opiates and pregnancy, 459
Opioid addicts, 18

Opioids, 5, 13
Oral pathology, 43
Outreach, 163

P

Parental attributes, 392
Parental separation, 77
Patenting, 352, 390
Patenting women, 381
Pathogenesis, 452
Patterns in smoking initiation, 40
Peer support, 166
Peer support groups, 159, 164
Perinatal addiction, 26
Personal problems, 310
Personality, 1, 3
Personality and addiction, 6
Personality factor questionnaire,
    22
Personality inventory, 23
Personality predictors, 363
"Postfeminist, " 242
Postmenopausal estrogen
    determinant, 198
Postmenopausal state, 197
Postmenopausal women, 202, 209
Posttraumatic stress disorder, 273
Posttreatment, 16
Pregnancy, 437, 445, 478
Pregnancy issues, 389
Prenatal alcohol exposure, 220
Prevention and treatment, 117
Prevention of smoking initiation in
    young women, 51
Prolactin, 199, 444, 450
Propanediol, 140
Psychiatric patients, 8
Psychological issues, 384
Psychopathology, 1, 79, 81, 342
Psychosocial sequelae, 288
Puritanical group ideal, 255